Athletic Training Clinical Workbook

A Guide to the Competencies

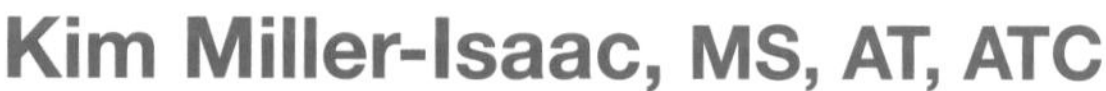
Kim Miller-Isaac, MS, AT, ATC
Assistant Professor
Sport Sciences
Wilmington College
Wilmington, OH

Melissa Noble, AT, ATC
Head Athletic Trainer, Fairlawn High School
Assistant Athletic Trainer, Sidney High School
Sports Medicine Program
Wilson Memorial Hospital
Sidney, OH

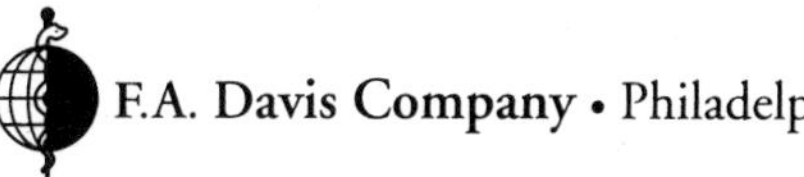
F.A. Davis Company • Philadelphia

F.A. Davis Company
1915 Arch Street
Philadelphia, PA 19103
www.fadavis.com

Printed in the United States of America

Last digit indicates print number: 10 9 8 7 6 5 4 3 2 1

Publisher: Quincy McDonald
Director of Content Development: George W. Lang
Developmental Editor: Joanna Cain
Art and Design Manager: Carolyn O'Brien

To

My loving husband Will,

Thank you for always believing in me and encouraging me to reach for the stars. Your unwavering support is priceless.

Mya,

Thanks for understanding and making me smile.

With love,
Kim

"You gain strength, courage, and confidence by every experience in which you really stop to look fear in the face. You must do the thing you think you cannot do."
—Eleanor Roosevelt

Thank you, Kim, for believing in me to co-write this workbook. You never gave up on me, which I am grateful for.
Thank you, Noble, for helping me see past my doubts, and encouraging, supporting, and above all, loving me through this journey.
Thank you, Kyle and Blake, for understanding during those times when Mommy needed to make time for writing. I love you both.
Thank you, Dad, for allowing me the opportunities to attend college and be a part of a profession that I truly enjoy. Wait until you see these flashcards!
Thank you, Mom, for making me a strong, independent woman. You always wanted your children to stand on their own two feet, and I am completing a journey that I never thought possible. Your love for the arts never went unheard or unnoticed.

Love,
Friend, wife, mother, and daughter,
Melissa

preface

In athletic training education, students must have a clinical education component where the knowledge and application of educational domains are integrated into real life situations. The students must be able to critically think and discern what is going on with an injured or ill athlete. The students have numerous classes teaching them foundational knowledge like the signs and symptoms of injuries, mechanisms of injuries, and treatments for injuries. When athletic trainers are presented with a situation, they must utilize all of their clinical knowledge regarding proper prevention, recognition, and rehabilitation management. Recently, the athletic training Board of Certification (BOC) has incorporated scenarios with corresponding questions on the certification exam in order to test students' ability to synthesize the foundational knowledge they have learned and to test the students' ability to apply this knowledge to real clinical scenarios. When an athlete is injured or sick, the athletic training student must be able to collect all of the necessary information, evaluate the problem, and deduce the assessment or diagnosis. This clinical reasoning skill is a difficult task for many athletic training students to master. The students may know the information, but they have difficulty putting it all together to gain a conclusion and thus a treatment plan.

This clinical workbook is a collaboration of clinical scenarios that, as a whole, touch on each educational domain within Athletic Training Programs (ATP) accredited by the Commission on Accreditation of Athletic Training Education (CAATE), thus enhancing the clinical education component of an ATP's curriculum. The goal of this workbook is to teach athletic training students how to formulate a mental checklist to identify an assessment or treatment plan when presented with a clinical scenario. This helps students develop their critical thinking skills, thus increasing their clinical competence in athletic training skills and improving their success rate on the BOC exam. The workbook may be used as a requirement for clinical practicum classes, as a supplement for classes, or in the clinical setting during student "downtime." This workbook is designed to parallel the fifth edition of the Athletic Training Education Competencies and to be used in conjunction with the foundational knowledge textbooks within ATP curriculums.

Audience

This product benefits professors, program preceptors, student athletic trainers, and Athletic Training Programs (ATPs). Professors can use this product as the required text for clinical practicum classes. The Commission on Accreditation of Athletic Training Education (CAATE) Standards for clinical education notes that athletic training students must have a clinical portion within their program and must have instruction and formal assessment of clinical skills prior to performing those skills on a patient. The workbook entries by the students can serve as another form of instruction and then can be reviewed by the professor, which will allow the professor to see the thought process of his or her students. This will then help the professor guide the students who may be struggling with their critical thinking processes.

A program preceptor can assess the Clinical Integration Proficiency (CIP) of athletic training students. The new CIPs are skills that students must demonstrate in the context of real patient care. The questions and tear-out flashcards found in this workbook will give the preceptors new ideas to spark conversations about clinical scenarios when actual scenarios may be few and far between in the clinical setting.

Students will be able to use this product for some of the same reasons as the preceptors. Frequently, in athletic training, students won't have the opportunity to observe injuries every day. Therefore, they can work through this workbook and flashcards to supplement a slow day in the field. Additionally, this product helps to develop their critical thinking skills to be a better athletic trainer and increases their confidence in decision-making involved in regard to patient care. This workbook may also improve students' success rate on the BOC exam because it covers scenarios from each educational domain that may possibly be covered in the scenario questions on the BOC exam.

This workbook is beneficial to the athletic training program as a whole by evaluating student learning and decision-making abilities. Initially, formal instruction and evaluation of knowledge and skill occurs in the core academic classes in the curriculum. However, this workbook serves as an opportunity to measure a student's ability to use classroom knowledge when considering a

Erin M. Jordan, MS, ATC/LAT
Clinical Instructor
Georgia Southern University
Statesboro, Georgia

Peter Koehneke, MS, ATC
Professor, Department of Kinesiology
Director, Athletic Training Education
Canisius College
Buffalo, New York

Joanne Klossner, PhD, LAT, ATC
Clinical Education Coordinator
Indiana University
Bloomington, Indiana

Justin E. Lehman, AT, CSCS
Assistant Athletic Trainer/Lecturer
Ohio Northern University
Ada, Ohio

Jack Winn Mansfield, EdD, ATC
Associate Professor of Athletic Training
Lincoln Memorial University
Harrogate, Tennessee

Jeff McKibben, MEd, ATC, LAT
Program Director, ELM
University of Central Oklahoma
Edmond, Oklahoma

Jamie Moul, EdD, LAT, ATC
Director, Athletic Training Education Program
Appalachian State University
Boone, North Carolina

Alison Jean Ness, MS, ATC, LAT
Assistant Athletic Trainer/Adjunct Faculty
Middle Tennessee State University
Murfreesboro, Tennessee

Jennifer O'Donoghue, PhD, LAT, ATC, CSCS
Associate Professor/Program Director
Barton College
Wilson, North Carolina

Pam Rast, PhD, LAT, ATC
Professor
Texas Wesleyan University
Fort Worth, Texas

Jaclyn Schwieterman, ATC
Assistant Professor
Marietta College
Marietta, Ohio

Brian D. Seiler, MS, ATC
Doctoral Assistant, Research and Education
University of South Carolina
Columbia, South Carolina

Justin Stanek, EdD, ATC
Clinical Education Coordinator
Illinois State University
Normal, Illinois

Abigail Sue Tibbetts, MS, ATC, LAT, PhD Candidate
Assistant Professor
Buena Vista University
Storm Lake, Iowa

Patricia M. Tripp, PhD, ATC, LAT, CSCS
Director, Undergraduate Athletic Training Education
University of Florida
Gainesville, Florida

Rhonda Verdegan, PhD, ATC, CSCS
Clinical Coordinator/Lecturer
University of Wisconsin
Stevens Point, Wisconsin

Katie M. Walsh, EdD, ATC, LAT
Director of Sports Medicine/Athletic Training
East Carolina University
Greenville, North Carolina

Kristi White, PhD, ATC
Program Director/Associate Professor
Angelo State University
San Angelo, Texas

Mike Wolhoy, MS, ATC/L
Head Athletic Trainer
Southwest Baptist University
Bolivar, Missouri

acknowledgments

We wish to thank our families and everyone that has believed in us from the beginning of this project. We owe deep gratitude to our students at Wilmington College who have given us inspiration and encouragement when the journey of writing this book looked so long and unattainable. The input and support of these students helped us complete this project.

We also wish to thank our colleagues who have written vignettes and provided advice and encouragement for our endeavor.

Wilmington College, Wilson Memorial Hospital, and Fairlawn High School deserve our gratitude for supporting our project throughout the process.

We would also like to express our sincere appreciation to Joanna Cain, Pamela Speh, and the editorial team at Auctorial Pursuits, Inc., that led us through this project with patience and encouragement. We also wish to thank F.A. Davis Publishers and their entire team for giving us this opportunity and helping us bring our vision to light.

abbreviations

AC: acromioclavicular
ACL: anterior cruciate ligament
AED: automated external defibrillator
ASIS: anterior superior iliac spine
AT: athletic trainer
ATP: athletic training program
BMI: body mass index
BOC: Board of Certification
CAATE: Commission on Accreditation of Athletic Training Education
CEU: continuing education unit
CMT: certified massage therapist
CPR: cardiopulmonary resuscitation
CSCS: certified strength and conditioning specialist
CT: computed tomography (tomographic)
DIP: distal interphalangeal
EAP: emergency action plan
EMS: emergency medical services
FDP: flexor digitorum profundus
FDS: flexor digitorum superficialis
GH: glenohumeral joint
HIPAA: Health Insurance Portability and Accountability Act
IP: interphalangeal
ITBS: iliotibial band syndrome
LCL: lateral collateral ligament
MCL: medial collateral ligament
MDI: metered-dose inhaler
MHR: maximum heart rate
MRI: magnetic resonance imaging
MRSA: methicillin-resistant *Staphylococcus aureus*
MTP: metatarsophalangeal
MTSS: medial tibial stress syndrome
NATA: National Athletic Trainers' Association
NCAA: National Collegiate Athletic Association
PCL: posterior cruciate ligament
PCS: postconcussion syndrome
PIP: proximal interphalangeal
PPAT: postprofessional program in athletic training
PRE: progressive resistive exercise
PSIS: posterior superior iliac spine
ROM: range of motion
SC: sternoclavicular
SCA: sudden cardiac arrest
SCM: sternocleidomastoid
SI: sacroiliac
TMJ: temporomandibular joint
UCL: ulnar collateral ligament

contents in brief

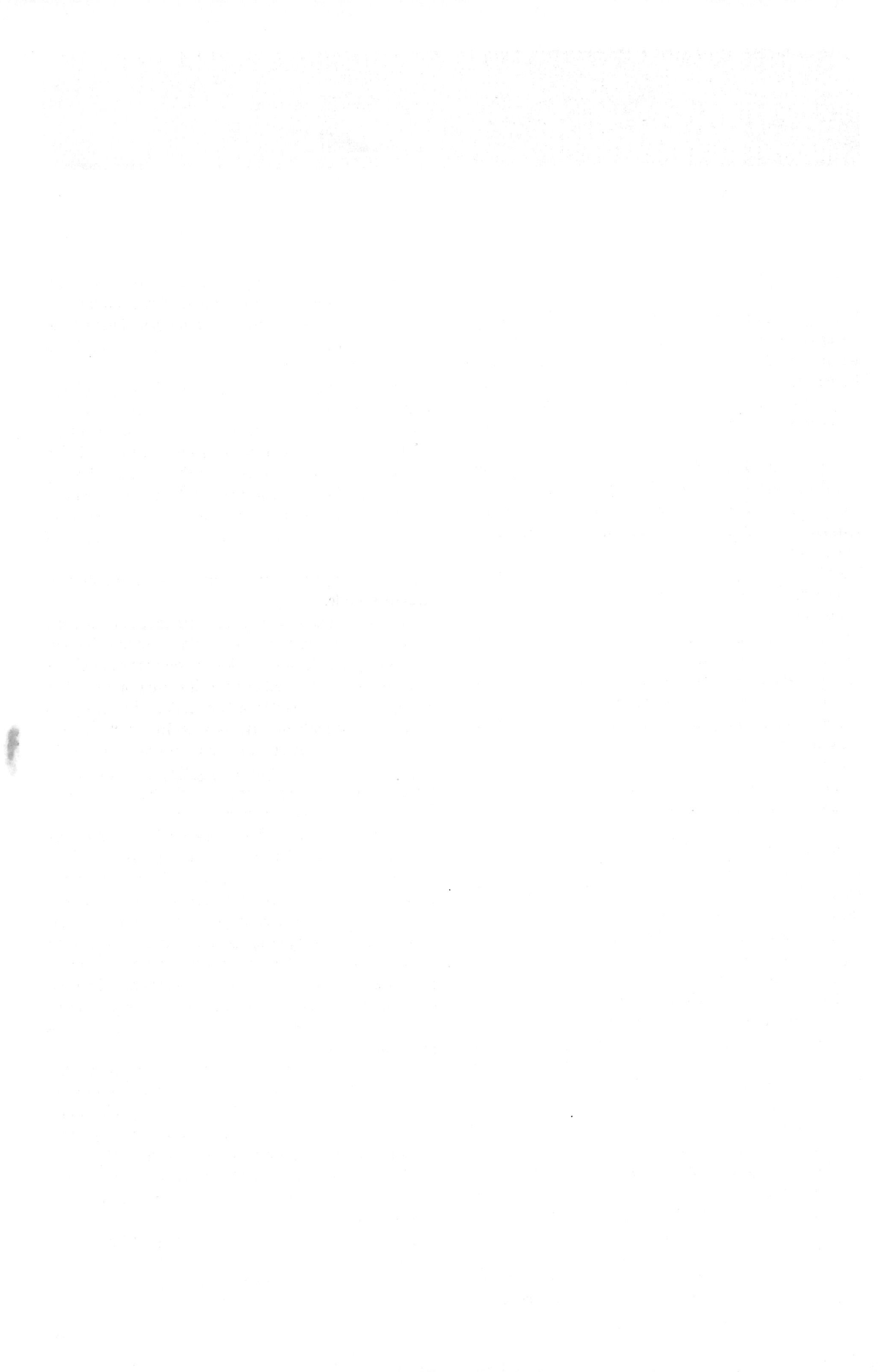

introduction

How to Use This Workbook

Each section of this workbook includes chapters that cover the athletic training educational domains and is written based on the fifth edition of the Athletic Training Education Competencies, which may be found here: http://www.nata.org/sites/default/files/5th-Edition Competencies-2011-PDF-Version.pdf. Within each chapter, the scenarios cover topics that athletic training students may encounter in the clinical setting. The scenarios are written to stand alone; therefore, they don't need to be completed in order. However, in each chapter model scenarios are included and outlined. These are example scenarios that lead the student through critical thinking exercises. Keep in mind that there may be variations in state laws and practices and variances in athletic training skills and protocols that may cause the answers to the practice questions to vary. Students should defer to their instructor for clarification or expansion on a topic; instructors should feel free to elaborate or add to the scenario's components. Information used to complete the scenarios should be gathered from textbooks and peer reviewed journal articles. Instructors can use their discretion as to what extent they require references for answers and the inclusion of evidence-based practice (e.g., evidence on sensitivity and specificity of special tests used). Repetition in component questions and content may be experienced because of the "pick and choose" nature of the chapter's scenarios as a learning tool. The workbook teaches the student to comprise a mental checklist to help identify an assessment or treatment plan when presented with a clinical scenario. This helps the student to become a better athletic trainer.

Each chapter begins with a vignette, or scenario, which is written by a clinician who has real world experience with that chapter's content. These experiences are meant to present the athletic training student with the information contained in the chapter and to show how this content is used by all professions under the athletic training umbrella. The intent is for the athletic training students to take something from the real world experiences and apply it to their future careers.

The learning outcomes present what the athletic training students will learn throughout the scenarios and activities in each chapter. They are based on the fifth edition of the Athletic Training Education Competencies. Following this section are the model scenarios and student scenarios. The model scenarios are formatted just like the student scenarios, but the model scenarios' activities are already completed. This serves as a template for students to follow while working through the subsequent student scenarios. The number of model and student scenarios vary depending on the complexity of each chapter's content.

The student scenarios are presented with blank answer spaces that the student is to complete. Various questions are presented after each scenario. The blank areas and/or bullets after the questions are to be filled in by the student. The number of bullets doesn't directly relate to the number of answers, but are to be used as a format guide. In some scenarios, students may write down more or fewer answers than the given number of bullets. Guidance for the assessment process and the scenario answers are provided in the corresponding instructor's guide.

The scenarios also include some special features: Brain Jolt, Conversation Buffer, and Treatment Detour. The Brain Jolts are bits of information that can help or "jolt" the student's memory and learning process. For example, in the injury evaluation section, the Brain Jolts are clues to the athlete's assessment. In other sections, the Brain Jolts serve as additional information to help signify important concepts or help the student with the transition from the assessment to the treatment plan. Conversation Buffers are written to give guidance with communication skills. This can pertain to communication between the athletic trainer and the coach, athlete, parent, or other medical personnel. A Treatment Detour is information that is related to the content of a particular scenario while presenting evidence-based information from published journal articles. These may include background information on a condition, new treatment protocols, or additional information that is useful for the clinician. It is a reminder that research is important to the profession and evidence-based practice helps to improve patient care.

The final aspect of the chapters is the knowledge checklist. This tool is based on the fifth edition of the Athletic Training Education Competencies, found in its entirety on NATA's website (http://www.nata.org/sites/default/files/5th-Edition-Competencies-2011-PDF-Version.pdf.). It can be used by instructors, preceptors, or peers to evaluate a student's proficiency of the chapter's content.

The back of the book includes tear-out flashcards. These flashcards encompass the content included in the scenarios. However, the flashcards are presented in a random order and can be used independently from the scenarios. The flashcards include information like signs and symptoms, special test results, vital sign values, or simple pictures or diagrams. The answers are presented on the back of each card. These flashcards have a rating system using stars as follows: 1 star signals a lower level or easier question; 2 stars signals a moderate level question; and 3 stars signals an upper level or difficult question. It is recommended that the students tear these flashcards out of the book, laminate them, and punch a hole in the corner of each card. Then the cards can be assembled on a key ring. This way, the flashcards are water resistant and more resilient so they may be kept in the student's or AT's medical kit. These flashcards are a simple way to spark conversation and quiz the student's knowledge of the content while in the clinical setting during "downtime" to further enhance learning and educational opportunities with peers and preceptors.

part one

Emergency Response Skills: Safety and Prevention

chapter 1

First Aid and Acute Care

chapter outline

athletic trainer's corner

Out there in the real world, one athletic training student experienced the following while being supervised by a certified athletic trainer:

During my senior year of college I was responsible for the volleyball team. During one of the matches, an opposing player began to bleed on the court. Although this wasn't a life-threatening emergency, it was still a good life lesson because I was not prepared for the situation. I had not obtained gauze and gloves to keep in my pockets prior to the game; therefore, I was in a panic trying to get the necessary items to deal with the player's injury. Once I was given permission from the referee to enter onto the court, I began to care for the athlete. I applied a gauze pad to the cut and applied pressure. I then had to observe the playing surface and her clothing for blood. All spots on the floor were cleaned with hydrogen peroxide, and the athlete had to change jerseys.

This situation taught me to always be prepared for an emergency. Gauze and gloves should be readily available at all times. Also, you should always make sure that emergency situations are discussed before the game along with your emergency action plan so that everyone working the game knows his or her specific role if something were to happen.

Mikaela Pope
Athletic training student
Wilmington College

learning outcomes

After working through this chapter, you will be able to:

1. Identify the components of an appropriate medical history.
2. Identify vital signs, as well as the process of monitoring these vital signs and identifying abnormal indicators.
3. Explain the warning signs of emergency medical conditions and appropriate treatments.
4. Explain the procedures for management of spinal and head injuries and injuries requiring first aid.

introduction

In the profession of athletic training, emergency response skills are crucial for your job responsibilities. Throughout this section, you will be presented with signs and symptoms of safety and prevention scenarios to help fine-tune your assessment skills. Beyond performing special tests and observing visual characteristics of the injured area, you need to determine quickly whether an injury is a medical emergency or is severe enough to prevent the athlete from returning to play or affect the athlete's activities of daily living. By implementing all the information obtained in the classroom about safety and prevention and then applying it by looking at the big picture in terms of what is going on with the athlete, you can quickly assess the situation, the injury, and the effective treatment to create the best possible outcome for the athlete.

MODEL SCENARIO 1: **DAVID BREYMEIR**

David Breymeir is a senior collegiate football player and is currently in the second week of twice-a-day practices. The athletic training staff is monitoring Mr. Breymeir daily because of his overweight status coming into camp and because his daily weigh-in and weigh-out amounts have become inconsistent, with more than 5% body weight loss from practices. One hour into today's practice, Mr. Breymeir begins exhibiting profuse sweating, dizziness, and disorientation. The athletic trainer removes him from the field. Once on the sideline, Mr. Breymeir's signs and symptoms also include pale skin, a rapid weak pulse (Fig. 1-1), and an elevated body temperature taken orally.

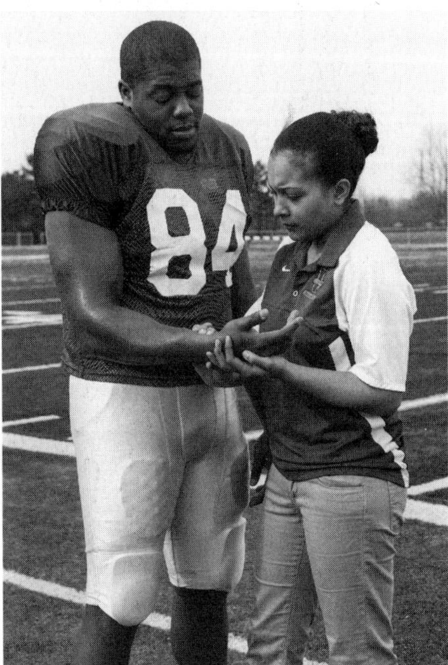

Figure 1-1: David Breymeir's current condition.

1. From the previous scenario, what do you know about Mr. Breymeir's condition?
    - *College football player in twice-a-day practices*
    - *Difficulty maintaining weight*
    - *Profuse sweating*
    - *Dizziness*
    - *Disorientation*
    - *Pale skin*
    - *Rapid weak pulse*
    - *Elevated body temperature*

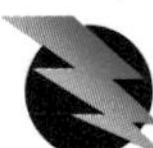

Brain Jolt
This condition can progress into a life-threatening emergency if not recognized early.

2. To effectively evaluate Mr. Breymeir's condition, you will need to gather additional information. What questions should you ask in addition to what is presented in this scenario?
    - *Is this condition a medical emergency?*
    - *Is there a risk of shock with this condition?*
    - *Are there any preexisting conditions or a history of medical conditions? If yes, what are they?*
    - *Has he been nauseated or vomiting?*
    - *What is his core temperature?*
    - *Is he hydrated?*
    - *Has he had any muscle cramping?*
    - *Has he eaten properly today?*
    - *Has the athlete been acclimated properly?*
3. Identify key terms and concepts and then research each to broaden your knowledge of first aid and acute care.
    - What is the most effective way to take a core body temperature? Explain the process.
      The most effective way to take a core body temperature is rectally. The athlete must be lying prone, and the

thermometer is lubricated with petroleum jelly. The buttocks are spread, and the thermometer is gently inserted into the rectum approximately 1 in. Hold onto the thermometer and leave it in place for 3 min. Remove gently and read the thermometer. Wash the thermometer with soap and water after each use.

- If Mr. Breymeir is vomiting, how should fluids be administered?
  If the athlete is vomiting, fluids cannot be administered orally. Fluids have to be administered by a physician intravenously.
- Where should Mr. Breymeir rest to be monitored?
  An athlete with these symptoms should be moved to a cool environment; inside an air-conditioned building or under a shade tree are two good examples.
- What techniques can be used to reduce core body temperature?
  Place ice bags or towels immersed in cool water in the axillas and around the neck, sponge cold water over the athlete's body, or do both. If the core temperature is dangerously high, the athlete can be submerged in cold water in a tub.
- List ways of preventing heat-related emergencies.
  Two ways to help prevent heat-related emergencies are (1) to use a wet bulb globe to monitor the temperature and the heat index and (2) to schedule practices or games before or after the hot and humid times of the day. In addition, ensure that the athletes are acclimatized properly and have them participate in a preseason conditioning program to improve their physical health. Make sure the athletes have unlimited access to water and minimize the clothing and equipment they wear on humid or hot days.

4. Based on the information that you currently have and what was provided by your instructor, what are the possible differential diagnoses for Mr. Breymeir's condition?
   Heat syncope
   Heat cramps
   Heat exhaustion
   Heat stroke

Why or why not?

For each assessment or diagnosis, write *why?* or *why not?* statements identifying why the information is correct or incorrect. Take details from your textbook, your own research, and data from Mr. Breymeir's scenario to help you formulate an answer.

1. *Mr. Breymeir does not have heat syncope. Dizziness is a symptom of heat syncope, but it also is in combination with fainting and nausea.*
2. *Mr. Breymeir does not have heat cramps. Heat cramps are muscle spasms that occur most often in the calf region of the leg. Profuse sweating is a precursor to heat cramps, but Mr. Breymeir did not have any type of muscle cramping.*
3. *Mr. Breymeir does have heat exhaustion. Heat exhaustion is brought on by dehydration. Mr. Breymeir had been having difficulty replacing his fluids before each practice, which left him with a water and electrolyte imbalance. Heat exhaustion can become a serious, life-threatening condition if the core body temperature is not reduced to less than 101°F and fluids are not able to replenish after vomiting.*
4. *Mr. Breymeir did not suffer a heat stroke. He did not have hot dry skin, a core body temperature greater than 102°F, or decreased sweating.*

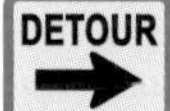

Treatment Detour

Many activity-related concussions occur each year. Research shows that concussions are associated with altered function of the autonomic nervous system (ANS). Exertional heat illness in athletes has also been associated with ANS dysfunction because the ANS controls the multi-organ system that regulates body temperature. Therefore, researchers conducted a study to determine whether there is an association between a history of concussion and previous symptoms of exertional heat illness. The study included 100 NCAA Division I athletes at one university. These athletes took an ImPACT test (ImPACT Applications, Pittsburgh, PA) to assess concussion history and then answered a questionnaire to assess history of symptoms associated with exertional heat illness. A statistically significant association was found between concussion history and several symptoms of exertional heat illness. The participants with a history of a concussion were more likely to report having previously experienced symptoms such as fatigue, muscle cramps, and lightheadedness when exercising in the heat. Although this study was retrospective and did not determine a cause-and-effect relationship, this knowledge may help athletic trainers to intervene more quickly based on an athlete's concussion history (Alosco, Knecht, Glickman, & Gunstad, 2012).

What do you think?

1. What is your assessment of Mr. Breymeir's condition?
   Answer: *Heat exhaustion*
2. Was your assessment of Mr. Breymeir's condition correct?
   Answer: *Yes*
3. If not, explain what you did incorrectly and how you could have performed a better assessment.

   Answer: ____________________

MODEL SCENARIO 2: BAUSTON QUILLEN

Bauston Quillen is a collegiate soccer player and an aggressive midfielder. This year, the college installed artificial turf on the soccer field. As Mr. Quillen is participating in a defensive practice drill, he slide tackles to redirect the ball. He slides on his left leg to stop the ball and redirects the ball to the opposite side of the field. Mr. Quillen immediately notices a burning sensation over the posterior lateral side of his left upper thigh. The athletic trainer examines the irritated area and notices that the first layer of skin has been removed (Fig. 1-2). The wound is bleeding and has a mild amount of edema.

1. From the previous scenario, what do you know about Mr. Quillen and his injury?
   - *Collegiate defensive soccer player*
   - *Playing on artificial turf*
   - *Slide tackles to redirect ball*
   - *Burning sensation on posterior lateral side of upper thigh*
   - *Wound bleeding, with mild amount of edema*
2. To evaluate Mr. Quillen's injury effectively, you will need to gather additional information. What questions should you ask in addition to what is presented in this model scenario?
   - *Is this injury a medical emergency?*
   - *Is there a risk of shock with this injury?*
   - *Are there any preexisting conditions or a history of injuries? If yes, what are they?*
   - *Is ecchymosis present?*
   - *Was Mr. Quillen wearing protective sliding shorts?*
   - *Is the burning sensation localized to just the site of the wound?*
   - *Is there any debris in the wound?*
   - *Are there any signs or symptoms of injury to other areas?*

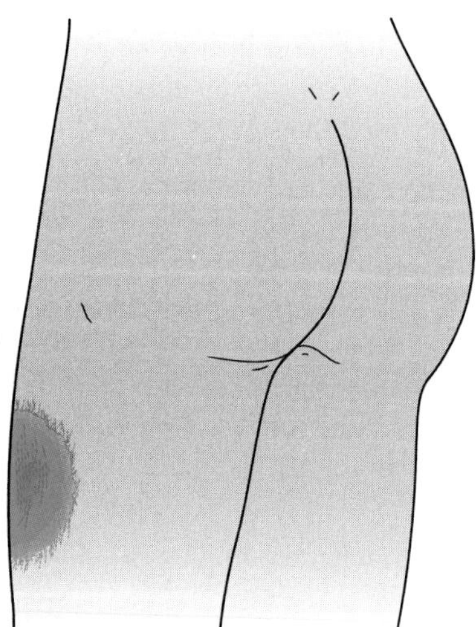

Figure 1-2: Bauston Quillen's wound.

3. Identify key terms and concepts and then research each to broaden your knowledge of first aid and acute care.
   - How should the wound be treated?
     The wound must be debrided and cleansed. The wound could possibly have small pieces of artificial turf embedded in it that need to be debrided with a brush or tweezers. Warm water and soap, along with sterile gauze, should be used during the cleansing process. Hydrogen peroxide should be applied over the affected area. If the wound becomes infected, a type of cleanser that focuses on reducing the risk of methicillin-resistant Staphylococcus aureus (MRSA) should be used because of the surface on which Mr. Quillen was playing when he was injured. Apply a triple-antibiotic ointment to the clean area to keep the skin moist. A sterile dressing should be applied after treatment.
   - How should the wound be covered? What instructions should be given to Mr. Quillen about caring for his wound himself?
     The wound should remain covered with a sterile gauze or dressing. Mr. Quillen should be instructed on how to clean the wound with warm, soapy water. A triple-antibiotic ointment should be applied to help with the healing process.
   - When Mr. Quillen returns for practice the following day, how should the wound be treated so that he can return back to activity?
     A sterile dressing should cover the wound, and the entire area should be covered with an Ace bandage wrap and sliding shorts. The purpose is to prevent the sterile dressing from coming off during practice. If the wound is sensitive to the touch or gets irritated during activity, adding a protective padding over the sterile gauze is also recommended.
   - Name the different types of wounds.
     Laceration
     Abrasion
     Puncture
     Avulsion
4. Based on the information you currently have and what was provided by your instructor, what are the differential diagnoses for Mr. Quillen's injury?
   Laceration
   Avulsion
   Abrasion
   Contact dermatitis

Why or why not?

For each assessment or diagnosis, write *why?* or *why not?* statements identifying why the information is correct or incorrect. Take details from your textbook, your own research, and data from Mr. Quillen's scenario to help you formulate an answer.

1. *Mr. Quillen does not have a laceration. Lacerations result from a sharp or pointed object penetrating the skin. Mr. Quillen did not come in contact with a sharp object.*
2. *Mr. Quillen does not have an avulsion wound. An avulsion results from a trauma that tears the skin away from or off the body.*
3. *Mr. Quillen does have an abrasion. Mr. Quillen's top layer of skin was scraped away when he slid on the artificial turf.*
4. *Mr. Quillen does not have contact dermatitis. Contact dermatitis is an allergic reaction to a wide variety of agents. The agents could be plants, topical medications, or chemicals. The time that it takes for contact dermatitis to develop can be 1 to 7 days. Onset is not immediate, as in Mr. Quillen's case.*

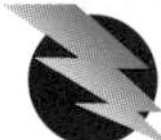

Brain Jolt
There is no need for stitches with this type of wound.

What do you think?

1. What is your assessment of Mr. Quillen's injury?
   Answer: *Abrasion*
2. Was your assessment of Mr. Quillen's injury correct?
   Answer: *Yes*
3. If not, please explain what you did incorrectly and how you could have performed a better assessment.

   Answer: ______________________________

STUDENT SCENARIO 1: WILLIAM SCHIPNER

William Schipner is a freshman college football player who is currently sidelined because of a MRSA infection. Mr. Schipner wears a protective knee brace every day and had an abrasion on the posterior side of the right knee. As a result of improper hygiene, the abrasion became infected with MRSA. Mr. Schipner is off practice this weekend and decides to go home to see his parents. Upon returning to campus on Monday, he is experiencing flu-like symptoms and is pale, sluggish, and dizzy. The posterior portion behind his right knee is bright red and hot to the touch. He notices a reddish line starting up his posterior thigh. He is concerned and decides to visit the campus physician. When Mr. Schipner is examined by the physician, he has a rapid weak pulse, and his blood pressure is 98/60 mm Hg. As Mr. Schipner stands up, he experiences syncope. He is immediately transported to the hospital (Fig. 1-3).

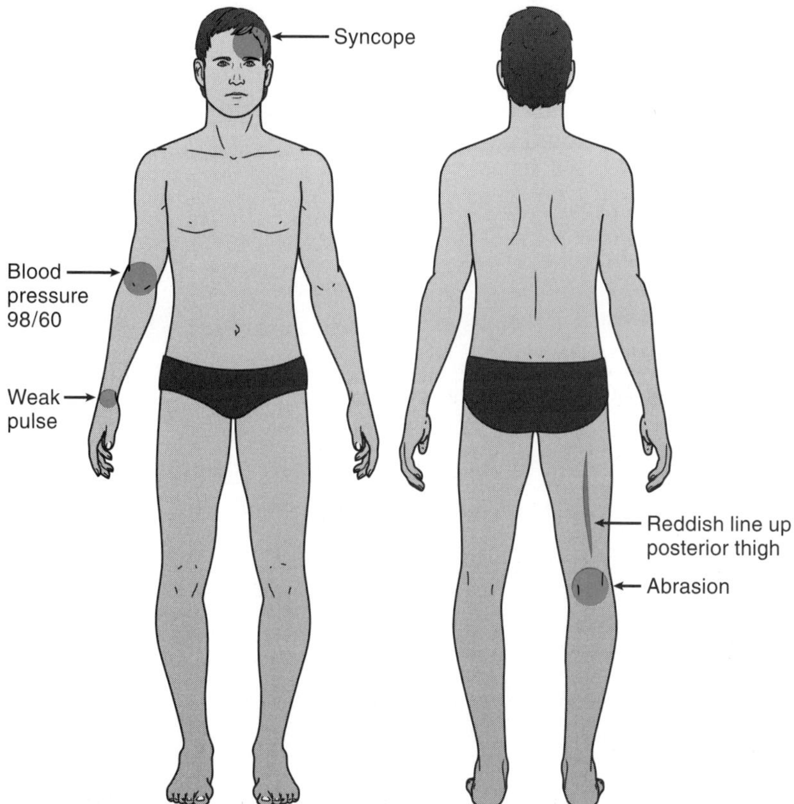

Figure 1-3: William Schipner's condition.

1. From the previous scenario, what do you know about Mr. Schipner's condition?

- ____________________
- ____________________
- ____________________
- ____________________

2. To effectively evaluate a condition like Mr. Schipner's, you would need to gather additional information. What questions would you ask in addition to what is presented in this scenario?

- ____________________
- ____________________
- ____________________
- ____________________

Brain Jolt
Monitoring of vital signs can provide significant information about a person's condition.

3. Identify key terms and concepts and then research each to broaden your knowledge of first aid and acute care.

- Define *MRSA* and explain the complications of this condition.

  Answer: ____________________
- Define *abrasion.*

  Answer: ____________________
- Could Mr. Schipner's flu-like symptoms be related to the spread of *MRSA* infection?

  Answer: ____________________
- What does the red line coming from the wound indicate?

  Answer: ____________________
- Define *syncope.*

  Answer: ____________________
- Identify vital signs and the normal ranges for each.

  Answer: ____________________

4. Based on the information you currently have and what was provided by your instructor, what are the differential diagnoses for Mr. Schipner's condition?

- ____________________
- ____________________
- ____________________
- ____________________
- ____________________

Why or why not?

For each assessment or diagnosis, write *why?* or *why not?* statements identifying why the information is correct or incorrect. Take details from your textbook, your own research, and data from Mr. Schipner's scenario to help you formulate an answer.

1. ____________________

2. ____________________

3. ____________________

4. ____________________

What do you think?

1. What is your assessment of Mr. Schipner's condition?

Answer: ____________________

2. Was your assessment correct for Mr. Schipner's condition?

Answer: ____________________

3. If not, explain what you did incorrectly and how you could have performed a better assessment.

Answer: ____________________

STUDENT SCENARIO 2: SHELBY NETZLEY

Shelby Netzley is a 15-year-old high school sophomore on the junior varsity volleyball team. The team has just finished playing an away game and is sitting in the stands waiting for the varsity game to begin. A fellow teammate's mother brought chocolate chip and peanut butter cookies. The girls pass around the container that holds both types of cookies. Ms. Netzley chooses a chocolate chip cookie. One hour into the varsity game, she notices that she is cool, clammy, and slightly perspiring. It is warm in the gym, but the symptoms begin to concern Ms. Netzley when she starts having trouble breathing and her lips begin to tingle and swell (Fig. 1-4). Ms. Netzley frantically talks to her coach and is advised to see the host athletic trainer. The athletic trainer asks Ms. Netzley questions pertaining to her history and takes her blood pressure, which is 85/60 mm Hg. Immediate actions are taken.

1. From the previous scenario, what do you know about Ms. Netzley's condition?
   - ______________________________
   - ______________________________
   - ______________________________
   - ______________________________

2. To effectively evaluate Ms. Netzley's condition, you will need to gather additional information. What questions should you ask in addition to what is presented in this scenario?
   - ______________________________
   - ______________________________
   - ______________________________
   - ______________________________

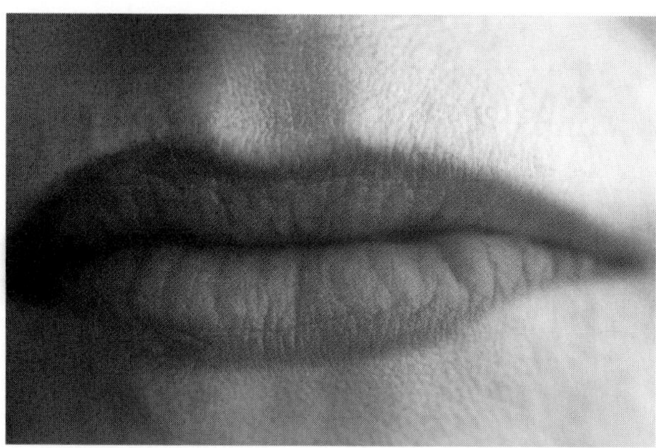

Figure 1-4: Shelby Netzley's lips. (© Thinkstock)

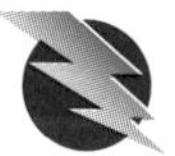

Brain Jolt

This type of reaction can be caused by food, insects, or inhaling dusts or pollens.

3. Identify key terms and concepts and then research each to broaden your knowledge of first aid and acute care.
   - Why would Ms. Netzley have cool, clammy skin and be slightly perspiring when she is not playing?

     Answer: ______________________________
   - What condition might a systolic blood pressure less than 90 mm Hg indicate?

     Answer: ______________________________
   - Based on the scenario, what immediate care should have been given?

     Answer: ______________________________

4. Based on the information you currently have and what was provided by your instructor, what are the possible differential diagnoses for Ms. Netzley's condition?
   - ______________________________
   - ______________________________
   - ______________________________
   - ______________________________

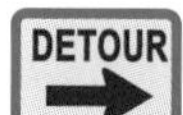

Treatment Detour

Epinephrine is the emergency treatment for severe allergic reactions. This medication comes in autoinjectors that will combat life-threatening symptoms, including hypotension, shock, and upper-airway obstruction resulting from such severe reactions. There are three brands of autoinjectors available: Epi-Pen, Adrenaclick, and Twinject. Each of these devices has a slightly different look, administration technique, and dose verification. It is important to be familiar with the devices used by your team or athletes. In addition, never inject epinephrine into a buttock or a vein; inject only into the anterolateral aspect of the thigh (Mohundro & Mohundro, 2010).

Why or why not?

For each assessment or diagnosis, write *why?* or *why not?* statements identifying why the information is correct or incorrect. Take details from your textbook, your own research, and data from Ms. Netzley's scenario to help you formulate an answer.

1. ______________________________

____

2. ______________________________

____

3. ______________________________

____

4. ______________________________

____

What do you think?

1. What is your assessment of Ms. Netzley's condition?

Answer: ______________________________

2. Was your assessment correct for Ms. Netzley's condition?

Answer: ______________________________

3. If not, explain what you did incorrectly and how you could have performed a better assessment.

Answer: ______________________________

STUDENT SCENARIO 3: ANDY WALLICK

Andy Wallick is a freshman collegiate soccer player who plays the position of goaltender. Mr. Wallick is acting unusual, seems disoriented, and complains of a headache. With 2 min left in the first half of the game, Mr. Wallick falls to the ground. When the athletic trainer approaches him, he is conscious, sweating, clenching his teeth, and drooling. Mr. Wallick is also posturing (Fig. 1-5). The athletic trainer makes sure that the area around Mr. Wallick is safe. His equipment is loosened, and his circulation, airway, and breathing are monitored.

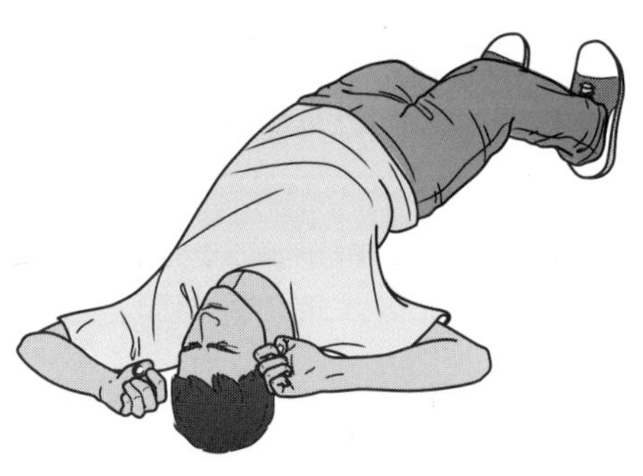

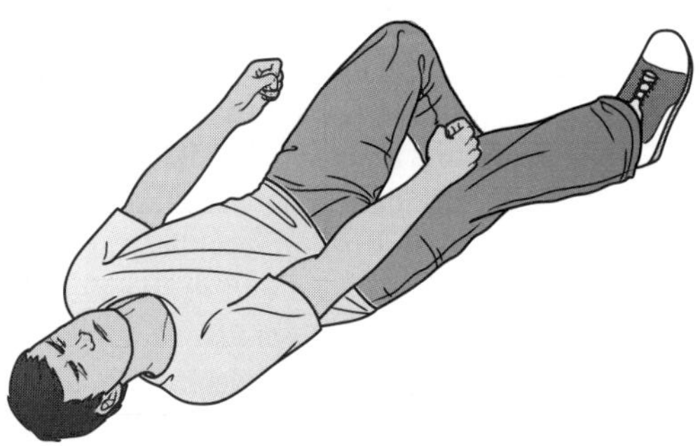

Figure 1-5: Andy Wallick's posturing.

1. From the previous scenario, what do you know about Mr. Wallick's condition?

- ______________________________

____

- ______________________________

____

- ______________________________

____

- ______________________________

____

2. To effectively evaluate Mr. Wallick's condition, you will need to gather additional information. What questions should you ask in addition to what is presented in this scenario?

- ______________________________

____

- ______________________________

____

- ______________________________

____

- ______________________________

____

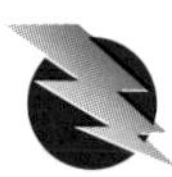

Brain Jolt

Do not restrain or put anything in the individual's mouth when caring for this disorder.

3. Identify key terms and concepts and then research each to broaden your knowledge of first aid and acute care.
   - A chronic condition would have been covered in what section of Mr. Wallick's physical?

     Answer: ____________________
   - Explain a plan of action once this episode ends.

     Answer: ____________________
   - Define *posturing*.

     Answer: ____________________
   - Is the length of the episode important?

     Answer: ____________________
   - Do the lengths of an athlete's episodes indicate anything?

     Answer: ____________________

Conversation Buffer

Episodes of this nature can have embarrassing side effects and serious complications. Therefore, it is important to communicate the importance of crowd control to the coaches and possibly teammates. It is also important to express the potential emergency outcomes of this episode, ensuring that those close to the patient understand the future plan to have him or her evaluated by a physician.

4. Based on the information you currently have and what was provided by your instructor, what are the possible differential diagnoses for Mr. Wallick's condition?
   - ____________________
   - ____________________
   - ____________________
   - ____________________

Why or why not?

For each assessment or diagnosis, write *why?* or *why not?* statements identifying why the information is correct or incorrect. Take details from your textbook, your own research, and data from Mr. Wallick's scenario to help you formulate an answer.

1. ____________________
2. ____________________
3. ____________________
4. ____________________

What do you think?

1. What is your assessment of Mr. Wallick's condition?

   Answer: ____________________
2. Was your assessment correct for Mr. Wallick's condition?

   Answer: ____________________
3. If not, explain what you did incorrectly and how you could have performed a better assessment.

   Answer: ____________________

STUDENT SCENARIO 4: LARRY HYNES

Larry Hynes is a collegiate football quarterback. During a play in the third quarter of the game, he maneuvers to pass the ball. Mr. Hynes is getting ready to release the ball when he is hit from the right side in the midback (Fig. 1-6). Mr. Hynes feels an instant, sharp pain at the site of impact, but he continues playing. He is evaluated after the game, and the athletic training staff believes that Mr. Hyne's injury is a contusion to the paraspinal muscles between T7 and T10. The athletic training staff has instructed him to ice the contused area. Two hours after the initial injury, Mr. Hynes notices that he is nauseated and dizzy. He palpates the area of the contusion and notices that his back muscles are rigid. Mr. Hynes has noticed hematuria when urinating.

1. From the previous scenario, what do you know about Mr. Hynes' injury?
   - ____________________
   - ____________________
   - ____________________
   - ____________________

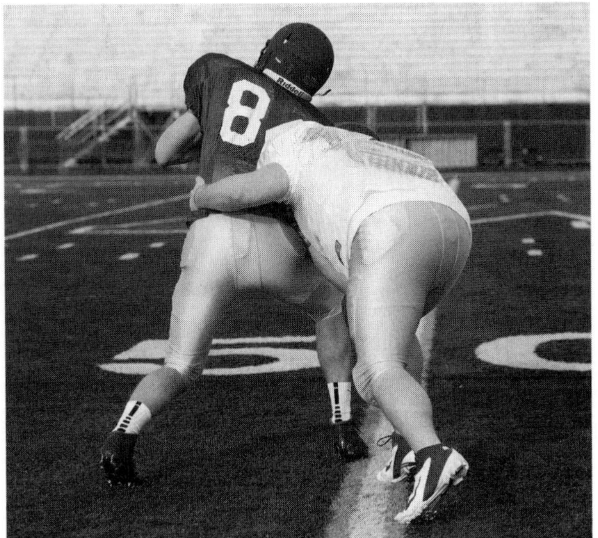

Figure 1-6: The hit to Larry Hynes.

2. To effectively evaluate Mr. Hynes' injury, you will need to gather additional information. What questions should you ask in addition to what is presented in this scenario?
   - ______________________________
   - ______________________________
   - ______________________________
   - ______________________________

3. Identify key terms and concepts and then research each to broaden your knowledge of first aid and acute care.
   - What anatomical structures are involved?

     Answer: ______________________________
   - What internal organ could have been injured with the direct hit on the right side of the body, between T7 and T10?

     Answer: ______________________________
   - Define *contusion*.

     Answer: ______________________________
   - Why are Mr. Hynes' back muscles rigid?

     Answer: ______________________________
   - Why may Mr. Hynes be experiencing nausea and dizziness?

     Answer: ______________________________
   - Define *hematuria*.

     Answer: ______________________________
   - What are the possible causes of hematuria?

     Answer: ______________________________

4. Based on the information you currently have and what was provided by your instructor, what are the possible assessments for Mr. Hynes' injury?
   - ______________________________
   - ______________________________
   - ______________________________
   - ______________________________

Brain Jolt

Hematuria, the result of a direct impact, can possibly mean an injury to a specific organ.

Why or why not?

For each assessment or diagnosis, write *why?* or *why not?* statements identifying why the information is correct or incorrect. Take details from your textbook, your own research, and data from Mr. Hynes' scenario to help you formulate an answer.

1. ______________________________
2. ______________________________
3. ______________________________
4. ______________________________

What do you think?

1. What is your assessment of Mr. Hynes' injury?

   Answer: ______________________________
2. Was your assessment correct for Mr. Hynes' injury?

   Answer: ______________________________
3. If not, explain what you did incorrectly and how you could have performed a better assessment.

   Answer: ______________________________

STUDENT SCENARIO 5: MARCUS WASHINGTON

Marcus Washington is a freshman on a college track team in Colorado. He is originally from Texas. Mr. Washington has been on the campus for 2 weeks when he notices a fever. He has been extremely fatigued recently, but attributed the fatigue and muscle weakness to the preconditioning track program and late-night studying sessions. Mr. Washington wakes up 2 days later with severe pain in his limbs and abdomen. When examining Mr. Washington, the athletic trainer notices that the upper-right quadrant of Mr. Washington's abdomen is point tender and rigid. Because of the fast onset of the symptoms and unfamiliarity with the patient, the athletic trainer references Mr. Washington's physical examination results and notes his African American family history. The athletic trainer refers Mr. Washington to the campus physician for blood work. The results identify abnormal red blood cells (Fig. 1-7), which is a source of concern for the campus physician.

1. From the previous scenario, what do you know about Mr. Washington's condition?
   - ______________________________
   - ______________________________
   - ______________________________
   - ______________________________

2. To effectively evaluate a condition such as Mr. Washington's, you would need to gather additional information. What questions would you ask in addition to what is presented in this scenario?
   - ______________________________
   - ______________________________
   - ______________________________
   - ______________________________

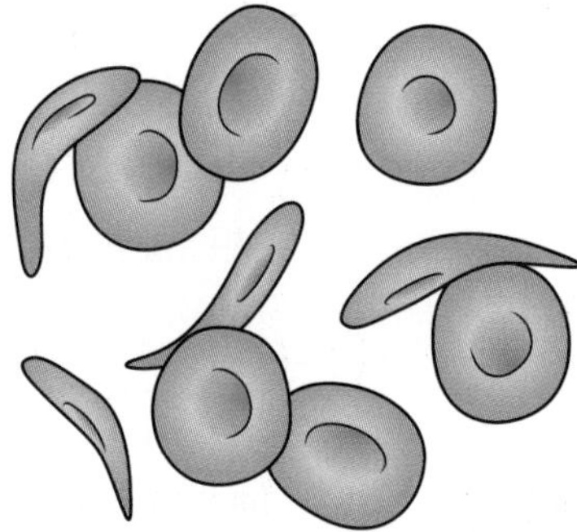

Figure 1-7: Marcus Washington's red blood cells.

3. Identify key terms and concepts and then research each to broaden your knowledge of first aid and acute care.
   - Identify the different quadrants of the abdomen and structures located in each.

     Answer: ______________________________
   - What could be causing Mr. Washington's abdominal rigidity?

     Answer: ______________________________
   - Explain the importance of knowing Mr. Washington's family history.

     Answer: ______________________________
   - Along with dehydration, could altitude be contributing to Mr. Washington's symptoms?

     Answer: ______________________________

Brain Jolt

This genetic defect disorder is more prominent in African American, Native American, and Mediterranean populations.

4. Based on the information you currently have and what was provided by your instructor, what are the possible differential diagnoses for Mr. Washington's condition?
   - ______________________________
   - ______________________________
   - ______________________________
   - ______________________________

Why or why not?

For each assessment or diagnosis, write *why?* or *why not?* statements identifying why the information is correct or incorrect. Take details from your textbook, your

own research, and data from Mr. Washington's scenario to help you formulate an answer.

1. ______________________________

____

2. ______________________________

____

3. ______________________________

____

4. ______________________________

____

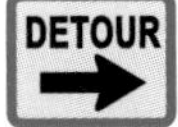

Treatment Detour

Sickle cell trait occurs in 8% of African Americans. Although most have no symptoms, there is a lack of research about the association of sickle cell trait with sudden death in athletes. A retrospective study by the United States Sudden Death in Athletes Registry from 1980 to 2010 found that 2,462 athlete deaths were recorded. Of these deaths, 23 African American deaths occurred in association with sickle cell trait in athletes aged 12 to 22 years. In addition, of the total number of deaths, 271 were African American football players, and 1 in 14 of these were associated with sickle cell trait. As a result, the Registry concluded that sickle cell trait can be associated with sudden death in athletes; therefore, extra precautions and knowledge of the condition can better prepare athletic trainers to monitor activity that might help to prevent sudden death from this condition (Harris, Haas, Eichner, & Maron, 2012).

What do you think?

1. What is your assessment of Mr. Washington's condition?

   Answer: ______________________________

2. Was your assessment correct for Mr. Washington's condition?

   Answer: ______________________________

3. If not, explain what you did incorrectly and how you could have performed a better assessment.

   Answer: ______________________________

STUDENT SCENARIO 6: JODI HUELSKAMP

Jodi Huelskamp is the head athletic trainer for a football team at a Division III college. This Saturday, the team will be traveling to a game 3 hours to the north. The expected high temperature for the November day is only 35°F, and there is rain in the forecast. Ms. Huelskamp is concerned about the prolonged exposure to the wind and low temperature. She instructs the athletic training students to dress accordingly. With 2 minutes remaining in the fourth quarter, an athletic training student comes to Ms. Huelskamp and complains of symptoms of tingling and pain in her toes. Ms. Huelskamp notices that the athletic training student's shoes and socks are wet. The student tells Ms. Huelskamp that her shoes got wet early in the first quarter with the muddy sidelines. Ms. Huelskamp has noted the weather conditions (35°F with a wind chill of 29°F and a rainy mist) and that there is unabsorbed water on the sidelines. As the game ends, Ms. Huelskamp takes the student into the locker room to examine her toes, revealing that they have a white, waxy appearance (Fig. 1-8). Ms. Huelskamp then takes the student's body temperature and discovers that it is 97.2°F. As a result, she decides to slowly begin the process of rewarming the student's toes.

1. What do you know about the athletic training student's condition?

   - ______________________________

     ____

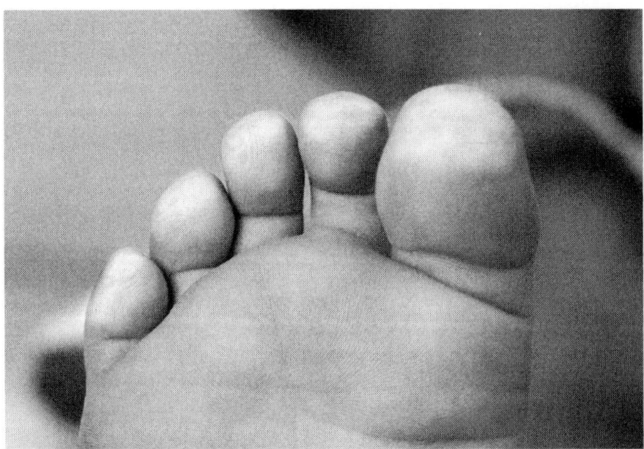

Figure 1-8: Jodi Huelskamp's toes. (© Medioimages/Photodisc © Thinkstock)

- ______________________________
- ______________________________
- ______________________________

2. To effectively evaluate the student's condition, you will need to gather additional information. What questions should you ask in addition to what is presented in this scenario?
   - ______________________________
   - ______________________________
   - ______________________________
   - ______________________________

Brain Jolt
This superficial condition involves only the skin and subcutaneous tissue.

3. Identify key terms and concepts and then research each to broaden your knowledge of first aid and acute care.
   - The tingling and pain in the athletic training student's toes could indicate what condition? Explain the condition.

     Answer: ______________________________
   - Why is the student taken into the locker room?

     Answer: ______________________________
   - With a core body temperature of 97.2°F, what cold-related condition can be ruled out?

     Answer: ______________________________
   - Explain various ways that Ms. Huelskamp can slowly rewarm the affected area.

     Answer: ______________________________
   - Why is it important to rewarm a cold-related condition slowly?

     Answer: ______________________________

4. Based on the information you currently have and what was provided by your instructor, what are the possible differential diagnoses for the athletic training student's condition?
   - ______________________________
   - ______________________________
   - ______________________________
   - ______________________________

Why or why not?

For each assessment or diagnosis, write *why?* or *why not?* statements identifying why the information is correct or incorrect. Take details from your textbook, your own research, and data from Ms. Huelskamp's scenario to help you formulate an answer.

1. ______________________________
2. ______________________________
3. ______________________________
4. ______________________________

What do you think?

1. What is your assessment of the athletic training student's condition?

   Answer: ______________________________
2. Was your assessment correct for the student's condition?

   Answer: ______________________________
3. If not, explain what you did incorrectly and how you could have performed a better assessment.

   Answer: ______________________________

STUDENT SCENARIO 7: STEVE MAXSON

Steve Maxson has 2 minutes left in the third period of a collegiate wrestling match. The opponent delivers a blunt force over Mr. Maxson's right zygomatic bone when Mr. Maxson is going for the opponent's legs. Mr. Maxson experiences an initial amount of pain around the zygomatic and eye orbit, and he has no eye diplopia. He has an excessive amount of external bleeding over the zygomatic bone. With protective gloves and sterile gauze, the athletic trainer applies direct pressure over the zygomatic bone to decrease the external bleeding. The wound is covered, with continuing direct pressure. Mr. Maxson is sent to the emergency department immediately to rule out a LeFort fracture (Fig. 1-9).

1. From the previous scenario, what do you know about Mr. Maxson's injury?
   - ______________________________
   - ______________________________
   - ______________________________
   - ______________________________

2. To effectively evaluate Mr. Maxson's injury, you will need to gather additional information. What questions should you ask in addition to what is presented in this scenario?
   - ______________________________
   - ______________________________
   - ______________________________
   - ______________________________

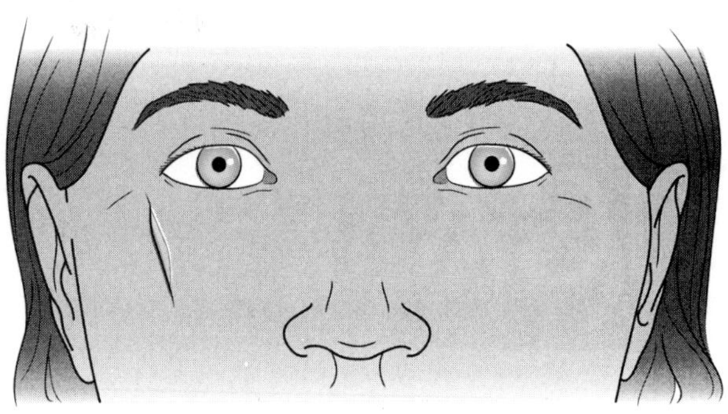

Figure 1-9: Steve Maxson's wound.

> ***Brain Jolt***
> *To prevent infection, avoid an excessive amount of wiping over the injured area.*

3. Identify key terms and concepts and then research each to broaden your knowledge of first aid and acute care.
   - How should external bleeding be controlled?

     Answer: ______________________________
   - Define *diplopia*.

     Answer: ______________________________
   - Explain a LeFort fracture.

     Answer: ______________________________
   - Is there any risk for a concussion? If so, why?

     Answer: ______________________________
   - Identify guidelines for the use of stitches or wound adhesive.

     Answer: ______________________________

4. Based on the information you currently have and what was provided by your instructor, what are the possible differential diagnoses for Mr. Maxson's injury?
   - ______________________________
   - ______________________________
   - ______________________________
   - ______________________________

Why or why not?

For each assessment or diagnosis, write *why?* or *why not?* statements identifying why the information is correct or incorrect. Take details from your textbook, your own research, and data from Mr. Maxson's scenario to help you formulate an answer.

1. ______________________________
2. ______________________________

3. ______________________________

____

4. ______________________________

____

What do you think?

1. What is your assessment of Mr. Maxson's injury?

   Answer: ______________________________

2. Was your assessment correct for Mr. Maxson's injury?

   Answer: ______________________________

3. If not, explain what you did incorrectly and how you could have performed a better assessment.

   Answer: ______________________________

STUDENT SCENARIO 8: REBEKA CROOKSHANK

Rebeka Crookshank is a collegiate volleyball player. She has a family history of vision loss and circulation problems in the lower extremities. The athletic trainer has noticed that Ms. Crookshank takes frequent restroom breaks during warm-ups. As the game begins, Ms. Crookshank is pale, her lips are turning a bluish color, and she is slightly nauseated. Ten minutes into the game, Ms. Crookshank begins to show signs of confusion. Although Ms. Crookshank is a senior collegiate volleyball player, she is suddenly unable to understand the volleyball rotation for serving. The athletic trainer removes Ms. Crookshank from the game and notices a fruity smell on her breath. Ms. Crookshank is taken to the athletic training room to be tested and monitored; she is also given a glucose tablet (Fig. 1-10).

1. From the previous scenario, what do you know about Ms. Crookshank's condition?

   - ______________________________
   - ______________________________
   - ______________________________
   - ______________________________

GLUCOSE TABLETS

Figure 1-10: Rebeka Crookshank's glucose tablets.

2. To evaluate Ms. Crookshank's condition effectively, you will need to gather additional information. What questions should you ask in addition to what is presented in this scenario?

   - ______________________________
   - ______________________________
   - ______________________________
   - ______________________________

Brain Jolt

This condition can be detected by using a "urine" strip, which will highlight imbalances.

3. Identify key terms and concepts and then research each to broaden your knowledge of first aid and acute care.
   - What can frequent urination indicate?

     Answer: ______________________________
   - Why is Ms. Crookshank given a glucose tablet? What might need to be identified before administering this tablet?

     Answer: ______________________________
   - What can the fruity smell on her breath indicate?

     Answer: ______________________________
   - Explain the difference between hyperglycemia and hypoglycemia. How does it apply to this scenario?

     Answer: ______________________________

- Explain different ways to prevent hypoglycemia during and after exercise.

  Answer: ____________________

- Explain the progression of symptoms if this condition remains untreated.

  Answer: ____________________

4. Based on the information you currently have and what was provided by your instructor, what are the possible differential diagnoses for Ms. Crookshank's condition?

   - ____________________
   - ____________________
   - ____________________
   - ____________________

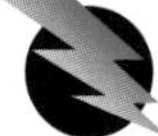

Conversation Buffer

It is important to understand the eating habits of patients with this condition. You must express the importance of proper eating habits and overall health to patients with this condition, so that they can avoid these types of episodes.

Why or why not?

For each assessment or diagnosis, write *why?* or *why not?* statements identifying why the information is correct or incorrect. Take details from your textbook, your own research, and data from Ms. Crookshank's scenario to help you formulate an answer.

1. ____________________
2. ____________________
3. ____________________
4. ____________________

What do you think?

1. What is your assessment of Ms. Crookshank's condition?

   Answer: ____________________

2. Was your assessment correct for Ms. Crookshank's condition?

   Answer: ____________________

3. If not, explain what you did incorrectly and how you could have performed a better assessment.

   Answer: ____________________

STUDENT SCENARIO 9: PETE OSBORNE

Pete Osborne is a senior high school football player. He sprints 5 yards and runs toward the center of the field to catch the ball. As Mr. Osborne turns to catch the ball, he is hit blindly from his left when rotating to continue running. From the impact of the hit, Mr. Osborne's head forcefully accelerates and then forcefully decelerates. He does not get up after being hit. Mr. Osborne is lying supine and conscious when the athletic training staff approaches him on the field. He has symptoms of a headache, dizziness, and tinnitus, and he does not have cervical spine tenderness. He is assisted off the field. Later, he is lucid and has an accurate memory, but is unable to return to the game because of concussion guidelines. One hour after the initial injury, Mr. Osborne is arriving home when he experiences a convulsion. The athletic trainer had instructed his parents about delayed symptoms, which would signify a medical emergency. They notice that his left pupil is dilated (Fig. 1-11), so they take their son to the hospital that is closest to their home.

Brain Jolt

The slow bleed and pressure make this injury a life-threatening emergency.

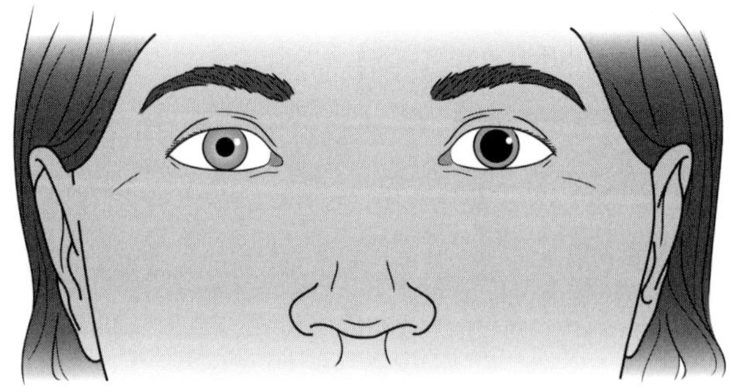

Figure 1-11: Pete Osborne's pupil.

1. From the previous scenario, what do you know about Mr. Osborne's injury?
   - ____________________
   - ____________________
   - ____________________
   - ____________________
2. To evaluate an injury like Mr. Osborne's effectively, you would need to gather additional information. What questions would you ask in addition to what is presented in this scenario?
   - ____________________
   - ____________________
   - ____________________
   - ____________________
3. Identify key terms and concepts and then research each to broaden your knowledge of first aid and acute care.
   - Define *convulsion*.

     Answer: ____________________
   - Define *tinnitus*.

     Answer: ____________________
   - What type of injury can cause Mr. Osborne's symptoms to be delayed?

     Answer: ____________________
   - Explain the process of acceleration and deceleration forces of the brain with a blunt force injury. Are there differences depending on the direction of the hit?

     Answer: ____________________
   - Why is only the left pupil dilated?

     Answer: ____________________
   - Explain what delayed symptoms would have been discussed with Mr. Osborne's parents.

     Answer: ____________________
   - What concussion guidelines does your institution mandate?

     Answer: ____________________
   - What would have changed with on-field management if Mr. Osborne had cervical spine pain? Explain.

     Answer: ____________________
4. Based on the information you currently have and what was provided by your instructor, what are the possible differential diagnoses for Mr. Osborne's injury?
   - ____________________
   - ____________________
   - ____________________
   - ____________________

Why or why not?

For each assessment or diagnosis, write *why?* or *why not?* statements identifying why the information is correct or incorrect. Take details from your textbook, your own research, and data from Mr. Osborne's scenario to help you formulate an answer.

1. ____________________
2. ____________________
3. ____________________
4. ____________________

What do you think?

1. What is your assessment of Mr. Osborne's injury?

   Answer: ____________________
2. Was your assessment correct for Mr. Osborne's injury?

   Answer: ____________________
3. If not, explain what you did incorrectly and how you could have performed a better assessment.

   Answer: ____________________

STUDENT SCENARIO 10: JONAS MARCELLA

Jonas Marcella is a collegiate track-and-field athlete who is traveling with his team to a competition 8 hours to the northwest. Upon arrival, Mr. Marcella notices that he has developed a headache. The headache persists through the evening, and he later develops a cough and occasional shortness of breath. The day of the competition, while getting taped to prevent injury, Mr. Marcella experiences symptoms of chest tightness, wheezing, and nausea. He does not have any symptoms of respiratory stridor, and he takes a short-acting beta-2 agonist (Fig. 1-12). He is then monitored in case any additional medical attention is needed.

1. From the previous scenario, what do you know about Mr. Marcella's condition?
   - ____________________
   - ____________________
   - ____________________
   - ____________________
2. To evaluate Mr. Marcella's condition effectively, you will need to gather additional information. What questions should you ask in addition to what is presented in this scenario?
   - ____________________
   - ____________________
   - ____________________
   - ____________________

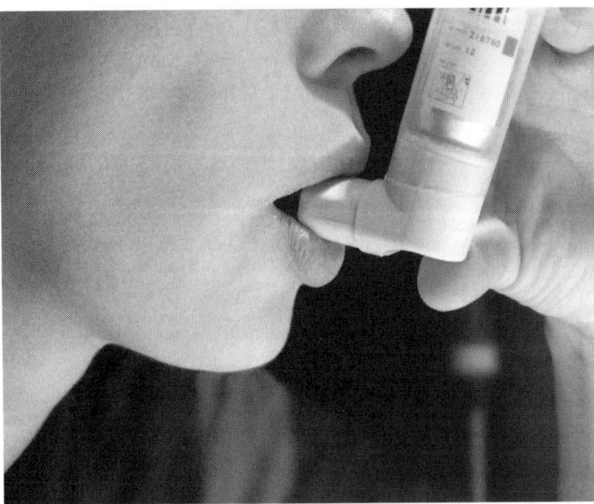

Figure 1-12: Jonas Marcella's medication. (© Thinkstock)

3. Identify key terms and concepts and then research each to broaden your knowledge of first aid and acute care.
   - Why is it important to take notice of the team traveling northwest or having a large barometric change?

     Answer: ____________________
   - Explain a respiratory stridor.

     Answer: ____________________
   - What is a short-acting beta-2 agonist? What is a commonly used brand?

     Answer: ____________________
   - How quickly will Mr. Marcella's medication start working to relieve his symptoms?

     Answer: ____________________
   - Will Mr. Marcella have to take the medication again before his competition?

     Answer: ____________________
   - How would you instruct a patient to use this medication?

     Answer: ____________________
   - When there is difficulty using this medication, what is the role of a spacer?

     Answer: ____________________
4. Based on the information you currently have and what was provided by your instructor, what are the possible differential diagnoses for Mr. Marcella's condition?
   - ____________________
   - ____________________
   - ____________________
   - ____________________

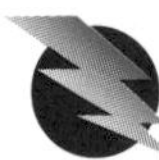

Brain Jolt

This respiratory disease can also be induced by exercise.

Why or why not?

For each assessment or diagnosis, write *why?* or *why not?* statements identifying why the information is correct or incorrect. Take details from your textbook, your own research, and data from Mr. Marcella's scenario to help you formulate an answer.

1. ______________________________

____

2. ______________________________

____

3. ______________________________

____

4. ______________________________

____

What do you think?

1. What is your assessment of Mr. Marcella's condition?

   Answer: ______________________________

2. Was your assessment correct for Mr. Marcella's condition?

   Answer: ______________________________

3. If not, explain what you did incorrectly and how you could have performed a better assessment.

   Answer: ______________________________

STUDENT SCENARIO 11: LANDON GRIMOND

Landon Grimond is a 13-year-old boy who plays quarterback for the junior high football team. During warm-ups, the team will practice various drills. Mr. Grimond is handing the ball to a running back when a fellow teammate directly hits him over the lateral side of his left quadriceps. Mr. Grimond feels a sharp pain and hears a loud crack, and he drops to the ground in extreme pain. The athletic trainer notices immediately that Mr. Grimond has a deformity at the midshaft of his femur, in addition to a left leg-length discrepancy because of the injury. The athletic trainer applies traction to the injured leg and instructs the coaching staff to retrieve the traction splint (Fig. 1-13), along with activating the emergency action plan.

1. From the previous scenario, what do you know about Mr. Grimond's injury?

   - ______________________________

     ____

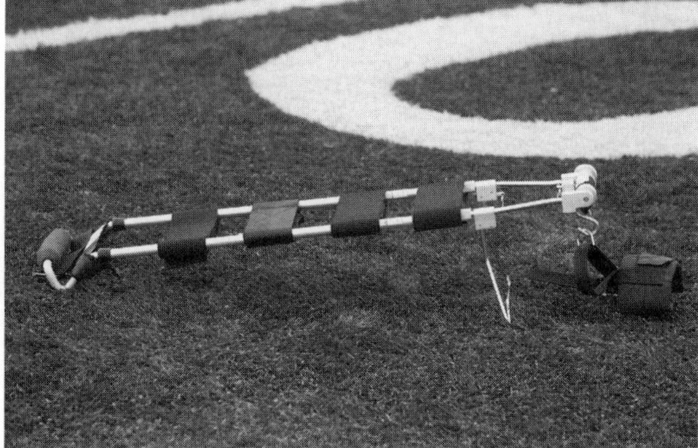

Figure 1-13: Landon Grimond's traction splint.

   - ______________________________

     ____

   - ______________________________

     ____

   - ______________________________

     ____

2. To effectively evaluate Mr. Grimond's injury, you will need to gather additional information. What questions should you ask in addition to what is presented in this scenario?

   - ______________________________

     ____

   - ______________________________

     ____

   - ______________________________

     ____

   - ______________________________

     ____

3. Identify key terms and concepts and then research each to broaden your knowledge of first aid and acute care.

   - What anatomical structures are involved?

     Answer: ______________________________

   - With noted deformity, why does the athletic trainer apply traction to this injury?

     Answer: ______________________________

- Where should traction be applied?

  Answer: ______________________
- Explain why Mr. Grimond has a leg-length discrepancy. Is this an anatomical discrepancy, a functional discrepancy, or neither? Explain.

  Answer: ______________________
- Describe other types of splints and when they are indicated.

  Answer: ______________________
- What are the guidelines when splinting an injury?

  Answer: ______________________
- Do these guidelines change if the injury is compound? If yes, explain.

  Answer: ______________________
- What vital signs should be assessed and where?

  Answer: ______________________

4. Based on the information you currently have and what was provided by your instructor, what are the possible differential diagnoses for Mr. Grimond's injury?

- ______________________
- ______________________
- ______________________
- ______________________

Conversation Buffer

This condition is extremely painful. It is important to talk continually with the athlete about the treatment being given. Sometimes it can be helpful to talk about something that takes the athlete's mind off the pain; this can ease the athlete and sometimes prevent shock. Be sure not to react with worry or surprise, which can evoke panic for the athlete.

Brain Jolt

If this injury is compound, control the bleeding first.

Why or why not?

For each assessment or diagnosis, write *why?* or *why not?* statements identifying why the information is correct or incorrect. Take details from your textbook, your own research, and data from Mr. Grimond's scenario to help you formulate an answer.

1. ______________________
2. ______________________
3. ______________________
4. ______________________

What do you think?

1. What is your assessment of Mr. Grimond's injury?

   Answer: ______________________
2. Was your assessment correct for Mr. Grimond's injury?

   Answer: ______________________
3. If not, explain what you did incorrectly and how you could have performed a better assessment.

   Answer: ______________________

knowledge checklist

Table 1-1 offers a checklist that can be used by a peer, instructor, or preceptor to evaluate each part of a first aid and acute care assessment. Use this table as a tool to ensure that the evaluation is complete and to assess your knowledge of the competencies that apply to this chapter.

TABLE 1-1 ■ First Aid and Acute Care Competency Checklist

	Proficient *Can demonstrate and execute the skill properly*	**Proficient With Assistance** *Can demonstrate and execute the skill with minimal guidance or tips*	**Not Proficient** *Unable to demonstrate and execute the skill properly; need to be reevaluated at another time after further study and practice*
Athlete's Health History			
Medical history			
History of injury or medical conditions			
Type of sport and position played			
Mechanisms of Injury			
How did the injury occur?			
Visual Observations			
Athlete's breathing			
Edema			
Ecchymosis			
Deformity			
Athlete's behavior			
Palpation			
Temperature change over the painful area; crepitus; deformity; intra-articular or extra-articular joint swelling			
Assess Vital Signs			
Neurological			
Reflexes			
Motor function			
Sensory function			
Cranial nerves			
Vascular			
Check pulse			
Capillary refill			
Administer First Aid			
Assess proper management of injury or bleeding (e.g., controlling bleeding, splinting, log roll, cervical spine stabilization)			
Final Assessment			
Sprain, strain, contusion, fracture, condition, severity; be sure to always compare bilaterally			
Proper Activation of EMS			

REFERENCES

Alosco, M. L., Knecht, K., Glickman, E., & Gunstad, J. (2012). History of concussion and exertional heat illness symptoms among college athletes. *International Journal of Athletic Therapy and Training, 17,* 22–27.

Gorse, K., Blanc, R., Feld, F., & Radelet, M. (2010). *Emergency care in athletic training.* Philadelphia, PA: F.A. Davis.

Harris, K. M., Haas, T. S., Eichner, E. R., & Maron, B. J. (2012). Sickle cell trait associated with sudden death in competitive athletes. *American Journal of Cardiology. 110,* 1185–1188.

Mohundro, B. L., & Mohundro, M. M. (2010). Important considerations when dispensing epinephrine auto-injector devices. *Pharmacy Times* [Online]. Retrieved from http://www.pharmacytimes.com/p2p/P2PEpinephrine-0910

National Athletic Training Association. (2011). *Athletic training education competencies* (5th ed.). Retrieved from http://www.nata.org/sites/default/files/5th-Edition-Competencies-2011-PDF-Version.pdf

Prentice, W. (2010). *Arnheim's principles of athletic training: A competency-based approach* (14th ed.). New York, NY: McGraw-Hill.

Starkey, C., Brown, S. D., & Ryan, J. (2010). *Examination of orthopedic and athletic injuries* (3rd ed.). Philadelphia, PA: F.A. Davis.

Venes, D. (Ed.). (2009). *Taber's cyclopedic medical dictionary* (21st ed.). Philadelphia, PA: F.A. Davis.

chapter 2

Emergency Responder

chapter outline

athletic trainer's corner

Out there in the real world, one athletic trainer experienced the following:

It is required by our state that every coach be certified in cardiopulmonary resuscitation (CPR) at the junior high and high school levels. Depending on the association in which the school system participates, the renewal process can be annual or biannual. One of my employers conducted CPR training for all coaches in August. Two weeks after one basketball coach completed our CPR course, he had to use CPR on a patron who was visiting the bank where he worked. The patron was an elderly woman who suffered a cardiac arrest. The coach was the first responder to the emergency and administered CPR until the paramedics arrived. Not only was it rewarding for the coach, who had just saved a life, but it was just as rewarding for me as an instructor. When you are employed in a medical profession, you must always expect that there is a possibility for using CPR. However, to be a loan officer in a bank and have to use those skills on an ordinary Saturday afternoon was impressive. The individuals you are teaching will only take the class as seriously as you present the material. You want those who attend your class to be just as passionate, educated, and comfortable with the skills that they have learned as you are being an instructor. Whether you are certified as a lay responder or a professional rescuer, you are saving lives. Each second counts, so be sure to teach so that the individuals understand this principle.

Melissa Noble, AT, ATC
American Red Cross Instructor
American Safety and Health Instructor
Wilson Memorial Hospital
Sidney, Ohio

learning outcomes

After working through this chapter, you will be able to:

1. Identify the components of a primary and secondary survey of a scene.
2. Explain the indications, guidelines, and supplies needed for equipment removal to access and maintain an airway.
3. Explain proper guidelines for maintaining neutral spine alignment for a spinal injury and identify the equipment and techniques used for cervical stabilization, spine boarding, and patient-transfer techniques.
4. Determine the situations when rescue breathing, cardiopulmonary resuscitation (CPR), or automated external defibrillator (AED) use is indicated following current accepted guidelines.

MODEL SCENARIO 1: VIVIAN O'TOOLE

Vivian O'Toole is an athletic trainer at the high school level. She is covering a girls' basketball game when she is asked by the athletic director to help assist an 65-year-old patron who has just inverted her right ankle while walking down the bleachers. As Ms. O'Toole is walking over to the injured patron, a basketball player goes up for a shot and her legs are taken out from underneath her. The player falls to the court, hitting her head on the gym floor. She is lying unconscious on the court, while the elderly patron is sitting on a bleacher holding her right ankle. Ms. O'Toole needs to decide her plan of action (Fig. 2-1).

1. Based on the previous scenario, what do you know about Ms. O'Toole's situation?
   - *An 65-year-old woman with an inverted right ankle*
   - *A high school basketball player who has hit her head on the gym floor and is unconscious*

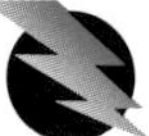

Brain Jolt
An on-the-field assessment is divided into two parts that give direction for emergency treatment.

2. To evaluate Ms. O'Toole's situation effectively, you will need to gather additional information. What questions should you ask in addition to what is presented in this scenario?
   - *Is this situation a medical emergency?*
   - *Is there a risk of shock in this situation?*
   - *Are there any preexisting conditions or a history of medical conditions that would influence this situation? If yes, what are they?*
   - *Does the basketball player have any severe external bleeding?*

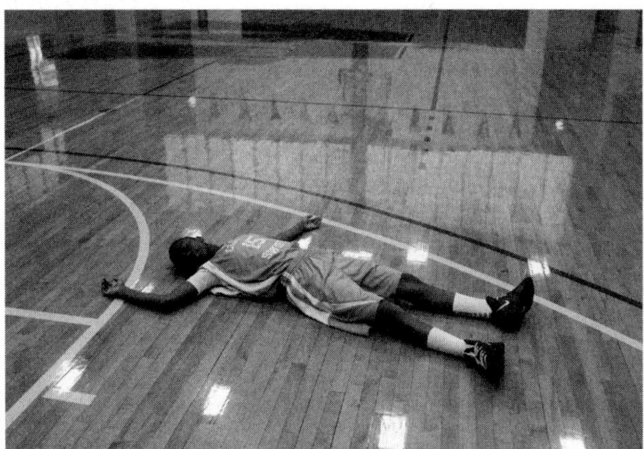

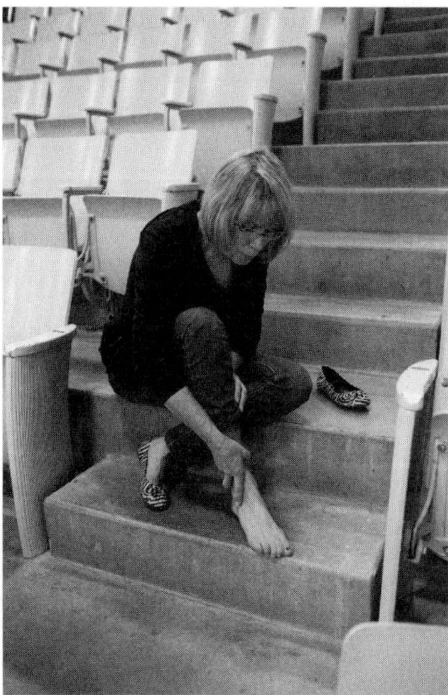

Figure 2-1: Vivian O'Toole's basketball player and elderly patron.

3. Identify key terms and concepts and then research each to broaden your knowledge of emergency care.
   - Explain an on-the-field assessment.
     An on-the-field assessment provides insight into the type of injury and how to prioritize the severity of the injury.
   - What does a primary survey evaluate or determine?
     The primary survey determines life-threatening emergencies or injuries.
   - What does a secondary survey evaluate or determine?
     The secondary survey provides information more specific to the injury. It is a more detailed look at the injury itself, once the injury has been ruled out as life threatening.
   - Does the age of the victim change the on-the-field assessment?
     The age of the victim does not change the primary survey. The life-threatening injuries have to be assessed first, regardless of the age of the victim.
4. Based on the information that you currently have and what was provided by your instructor, what are the possible actions for Ms. O'Toole's situation?
   Primary survey
   Secondary survey
   Complete medical history

Why or why not?

For each possible action, write *why?* or *why not?* statements identifying why the information is correct or incorrect. Take details from your textbook, your own research, and data from Ms. O'Toole's scenario to help formulate an answer.

1. *In this scenario, Ms. O'Toole must focus on the process of a primary survey. The athletic trainer has to assess which injury, either the inverted ankle or the head trauma, requires immediate medical attention.*
2. *In this scenario, Ms. O'Toole is not focusing on a secondary survey. A secondary survey examines the specific injury and the history or mechanism of the injury.*
3. *In this scenario, Ms. O'Toole is not focusing on a complete medical history. A complete medical history is often obtained during a physical examination, and this does not occur with this situation at this point.*

What do you think?

1. What is your plan of action for Ms. O'Toole's situation?
   Answer: *Primary survey*
2. Was your plan of action for Ms. O'Toole's situation correct?
   Answer: *Yes*
3. If not, explain what you did incorrectly and how you could have performed better.
   Answer: ______________________________

MODEL SCENARIO 2: SCOTT ALTENBURG

Scott Altenburg is a collegiate athletic trainer. He is covering a football game when a player falls on the field. When Mr. Altenburg approaches the football player and performs a primary survey, he sees that the supine football player is unconscious and unresponsive. He immediately instructs the football coach to retrieve the AED. Mr. Altenburg has the senior athletic training student stabilize the cervical spine because he has to remove a piece of protective equipment using the trainer's angel. This removal is necessary if emergency respiration treatment has to be performed. The football team currently has two different types of helmets—one with loop straps (traditional helmet) and the other with a quick-release mechanism (revolution helmet). Each type requires a different tool for removal. The fastener for this football player's helmet is a loop strap (Fig. 2-2).

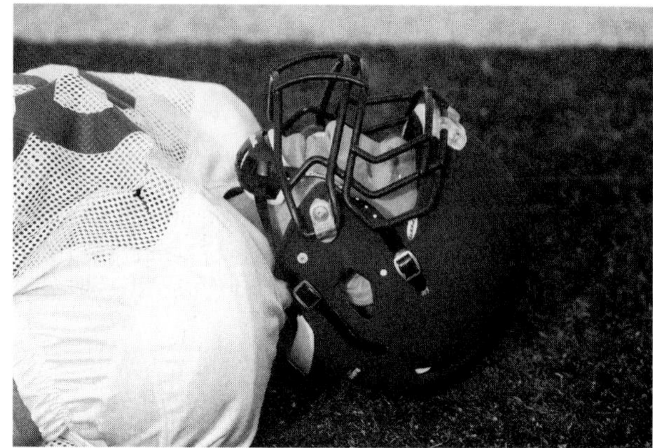

Figure 2-2: Scott Altenburg's traditional helmet with loop straps.

1. Based on the previous scenario, what do you know about Mr. Altenburg's situation?
   - *Unresponsive and unconscious football player*
   - *AED retrieved*
   - *Removed piece of equipment that could obstruct emergency respiratory care*
   - *Different types of helmet clip fasteners*
2. To evaluate Mr. Altenburg's situation effectively, you will need to gather additional information. What

questions should you ask in addition to what is presented in this scenario?

- *Is this situation a medical emergency?*
- *Is there a risk of shock in this situation?*
- *Are there any preexisting conditions or a history of medical conditions that would influence this situation? If yes, what are they?*
- *Is there any family history of concern?*
- *What was the mechanism of injury?*
- *Could there be an obstructed airway?*

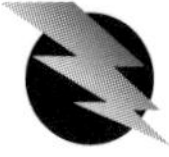

Brain Jolt

Regardless of the respiratory status, this piece of equipment should always be removed when emergency care is needed.

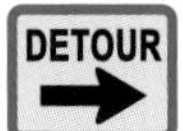

Treatment Detour

In the case of spinal emergencies with football players, research shows that only the face mask should be removed to maintain proper spinal alignment. There are also many techniques to remove a face mask depending on the type of helmet. This study compares the effectiveness of removing a face mask from a new helmet with a quick-release mechanism and one with traditional loop straps, screws, or T-nuts. When assessing the effectiveness of face mask removal, the removal time, amount of head movement, and ease of removal are investigated. The results of this study show that face mask removal was most effective with helmets that required only an electric screwdriver or the specific tool needed for the quick-release mechanism. These face mask removals were faster, had less head motion, and were easier for the athletic trainers when compared with the helmets that required cutting loop straps. It was also noted that the athletic trainers had trouble cutting the loop straps, which could prove to be a concern if this skill is not practiced regularly. These results are important because they show that practice is essential to be effective at face mask removal with any technique and also that athletic trainers must be familiar with the type of helmet they will see most often (Swartz, Belmore, Decoster, & Armstrong, 2010).

3. Identify key terms and concepts and then research each to broaden your knowledge of emergency care.

- Is the check, call, and care sequence executed correctly in this scenario? Explain.
  Mr. Altenburg performs a primary survey, assessing the scene and the level of consciousness of the athlete. 9-1-1 should have been the next step in the check, call, and care sequence. Mr. Altenburg cared for the victim properly but did not have emergency personnel activated.
- When caring for a football player, does the helmet need to be removed?
  A football player's helmet is never removed for fear of a cervical spine injury. If a cervical spine injury is present, the spinal column must stay in a straight line. If the helmet is removed, the athlete's cervical spine will fall back into extension.
- If for some reason a football helmet has to be removed, what other piece of equipment should also be removed? Why?
  If an athlete's helmet has to be removed, the shoulder pads must also be removed to ensure that the cervical spine stays as straight as possible.
- Explain the AED.
  The AED is a portable device that is used when abnormal heart rhythms are suspected, such as during a cardiac arrest. The AED will deliver an electric shock if an abnormal heart rhythm is detected. It is simple enough that any person, professional or lay, can use it.
- Describe a trainer's angel. Are there other tools that could be used to remove the helmet fasteners?
  A trainer's angel is a cutting device used to remove a face mask. It is a handheld device for cutting away a clip on a helmet. Its razor-sharp edges go above and below the clip. When its handles are squeezed together, it cuts down through the clip of the helmet. A similar device is pruning shears. Electric screwdrivers can also be used, but their batteries must be charged. The revolution helmet clips require a device that is pushed into the bolt of the clip to have it pop off the clip. Athletic trainers must be sure that the special tool for the revolution clips is always accessible.

4. Based on the information that you currently have and what was provided by your instructor, what are the possible actions for Mr. Altenburg's situation?
Shoulder pad removal
Face mask removal
Cowboy collar removal
Knee brace removal

Why or why not?

For each possible action, write *why?* or *why not?* statements identifying why the information is correct or incorrect. Take details from your textbook, your own research, and data from Mr. Altenburg's scenario to help you formulate an answer.

1. *The scenario is not focusing on shoulder pad removal. The shoulder pads will not obstruct respiratory care and should remain on the athlete. The only time the shoulder pads are to be cut away and removed is in conjunction with the helmet being removed.*

2. *The scenario is implying that the face mask be removed. The face mask does obstruct respiratory care. If the athletic trainer had to administer resuscitation breaths,* *the face mask would block the process. The face mask should be removed whether the athlete is conscious or unconscious. You never know when emergency respiratory care will be needed.*

3. *The scenario is not focusing on the removal of the cowboy collar. The cowboy collar should remain in place to ensure that the cervical spine does not fall back into extension.*
4. *The scenario is not focusing on a knee brace removal. A knee brace will not interfere with emergency respiratory care.*

What do you think?

1. What is your plan of action for Mr. Altenburg's situation?
   Answer: *Face mask removal*
2. Was your plan of action for Mr. Altenburg's situation correct?
   Answer: *Yes*
3. If not, please explain what you did incorrectly and how you could have performed better.

   Answer: ______________________

STUDENT SCENARIO 1: PHILLIP PIERRI

Phillip Pierri is a collegiate football player who plays wide receiver. Mr. Pierri's route is to sprint 15 yards and then cut toward the center of the field to catch the ball. As Mr. Pierri extends up to catch the ball, an opposing player hits him in the back. Mr. Pierri falls at an odd angle onto his left shoulder and neck and immediately goes limp. He is lying supine and unconscious when the athletic training staff approaches him on the field. It is noted that Mr. Pierri is unresponsive and is not breathing. 9-1-1 is activated, and Mr. Pierri's head is immediately stabilized. The head athletic trainer removes Mr. Pierri's face mask, and the shoulder pads are cut away but not removed. The jaw thrust maneuver (Fig. 2-3) is performed to open his airway. This maneuver proves to be effective, and the athletic trainer inserts an airway adjunct. The athlete's gag reflex is absent.

1. Based on the previous scenario, what do you know about Mr. Pierri's situation?
   - ______________________
   - ______________________
   - ______________________
   - ______________________

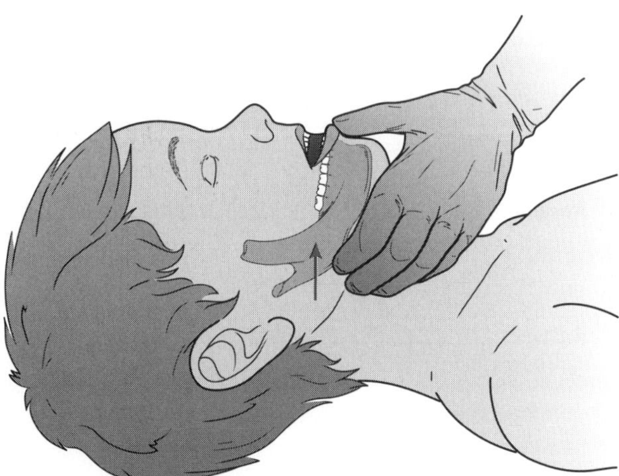

Figure 2-3: Phillip Pierri's jaw thrust maneuver.

2. To evaluate Mr. Pierri's situation effectively, you will need to gather additional information. What questions should you ask in addition to what is presented in this scenario?
   - ______________________
   - ______________________
   - ______________________
   - ______________________

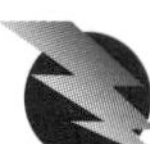

Brain Jolt
The presence or absence of a gag reflex will help you decide which airway device to use.

3. Identify key terms and concepts and then research each to broaden your knowledge of emergency care.
   - Why is Mr. Pierri's head stabilized?

     Answer: ______________________
   - Explain the jaw thrust maneuver.

     Answer: ______________________
   - Why was this technique used in this scenario?

     Answer: ______________________

- Identify the different airway adjuncts and indications for their use.

  Answer: ______________________________

- Do airway adjuncts come in different sizes? Explain how to size each device.

  Answer: ______________________________

- Are there contraindications for using airway adjuncts? Explain.

  Answer: ______________________________

Conversation Buffer

It is important to have a good relationship with your local emergency medical services (EMS) crew. When an emergency injury occurs, time is of the essence. Therefore, it is vital for the EMS crew and the athletic training staff members to be on the same page for injury management. A good way to ensure this is to meet with the crew to discuss patient management before the season or game.

4. Based on the information that you currently have and what was provided by your instructor, what are the possible actions for Mr. Pierri's situation?

   - ______________________________
   - ______________________________
   - ______________________________
   - ______________________________

Treatment Detour

DETOUR

Most injuries that occur during athletic events are minor; however, life-threatening emergencies can and do occur, and emergency plans need to be in place. Emergency situations will include EMS; therefore, it is vital to have a plan that is supported by the EMS staff members. It has been reported that 42% of athletic trainers have been a part of at least one dispute with EMS while on the field caring for an injured athlete, especially regarding helmet and face mask removal. A qualitative study identified EMS perceptions of an athletic trainer's role in emergencies as well as what can be done to improve the working relationship between the two professionals. There was evidently a lack of understanding of the athletic trainer's role in providing care in general and in an emergency situation in particular. EMS staff members also did not understand the professional training that athletic trainers receive or their qualifications to assist in an emergency situation. One EMS participant stated that communication from an athletic trainer before a game or season is helpful. It is important to have annual meetings and emergency rehearsals of the plan of action so that there is a clear plan of action for both parties involved. Ultimately, there needs to be more education regarding the athletic trainer's professional role and open communication to ensure optimal patient care and injury management in an emergency situation (Mazerolle, Pagnotta, Applegate, Casa, & Maresh, 2012).

Why or why not?

For each possible action, write *why?* or *why not?* statements identifying why the information is correct or incorrect. Take details from your textbook, your own research, and data from Mr. Pierri's scenario to help you formulate an answer.

1. ______________________________
2. ______________________________
3. ______________________________
4. ______________________________

What do you think?

1. What is your plan of action for Mr. Pierri's situation?

   Answer: ______________________________

2. Was your plan of action for Mr. Pierri's situation correct?

   Answer: ______________________________

3. If not, explain what you did incorrectly and how you could have performed better.

   Answer: ______________________________

STUDENT SCENARIO 2: DEANNA HAMMEL

Deanna Hammel is a collegiate athletic trainer covering a cross-country track meet. The temperature is unseasonably hot and humid for October. Ms. Hammel is contacted on the radio by her senior athletic training student that a female runner has collapsed at the 4-km mark on the trail. The runner is hyperventilating but shows no signs of apnea. Ms. Hammel instructs the athletic training student to monitor the female athlete and to obtain a medical history until she and the other students arrive. The female runner has a history of asthma. Ms. Hammel discusses with the accompanying athletic training student which oxygen-delivery device would be most appropriate for the conscious female runner and the appropriate flow rate for delivering the oxygen (Fig. 2-4).

1. Based on the previous scenario, what do you know about Ms. Hammel's situation?
   - ______________________________
   - ______________________________
   - ______________________________
   - ______________________________

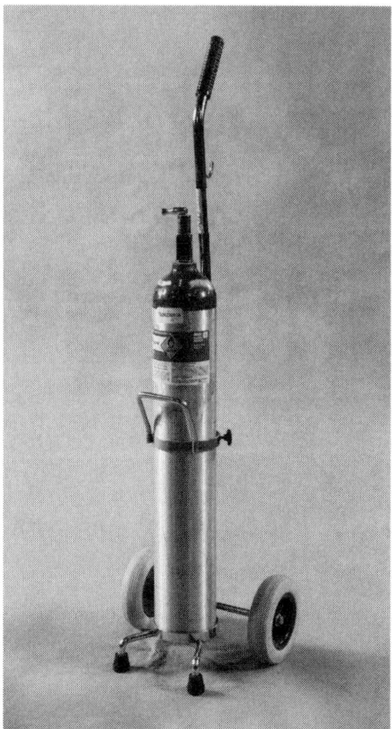

Figure 2-4: Deanna Hammel's oxygen tank.

2. To evaluate Ms. Hammel's situation effectively, you will need to gather additional information. What questions should you ask in addition to what is presented in this scenario?
   - ______________________________
   - ______________________________
   - ______________________________
   - ______________________________

Brain Jolt

A full oxygen tank should read 2000 psi.

3. Identify key terms and concepts and then research each to broaden your knowledge of emergency care.
   - Define *asthma*.

     Answer: ______________________________
   - Why is the course of emergency care for Ms. Hammel to receive oxygen?

     Answer: ______________________________
   - Is asthma a contraindication for receiving oxygen? Are there specific parameters?

     Answer: ______________________________
   - Describe the different types of oxygen-delivery devices. What are the flow rates for each?

     Answer: ______________________________
   - Define *hyperventilation*.

     Answer: ______________________________
   - Define *apnea*.

     Answer: ______________________________
   - Explain how you are able to identify an oxygen tank.

     Answer: ______________________________
   - What is the regulator on the oxygen tank? What are the various parts of the regulator?

     Answer: ______________________________

4. Based on the information that you currently have and what was provided by your instructor, what are the possible actions for Ms. Hammel's situation?

- ____________________
- ____________________
- ____________________
- ____________________

Why or why not?

For each possible action, write *why?* or *why not?* statements identifying why the information is correct or incorrect. Take details from your textbook, your own research, and data from Ms. Hammel's scenario to help you formulate an answer.

1. ____________________
2. ____________________
3. ____________________
4. ____________________

What do you think?

1. What is your plan of action for Ms. Hammel's situation?

   Answer: ____________________

2. Was your plan of action for Ms. Hammel's situation correct?

   Answer: ____________________

3. If not, explain what you did incorrectly and how you could have performed better.

   Answer: ____________________

STUDENT SCENARIO 3: MITT WIMBLED

Mitt Wimbled is a certified athletic trainer for a college lacrosse team. Mr. Wimbled is covering a lacrosse game when a player suddenly collapses. When approaching the player, he notices that the athlete is unconscious and unresponsive. Mr. Wimbled instructs the coach to call 9-1-1, and the athletic trainer from the opposing team helps to stabilize the player's cervical spine. Mr. Wimbled assesses the circulation, airway, and breathing and finds that there is neither breath nor signs of life. Mr. Wimbled cuts the face mask away from the helmet, cuts the shoulder pads but does not remove them, and then performs a jaw thrust maneuver to open the airway. Mr. Wimbled begins CPR and begins using an available device (Fig. 2-5).

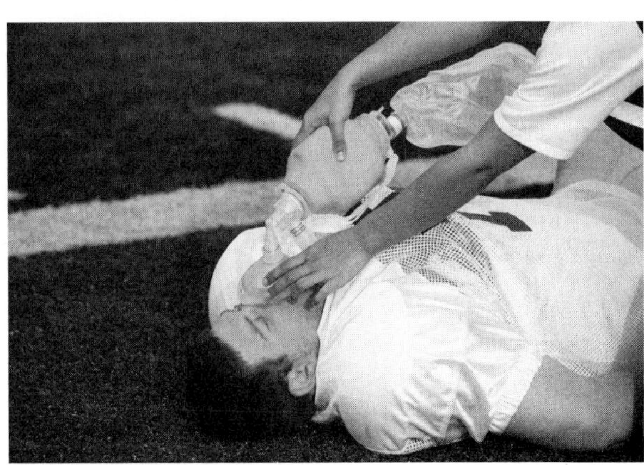

Figure 2-5: Mitt Wimbled's available device.

1. Based on the previous scenario, what do you know about Mr. Wimbled's situation?

- ____________________
- ____________________
- ____________________
- ____________________

2. To evaluate Mr. Wimbled's situation effectively, you will need to gather additional information. What questions should you ask in addition to what is presented in this scenario?

- ____________________
- ____________________
- ____________________

- ______________________________________

____

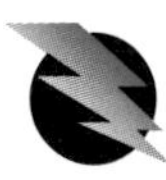

Brain Jolt
This device must have a good seal around the nose and mouth and deliver a higher concentration of oxygen.

3. Identify key terms and concepts and then research each to broaden your knowledge of emergency care.
   - Which electrical device was omitted during the primary survey?

     Answer: ______________________
   - Why did Mr. Wimbled remove the face mask?

     Answer: ______________________
   - Explain the jaw thrust maneuver. When is it recommended?

     Answer: ______________________
   - What are the current guidelines for CPR?

     Answer: ______________________
   - How many cycles are completed in 1 minute of care?

     Answer: ______________________
   - What are the current guidelines for two-person CPR?

     Answer: ______________________
   - How deep are the compressions for adult CPR?

     Answer: ______________________
4. Based on the information that you currently have and what was provided by your instructor, what are the possible actions for Mr. Wimbled's situation?
   - ______________________________________

     ____
   - ______________________________________

     ____
   - ______________________________________

     ____
   - ______________________________________

     ____

Why or why not?

For each possible action, write *why?* or *why not?* statements identifying why the information is correct or incorrect. Take details from your textbook, your own research, and data from Mr. Wimbled's scenario to help you formulate an answer.

1. ______________________________________

   ____
2. ______________________________________

   ____
3. ______________________________________

   ____
4. ______________________________________

   ____

What do you think?

1. What is your plan of action for Mr. Wimbled's situation?

   Answer: ______________________
2. Was your plan of action for Mr. Wimbled's situation correct?

   Answer: ______________________
3. If not, explain what you did incorrectly and how you could have performed better.

   Answer: ______________________

STUDENT SCENARIO 4: MELANIE PARLIN

Melanie Parlin is a collegiate athletic trainer traveling home with the wrestling team from a conference 3 hours to the south. One inch of snow has accumulated on the roads within 2 hours. As the snow continues, Ms. Parlin hears the bus driver mention his concern about the road conditions. She is awakened suddenly by a loud crash and is thrown from her seat. Ms. Parlin knows that she is the only trained medical personnel on the bus. The head coach has had a basic CPR and first aid course. Along with the head coach and herself, the wrestling team has a roster of 15 people. She must assess the scene and injuries. Before she does, Ms. Parlin has to ensure her safety. Once she has done so, Ms. Parlin calls 9-1-1 (Fig. 2-6). She still needs to triage the injuries for treatment.

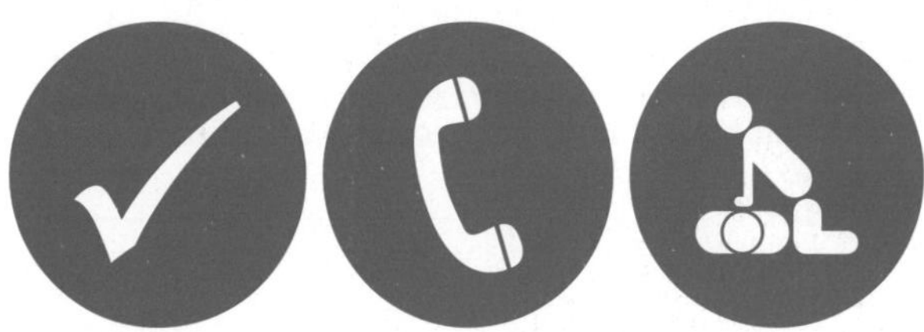

Figure 2-6: Melanie Parlin's emergency care sequence.

1. Based on the previous scenario, what do you know about Ms. Parlin's situation?
   - ______________________________
   - ______________________________
   - ______________________________
   - ______________________________

Brain Jolt
Be educated on the emergency care sequence and how it applies to specific emergency situations and age groups.

2. To evaluate Ms. Parlin's situation effectively, you will need to gather additional information. What questions should you ask in addition to what is presented in this scenario?
   - ______________________________
   - ______________________________
   - ______________________________
   - ______________________________

3. Identify key terms and concepts and then research each to broaden your knowledge of emergency care.
   - What type of questions should Ms. Parlin ask herself when ensuring her safety and the safety of the other passengers?

     Answer: ______________________________
   - What type of information should Ms. Parlin give when calling 9-1-1?

     Answer: ______________________________
   - How could the head coach help to assist in caring for the injured athletes?

     Answer: ______________________________
   - Define *triage*.

     Answer: ______________________________
   - What type of injury would be treated first?

     Answer: ______________________________
   - What are the emergency action steps? Do they vary depending with the type of emergency and the age group?

     Answer: ______________________________

4. Based on the information that you currently have and what was provided by your instructor, what are the first possible actions for Ms. Parlin's situation?
   - ______________________________
   - ______________________________
   - ______________________________
   - ______________________________

Why or why not?

For each possible action, write *why?* or *why not?* statements identifying why the information is correct or incorrect. Take details from your textbook, your own research, and data from Ms. Parlin's scenario to help you formulate an answer.

1. ______________________________
2. ______________________________
3. ______________________________
4. ______________________________

What do you think?

1. What is your plan of action for Ms. Parlin's situation?

   Answer: ______________________________
2. Was your plan of action for Ms. Parlin's situation correct?

   Answer: ______________________________
3. If not, explain what you did incorrectly and how you could have performed a better assessment.

   Answer: ______________________________

STUDENT SCENARIO 5: CARTER SHERRICK

Carter Sherrick is an athletic trainer for a Little League baseball team. After a hit ball, the third baseman is watching the ball but then briefly checks to see whether the second base runner is advancing. Within that second, the ball misses his glove and hits him in the center of his sternum (Fig. 2-7), and he collapses on the field. Mr. Sherrick assesses the athlete's responsiveness and immediately calls 9-1-1. The athlete is in sudden cardiac arrest because of commotio cordis. Mr. Sherrick knows that for every minute without adequate blood flow and oxygen, 10% of the athlete's life is decreased. He starts CPR while awaiting the next step.

Brain Jolt
This portable device can detect heart arrhythmias.

1. From the previous scenario, what do you know about Mr. Sherrick's situation?
   - ______________________________
   - ______________________________
   - ______________________________
   - ______________________________

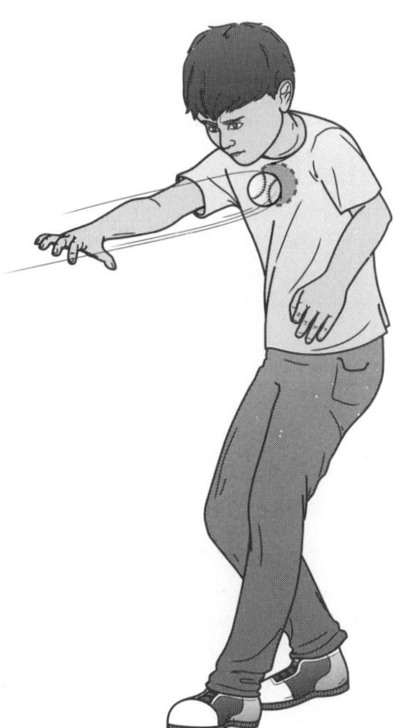

Figure 2-7: Carter Sherrick's mechanism of injury.

2. To evaluate Mr. Sherrick's situation effectively, you will need to gather additional information. What questions should you ask in addition to what is presented in this scenario?
   - ______________________________
   - ______________________________
   - ______________________________
   - ______________________________
3. Identify key terms and concepts and then research each to broaden your knowledge of emergency care.
   - Define *cardiac arrest.*

     Answer: ______________________________
   - Define *commotio cordis.*

     Answer: ______________________________
   - Define *CPR.*

     Answer: ______________________________
   - Explain the current parameters for CPR.

     Answer: ______________________________
   - What is the purpose of CPR?

     Answer: ______________________________
   - What additional equipment is needed in conjunction with CPR?

     Answer: ______________________________
   - What are the parameters for this device? What are the indications and contraindications?

     Answer: ______________________________
4. From the information that you currently have and from what was provided by your instructor, what are the possible actions for Mr. Sherrick's situation?
   - ______________________________
   - ______________________________
   - ______________________________
   - ______________________________

Why or why not?

For each possible action, write *why?* or *why not?* statements identifying why the information is correct or incorrect. Take details from your textbook, your own research, and data from Mr. Sherrick's scenario to help you formulate an answer.

1. ______________________________

____

2. ______________________________

____

3. ______________________________

____

4. ______________________________

____

Conversation Buffer

A situation like this is serious and obviously frightening for everyone present. It is important to discuss an emergency action plan with all personnel working with athletes and to have someone controlling the crowd while care is being given. This person can explain to the parents or guardian what steps are being taken and can try to keep them calm. If bystanders interrupt the care being given, the athlete's condition could be affected.

Treatment Detour

There has been increased awareness of sudden cardiac arrest (SCA) in athletes, and the need to prevent catastrophic sudden cardiac death has increased the importance of the quick availability of AEDs. In the event of SCA, the survival rates decrease by 7% to 10% with each minute without defibrillation after the time of collapse. The goal is to have a shock administered in less than 3 to 5 minutes after the collapse. This study investigated the prevalence, location, and past use of AEDs at NCAA Division II and III institutions. Of the 254 institutions that returned surveys, 205 had at least one AED in the athletic setting, typically placed in the athletic training room, which is less than the number reported at Division I schools. There were 12 reports of the AED being used for SCA: eight older non-athletes, two intercollegiate athletes, and two students. In these cases, there was a 33% survival rate to hospital discharge. These types of emergencies do happen, and the best way to save a life is to have an AED readily available (Drezner, Rogers, & Horneff, 2011).

What do you think?

1. What is your plan of action for Mr. Sherrick's situation?

   Answer: ______________________________

2. Was your plan of action for Mr. Sherrick's situation correct?

   Answer: ______________________________

3. If not, explain what you did incorrectly and how you could have performed better.

   Answer: ______________________________

STUDENT SCENARIO 6: PAUL AMSDEN

Paul Amsden is the goalkeeper for his high school soccer team. During the warm-up for each game, he chews two pieces of gum for good luck. Mr. Amsden dives for a ball and has to roll supine to catch it. As a result, he swallows his gum and begins forcefully coughing. A fellow teammate alerts the athletic trainer, who is familiar with Mr. Amsden's pregame routine. The athletic trainer encourages him to continue coughing. Mr. Amsden begins to gasp for air and stops coughing, giving the universal sign for choking (Fig. 2-8); 9-1-1 is called. The athletic trainer performs a sequence of life-saving techniques to hopefully expel the object. When the athletic trainer is standing behind Mr. Amsden, Mr. Amsden is 1 foot taller.

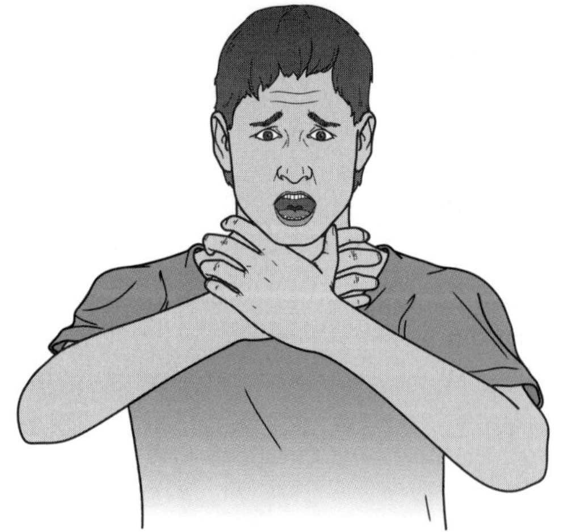

Figure 2-8: Paul Amsden's universal sign of choking.

1. From the previous scenario, what do you know about Mr. Amsden's situation?
   - ______________________________
   - ______________________________
   - ______________________________
   - ______________________________

2. To evaluate Mr. Amsden's situation effectively, you will need to gather additional information. What questions should you ask in addition to what is presented in this scenario?
   - ______________________________
   - ______________________________
   - ______________________________
   - ______________________________

Brain Jolt
Always receive consent when treating any conscious adult victim.

3. Identify key terms and concepts and then research each to broaden your knowledge of emergency care.
   - Why is Mr. Amsden encouraged to continue to cough?

     Answer: ______________________________
   - What signs will Mr. Amsden exhibit to indicate that he is no longer able to expel the object on his own?

     Answer: ______________________________
   - What is the sequence that the athletic trainer follows to help expel the lodged object?

     Answer: ______________________________
   - What can be done if there is a height difference? What if this scenario involved a child?

     Answer: ______________________________

4. From the information that you currently have and from what was provided by your instructor, what are the possible actions for Mr. Amsden's situation?
   - ______________________________
   - ______________________________
   - ______________________________
   - ______________________________

Why or why not?

For each possible action, write *why?* or *why not?* statements identifying why the information is correct or incorrect. Take details from your textbook, your own research, and data from Mr. Amsden's scenario to help you formulate an answer.

1. ______________________________
2. ______________________________
3. ______________________________
4. ______________________________

What do you think?

1. What is your plan of action for Mr. Amsden's situation?

   Answer: ______________________________
2. Was your plan of action for Mr. Amsden's situation correct?

   Answer: ______________________________
3. If not, explain what you did incorrectly and how you could have performed better.

   Answer: ______________________________

STUDENT SCENARIO 7: CARLOS MACCHIATO

Carlos Macchiato is a senior on his high school football team and plays quarterback. With 2 minutes left in the fourth quarter, Mr. Macchiato is passing the ball to the right side of the field when he is hit from the left side. He goes down and does not get back up. Upon approaching Mr. Macchiato, the athletic trainer recognizes that he is lying prone and limp but conscious. Manual stabilization is applied immediately to Mr. Macchiato's helmet. Mr. Macchiato is unable to move his legs and has neck pain. The athletic training staff performs a log roll (Fig. 2-9) to further evaluate him. They remove his face mask, perform a secondary survey, and take the next step.

1. From the previous scenario, what do you know about Mr. Macchiato's situation?
   - ______________________________
   - ______________________________
   - ______________________________
   - ______________________________

2. To evaluate Mr. Macchiato's situation effectively, you will need to gather additional information. What questions should you ask in addition to what is presented in this scenario?
   - ______________________________
   - ______________________________
   - ______________________________
   - ______________________________

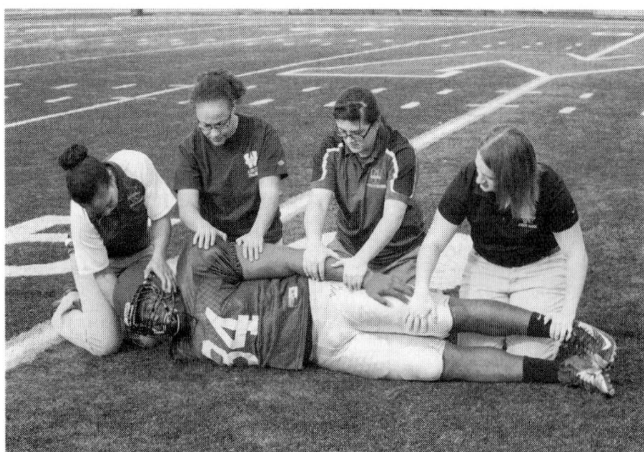

Figure 2-9: Carlos Macchiato's log roll technique.

Brain Jolt

When performing the log roll technique, be sure to have the correct number of people to help stabilize the body when rolling from prone to supine.

3. Identify key terms and concepts and then research each to broaden your knowledge of emergency care.
   - What was determined in the primary survey?

     Answer: ______________________________
   - Explain manual stabilization.

     Answer: ______________________________
   - Why is the face mask removed?

     Answer: ______________________________
   - What is involved in the secondary survey?

     Answer: ______________________________
   - Describe the log roll technique. How many people should assist with this maneuver?

     Answer: ______________________________
   - What other techniques can be used? Can these be used with an athlete lying prone?

     Answer: ______________________________

4. From the information that you currently have and what was provided by your instructor, what are the possible actions for Mr. Macchiato's situation?
   - ______________________________
   - ______________________________
   - ______________________________
   - ______________________________

Why or why not?

For each possible action, write *why?* or *why not?* statements identifying why the information is correct or incorrect. Take details from your textbook, your own research, and data from Mr. Macchiato's scenario to help you formulate an answer.

1. ____

____

2. ____

____

3. ____

____

4. ____

____

What do you think?

1. What is your plan of action for Mr. Macchiato's situation?

   Answer: ____

2. Was your plan of action for Mr. Macchiato's situation correct?

   Answer: ____

3. If not, explain what you did incorrectly and how you could have performed better.

   Answer: ____

STUDENT SCENARIO 8: WALTER WASSON

Walter Wasson works at a local high school as an athletic trainer and is covering a boys' basketball game. Two minutes into the fourth quarter, an overweight official collapses on the court. Mr. Wasson surveys the scene, puts on his personal protective equipment, and assesses the official's level of responsiveness and consciousness. Mr. Wasson instructs the athletic director to call 9-1-1 and to retrieve the AED. Mr. Wasson begins CPR until the AED is retrieved from the hallway. Once the official's heart rhythm is analyzed, a shock is indicated and delivered (Fig. 2-10). The official begins to show signs of life, and Mr. Wasson puts him in a position for monitoring.

1. From the previous scenario, what do you know about Mr. Wasson's situation?

   - ____

     ____

   - ____

     ____

   - ____

     ____

   - ____

     ____

Figure 2-10: Walter Wasson's CPR with an AED.

2. To evaluate Mr. Wasson's situation effectively, you will need to gather additional information. What questions should you ask in addition to what is presented in this scenario?

   - ____

     ____

   - ____

     ____

   - ____

     ____

   - ____

     ____

Brain Jolt

The modified HAINES position is used to monitor someone with suspected spinal injury.

3. Identify key terms and concepts and then research each to broaden your knowledge of emergency care.
   - Why does Mr. Wasson survey the scene?

     Answer: ____
   - What type of protective equipment would Mr. Wasson be using?

     Answer: ____
   - What is the AED? Explain how it works and how it is applied to the patient.

     Answer: ____
   - Explain the modified HAINES position.

     Answer: ____
   - How would this situation change if Mr. Wasson were alone?

     Answer: ____

4. From the information that you currently have and from what was provided by your instructor, what are the possible actions for Mr. Wasson's situation?
   - ______________________________
   - ______________________________
   - ______________________________
   - ______________________________

Why or why not?

For each possible action, write *why?* or *why not?* statements identifying why the information is correct or incorrect. Take details from your textbook, your own research, and data from Mr. Wasson's scenario to help you formulate an answer.

1. ______________________________
2. ______________________________
3. ______________________________
4. ______________________________

What do you think?

1. What is your assessment of Mr. Wasson's situation?

   Answer: ______________________________

2. Was your assessment correct for Mr. Wasson's situation?

   Answer: ______________________________

3. If not, explain what you did incorrectly and how you could have performed better.

   Answer: ______________________________

STUDENT SCENARIO 9: AMANDA CLECKNER

Amanda Cleckner is covering a women's soccer game. She is taping some of the athletes' ankles when a female soccer player begins coughing forcefully. The female athlete had been eating a piece of hard candy. Ms. Cleckner encourages the athlete to continue coughing. The athlete stops coughing, struggles to breathe, and is unable to speak. Ms. Cleckner obtains consent to treat from the conscious athlete. Ms. Cleckner delivers five back blows and five abdominal thrusts to expel the object. This technique is unsuccessful, and the athlete becomes unconscious. Ms. Cleckner lowers the athlete to the floor and performs a head-tilt/chin-lift maneuver (Fig. 2-11). Ms. Cleckner tries to ventilate the athlete's lungs but is unsuccessful, even after repositioning the head. Ms. Cleckner proceeds with the proper technique.

Brain Jolt
Perform a finger sweep during this technique only when you see an object.

1. From the previous scenario, what do you know about Ms. Cleckner's situation?
   - ______________________________
   - ______________________________
   - ______________________________
   - ______________________________

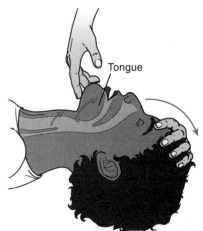

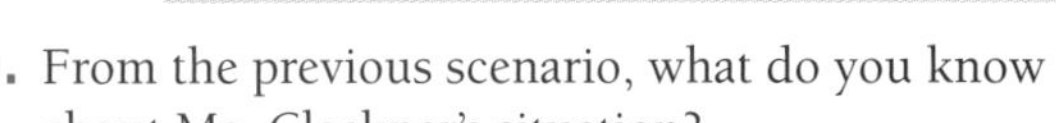

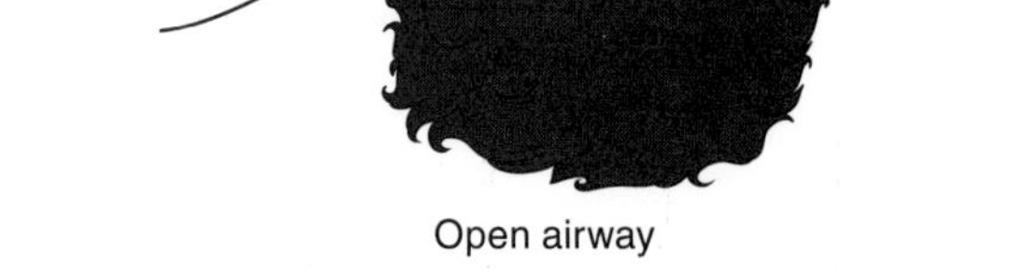

Figure 2-11: Amanda Cleckner's head-tilt/chin-lift maneuver.

2. To evaluate Ms. Cleckner's situation effectively, you will need to gather additional information. What questions should you ask in addition to what is presented in this scenario?

- ____________________
- ____________________
- ____________________
- ____________________

3. Identify key terms and concepts and then research each to broaden your knowledge of emergency care.
   - Why does Ms. Cleckner encourage the athlete to cough?

     Answer: ____________________
   - Why is it important to obtain consent to treat? Do you need consent with an unconscious victim?

     Answer: ____________________
   - If the victim is a child, how does this change your plan of action?

     Answer: ____________________
   - What is the importance of the back blows and abdominal thrusts?

     Answer: ____________________
   - What is the head-tilt/chin-lift maneuver? Why does Ms. Cleckner have to reposition the head?

     Answer: ____________________
   - Explain a finger sweep during this technique.

     Answer: ____________________

4. From the information that you currently have and from what was provided by your instructor, what are the possible actions for Ms. Cleckner's situation?

- ____________________
- ____________________
- ____________________
- ____________________

Why or why not?

For each possible action, write *why?* or *why not?* statements identifying why the information is correct or incorrect. Take details from your textbook, your own research, and data from Ms. Cleckner's scenario to help you formulate an answer.

1. ____________________
2. ____________________
3. ____________________
4. ____________________

What do you think?

1. What is your plan of action for Ms. Cleckner's situation?

   Answer: ____________________
2. Was your plan of action for Ms. Cleckner's situation correct?

   Answer: ____________________
3. If not, explain what you did incorrectly and how you could have performed better.

   Answer: ____________________

knowledge checklist

Table 2-1 offers a checklist that may be used by a peer, instructor, or preceptor to evaluate skills in emergency care. Use this checklist as a tool to ensure that the evaluation is complete and to assess your knowledge of the competencies that apply to this chapter.

TABLE 2-1 ■ Emergency Responder Competency Checklist

	Proficient *Can demonstrate and execute the skill properly*	**Proficient With Assistance** *Can demonstrate and execute the skill with minimal guidance or tips*	**Not Proficient** *Unable to demonstrate and execute the skill properly; needs to be reevaluated at another time after further study and practice*
Athlete's Health History			
Medical history			
History of injury or medical conditions			
Type of sport and position played			
Mechanisms of Injury			
How did the injury occur?			
Primary Survey			
Secondary Survey			
Conscious choking			
Unconscious choking			
Checking unconscious athlete			
CPR			
AED			
Airway adjuncts			
Oxygen administration			
Patient-transfer techniques			
Spinal-injury management • Equipment removal • Spine boarding			

REFERENCES

Drezner, J. A., Rogers, K. J., & Horneff, J. G. (2011). Automated external defibrillators use at NCAA Division II and III universities. *British Journal of Sports Medicine, 45*, 1174–1178.

Gorse, K., Blanc, R., Feld, F., & Radelet, M. (2010). *Emergency care in athletic training*. Philadelphia, PA: F.A. Davis.

Mazerolle, S. M., Pagnotta, K. D., Applegate, K. A., Casa, D. J., & Maresh, C. M. (2012). The athletic trainer's role in providing emergency care in conjunction with the emergency medical services. *International Journal of Athletic Therapy and Training*, March, 39–44.

National Athletic Training Association. (2011). *Athletic training education competencies* (5th ed.). Retrieved from http://www.nata.org/sites/default/files/5th-Edition-Competencies-2011-PDF-Version.pdf

Prentice, W. (2010). *Arnheim's principles of athletic training: A competency-based approach* (14th ed.). New York, NY: McGraw-Hill.

Starkey, C., Brown, S. D., & Ryan, J. (2010). *Examination of orthopedic and athletic injuries* (3rd ed.). Philadelphia, PA: F.A. Davis.

Swartz, E. E., Belmore, K., Decoster, L. C., & Armstrong, C. W. (2010). Emergency face-mask removal effectiveness: A comparison of traditional and nontraditional football helmet face-mask attachment systems. *Journal of Athletic Training*, 45, 560–569.

Venes, D. (Ed.). (2009). *Taber's cyclopedic medical dictionary* (21st ed.). Philadelphia, PA: F.A. Davis.

chapter 3

Injury Prevention and Safety

chapter outline

athletic trainer's corner

Out there in the real world, one athletic training student experienced the following while being supervised by a certified athletic trainer:

As an athletic training student, taping was always a skill that I overlooked. I never really realized how important it was until one specific event. I was working in the athletic training room one day my sophomore year when one of the football players needed his hand, wrist, and thumb taped. I was always the one who tried to avoid a situation if I wasn't comfortable with what the athlete needed, but this time I couldn't. The athlete could tell that I was nervous and hesitant with what I was doing, and I think it made him nervous as well. I finished the tape job, which didn't look terrible, but it definitely could have been better. The athlete went out to practice and about 30 minutes later he had cut it off and one of the senior students retaped his hand, wrist, and thumb. I knew then that I needed to practice my tape jobs more and make sure that I was confident in performing each of them. If the athlete knows you are confident in what you are doing, he or she will be more confident with you taping him or her before practice and games. I made sure that I practiced my tape jobs, and didn't just focus on one specific area so that when a situation came up I wouldn't be unsure of myself. Being confident in what you know makes things easier when an athlete needs something done and you can step up and do it without any question or doubt. In this case it was just a simple tape job that I wasn't comfortable with, but you never know how serious the situation could be, and you don't want to be the one who treats an athlete improperly.

Shauna Ward
Athletic Training Student
Wilmington College

learning outcomes

After working through this chapter, you will be able to:

1. Identify the guidelines for fitting and maintaining protective equipment.
2. Identify indications and techniques for using preventative taping and wrapping.
3. Explain the current practice guidelines for activities in extreme weather conditions and interpreting weather data and indicators.
4. Explain the components needed to prevent environmental heat illness.

MODEL SCENARIO 1: ALLEN HOERSTEIN

Allen Hoerstein is the kicker on the football team and has a mild right hip flexor strain (Fig. 3-1). He has been attending rehabilitation sessions daily since he injured his hip flexor and is progressing well. Throughout rehabilitation, Mr. Hoerstein's chief complaint is that his right leg lags upon hip flexion when practicing the motion of kicking the ball. He states that it feels "slow." The athletic trainer wants to apply a wrap technique that could assist Mr. Hoerstein with this motion.

1. Based on this scenario, what do you know about Mr. Hoerstein's condition?
   - *Football kicker*
   - *Right hip flexor strain*
   - *Still has mild pain with hip extension*
   - *Athletic trainer wants to use a technique to assist with hip flexion*

Brain Jolt

This technique can assist with hip extension or hip flexion depending on how it is applied.

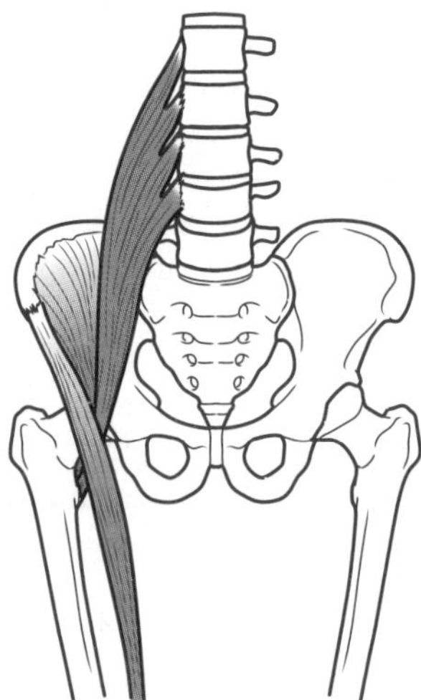

Figure 3-1: Allen Hoerstein's hip flexor muscle group.

2. To evaluate Mr. Hoerstein's condition effectively, you will need to gather additional information. What questions should you ask in addition to what is presented in this scenario?
   - *Are there any preexisting injuries or is there a history of medical conditions? If yes, what are they?*
   - *In the initial examination, was any posterior musculature weakness or injury present?*
   - *What was the mechanism of injury?*
   - *How long ago did the injury occur?*
   - *What is Mr. Hoerstein's range of motion (ROM) and strength at the hip compared bilaterally?*
3. Identify key terms and concepts and then research each to broaden your knowledge of injury prevention and safety.
   - Explain signs and symptoms of a hip flexor strain.

     Signs and symptoms of a hip flexor strain include anterior pain often located at the anterior superior iliac spine (ASIS), along with pain with hip flexion. The athlete will have a strength deficit with active resistive exercises. Ecchymosis can occur, but it depends on the severity and mechanism of the injury.
   - What are the hip flexor muscles?

     The iliopsoas and the rectus femoris.
   - What materials will most likely be used to assist with hip flexion in this scenario? Explain the length and size of the material used.

     An elastic bandage will be used to wrap Mr. Hoerstein's hip. A double-length elastic bandage is recommended to cover or wrap around the hip joint two to three times.
   - Describe how a hip spica would be applied to assist someone with hip flexion.

     The elastic bandage will start at the anterior part of the right ASIS bony landmark. Wrapping right and posterior, the elastic bandage will go around the athlete's posterior, coming in front and across the right quadriceps. The elastic bandage will wrap behind the right hamstring and then be pulled up into hip flexion. This process will be done until the elastic bandage used can be secured with tape. The leg should be relaxed and slightly flexed. The hip does not have to be internally or externally rotated.

- Describe how a hip spica would be applied to assist someone with hip extension.

The elastic wrap would still start over the right ASIS bony landmark for a right side injury. The elastic bandage would wrap left and posterior around Mr. Hoerstein. The wrap would come across the ASIS bony landmark and be directed down over the right quadriceps, then pull the wrap posterior or into extension. The leg should be extended with the hip in slight external rotation.

4. Based on the information that you currently have and what was provided by your instructor, what are the possible techniques used for Mr. Hoerstein's condition?

Neoprene sleeve
Hip spica with hip extension as the focus
Hip spica with hip flexion as the focus
Quadriceps wrap

Why or why not?

For each technique, write *why?* or *why not?* statements identifying why the information is correct or incorrect. Take details from your textbook, your own research, and data from Mr. Hoerstein's scenario to help you formulate an answer.

1. *Mr. Hoerstein is not going to use a neoprene sleeve, because the sleeve will not assist with hip flexion and does not go around the hip. It surrounds only the quadriceps.*
2. *Mr. Hoerstein is not going to have a hip spica focusing on hip extension applied because weakness is occurring during the follow-through of his kicking motion. Going from extension to flexion is where the weakness and "slow" feeling is noted.*
3. *Mr. Hoerstein is going to have a hip spica applied that will help with hip flexion. Mr. Hoerstein is weak with hip flexion and needs the extra assistance to complete the range of motion for his kicking.*
4. *Mr. Hoerstein is not going to have a quadriceps wrap applied, because the wrap will not assist with hip flexion and does not go around the hip. It surrounds only the quadriceps.*

What do you think?

1. What is your plan of action for Mr. Hoerstein's condition?
   Answer: *Hip spica with hip flexion as the focus*
2. Was your plan of action for Mr. Hoerstein's condition correct?
   Answer: *Yes*
3. If not, explain what you did incorrectly and how you could have performed better.
   Answer: ________________________________

MODEL SCENARIO 2: RICK SLAYTON

Rick Slayton is a certified athletic trainer at the high school level. He is covering a championship baseball game at home. The sky is quickly becoming dark, and it is extremely windy. The game is in the second inning when the lightning detector (Fig. 3-2) goes off, signifying a threat of severe weather ranging about 20 miles away. Mr. Slayton checks the weather service on his smartphone to see what is developing on the radar.

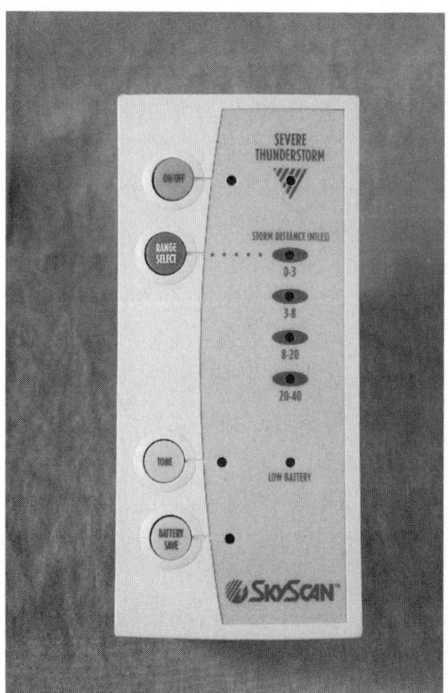

Figure 3-2: Rick Slayton's lightning detector.

1. Based on this scenario, what do you know about Mr. Slayton's situation?
   - *Home baseball game*
   - *Dark sky, windy*
   - *Lightning 20 miles away*
   - *Checking weather service radar*

2. To evaluate Mr. Slayton's situation effectively, you will need to gather additional information. What questions should you ask in addition to what is presented in this scenario?
   - *Have the athletic trainer and head coach reviewed an emergency action plan?*
   - *What types of facilities are available where the game is being played?*
   - *What advisories has the weather service indicated?*
3. Identify key terms and concepts and then research each to broaden your knowledge of injury prevention and safety.
   - When are outside activities canceled and everyone evacuated to safety?
     If lightning is detected within 6 miles or less, then the team will have to evacuate the field.
   - If a school does not have a lightning detector, what theory can a person use to ensure safety in a springtime storm?
     If a school does not have a lightning detector, the staff can use the flash-to-bang theory.
   - Explain the flash-to-bang theory.
     The flash-to-bang theory involves counting how many seconds it takes to hear thunder after lightning is detected and seen. Divide that amount of time by five to determine the distance in miles.
   - In severe weather, where should an outside athletic event be evacuated?
     An outside event should be directed to an inside facility or to parked cars.
   - If there is not an available inside facility, what should Mr. Slayton direct the teams to do?
     If an inside shelter or parked car is not available, have the team go to a low-lying area and crouch down, in a ditch if possible. Do not have the team stand around any trees, do not allow an athlete to lie down, and avoid standing water.
   - What are the return-to-play guidelines for a storm?
     The teams can return to play 30 minutes after the last lightning strike or sound of thunder.
   - Is Mr. Slayton responsible for the safety of the team in severe weather?
     Yes, Mr. Slayton is responsible for advising the coach and officials of the weather threats and the procedures to follow.
4. Based on the information that you currently have and what was provided by your instructor, what are the possible actions for Mr. Slayton's situation?
   Continue to allow the team to play while assessing the situation.
   Evacuate the team immediately and monitor the weather.
   Cancel the game immediately.

Why or why not?

For each possible action, write *why?* or *why not?* statements identifying why the information is correct or incorrect. Take details from your textbook, your own research, and data from Mr. Slayton's scenario to help you formulate an answer.

1. *Mr. Slayton should continue to allow the team to play while assessing the situation and checking the weather service radar. At this time, he should make the coach aware of the possible threat while he is verifying the lightning detector's accuracy.*
2. *Mr. Slayton should not evacuate the team until he is sure of the conditions and has confirmed the lightning detector's accuracy with the weather service; however, this action could become necessary quickly.*
3. *Mr. Slayton should not cancel the game immediately. First, the officials must "call" the game on the advice of the athletic trainer. In addition, even if severe weather is confirmed, the teams can return to play 30 minutes after the last lightning strike, because spring storms can end fairly quickly. Canceling the game at this time would be premature.*

Conversation Buffer

Sometimes weather issues can be an area of conflict between coaches and athletic trainers. Before the season begins, it is important to talk with your coaches about the guidelines for severe weather safety and the parameters for returning to play. This can help to resolve confusion when an event occurs. Having a weather policy written and outlined to supporting staff can help to reduce any confusion during the threat of unpredictable weather.

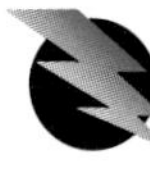

Brain Jolt

Storms can move in fast, so it is important to be aware of the weather and have a plan to get the teams to safety.

What do you think?

1. What is your plan of action for Mr. Slayton's situation?
   Answer: *Continue to allow the teams to play while assessing the situation.*
2. Was your plan of action for Mr. Slayton's situation correct?
   Answer: *Yes*
3. If not, please explain what you did incorrectly and how you could have performed a better assessment.

   Answer: ____________________

STUDENT SCENARIO 1: HERMAN MEKELBURG

Herman Mekelburg is a certified athletic trainer at the high school level. He has recently had four football players sustain concussions and is attributing the injuries to improperly fitted helmets. Mr. Mekelburg approaches the head football coach with his concerns. The coach assures him that the helmets are properly sized and fitted and demonstrates how he fits a helmet (Fig. 3-3). The coach explains that the helmet should come down below the base of the skull posteriorly and meet the eyebrow line anteriorly. The coach states that he will occasionally switch cheek pads to make the helmets fit more players. The coach shows Mr. Mekelburg that he allows the snugness of the helmet to be judged by inserting his fifth finger between the head and the helmet liner. The coach also states that his budget only allows for half of the helmets to be reconditioned each year, so he takes the other helmets home to be painted and go unnoticed.

1. Based on this scenario, what do you know about Mr. Mekelburg's situation?
   - ______________________
   - ______________________
   - ______________________
   - ______________________

2. To evaluate Mr. Mekelburg's situation effectively, you will need to gather additional information. What questions should you ask in addition to what is presented in this scenario?
   - ______________________
   - ______________________
   - ______________________
   - ______________________

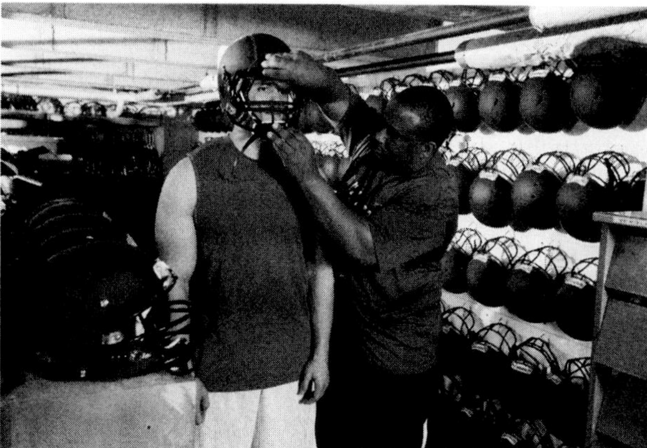

Figure 3-3: Herman Mekelburg's helmet fitting.

> ***Brain Jolt***
> *A helmet's certification is valid only if the helmet is fitted properly.*

3. Identify key terms and concepts and then research each to broaden your knowledge of injury prevention and safety.
   - What anatomical landmarks are important for helmet fitting?

     Answer: ______________________
   - Where should a properly fitting helmet extend to posteriorly?

     Answer: ______________________
   - What is the anterior point of reference for a helmet? How should it be sized from that point of reference?

     Answer: ______________________
   - What is the norm for how far the face mask should be from the face?

     Answer: ______________________
   - How do you check for snugness of a helmet?

     Answer: ______________________
   - If a helmet shifts on a player's head, how do you fix the problem?

     Answer: ______________________
   - What keeps a helmet from shifting anteriorly and posteriorly? Are there different types?

     Answer: ______________________
   - What certification is needed for football helmets?

     Answer: ______________________
   - Is the mouthguard part of the necessary football equipment? How do you fit a mouthguard?

     Answer: ______________________

4. Based on the information that you currently have and what was provided by your instructor, what are the possible actions for Mr. Mekelburg's situation?
   - ______________________

- ______
- ______
- ______

3. ______
4. ______

What do you think?

1. What is your plan of action for Mr. Mekelburg's situation?

   Answer: ______

2. Was your plan of action correct for Mr. Mekelburg's situation?

   Answer: ______

3. If not, explain what you did incorrectly and how you could have performed better.

   Answer: ______

Why or why not?

For each possible action, write *why?* or *why not?* statements identifying why the information is correct or incorrect. Take details from your textbook, your own research, and data from Mr. Mekelburg's scenario to help you formulate an answer.

1. ______
2. ______

STUDENT SCENARIO 2: KELLY BELCHER

Kelly Belcher is a high school athletic trainer. One of her female soccer players has just been released by the team orthopedist to return to functional activities after sustaining a grade 2 medial collateral ligament sprain 4 weeks earlier. However, the physician is requiring the athlete to wear a hinged knee brace (Fig. 3-4) for support. The female soccer player comes to Ms. Belcher with concerns about how her brace is fitting. The brace continues to slide down at practice, and the player states that it is pinching and rubbing in her popliteal fossa. Upon inspection, Ms. Belcher notices that the anterior hole does not align with the correct bony anatomy, along with the medial and lateral supports over the joint line.

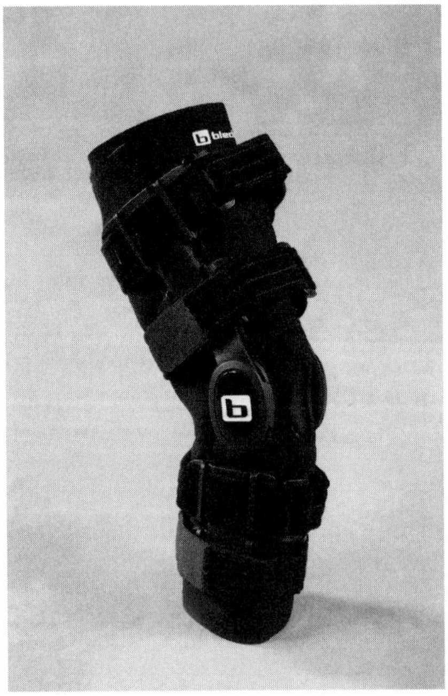

Figure 3-4: Kelly Belcher's hinged knee brace.

1. Based on this scenario, what do you know about Ms. Belcher's situation?
   - ______
   - ______
   - ______
   - ______
2. To evaluate Ms. Belcher's situation effectively, you will need to gather additional information. What questions should you ask in addition to what is presented in this scenario?
   - ______
   - ______

- ______________________________

  ____
- ______________________________

  ____

DETOUR

Treatment Detour

Epidemiologic studies have found that injuries to the knee are the most common injury keeping athletes from play. Therefore, numerous knee braces have been developed to help athletes return to play and to help reduce injury. However, with so many choices, researchers wonder which brace is best and which brace will be most effective on functional performance. A study was performed with 24 subjects examining five different DonJoy braces with a testing protocol including dynamic balance, jumping performance, proprioception, coordination, and maximal force. It was concluded that the hinged "H" buttress used for knee support was the best brace for balance, and the DonJoy Drytex economy hinged knee brace was the best for proprioception and maximal force. There were no significant differences with vertical jump or coordination. With many braces on the market, it is essential to fit the brace properly and to choose the one that is the best for the individual goal (Baltaci, Aktas, Camci, Oksuz, Yildiz, & Kalaycioglu, 2011).

Brain Jolt

An increase or decrease in a muscle's girth can affect the fit of a sized knee brace.

3. Identify key terms and concepts and then research each to broaden your knowledge of injury prevention and safety.
   - Are there different types of athletic knee braces? Explain each and its function.

     Answer: ______________________________
   - How do you fit a knee brace, and what landmarks are important?

     Answer: ______________________________
   - Why might the female soccer player's brace be slipping and rubbing?

     Answer: ______________________________
   - What bony anatomy is not properly fitting in the anterior hole on the brace?

     Answer: ______________________________

4. Based on the information that you currently have and what was provided by your instructor, what are the possible actions for Ms. Belcher's situation?
   - ______________________________

     ____
   - ______________________________

     ____
   - ______________________________

     ____
   - ______________________________

     ____

Why or why not?

For each possible action, write *why?* or *why not?* statements identifying why the information is correct or incorrect. Take details from your textbook, your own research, and data from Ms. Belcher's scenario to help you formulate an answer.

1. ______________________________

   ____
2. ______________________________

   ____
3. ______________________________

   ____
4. ______________________________

   ____

What do you think?

1. What is your plan of action for Ms. Belcher's situation?

   Answer: ______________________________
2. Was your plan of action correct for Ms. Belcher's situation?

   Answer: ______________________________
3. If not, explain what you did incorrectly and how you could have performed better.

   Answer: ______________________________

STUDENT SCENARIO 3: MARIE SCHIPPER

Marie Schipper is a college freshman who runs cross-country. She has experienced discomfort with both of her feet during her high school career. To provide temporary relief, Ms. Schipper would use off-the-shelf foot orthotics. The athletic trainer at her college requires all the distance runners to be examined by a podiatrist at the start of the season. The podiatrist examines Ms. Schipper, focusing on her prior history, structural deformities, and shoe wear patterns. The podiatrist diagnoses pes planus (Fig. 3-5) and then takes a mold of her feet, using a casting material. The podiatrist talks to the athletic trainer and Ms. Schipper about various materials that can be added to her running shoes to help correct the pes planus.

1. Based on this scenario, what do you know about Ms. Schipper's condition?
   - ______________________________________
   - ______________________________________
   - ______________________________________
   - ______________________________________
2. To evaluate Ms. Schipper's condition effectively, you will need to gather additional information. What questions should you ask in addition to what is presented in this scenario?
   - ______________________________________
   - ______________________________________
   - ______________________________________
   - ______________________________________

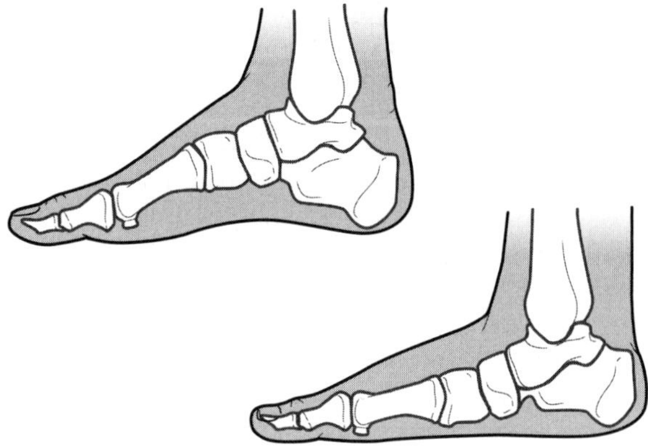

Figure 3-5: Marie Schipper's pes planus.

Brain Jolt

When assessing for treatment options for pes planus, be sure to address the athlete in the weight-bearing and non–weight-bearing stance.

3. Identify key terms and concepts and then research each to broaden your knowledge of injury prevention and safety.
   - Explain the pes planus condition.

     Answer: ______________________________
   - Why would the podiatrist be concerned about Ms. Schipper's foot history?

     Answer: ______________________________
   - What structural deformities would the podiatrist be looking for?

     Answer: ______________________________
   - Explain anterior, posterior, medial, and lateral shoe pattern wear on the sole.

     Answer: ______________________________
   - What are different types of materials that can be added to Ms. Schipper's shoes to help correct her pes planus?

     Answer: ______________________________
   - When adding materials to a shoe, does the insole remain inside the shoe or is it removed?

     Answer: ______________________________
4. Based on the information that you currently have and what was provided by your instructor, what are the possible actions for Ms. Schipper's condition?
   - ______________________________________
   - ______________________________________
   - ______________________________________
   - ______________________________________

Why or why not?

For each possible action, write *why?* or *why not?* statements identifying why the information is correct or incorrect. Take details from your textbook, your own research, and data from Ms. Schipper's scenario to help you formulate an answer.

1. ______________________________

____

2. ______________________________

____

3. ______________________________

____

4. ______________________________

____

What do you think?

1. What is your plan of action for Ms. Schipper's condition?

   Answer: ______________________________

2. Was your plan of action correct for Ms. Schipper's condition?

   Answer: ______________________________

3. If not, explain what you did incorrectly and how you could have performed better.

   Answer: ______________________________

STUDENT SCENARIO 4: NELSON SCHLIMMER

Nelson Schlimmer is a high school athletic trainer. It is the second week of twice daily practices for the football team, and he is concerned about the environmental conditions and preventing heat illnesses at the 11:00 a.m. August practice. The head football coach has planned on the team being in full pads for a day of hard hitting. Mr. Schlimmer uses a sling psychrometer (Fig. 3-6a and 3-6b) and obtains a wet bulb globe temperature. The heat category is a three.

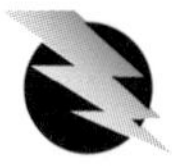

Brain Jolt

The wet and dry readings can be done digitally or by slinging a device around in the air.

1. Based on this scenario, what do you know about Mr. Schlimmer's situation?

   - ______________________________

     ____

   - ______________________________

     ____

   - ______________________________

     ____

   - ______________________________

     ____

2. To evaluate Mr. Schlimmer's situation effectively, you will need to gather additional information. What questions should you ask in addition to what is presented in this scenario?

   - ______________________________

     ____

   - ______________________________

     ____

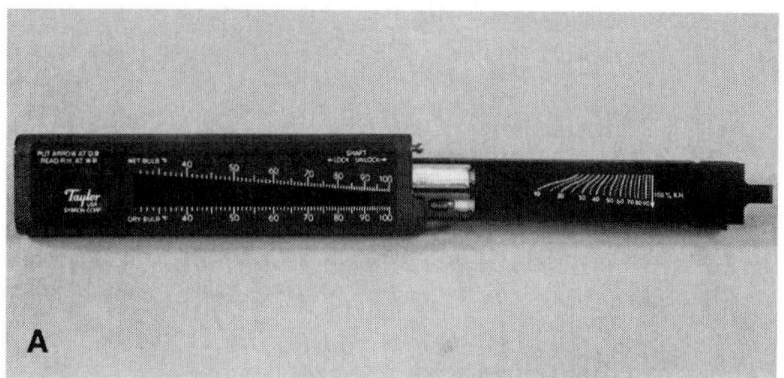

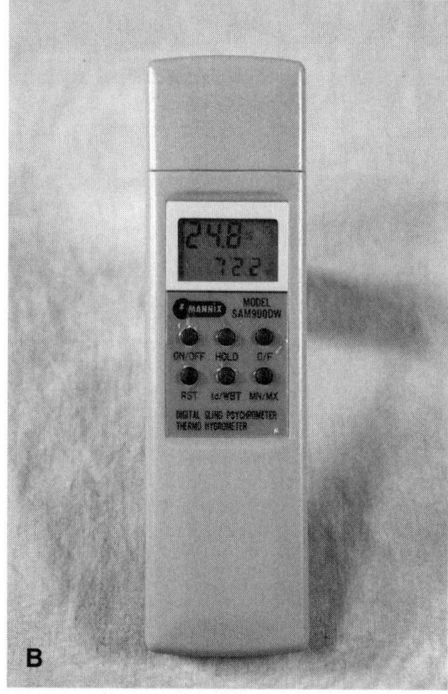

Figure 3-6: Nelson Schlimmer's sling psychrometer.

- ______________________________
- ______________________________

3. Identify key terms and concepts and then research each to broaden your knowledge of injury prevention and safety.
   - What does the heat index measure?

     Answer: ______________________________
   - Explain different types of heat illnesses.

     Answer: ______________________________
   - Is it important to have both a dry and wet air temperature reading?

     Answer: ______________________________
   - What is the universal formula for the wet and dry readings to determine heat categories?

     Answer: ______________________________
   - Explain the heat categories and advised restrictions based on each category.

     Answer: ______________________________
   - Give examples of other hot weather activity restrictions.

     Answer: ______________________________
4. Based on the information that you currently have and what was provided by your instructor, what are the possible actions for Mr. Schlimmer's situation?
   - ______________________________
   - ______________________________
   - ______________________________
   - ______________________________

Conversation Buffer

A heat illness can turn into a medical emergency quickly. It is important to monitor daily temperature and humidity readings. Heat restrictions should be discussed with the head football coach at the beginning of the season, along with ways the risk can be reduced using proper water breaks, equipment and uniform conditions, and different practice times. This open communication can help to ensure athletes' safety.

Why or why not?

For each possible action, write *why?* or *why not?* statements identifying why the information is correct or incorrect. Take details from your textbook, your own research, and data from Mr. Schlimmer's scenario to help you formulate an answer.

1. ______________________________
2. ______________________________
3. ______________________________
4. ______________________________

What do you think?

1. What is your plan of action for Mr. Schlimmer's situation?

   Answer: ______________________________
2. Was your plan of action correct for Mr. Schlimmer's situation?

   Answer: ______________________________
3. If not, explain what you did incorrectly and how you could have performed better.

   Answer: ______________________________

STUDENT SCENARIO 5: MIQUEL TOOPES

Miquel Toopes is the goalie on the college soccer team. During today's tournament game, he dives and extends to his right to deflect a ball from going into the goal. Mr. Toopes comes down hard onto his right iliac crest. Mr. Toopes presents with point tenderness, edema, and ecchymosis over the right iliac crest. The athletic trainer examines Mr. Toopes' right hip and diagnoses a hip pointer (Fig. 3-7). The team is to play another tournament game tomorrow. Mr. Toopes' hip strength is comparable bilaterally. Mr. Toopes is cleared to play by the athletic trainer, as long as the right iliac crest is protected. The athletic trainer must protect this injury.

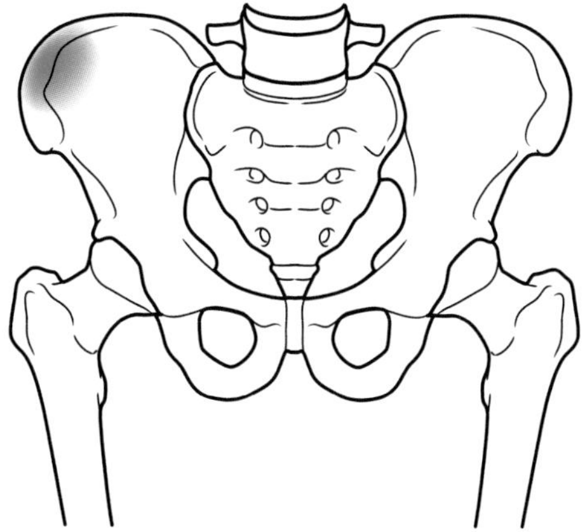

Figure 3-7: Miquel Toopes' hip pointer.

1. Based on this scenario, what do you know about Mr. Toopes' injury?
   - ______________________________
   - ______________________________
   - ______________________________
   - ______________________________

2. To evaluate Mr. Toopes' injury effectively, you will need to gather additional information. What questions should you ask in addition to what is presented in this scenario?
   - ______________________________
   - ______________________________
   - ______________________________
   - ______________________________

3. Identify key terms and concepts and then research each to broaden your knowledge of injury prevention and safety.
   - Explain the signs and symptoms of a hip pointer.

     Answer: ______________________________
   - Explain how to test hip strength and what directions are tested.

     Answer: ______________________________
   - What can be used to protect this injury?

     Answer: ______________________________
   - What is the goal of the protective technique chosen?

     Answer: ______________________________
   - What are the pros and cons of each protective technique?

     Answer: ______________________________

Brain Jolt
When protecting an injury, mobility of the athlete and stability of the protective device must be considered.

4. Based on the information that you currently have and what was provided by your instructor, what are the possible actions for Mr. Toopes' injury?
   - ______________________________
   - ______________________________
   - ______________________________
   - ______________________________

Why or why not?

For each possible action, write *why?* or *why not?* statements identifying why the information is correct or incorrect. Take details from your textbook, your own research, and data from Mr. Toopes' scenario to help you formulate an answer.

1. ______________________________
2. ______________________________
3. ______________________________
4. ______________________________

What do you think?

1. What is your plan of action for Mr. Toopes' injury?

   Answer: ______________________________
2. Was your plan of action correct for Mr. Toopes' injury?

   Answer: ______________________________
3. If not, explain what you did incorrectly and how you could have performed better.

   Answer: ______________________________

STUDENT SCENARIO 6: SANDRA EHRICH

Sandra Ehrich is the collegiate head athletic trainer for the football team. The football team is reporting for preseason training. She has met with the head football coach to discuss the team's acclimation schedule. The team will have a different set of daily rules pertaining to their equipment to follow for the first week of practice. Ms. Ehrich has also reviewed with the head football coach the team's hydration requirements and acclimation guidelines to ensure a safe training camp. Ms. Ehrich bases her acclimation schedule on the National Athletic Trainer's Association (NATA) position statement for hydration and acclimation. She will also talk to the players about guidelines for appropriate fluid replacement and weight loss (Fig. 3-8).

1. Based on this scenario, what do you know about Ms. Ehrich's situation?
   - ______________________________
   - ______________________________
   - ______________________________
   - ______________________________

2. To evaluate Ms. Ehrich's situation effectively, you will need to gather additional information. What questions should you ask in addition to what is presented in this scenario?
   - ______________________________
   - ______________________________
   - ______________________________
   - ______________________________

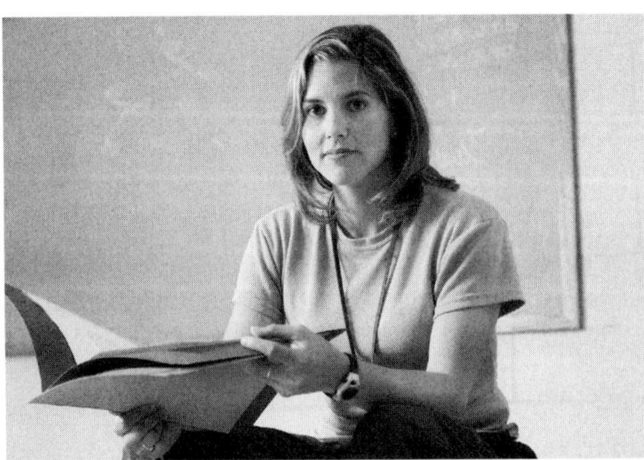

Figure 3-8: Sandra Ehrich's preseason training camp. (© Hemera Technologies © Thinkstock)

Treatment Detour

An observational study examined 25 heat-acclimatized adolescent boys (14 to 16 years old) who practiced outdoors in late August. These football players practiced once per day for the first 5 days, twice a day for days 6 and 7, and once per day on days 8 through 10. The maximum wet bulb globe temperature averaged 23°C. Various outcomes were measured including fluid consumption, forearm sweat composition, and sweat rate, and the athletes completed a questionnaire testing their knowledge of hydration and heat illness. It was concluded that previously heat-acclimatized adolescent boys can safely complete preseason football training in moderate environmental conditions if practice guidelines are followed. It was also noted that the athletes replaced fluids in practice adequately but did not hydrate properly outside of practice. This study shows that an emphasis on athlete education is needed and that athletic trainers need to enforce strict practice guidelines pertaining to work-to-rest ratios appropriate for the environmental conditions present to maintain safe preseason training (Yeargin et al., 2010).

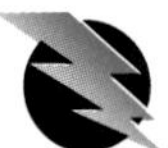

Brain Jolt

A preseason conditioning program should occur before the first day of practice to help ease the acclimation process.

3. Identify key terms and concepts and then research each to broaden your knowledge of injury prevention and safety.
   - Explain the NATA position statement on hydration and acclimation.

     Answer: ______________________________
   - Explain the acclimation process pertaining to the type of equipment that the football players will wear each day during the first week.

     Answer: ______________________________
   - Why are weight charts important? Explain the concern about a weight loss of 5% or more during a practice.

     Answer: ______________________________

- How much fluid should an athlete consume for every pound of body weight lost?

  Answer: ______

- What beverages should be used for fluid replacement?

  Answer: ______

- In reference to proper fluid replacement, can an athlete's urine color be important to note? Explain the meaning of dark to light urine color.

  Answer: ______

- What other guidelines should be discussed?

  Answer: ______

4. Based on the information that you currently have and what was provided by your instructor, what are the possible actions for Ms. Ehrich's situation?

- ______
- ______
- ______
- ______

Why or why not?

For each topic of discussion, write *why?* or *why not?* statements identifying why the information is correct or incorrect. Take details from your textbook, your own research, and data from Ms. Ehrich's scenario to help you formulate an answer.

1. ______
2. ______
3. ______
4. ______

What do you think?

1. What is your plan of action for Ms. Ehrich's situation?

   Answer: ______

2. Was your plan of action correct for Ms. Ehrich's situation?

   Answer: ______

3. If not, explain what you did incorrectly and how you could have performed better.

   Answer: ______

STUDENT SCENARIO 7: LORI JANS

Lori Jans is a college softball player. She is running to second base, slides, and forces her right ankle into eversion when tagging the base. The athletic trainer diagnoses a grade 1 eversion ankle sprain (Fig. 3-9). She is expected to return to play when symptoms subside, approximately 1 week. One week after the injury, Ms. Jans is cleared to return back to limited play. She is instructed to have a technique applied daily to help prevent the eversion movement. Ms. Jans overhears the head athletic trainer discussing with the athletic training students the proper preparation, rules for application, and proper technique for caring for an injured ankle when returning to play.

1. Based on this scenario, what do you know about Ms. Jans' injury?

- ______
- ______

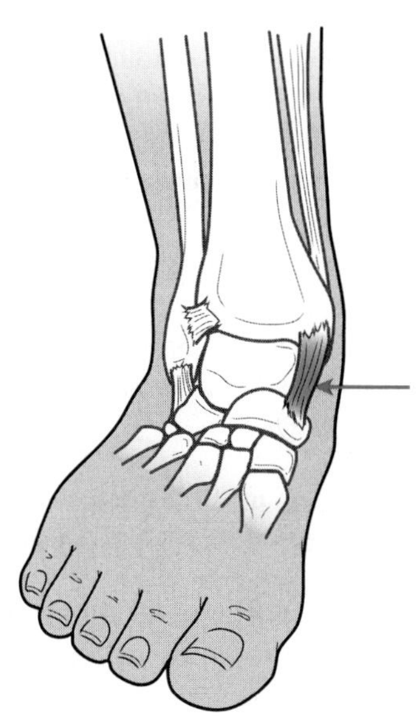

Figure 3-9: Lori Jans' eversion ankle sprain.

- ______________________________________
- ______________________________________

2. To evaluate Ms. Jans' injury effectively, you will need to gather additional information. What questions should you ask in addition to what is presented in this scenario?
   - ______________________________________
   - ______________________________________
   - ______________________________________
   - ______________________________________

DETOUR

Treatment Detour

Twenty percent of athletic injuries are to the ankle, and 33% to 73% of these injuries are ankle sprains. Many of the athletes who have ankle sprains experience frequent recurrence and functional instability. The objective of this study was to compare the literature to determine whether wearing an ankle brace or taping the ankle improves proprioception acuity when compared with no tape or a brace in those with a history of an ankle sprain or instability. Eighteen studies were included. Although each study had various findings, some with better proprioception in the taped or braced condition and some with worse results, the overall conclusion was that there was no significant difference in proprioception acuity in participants with a history of ankle sprains when taped or braced. However, the authors conclude that it is important to note that this should not discourage the use of taping or bracing, because research does support the use of these techniques in injury prevention (Raymond, Nicholson, Hiller, & Refshauge, 2012).

Brain Jolt

To support an injured ankle for return to play, be sure to position the ankle properly for stabilization.

3. Identify key terms and concepts and then research each to broaden your knowledge of injury prevention and safety.
   - Explain symptoms of a grade 1 ankle sprain. What are the return-to-play requirements for a grade 1 ankle sprain?

     Answer: ______________________________________
   - What methods could be used for ankle support? What are the pros and cons of each method?

     Answer: ______________________________________
   - Explain how to apply each supportive technique.

     Answer: ______________________________________
   - For an ankle eversion injury, how should the ankle be positioned when stabilizing?

     Answer: ______________________________________
4. Based on the information that you currently have and what was provided by your instructor, what are the possible actions for Ms. Jans' injury?
   - ______________________________________
   - ______________________________________
   - ______________________________________
   - ______________________________________

Why or why not?

For each possible action, write *why?* or *why not?* statements identifying why the information is correct or incorrect. Take details from your textbook, your own research, and data from Ms. Jans' scenario to help you formulate an answer.

1. ______________________________________
2. ______________________________________
3. ______________________________________
4. ______________________________________

What do you think?

1. What is your plan of action for Ms. Jans' injury?

   Answer: ______________________________________
2. Was your plan of action correct for Ms. Jans' injury?

   Answer: ______________________________________
3. If not, explain what you did incorrectly and how you could have performed better.

   Answer: ______________________________________

STUDENT SCENARIO 8: KIM PADGITT

Kim Padgitt is a freshman in college. During her second week on campus, Ms. Padgitt is expected to have a physical examination to be cleared for participation for a college club team. The first station of the examination process involves a review of her medical history and the questionnaire she has completed. Ms. Padgitt has reported that she is nauseated frequently. Next, the team physician questions her and expresses concern when syncope is detected in her medical history. The nausea and syncope are noted, and Ms. Padgitt is not cleared for participation until further examination (Fig. 3-10).

1. Based on this scenario, what do you know about Ms. Padgitt's condition?
   - ____________________
   - ____________________
   - ____________________
   - ____________________

2. To evaluate Ms. Padgitt's condition effectively, you will need to gather additional information. What questions should you ask in addition to what is presented in this scenario?
   - ____________________
   - ____________________
   - ____________________
   - ____________________

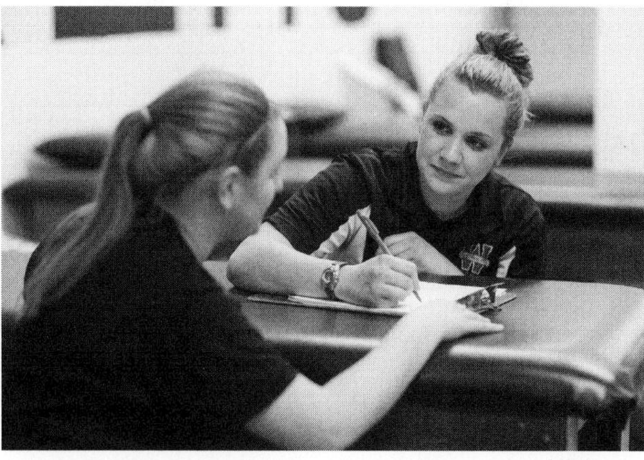

Figure 3-10: Kim Padgitt's preparticipation examination.

Brain Jolt

A thorough physical and medical history can identify a health risk in an athlete that could be dismissed as normal or unimportant.

3. Identify key terms and concepts and then research each to broaden your knowledge of injury prevention and safety.
   - Is the physical examination form universal? What other areas of screening does it address?

     Answer: ____________________
   - What is the station method for physical examinations?

     Answer: ____________________
   - Define *syncope.*

     Answer: ____________________
   - What could syncope and nausea possibly indicate? Why is it important to be thorough when completing the history portion of the form?

     Answer: ____________________
   - What other indicators should be noted from a physical form?

     Answer: ____________________

4. Based on the information that you currently have and what was provided by your instructor, what are the possible actions for Ms. Padgitt's condition?
   - ____________________
   - ____________________
   - ____________________
   - ____________________

Why or why not?

For each possible action, write *why?* or *why not?* statements identifying why the information is correct or incorrect. Take details from your textbook, your own research, and data from Ms. Padgitt's scenario to help you formulate an answer.

1. ____________________

2. ______________________________

____

3. ______________________________

____

4. ______________________________

____

What do you think?

1. What is your plan of action for Ms. Padgitt's condition?

   Answer: ______________________

2. Was your plan of action correct for Ms. Padgitt's condition?

   Answer: ______________________

3. If not, explain what you did incorrectly and how you could have performed better.

   Answer: ______________________

STUDENT SCENARIO 9: CINDY GIFFLE

Cindy Giffle is a cross-country runner. Upon evaluation by an athletic trainer, she is noted as having a weak left quadriceps and anterior knee pain. Ms. Giffle has been working on her quadriceps weakness with a weekly strengthening program, but she is continually having pain. The athletic trainer wants her to come in before practice for a reevaluation. Upon closer investigation, it is noted that Ms. Giffle has a patellar tracking issue. In addition to her medial quadriceps weakness, her patella is being pulled laterally (Fig. 3-11) as a result of this weakness and a tight iliotibial band. The athletic trainer wants to give Ms. Giffle something to assist with this tracking issue to help realign the patella during rehab.

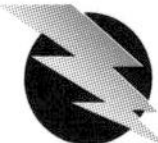

Brain Jolt
Lateral patellar tracking can be a result of a weak vastus medialis oblique muscle.

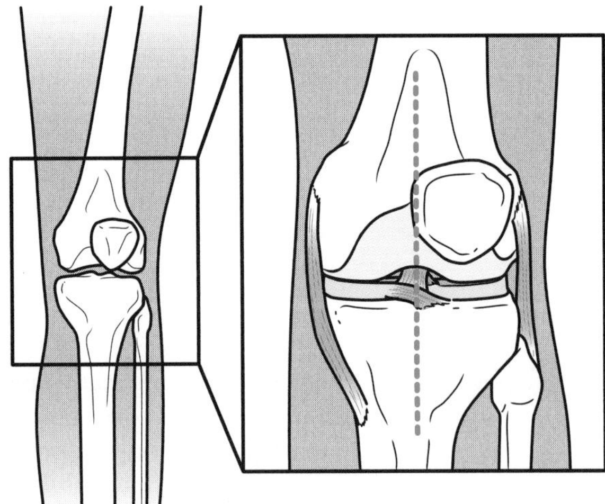

Figure 3-11: Cindy Giffle's lateral patellar tracking.

1. Based on this scenario, what do you know about Ms. Giffle's condition?
   - ______________________________
   - ______________________________
   - ______________________________
   - ______________________________

2. To evaluate Ms. Giffle's condition effectively, you will need to gather additional information. What questions should you ask in addition to what is presented in this scenario?
   - ______________________________
   - ______________________________
   - ______________________________
   - ______________________________

3. Identify key terms and concepts and then research each to broaden your knowledge of injury prevention and safety.
   - What are the signs and symptoms of patellofemoral syndrome?

     Answer: ______________________

- What other patellar alignment or tracking positions are there?

  Answer: ______________________________

- Explain the different types of patellofemoral alignment techniques.

  Answer: ______________________________

- What are the pros and cons of each technique?

  Answer: ______________________________

- What materials are needed for each technique?

  Answer: ______________________________

4. Based on the information that you currently have and what was provided by your instructor, what are the possible actions for Ms. Giffle's condition?

- ______________________________
  ____
- ______________________________
  ____
- ______________________________
  ____
- ______________________________
  ____

Why or why not?

For each possible action, write *why?* or *why not?* statements identifying why the information is correct or incorrect. Take details from your textbook, your own research, and data from Ms. Giffle's scenario to help you formulate an answer.

1. ______________________________
   ____
2. ______________________________
   ____
3. ______________________________
   ____
4. ______________________________
   ____

What do you think?

1. What is your plan of action for Ms. Giffle's condition?

   Answer: ______________________________

2. Was your plan of action correct for Ms. Giffle's condition?

   Answer: ______________________________

3. If not, explain what you did incorrectly and how you could have performed better.

   Answer: ______________________________

knowledge checklist

Table 3-1 offers a checklist that can be used by a peer, instructor, or preceptor to evaluate your knowledge of injury prevention and safety. Use this checklist as a tool to ensure that the evaluation is complete and to assess your knowledge of the competencies that apply to this chapter.

TABLE 3-1 ■ Injury Prevention and Safety Competency Checklist

	Proficient *Can demonstrate and execute the skill properly*	**Proficient With Assistance** *Can demonstrate and execute the skill with minimal guidance or tips*	**Not Proficient** *Unable to demonstrate and execute the skill properly; needs to be reevaluated at another time after further study and practice*
Athlete's Health History			
Medical history			
History of injury or medical conditions			
Type of sport and position played			
Mechanisms of Injury			
How did/does the injury occur?			
Indications and techniques for preventative taping techniques			
Indications and techniques for preventative wrapping techniques			
Guidelines for fitting and maintaining protective equipment			
Guidelines for activities in extreme weather and interpreting weather indicators			
Guidelines for preventing environmental heat illness			
Guidelines for performing preparticipation physicals			

REFERENCES

Baltaci, G., Aktas, G., Camci, E., Oksuz, S., Yildiz, S., & Kalaycioglu, T. (2011). The effect of prophylactic knee bracing on performance: Balance, proprioception, coordination, and muscular power. *Knee Surgery, Sports Traumatolog, Arthroscopy, 19*, 1722–1728.

Beam, J. W. (2006). *Orthopedic taping, wrapping, bracing and padding*. Philadelphia, PA: F.A. Davis.

National Athletic Training Association. (2011). *Athletic training education competencies* (5th ed.). Retrieved from http://www.nata.org/sites/default/files/5th-Edition-Competencies-2011-PDF-Version.pdf

Prentice, W. (2010). *Arnheim's principles of athletic training: A competency-based approach* (14th ed.). New York, NY: McGraw-Hill.

Raymond, J., Nicholson, L. L., Hiller, C. E., & Refshauge, K. M. (2012). The effect of ankle taping or bracing on proprioception in functional ankle instability: A systematic review and meta-analysis. *Journal of Science and Medicine in Sport, 15*, 386–392.

Starkey, C., Brown, S. D., & Ryan, J. (2010). *Examination of orthopedic and athletic injuries* (3rd ed.). Philadelphia, PA: F.A. Davis.

Venes, D. (Ed.). (2009). *Taber's cyclopedic medical dictionary* (21st ed.). Philadelphia, PA: F.A. Davis.

Yeargin, S. W., Casa, D. J., Judelson, D. A., McDermott, B. P., Ganio, M. S., Lee, E. C., Lopez, R. M., Stearns, R. L., Anderson, J. M., Armstrong, L. E., Kraemer. W. J., & Maresh, C. M. (2010). Thermoregulatory responses and hydration practices in heat-acclimatized adolescents during preseason high school football. *Journal of Athletic Training, 45*, 136–146.

part two

Athletic Injury Evaluation

chapter 4

Lower Extremity: The Ankle and Foot

chapter outline

athletic trainer's corner

Out there in the real world, one athletic training student experienced the following while being supervised by a certified athletic trainer:

The band has just played "The Star-Spangled Banner" on a warm Friday night, and the announcer is introducing the visiting football team. I can feel the excitement rising as the home team is announced. The crowd leaps to its feet, roaring with cheers as the home players jog onto the field. I have always said that the thrill of a Friday night football game is infectious. In the first half of the game, the home team's senior running back goes down with an injury. The referee signals for the athletic trainer to approach the field. I look around for that person, and then remember that it is, in fact, me. I'm a new college graduate, and am now the certified athletic trainer who cares for the home team. I run to the injured athlete and realize that I'm going to have two obstacles to overcome. First, this is the biggest injury of the year that I've experienced (a lateral malleolus fracture); second, this athlete is hearing impaired. I ask the coaches to retrieve the athlete's hearing aids from his bag so that we can decrease the present language barrier. After calming the athlete and explaining to him, the coach, and his parents the course of action, he is transported to the nearest hospital.

Every injury is different. The athlete's pain level, the injury's severity, and any other handicaps that can enter the equation affect your actions. The course of action will not always be the same. Being a new, certified athletic trainer at the time, this experience was frightening for me. My advice to you is to make sure you learn as much as you can about the athletes you care for, always keep current with the latest athletic training techniques, and continually improve your evaluation skills.

Melissa Noble, AT, ATC
Head Athletic Trainer, Fairlawn High School
Assistant Athletic Trainer, Sidney High School
Wilson Memorial Hospital

learning outcomes

After working through this chapter, you will be able to:

1. Verbalize the questions to use when obtaining a thorough medical history for an assessment.
2. Describe the principles of body movement at the ankle and foot and the various mechanisms of injury that affect the ankle and foot.
3. Compare and contrast the findings of various special tests and the role of diagnostic tests used during an ankle and foot evaluation.
4. Explain the medical terminology associated with the assessment of musculoskeletal injuries.
5. Verbalize the standard procedures used for a clinical evaluation of the ankle and foot and interpret the findings for differential diagnoses.

introduction

The athletic training profession inevitably involves many ankle and foot injuries, which are common with weight-bearing exercise. This chapter presents many signs and symptoms of ankle and foot injuries to help you fine-tune your assessment skills. Beyond performing special tests and observing visual characteristics of the injured area, you need to determine quickly whether the injury is severe enough to prevent the athlete from returning to play or to affect the athlete's activities of daily living. By implementing all the information you have learned in the classroom and then applying it in terms of what is going on with the athlete, you can quickly determine the injury type and the effective treatment for the injury to create the best possible outcome for the athlete.

MODEL SCENARIO 1: BRANDON GOODWIN

Brandon Goodwin sees a certified athletic trainer because he has an injured right foot. He had prior pain with his right big toe for 2 to 3 weeks. When Mr. Goodwin high jumps, he experiences pain in his right foot each time he pushes off the ground. He recently purchased a more flexible jumping shoe, thinking that this might reduce the irritation; however, the new shoes have less cushioning and Mr. Goodwin still experiences pain while jumping. Mr. Goodwin has edema on the dorsal and plantar side of the right foot located over the metatarsophalangeal (MTP) joint of the great toe. He is moderately point tender around the MTP joint (Fig. 4-1) and sesamoid bones. Mr. Goodwin has a bunion on the right great toe.

1. Based on this scenario, what do you know about Mr. Goodwin's injury?
   - *Male athlete*
   - *High jumper*
   - *Point tender over MTP joint and sesamoid bones*
   - *Chronic mechanism of injury, because it occurred 2 to 3 weeks ago*
   - *Bunion on right great toe*
   - *Edema around the MTP joint on the dorsal and plantar surface*
   - *Changed footwear*

Figure 4-1: Brandon Goodwin's location of point tenderness.

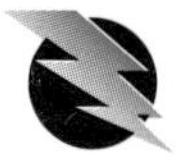

Brain Jolt
This injury can sometimes be treated with a steel shoe insert.

2. To evaluate Mr. Goodwin's injury effectively, you will need to gather additional information. What questions should you ask in addition to what is presented in this scenario?
   - *Is this a medical emergency?*
   - *Are there preexisting injuries? If yes, what are they?*
   - *Are there any special tests that are important to perform? If yes, elaborate.*
   - *Are the results of the special tests positive or negative, and what does that indicate?*
   - *Are there gait irregularities?*
   - *Are there arch irregularities?*
   - *Is there limited passive or active ROM in the great toe?*
   - *What is the strength at the great toe?*
   - *Is ecchymosis present?*
3. Identify key terms and concepts, and then research each to broaden your knowledge about ankle and foot injuries.
   - What anatomical structures are involved?
     MTP joint
     Sesamoid bones

Flexors of the great toe
Extensors of the great toe

- Define *dorsal*.
  Directional term meaning "top of the foot"
- Define *plantar*.
  Directional term meaning "bottom of the foot"
- What is the metatarsophalangeal joint?
  The union between the distal end of the metatarsal and the proximal end of the phalange
- What are sesamoid bones?
  Floating bones located on the plantar side of the MTP joint embedded in the flexor and adductor tendons of the great toe
- What is a bunion?
  Hallus valgus deformity; structural forefoot varus in which the first ray tends to point outward
- Is the footwear change important to note?
  Yes, the footwear change is important because it could be altering his foot positioning or could be an improper shoe fit for his foot, causing pain
- In what position are the toes when he is "pushing off"?
  Toe extension

4. Based on the information that you currently have and what was provided by your instructor, what are the possible differential diagnoses for Mr. Goodwin's injury?
   Bunion
   Sesamoiditis
   Turf toe
   Hallux rigidus

Why or why not?

For each assessment or diagnosis, write *why?* or *why not?* statements identifying why the information is correct or incorrect. Take details from your textbook, your own research, and data from Mr. Goodwin's scenario to help you formulate an answer.

1. *Mr. Goodwin's bunion is preexisting. The edema is already present, and bunions do not typically produce pain; therefore, the bunion is not the cause of the present injury and pain.*
2. *Mr. Goodwin does not seem to have sesamoiditis, because he has pain and swelling that sits on the dorsal surface of the foot and the sesamoid bones are on the plantar surface of the foot.*
3. *Mr. Goodwin seems to have turf toe, demonstrated by the pattern of swelling on the dorsal and plantar surface of the foot. The pain occurs with pushing off of the great toe, which hyperextends the joint.*
4. *Mr. Goodwin does not have hallux rigidus because he has full range of motion at his joint.*

What do you think?

1. What is your assessment of Mr. Goodwin's injury?
   Answer: *Turf toe*
2. Was your assessment of Mr. Goodwin's injury correct?
   Answer: *Yes*
3. If not, explain what you did incorrectly and how you could have performed a better assessment.

   Answer: ________________________________

MODEL SCENARIO 2: MELISSA GIBHART

Melissa Gibhart is a softball player currently in preseason. Ms. Gibhart had a busy offseason, which prevented her from doing any of the workouts that the coach assigned. During the first few days of running, she notices bilateral gastrocnemius tightness. Ms. Gibhart routinely stretches before practice, but never after practice. She states that most of her discomfort occurs when she pushes off her toes while running (Fig. 4-2). After practice, she experiences a stabbing pain on the plantar surface of her right calcaneous, and the pain continues into the next day. The pain is not bilateral. One thing to note is that Ms. Gibhart has new softball cleats that are rigid, and it has been a wet spring season with a soft and slippery playing field. Radiographs are taken to determine the origin of Ms. Gibhart's pain.

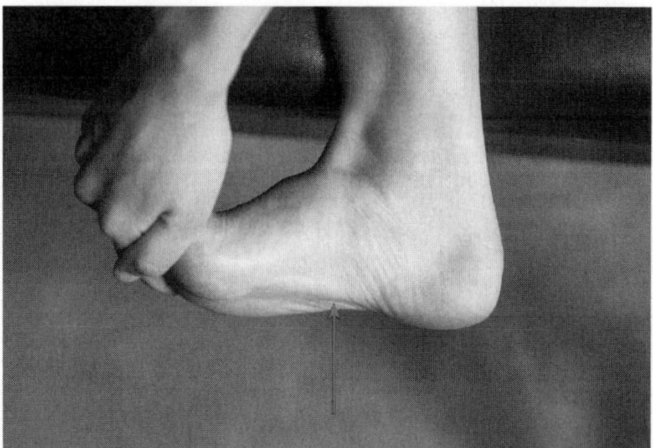

Figure 4-2: Melissa Gibhart's point of pain.

1. Based on this scenario, what do you know about Ms. Gibhart's injury?
   - *Female athlete*
   - *Softball player*
   - *Tight bilateral gastrocnemius*
   - *Chronic mechanism of injury*
   - *Discomfort in the right foot when pushing off toes*
   - *Pain on plantar surface of calcaneus after activity, lasting until next day*
   - *Soft and slippery playing surface*
   - *Has changed footwear*
   - *Foot pain not bilateral*
   - *Has not been conditioning*
2. To evaluate Ms. Gibhart's injury effectively, you will need to gather additional information. What questions should you ask in addition to what is presented in this scenario?
   - *Is this a medical emergency?*
   - *Are there preexisting injuries? If yes, what are they?*
   - *Are there any special tests that are important to perform? If yes, elaborate.*
   - *Are the results of the special tests positive or negative? What do the results indicate?*
   - *Are there gait irregularities?*
   - *What structures are point tender?*
   - *Is there limited passive or active ROM in the foot?*
   - *What is the strength at the foot?*
   - *What type of pain is it? For example, is the pain sharp, dull, or throbbing?*

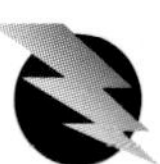

Brain Jolt
The patient's pain often becomes worse with the first initial steps after sitting for a prolonged period of time or when getting out of bed in the morning.

3. Identify key terms and concepts, and then research each to broaden your knowledge about ankle and foot injuries.
   - What anatomical structures are involved?
     Plantar fascia
     Gastrocnemius
     Soleus
     Transverse metatarsal arch
     Medial longitudinal arch
     Lateral longitudinal arch
   - Define *bilateral.*
     Affecting or relating to two sides.
   - In this scenario, does gastrocnemius tightness play a role in the pain?
     It could play a role because the gastrocnemius and soleus insert into the Achilles tendon, which is connected to the plantar fascia that then runs across the plantar surface of the foot.
   - Why is proper footwear important?
     The rigidity of the shoe provides limited motion and is causing her gait to change.
   - Why is the condition of the playing field surface important?
     Because the playing surface is slippery and wet, Ms. Gibhart's foot has to stabilize more, leading to increased stress and pain.
4. Based on the information that you currently have and what was provided by your instructor, what are the possible differential diagnoses for Ms. Gibhart's injury?
   Calcaneal exostosis
   Plantar fasciitis
   Medial longitudinal arch strain
   Achilles tendonitis

Why or why not?

For each assessment or diagnosis, write *why?* or *why not?* statements identifying why the information is correct or incorrect. Take details from your textbook, your own research, and data from Ms. Gibhart's scenario to help you formulate an answer.

1. *Ms. Gibhart does not have a calcaneal exostosis because it did not show on the radiograph. If she did have a calcaneal exostosis, her pain would be constant with walking and activity.*
2. *Ms. Gibhart seems to have plantar fasciitis because she has pain before and after practice, localized pain on her calcaneus that extends to her metatarsal heads, and tight gastrocnemii that exacerbate the problem.*
3. *Ms. Gibhart does not have a medial longitudinal arch strain because her pain is over the calcaneal region and not on the medial aspect of the foot.*
4. *Ms. Gibhart does not have Achilles tendonitis because her Achilles tendon is not thickened or inflamed.*

What do you think?

1. What is your assessment of Ms. Gibhart's injury?
   Answer: *Plantar fasciitis*
2. Was your assessment of Ms. Gibhart's injury correct?
   Answer: *Yes*
3. If not, explain what you did incorrectly and how you could have performed a better assessment.
   Answer: ______________________________

MODEL SCENARIO 3: MYA JACKSON

Mya Jackson is a high school swimmer. Observing Ms. Jackson one day at swim practice, you see her jump into the pool around the transition area from shallow to deep water. As her left calcaneus hits the bottom of the pool, you see Ms. Jackson pop out of the water quickly, appearing to be in pain. As she begins to climb up the steps to exit the pool, Ms. Jackson states that she cannot bear any weight on her left foot. You assist her to the treatment table without letting her bear any weight on her left foot. Upon evaluation, Ms. Jackson is point tender posterior to the medial malleolus and in the talar dome (Fig. 4-3). Once Ms. Jackson's initial pain subsides, she has limited range of motion (ROM) with plantar flexion and dorsiflexion. Ms. Jackson's strength in her left foot is a 3/5 with plantar flexion and dorsiflexion. Ms. Jackson is still unable to bear any weight on her left foot after rest.

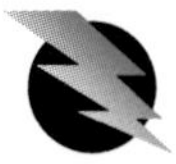

Brain Jolt

This injury is often overlooked and can lead to avascular necrosis if not treated properly.

1. Based on this scenario, what do you know about Ms. Jackson's injury?
   - *Female athlete*
   - *Swimmer*
   - *Jumped into too shallow water in swimming pool (mechanism of injury)*
   - *Unable to bear weight*
   - *Limited ROM and strength*
   - *Point tender posterior to medial malleolus and talar dome*
2. To evaluate Ms. Jackson's injury effectively, you will need to gather additional information. What questions should you ask yourself in addition to what is presented in this scenario?
   - *Is this a medical emergency?*
   - *Are there preexisting injuries? If yes, what are they?*
   - *Are there any special tests that are important to perform? If yes, elaborate.*
   - *Are the results of the special tests negative or positive? What does each indicate?*
   - *Were any pops, cracks, or snaps heard?*
   - *Is there any numbness or paraesthesia?*
   - *What type of pain is it? For example, is the pain sharp, dull, or throbbing?*
3. Identify key terms and concepts, and then research each to broaden your knowledge about ankle and foot injuries.
   - What anatomical structures are involved?

     Medial malleolus
     Calcaneus
     Tibia
     Fibula
     Cuboid
     Navicular
     Talus
     Deltoid ligament
     Spring (calcaneonavicular) ligament
   - Define *posterior.*

     Directional term meaning "behind"
   - Describe the different types of pain and what each indicate.

     Sharp pain indicates a fracture.
     Pins and needles or numbness indicates nerve pathology.
     Sharp and localized stinging indicates an acute injury.
     Aching or throbbing indicates a chronic or post injury (few days old).
     Radiating pain indicates pain dissipating away from the injured area along a nerve or along the length of a muscle.
4. Based on the information that you currently have and what was provided by your instructor, what are the possible differential diagnoses for Ms. Jackson's injury?

   Calcaneus fracture
   Talus fracture
   Medial ankle sprain

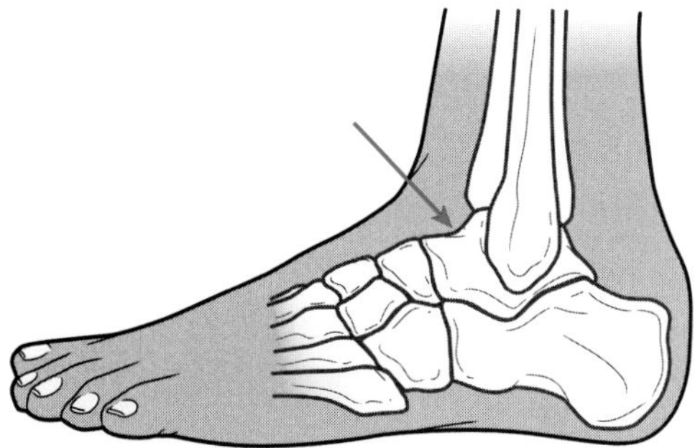

Figure 4-3: Mya Jackson's point of pain.

Why or why not?

For each assessment or diagnosis, write *why?* or *why not?* statements identifying why the information is correct or incorrect. Take details from your textbook, your own research, and data from Ms. Jackson's scenario to help you formulate an answer.

1. *It does not appear that Ms. Jackson has a calcaneal fracture because her pain is not over her calcaneus. The pain is more medial and occurs in the talar dome.*
2. *It appears that Ms. Jackson has a talus fracture because she is point tender posterior to the medial malleolus and in the talar dome, which indicates that the talus is affected. In addition, a tap test is positive for pain.*

3. *Ms. Jackson does not have a medial ankle sprain because she is not point tender over the deltoid or spring (calcaneonavicular) ligament, the talar tilt test is negative, and her ROM and strength are good.*

What do you think?

1. What is your assessment of Ms. Jackson's injury?
   Answer: *Talus fracture*
2. Was your assessment of Ms. Jackson's injury correct?
   Answer: *Yes*
3. If not, explain what you did incorrectly and how you could have performed a better assessment.

   Answer: ______________________________

STUDENT SCENARIO 1: **SAM CARROL**

Sam Carrol is a senior football player who plays the position of linebacker. During today's practice, Mr. Carrol is practicing taking on-cut blocks. He grasps his opponent, pushes the player back while raising forcefully on his toes, and cuts to the side. He feels a pop over the dorsal surface of the left foot. On examination, he is point tender over the medial dorsal aspect of the foot and is having trouble bearing weight on his foot. After the injury, Mr. Carrol experiences localized edema over the proximal aspect of first and second metatarsals (Fig. 4-4).

1. Based on this scenario, what do you know about Mr. Carrol's injury?
   - plant & cut mechanism + calf raise
   - "pop" felt
   - (L) side, point tender over medial dorsal side PWB
   - edema over

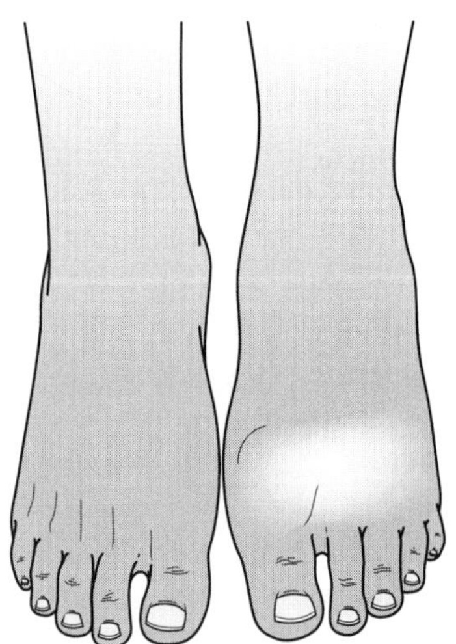

Figure 4-4: Sam Carrol's edema.

2. To evaluate Mr. Carrol's injury effectively, you will need to gather additional information. What questions should you ask in addition to what is presented in this scenario?
   - ______________________________
   - ______________________________
   - ______________________________
   - ______________________________

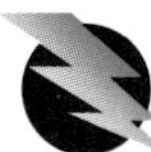

Brain Jolt

Remember that an on-field evaluation has fewer steps than your evaluation that occurs on the sidelines or in the athletic training room. When on the field, you need to determine the pertinent actions to get the athlete off the field safely without further exacerbating the injury.

3. Identify key terms and concepts, and then research each to broaden your knowledge about ankle and foot injuries.
   - What anatomical structures are involved?

     Answer: ______________________________
   - Define *dorsum*.

     Answer: ______________________________
   - Define *inversion*.

     Answer: ______________________________
   - Define *proximal*.

     Answer: ______________________________
   - What does *localized edema* mean?

     Answer: ______________________________
   - Why is it important to have an understanding of football terminology?

     Answer: ______________________________

4. Based on the information that you currently have and what was provided by your instructor, what are the possible differential diagnoses for Mr. Carrol's injury?

- ______________________________
- ______________________________
- ______________________________
- ______________________________

Why or why not?

For each assessment or diagnosis, write *why?* or *why not?* statements identifying why the information is correct or incorrect. Take details from your textbook, your own research, and data from Mr. Carrol's scenario to help you formulate an answer.

1. ______________________________
2. ______________________________
3. ______________________________
4. ______________________________

What do you think?

1. What is your assessment of Mr. Carrol's injury?

   Answer: ______________________________

2. Was your assessment of Mr. Carrol's injury correct?

   Answer: ______________________________

3. If not, explain what you did incorrectly and how you could have performed a better assessment.

   Answer: ______________________________

STUDENT SCENARIO 2: ERICA NEPTUNE

Erica Neptune is a cross-country and track runner who averages 30 to 40 miles per week. Sometimes her runs involve uneven terrain. Rain has caused the ground to become considerably soft. As Ms. Neptune is running up a hill, the ground gives way, causing her to slip. She feels her left ankle invert and immediately experiences ankle pain. As a result, she has difficulty bearing weight and walks with a limp. She also waits to visit the certified athletic trainer until the following day. On examination, she exhibits a moderately altered gait, moderate edema, and mild eccyhmosis over her left ankle (Fig. 4-5). She has no history of ankle injuries.

1. Based on this scenario, what do you know about Ms. Neptune's injury?

- ______________________________
- ______________________________
- ______________________________
- ______________________________

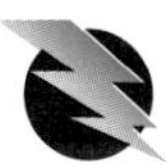

Brain Jolt

The injured structure is one of the most frequently injured structures in the ankle, and it prevents anterior movement of the ankle joint.

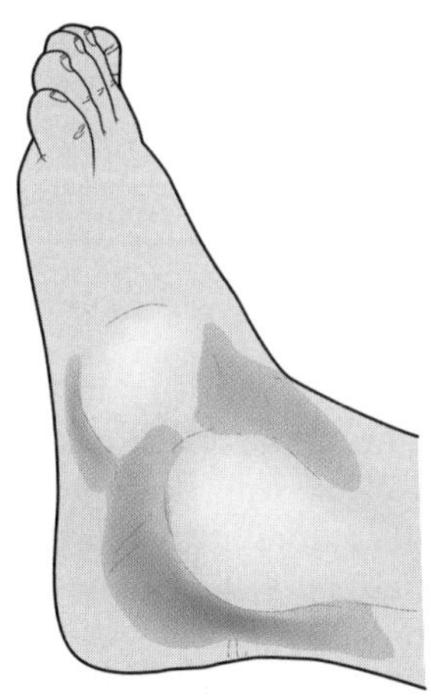

Figure 4-5: Erica Neptune's ankle.

2. To evaluate Ms. Neptune's injury effectively, you will need to gather additional information. What questions should you ask in addition to what is presented in this scenario?
   - ______________________________
   - ______________________________
   - ______________________________
   - ______________________________
3. Identify key terms and concepts, and then research each to broaden your knowledge about ankle and foot injuries.
   - What anatomical structures are involved?

     Answer: ______________________________
   - Define *eversion*.

     Answer: ______________________________
   - Define *lateral*.

     Answer: ______________________________
   - Define *ecchymosis*.

     Answer: ______________________________
   - Do different running terrains affect the body?

     Answer: ______________________________
   - Did seeing the athletic trainer the following day affect her injury negatively?

     Answer: ______________________________
4. Based on the information that you currently have and what was provided by your instructor, what are the possible differential diagnoses for Ms. Neptune's injury?
   - ______________________________
   - ______________________________
   - ______________________________
   - ______________________________

Why or why not?

For each assessment or diagnosis, write *why?* or *why not?* statements identifying why the information is correct or incorrect. Take details from your textbook, your own research, and data from Ms. Neptune's scenario to help you formulate an answer.

1. ______________________________
2. ______________________________
3. ______________________________
4. ______________________________

What do you think?

1. What is your assessment of Ms. Neptune's injury?

   Answer: ______________________________
2. Was your assessment of Ms. Neptune's injury correct?

   Answer: ______________________________
3. If not, explain what you did incorrectly and how you could have performed a better assessment.

   Answer: ______________________________

STUDENT SCENARIO 3: BOBBY EVANS

Bobby Evans is a running back on the high school football team. During the fourth quarter of the game, Mr. Evans receives the ball, runs up the middle of the field, and is tackled from his right side. His left foot is planted on the field and rolls from inversion to eversion (Fig. 4-6). As the ankle everts, the opponent's weight comes down on Mr. Evans' ankle. Mr. Evans feels a pop, and the opposing player states that he heard the pop as the play ended. Mr. Evans is in severe pain. There is no deformity, but he is carried off the field because of the pain.

1. Based on this scenario, what do you know about Mr. Evans' injury?
   - ______________________________

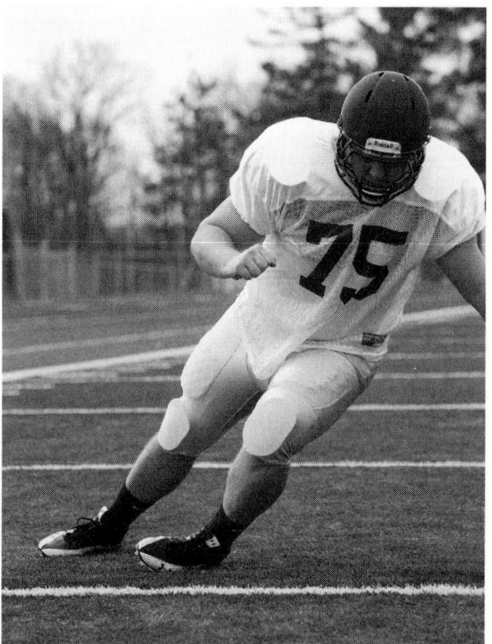

Figure 4-6: Bobby Evans' mechanism of injury.

- ______________________________
  ____
- ______________________________
  ____
- ______________________________
  ____

2. To evaluate Mr. Evans' injury effectively, you will need to gather additional information. What questions should you ask in addition to what is presented in this scenario?
   - ______________________________
     ____
   - ______________________________
     ____
   - ______________________________
     ____
   - ______________________________
     ____
3. Identify key terms and concepts, and then research each to broaden your knowledge about ankle and foot injuries.
   - What anatomical structures are involved?

     Answer: ______________________________
   - Define *inversion.*

     Answer: ______________________________
   - Define *eversion.*

     Answer: ______________________________
   - What might hearing a "pop" sound indicate?

     Answer: ______________________________

Brain Jolt

Be sure that before removing the shoe from an injured ankle, any possible deformity has been ruled out.

4. From the information you currently have and from what was given to you by your instructor, what are the possible differential diagnoses for Mr. Evans' injury?
   - ______________________________
     ____
   - ______________________________
     ____
   - ______________________________
     ____
   - ______________________________
     ____

Why or why not?

For each assessment or diagnosis, write *why?* or *why not?* statements identifying why the information is correct or incorrect. Take details from your textbook, your own research, and data from Mr. Evans' scenario to help you formulate an answer.

1. ______________________________
   ____
2. ______________________________
   ____
3. ______________________________
   ____
4. ______________________________
   ____

What do you think?

1. What is your assessment of Mr. Evans' injury?

   Answer: ______________________________
2. Was your assessment of Mr. Evans' injury correct?

   Answer: ______________________________
3. If not, explain what you did incorrectly and how you could have performed a better assessment.

   Answer: ______________________________

STUDENT SCENARIO 4: DARREN JORDAN

Darren Jordan is a first baseman and designated hitter on his baseball team. Mr. Jordan hits the ball into the outfield between shortstop and third base. Upon approaching second base, Mr. Jordan notices the ball being thrown to the shortstop. Mr. Jordan quickly slides into second base on his right hip and feet first. His left foot catches the base as he attempts to stand during the slide, causing his left foot to forcefully dorsiflex and invert (Fig. 4-7). Mr. Jordan is unable to continue the game because of lateral ankle pain while weight-bearing. Edema develops over the lateral region of the malleolus and lateral side of the lower leg. He is unable to actively dorsiflex his left foot. Mr. Jordan has a history of lateral ankle sprains.

1. Based on this scenario, what do you know about Mr. Jordan's injury?
   - ______________________________
   - ______________________________
   - ______________________________
   - ______________________________

2. To evaluate Mr. Jordan's injury effectively, you will need to gather additional information. What questions should you ask in addition to what is presented in this scenario?
   - ______________________________
   - ______________________________
   - ______________________________
   - ______________________________

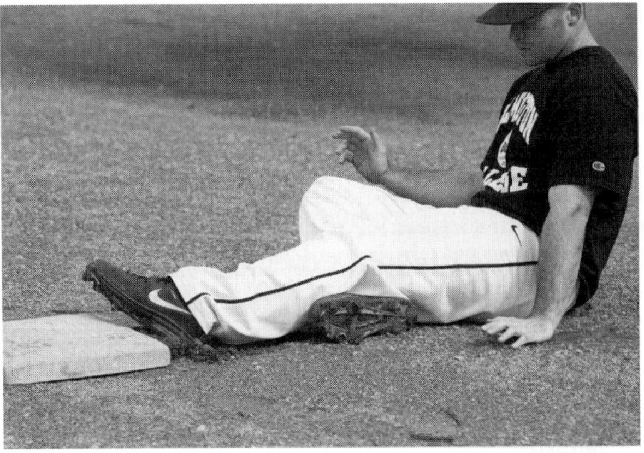

Figure 4-7: Darren Jordan's mechanism of injury.

Brain Jolt
A loss of function does not always indicate a fracture. Rely on your special tests to direct you.

3. Identify key terms and concepts, and then research each to broaden your knowledge about ankle and foot injuries.
   - What anatomical structures are involved?

     Answer: ______________________________
   - Define *dorsiflexion.*

     Answer: ______________________________
   - Define *eversion.*

     Answer: ______________________________
   - Why is noting the pattern and location of edema important?

     Answer: ______________________________
   - Does lack of active ROM indicate an avulsion?

     Answer: ______________________________
   - What is a designated hitter?

     Answer: ______________________________

4. Based on the information that you currently have and what was provided by your instructor, what are the possible differential diagnoses for Mr. Jordan's injury?
   - ______________________________
   - ______________________________
   - ______________________________
   - ______________________________

Why or why not?

For each assessment or diagnosis, write *why?* or *why not?* statements identifying why the information is correct or incorrect. Take details from your textbook, your own research, and data from Mr. Jordan's scenario to help you formulate an answer.

1. ______________________________

2. ______________________________

____

3. ______________________________

____

4. ______________________________

____

What do you think?

1. What is your assessment of Mr. Jordan's injury?

   Answer: ______________________________

2. Was your assessment of Mr. Jordan's injury correct?

   Answer: ______________________________

3. If not, explain what you did incorrectly and how you could have performed a better assessment.

   Answer: ______________________________

Conversation Buffer

This type of injury can have a slow recovery rate as a result of repetitive separation at the involved joint. Therefore, you need to be realistic with the patient and coach about expectations regarding the athlete's return to play. Although the severity of the injury might not seem substantial, surgery and a lengthy rehabilitation may be necessary in the future.

STUDENT SCENARIO 5: MANDY DUNLAP

Mandy Dunlap plays forward on the women's soccer team. As twice daily practices begin, Ms. Dunlap complains of a burning sensation on the plantar surface of her right foot during practice. She explains that she experienced right plantar foot pain while working this summer as an office secretary. The prior pain occurred only when she put on her dress shoes for work and with extensive standing at work. Ms. Dunlap's pain is located on the plantar surface of the right foot, around the third and fourth metatarsal heads (Fig. 4-8). Ms. Dunlap experiences some relief when not bearing weight. Ms. Dunlap has a history of a fallen transverse arch that produces pain when standing and hyperextending her toes.

1. Based on this scenario, what do you know about Ms. Dunlap's injury?

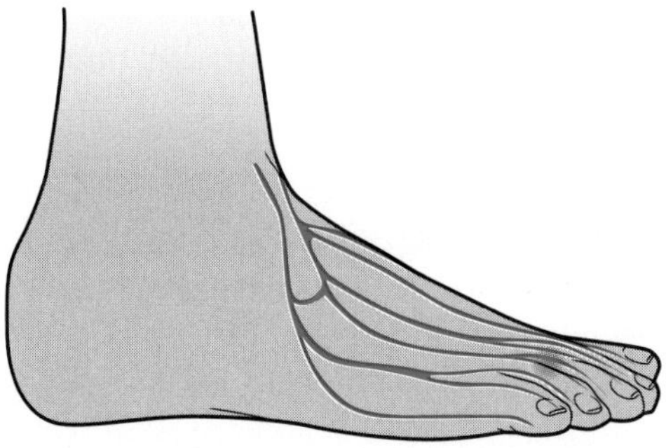

   - ______________________________

     ____

   - ______________________________

     ____

   - ______________________________

     ____

   - ______________________________

     ____

Figure 4-8: Mandy Dunlap's point of pain.

2. To evaluate Ms. Dunlap's injury effectively, you will need to gather additional information. What questions should you ask in addition to what is presented in this scenario?

   - ______________________________

     ____

   - ______________________________

     ____

   - ______________________________

     ____

   - ______________________________

     ____

3. Identify key terms and concepts, and then research each to broaden your knowledge about ankle and foot injuries.

   - What anatomical structures are involved?

     Answer: ______________________________

   - What muscles are involved in hyperextension of the toes?

     Answer: ______________________________

   - Define *plantar surface.*

     Answer: ______________________________

- Define *hyperextension*.

  Answer: ________________________________

- What is a transverse arch?

  Answer: ________________________________

- How could Ms. Dunlap's summer job have affected her injury? What does the plantar surface burning sensation possibly indicate?

  Answer: ________________________________

> **Brain Jolt**
> *The athlete's type of pain can guide you to the structure injured.*

4. Based on the information you currently have and what was provided by your instructor, what are the possible differential diagnoses for Ms. Dunlap's injury?

- ________________________________
- ________________________________
- ________________________________
- ________________________________

Why or why not?

For each assessment or diagnosis, write *why?* or *why not?* statements identifying why the information is correct or incorrect. Take details from your textbook, your own research, and data from Ms. Dunlap's scenario to help you formulate an answer.

1. ________________________________

2. ________________________________

3. ________________________________

4. ________________________________

What do you think?

1. What is your assessment of Ms. Dunlap's injury?

Answer: ________________________________

2. Was your assessment of Ms. Dunlap's injury correct?

Answer: ________________________________

3. If not, explain what you did incorrectly and how you could have performed a better assessment.

Answer: ________________________________

STUDENT SCENARIO 6: STEPHANIE MAPES

Stephanie Mapes is a member of the equestrian team at her college and has been showing horses since the age of 8. Ms. Mapes is aware of the dangers of working with animals, as she has a history of being kicked in the shins, stepped on, and bitten. She is currently training a new Arabian horse that has been brought to the college stables. As she is leading the horse from the stall, the door slams shut, spooking the horse and causing it to rear up and land on the lateral side of Ms. Mapes' right foot while in slight plantar flexion. Ms. Mapes limps as she guides the horse into the stall. As with her prior injuries, she has an altered gait for a couple of weeks, hoping the injury will improve. Ms. Mapes notices localized edema over the dorsal lateral side of the right foot and is point tender over the dorsal lateral bony process (Fig. 4-9).

1. Based on this scenario, what do you know about Ms. Mapes' injury?

- ________________________________

- ________________________________
- ________________________________

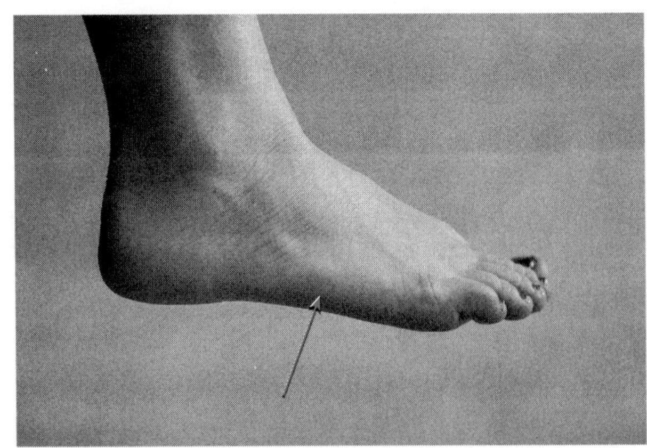

Figure 4-9: Stephanie Mapes' point of pain.

- ______________________________
  ____

2. To evaluate Ms. Mapes' injury effectively, you will need to gather additional information. What questions should you ask in addition to what is presented in this scenario?
   - ______________________________
     ____
   - ______________________________
     ____
   - ______________________________
     ____
   - ______________________________
     ____

Brain Jolt
This injury has a tendency to cause lingering pain without many other symptoms as a result of its healing process and its non-union characteristics.

3. Identify any key terms and concepts and research each to broaden your knowledge about ankle and foot injuries.
   - What anatomical structures are involved?

     Answer: ______________________________
   - Define *edema.*

     Answer: ______________________________
   - Define *dorsal.*

     Answer: ______________________________
   - What is the difference between acute edema and chronic edema?

     Answer: ______________________________
   - What bony process is located on the lateral dorsal side of the foot?

     Answer: ______________________________
   - Are there dangers in having an altered gait for an extended amount of time? If yes, what are they?

     Answer: ______________________________
4. From the information you currently have and from what was given to you by your instructor, what are the possible differential diagnoses for Ms. Mapes' injury?
   - ______________________________
     ____
   - ______________________________
     ____
   - ______________________________
     ____
   - ______________________________
     ____

Why or why not?

For each assessment or diagnosis, write *why?* or *why not?* statements identifying why the information is correct or incorrect. Take details from your textbook, your own research, and data from Ms. Mapes' scenario to help you formulate an answer.

1. ______________________________
   ____
2. ______________________________
   ____
3. ______________________________
   ____
4. ______________________________
   ____

What do you think?

1. What is your assessment of Ms. Mapes' injury?

   Answer: ______________________________
2. Was your assessment of Ms. Mapes' injury correct?

   Answer: ______________________________
3. If not, explain what you did incorrectly and how you could have performed a better assessment.

   Answer: ______________________________

STUDENT SCENARIO 7: CALEB COX

Caleb Cox is a former college football player. He continues to be committed to maintaining his health and developing his athletic ability, and he lifts weights regularly and plays flag football on weekends, resulting in overly developed calf muscles. However, Mr. Cox does not stretch regularly to enhance his training and prevent injury. During a flag football game, Mr. Cox runs up the middle of the field with the ball. A fellow player falls backwards onto Mr. Cox, forcing his left knee straight as he continues moving forward while pushing off his left foot. Mr. Cox feels a sudden "pop" posteriorly in his lower left leg as though he has been kicked. The pain is excruciating but subsides 15 minutes later. Mr. Cox is able to partially perform active dorsiflexion with his left foot, but is unable to perform active plantar flexion. He exhibits some deformity of his lower left leg (Fig. 4-10) and edema over the gastrocnemius region. When Mr. Cox was in high school and college, he had a history of lateral ankle sprains and Achilles tendonitis.

1. Based on this scenario, what do you know about Mr. Cox's injury?

    - ____
    - ____
    - ____
    - ____

2. To evaluate Mr. Cox's injury effectively, you will need to gather additional information. What questions should you ask in addition to what is presented in this scenario?

    - ____
    - ____
    - ____
    - ____

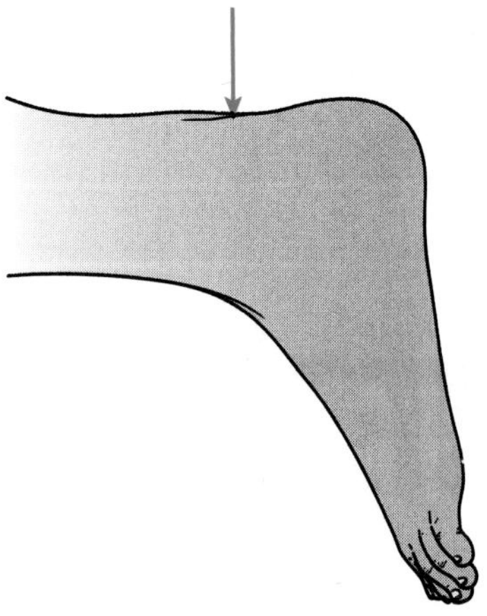

Figure 4-10: Caleb Cox's posterior leg.

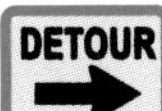

Treatment Detour

When athletes sustain this injury, they often suffer from residual weakness and decreased function. Research shows that early immobilization is beneficial for this injury whether it is ultimately treated surgically or conservatively. Although the best method for treatment of this injury is still unknown, there is a considerable risk of reinjury after healing from this injury (Nilsson-Helander et al., 2010).

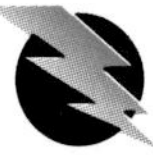

Brain Jolt

This injury is a medical emergency that requires immediate splinting of the foot in plantar flexion.

3. Identify key terms and concepts, and then research each to broaden your knowledge about ankle and foot injuries.
    - What anatomical structures are involved?

      Answer: ________________________________
    - What muscles attach to the Achilles tendon?

      Answer: ________________________________
    - Define *plantar flexion.*

      Answer: ________________________________
    - Define *dorsiflexion.*

      Answer: ________________________________
    - What is Achilles tendonitis?

      Answer: ________________________________
    - Define *edema.*

      Answer: ________________________________
    - Why is a lack of flexibility important to know in the assessment of this injury?

      Answer: ________________________________
    - Why did Mr. Cox's pain subside shortly after his injury?

      Answer: ________________________________

4. Based on the information that you currently have and what was provided by your instructor, what are the possible differential diagnoses for Mr. Cox's injury?

    - ____
    - ____
    - ____
    - ____

Conversation Buffer
When this injury occurs, the patient will often describe the sound as a gunshot, because of the tensile force. Therefore, depending on its severity, this injury can produce significant deformity. Try to keep your athlete calm by discussing something off the topic at hand and maintain crowd control.

Why or why not?

For each assessment or diagnosis, write *why?* or *why not?* statements identifying why the information is correct or incorrect. Take details from your textbook, your own research, and data from Mr. Cox's scenario to help you formulate an answer.

1. ______________________________

2. ______________________________

3. ______________________________

4. ______________________________

What do you think?

1. What is your assessment of Mr. Cox's injury?

   Answer: ______________________________

2. Was your assessment of Mr. Cox's injury correct?

   Answer: ______________________________

3. If not, explain what you did incorrectly and how you could have performed a better assessment.

   Answer: ______________________________

STUDENT SCENARIO 8: HILARY SMITH

Hilary Smith is a freshman high school soccer player in her first year playing soccer. She is excited about getting a uniform, new cleats, and shin guards. The first few weeks of practice are hard, but Ms. Smith is beginning to feel comfortable with her team. Ms. Smith has started experiencing pain located on the posterior aspect of her left foot when she wears her cleats. The edema is localized and feels watery at the Achilles tendon (Fig. 4-11). Ms. Smith's gait is altered because of irriation when she wears shoes. Ms. Smith's parents mention to her that she needs to stretch her gastrocnemius muscles.

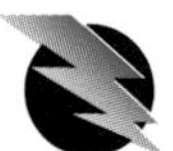

Brain Jolt
The shoe friction is causing the fluid-filled shock absorber to become irritated.

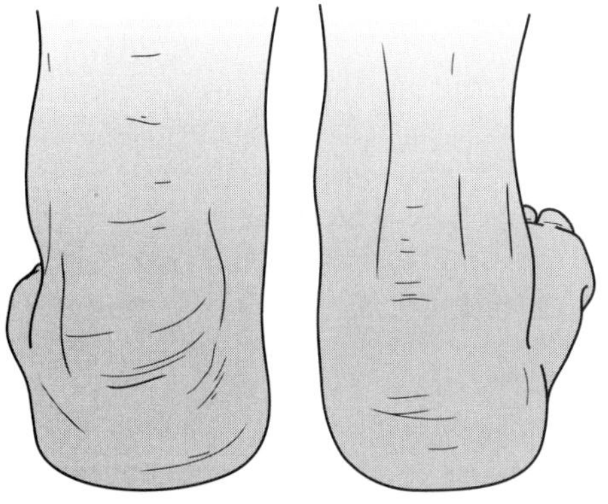

Figure 4-11: Hilary Smith's point of pain and edema.

1. Based on this scenario, what do you know about Ms. Smith's injury?

   - ______________________________
   - ______________________________
   - ______________________________
   - ______________________________

2. To evaluate Ms. Smith's injury effectively, you will need to gather additional information. What questions should you ask in addition to what is presented in this scenario?

   - ______________________________
   - ______________________________
   - ______________________________
   - ______________________________

3. Identify key terms and concepts, and then research each to broaden your knowledge about ankle and foot injuries.
   - What anatomical structures are involved?

     Answer: ________________

   - Why does Ms. Smith's edema look different?

     Answer: ________________

   - Why is Ms. Smith's new gear important to consider in the assessment of this injury?

     Answer: ________________

   - Why would Ms. Smith experience pain wearing shoes?

     Answer: ________________

4. Based on the information that you currently have and what was provided by your instructor, what are the possible differential diagnoses for Ms. Smith's injury?
   - ________________
   - ________________
   - ________________
   - ________________

Why or why not?

For each assessment or diagnosis, write *why?* or *why not?* statements identifying why the information is correct or incorrect. Take details from your textbook, your own research, and data from Ms. Smith's scenario to help you formulate an answer.

1. ________________
2. ________________
3. ________________
4. ________________

What do you think?

1. What is your assessment of Ms. Smith's injury?

   Answer: ________________

2. Was your assessment of Ms. Smith's injury correct?

   Answer: ________________

3. If not, explain what you did incorrectly and how you could have performed a better assessment.

   Answer: ________________

STUDENT SCENARIO 9: DJ VAUGHN

DJ Vaughn is an active 12-year-old who participates in basketball, soccer, baseball, and swimming. DJ is 4 feet, 5 inches tall, and his growth rate is normal on the growth chart. Throughout his soccer season, he has complained periodically of pain on his left calcaneus. The pain becomes more consistent toward the end of the soccer season and continues into basketball season. DJ experiences pain only when playing a sport. He is instructed by his parents to do towel stretching, but this seems to exacerbate the pain. He now notices a minor deformity and edema at the back of his left calcaneus (Fig. 4-12).

1. Based on this scenario, what do you know about DJ's injury?
   - ________________
   - ________________
   - ________________
   - ________________

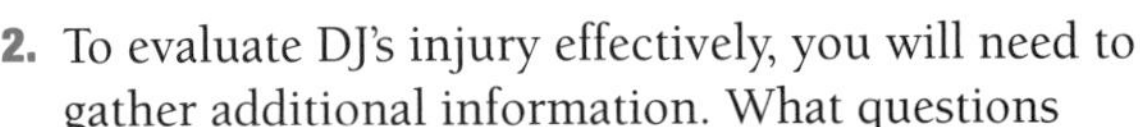

2. To evaluate DJ's injury effectively, you will need to gather additional information. What questions

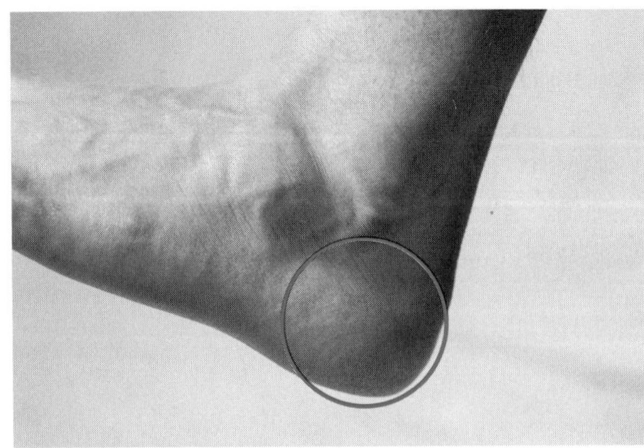

Figure 4-12: DJ Vaughn's point of pain.

should you ask in addition to what is presented in this scenario?

- ______________________________
  ____
- ______________________________
  ____
- ______________________________
  ____

DETOUR

Treatment Detour

Foot and ankle injuries are the second most common injuries seen in young athletes. Proposed etiologies include rapid growth, heredity, anatomic characteristics, trauma, overuse, and defects in vascular supply. This injury is most common in children between 8 and 12 years old and accounts for more than 8% of overuse injuries in adolescents. Previously, this injury was thought to result from traction, but new research indicates that it actually results from chronic repetitive compression (Gillespie, 2010).

Brain Jolt

This injury is comparable to Osgood-Schlatter disease. Be sure to look for a bump or deformity.

3. Identify key terms and concepts, and then research each to broaden your knowledge about ankle and foot injuries.

- What anatomical structures are involved?

  Answer: ______________________________
- Define *edema.*

  Answer: ______________________________
- What are towel stretches and why can they cause pain?

  Answer: ______________________________
- Why is it important to know the adolescent growth chart?

  Answer: ______________________________
- Describe the appearance of a calcaneal deformity.

  Answer: ______________________________
- What risk factors do younger athletes face with ankle and foot injuries?

  Answer: ______________________________

4. From the information you currently have and from what was given to you by your instructor, what are the possible differential diagnoses for DJ's injury?

- ______________________________
  ____
- ______________________________
  ____
- ______________________________
  ____
- ______________________________
  ____

Why or why not?

For each assessment or diagnosis, write *why?* or *why not?* statements identifying why the information is correct or incorrect. Take details from your textbook, your own research, and data from DJ's scenario to help you formulate an answer.

1. ______________________________
____

2. ______________________________
____

3. ______________________________
____

4. ______________________________
____

What do you think?

1. What is your assessment of DJ's injury?

Answer: ______________________________

2. Was your assessment of DJ's injury correct?

Answer: ______________________________

3. If not, explain what you did incorrectly and how you could have performed a better assessment.

Answer: ______________________________

STUDENT SCENARIO 10: ALEX BARTON

Alex Barton is a college sophmore who participates in intramural activities. Mr. Barton was a cross-country athlete in high school and has no history of injury. The intramural basketball team is midway through the season when Mr. Barton notices pain on the plantar surface of his right foot (Fig. 4-13). The majority of pain occurs while pushing off his right foot. Upon examination by the certified athletic trainer, Mr. Barton has point tenderness localized at the plantar surface of the great toe near the metatarsophalangeal joint. The athletic trainer also notices a large callus on the ball of Mr. Barton's right foot.

1. Based on this scenario, what do you know about Mr. Barton's injury?
   - ____________________
   - ____________________
   - ____________________

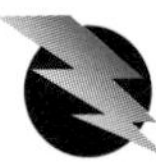

Brain Jolt
Those with this injury often have pes cavus.

2. To evaluate Mr. Barton's injury effectively, you will need to gather additional information. What questions should you ask in addition to what is presented in this scenario?
   - ____________________
   - ____________________
   - ____________________
   - ____________________

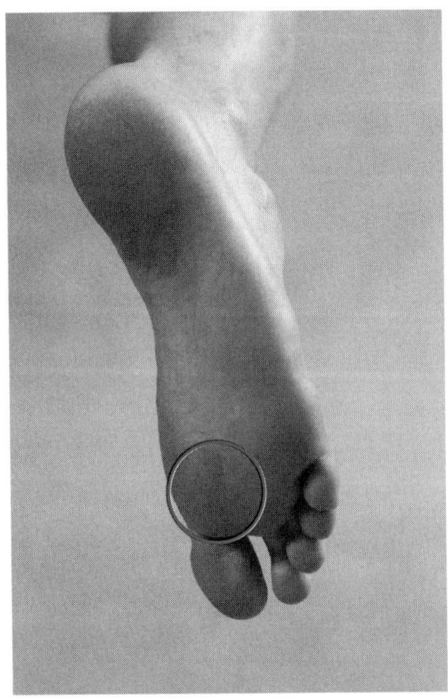

Figure 4-13: Alex Barton's point of pain.

3. Identify key terms and concepts, and then research each to broaden your knowledge about ankle and foot injuries.
   - What anatomical structures are involved?

     Answer: ____________________
   - Define *plantar surface.*

     Answer: ____________________
   - Why is a callus important in the assessment of this injury?

     Answer: ____________________
4. Based on the information that you currently have and what was provided by your instructor, what are the possible differential diagnoses for Mr. Barton's injury?
   - ____________________
   - ____________________
   - ____________________
   - ____________________

Why or why not?

For each assessment or diagnosis, write *why?* or *why not?* statements identifying why the information is correct or incorrect. Take details from your textbook, your own research, and data from Mr. Barton's scenario to help you formulate an answer.

1. ____________________
2. ____________________
3. ____________________
4. ____________________

What do you think?

1. What is your assessment of Mr. Barton's injury?

   Answer: ______________________________

2. Was your assessment of Mr. Barton's injury correct?

   Answer: ______________________________

3. If not, explain what you did incorrectly and how you could have performed a better assessment.

   Answer: ______________________________

knowledge checklist

Table 4-1 offers a checklist that can be used by a peer, instructor, or preceptor to evaluate each part of a foot and ankle assessment. Use this checklist as a tool to ensure that the evaluation is complete and to assess your knowledge of the competencies that apply to this chapter.

TABLE 4-1 ■ Ankle and Foot Assessment Competency Checklist

	Proficient *Can demonstrate and execute the skill properly*	**Proficient With Assistance** *Can demonstrate and execute the skill with minimal guidance or tips*	**Not Proficient** *Unable to demonstrate and execute the skill properly; need to be reevaluated at another time after further study and practice*
Athlete's Health History			
Medical history			
History of ankle and foot injury			
Type of sport and position played			
When did the injury occur?			
Mechanisms of Injury			
How did the injury occur?			
When does the pain occur?			
What makes the pain better or worse?			
Was the athlete's ankle or foot forced into an unusual direction?			
Was the athlete's foot planted?			
Were any pops, cracks, or snaps heard?			
Does the athlete experience pain going up or down stairs?			
How did the athlete's ankle and foot look at the time the injury occurred?			
Visual Observations			
Gait			
Edema			
Ecchymosis			
Deformity			
Palpation *Temperature change over the painful area; crepitus; deformity; intra-articular or extra-articular joint swelling; changes within the muscle fibers*			
Lateral malleolus			
Medial malleolus			
Styloid process of the fifth metatarsal			
Sinus tarsi			
Dome of the talus			
Sesamoid bones			
Metatarsal heads			
Anterior tuberosity of the calcaneus			
Sustentaculum tali			
Peroneal tubercle			

Continued

TABLE 4-1 ■ Ankle and Foot Assessment Competency Checklist—cont'd

	Proficient	Proficient With Assistance	Not Proficient
Anterior compartment muscles			
Posterior superficial compartment muscles			
Posterior deep compartment muscles			
Lateral compartment muscles			
Achilles tendon			
Plantar fascia			
Retrocalcaneal bursa			
Four arches of the foot			
Anterior tibiofibular ligament			
Lateral talocalcaneal ligament			
Calcaneofibular ligament			
Posterior talofibular ligament			
Bifurcated ligament			
Syndesmosis			
Deltoid ligament			
Calcaneonavicular (spring) ligament			
Posterior talotibial ligament			
Posterior talocalcaneal ligament			
Range of Motion			
Passive or active			
Flexion of toes			
Extension of toes			
Dorsiflexion			
Plantar flexion			
Eversion			
Inversion			
Strength			
Grade through manual muscle tests			
Flexion			
Extension			
Inversion			
Eversion			
Special Tests			
Anterior drawer test			
Forefoot stress test			
Tap, percussion, bump test			
Talar tilt test			
Peroneal subluxation test			
Compression test			
Homan's test			
Interdigital neuroma test			
Kleiger's test			
Tinel's sign			
Morton's test			
Thompson test			
Valgus stress test (metatarsophalangeal and interphalangeal joints)			
Varus stress test (metatarsophalangeal and interphalangeal joints)			

TABLE 4-1 ■ Ankle and Foot Assessment Competency Checklist—cont'd

	Proficient	Proficient With Assistance	Not Proficient
Neurological			
L4–S2 nerve roots			
Achilles reflex			
Vascular			
Dorsal pedal pulse			
Posterior tibial pulse			
Popliteal pulse			
Capillary refill			
Final Assessment			
Sprain; strain; contusion; fracture; condition; severity			

*Be sure to always compare bilaterally.

REFERENCES

Gillespie, H. (2010). Osteochondroses and apophyseal injuries of the foot in the young athlete. *Current Sports Medicine Reports, 9,* 265–268.

National Athletic Training Association. (2011). *Athletic training education competencies* (5th ed.). Retrieved from http://www.nata.org/sites/default/files/5th-Edition-Competencies-2011-PDF-Version.pdf

Nilsson-Helander, K., Silbernagel, K. G., Thomeé, R., Faxén, E., Olsson, N., Eriksson, B. I., & Karlsson, J. (2010). A randomized, controlled study comparing surgical and nonsurgical treatments using validated outcome measures. *American Journal of Sports Medicine, 38,* 2186–2193.

Prentice, W. (2010). *Arnheim's principles of athletic training: A competency-based approach* (14th ed.). New York, NY: McGraw-Hill.

Starkey, C., Brown, S. D., & Ryan, J. (2010). *Examination of orthopedic and athletic injuries* (3rd ed.). Philadelphia, PA: F.A. Davis.

Venes, D. (Ed.) (2009). *Taber's cyclopedic medical dictionary* (21st ed.). Philadelphia, PA: F.A. Davis.

chapter 5

Lower Extremity: The Knee

chapter outline

athletic trainer's corner

Out there in the real world, one athletic trainer experienced the following:

Being an athletic trainer comes with its ups and downs. There are days when you are able to improve an athlete's condition and give him the good news that he can play in the big game. But the lows of the profession hit when you have to tell an athlete that he is out of the sport indefinitely. I remember a situation like this as though it were yesterday. I attended an away football game where one of my players leaped up to catch a ball, and when he landed on the playing field his knee buckled. I experienced a horrible feeling of dread as I ran onto the field to perform a Lachman and Valgus stress test, which were both grossly positive. A magnetic resonance image and a physician's examination confirmed the diagnosis. I just knew the player would undergo knee surgery within the week, causing his career to come to an abrupt end.

Kim Isaac, MS, AT, ATC
Assistant Professor
Assistant Athletic Trainer
Wilmington College
Wilmington, Ohio

learning outcomes

After working through this chapter, you will be able to:

1. Verbalize the questions to use when obtaining a thorough medical history for an assessment.
2. Describe the principles of body movement at the knee and the various mechanisms of injury that affect the knee.
3. Compare and contrast the findings of various special tests and the role of diagnostic tests used during a knee evaluation.
4. Explain the medical terminology associated with the assessment of musculoskeletal injuries.
5. Verbalize the standard procedures used for a clinical evaluation of the knee and interpret the findings for differential diagnoses.

MODEL SCENARIO 1: DAN MUELLER

Dan Mueller has an altered gait and moderate pain in his left knee. He states that when he was playing shortstop in the baseball game yesterday, he hurt his left knee while fielding a ground ball. Mr. Mueller aggressively lunged forward to catch a wild hit, took a misstep, fell, and hit the ground hard with his left knee flexed to 90 degrees (Fig. 5-1). Mr. Mueller has no history of injuries to his left knee. Mr. Mueller is having a hard time walking, which is apparent from his disrupted gait. He says most of his knee pain is located posteriorly. Upon observation of his left knee, you notice that there is moderate edema located in the popliteal fossa, no visual deformity, and no ecchymosis when compared bilaterally.

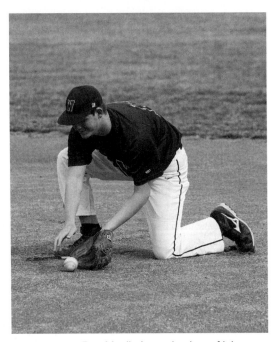

Figure 5-1: Dan Mueller's mechanism of injury.

1. Based on this scenario, what do you know about Mr. Mueller's injury?
   - *Male athlete*
   - *Baseball shortstop*
   - *Injury occurred at least 24 hours ago*
   - *Mechanism of injury includes hitting a flexed knee on the ground with force*
   - *No previous knee injury*
   - *Apparent limp when ambulating*
   - *Moderate edema posteriorly in popliteal fossa region compared bilaterally*
   - *No visual deformity*
   - *No ecchymosis*
   - *Posterior knee pain*
2. To evaluate Mr. Mueller's injury effectively, you will need to gather additional information. What questions should you ask in addition to what is presented in this scenario?
   - *Is this injury a medical emergency?*
   - *Are there preexisting injuries? If yes, what are they?*
   - *Are there any special tests that are important to perform? If yes, elaborate.*
   - *Are the results of the special tests positive or negative? What does each result indicate?*
   - *Is there passive or active range of motion (ROM) in the knee?*
   - *What is the strength at the knee?*
   - *Were any pops, cracks, or snaps heard?*
   - *Does the knee feel unstable?*
   - *Where is the most tender point?*

Brain Jolt

The injured structure prevents posterior translation of the tibia.

Conversation Buffer

When asking an athlete about the location of pain, you may frequently receive an answer that is not specific; therefore, this information might not be helpful to you. The athlete may motion around his or her entire knee without pointing to a specific area. To focus your assessment, ask the athlete to use one finger to point to where it hurts the most. This method provides a starting point for your assessment.

3. Identify key terms and concepts, and then research each to broaden your knowledge of knee injuries.
   - What anatomical structures are involved?
     PCL
     Tibia
     Patella
     Femur
     Popliteal fossa
   - Define *bilateral.*
     Directional term meaning "both sides"
   - Define *posterior.*
     Directional term meaning "in back of" or "behind"
   - Define *ecchymosis.*
     Discoloration of the skin, bruising
   - What is the tibial tuberosity?
     A bony landmark on the tibia where the patellar tendon attaches
   - What are the ligamentous structures of the knee?
     The anterior cruciate ligament (ACL), posterior cruciate ligament (PCL), medial collateral ligament (MCL), lateral collateral ligament (LCL)
4. Based on the information that you currently have and what was provided by your instructor, what are the possible differential diagnoses for Mr. Mueller's injury?
   ACL injury
   Sprained posterior capsule
   Bone bruise to the tibial tuberosity
   PCL injury
   Muscle strain (hamstring or gastrocnemius)

Why or why not?

For each assessment or diagnosis, write *why?* or *why not?* statements identifying why the information is correct or incorrect. Take details from your textbook, your own research, and data from Mr. Mueller's scenario to help you formulate an answer.

1. *Mr. Mueller does not have an ACL injury because the Lachman and anterior drawer tests are negative. Mr. Mueller's posterior pain is not consistent with an ACL injury.*
2. *Mr. Mueller has a posterior capsule sprain in addition to a PCL injury as a result of the mechanism of injury and because the posterior drawer test is positive for pain and laxity.*
3. *Mr. Mueller does not have a bone bruise from the fall because his pain is in the posterior knee, and he is not point tender over the anterior knee.*
4. *Mr. Mueller has a grade 2 sprain to the PCL as a result of the mechanism of injury and because the posterior drawer test is positive for laxity and has an end feel, and Mr. Mueller's pain is in the posterior knee.*
5. *Mr. Mueller does not have a muscle strain because his strength is good and equal bilaterally, and he is not point tender over the tendons or muscle belly.*

What do you think?

1. What is your assessment of Mr. Mueller's injury?
   Answer: *Posterior capsule and PCL sprain*
2. Was your assessment of Mr. Mueller's injury correct?
   Answer: *Yes*
3. If not, explain what you did incorrectly and how you could have performed a better assessment.

Answer: ______________________________

MODEL SCENARIO 2: **DON SMITSON**

Don Smitson, a cross-country runner, comes to you 3 weeks into the cross-country season complaining of knee pain. He states that the pain occurs only during and after practice. The discomfort began at the start of the season. He is still able to give 100% effort in practice, but he experiences chronic pain. All his pain is located anteriorly in the left knee. Mr. Smitson is point tender at the inferior pole of the patella and over the patellar tendon (Fig. 5-2). He experiences pain over the patella and into the patellar tendon when he is asked to contract his left quadriceps muscle. Mr. Smitson has no history of injury to this knee. When compared bilaterally, there is mild edema near the tibial tuberosity and no deformity of the patella or near the tibial tuberosity.

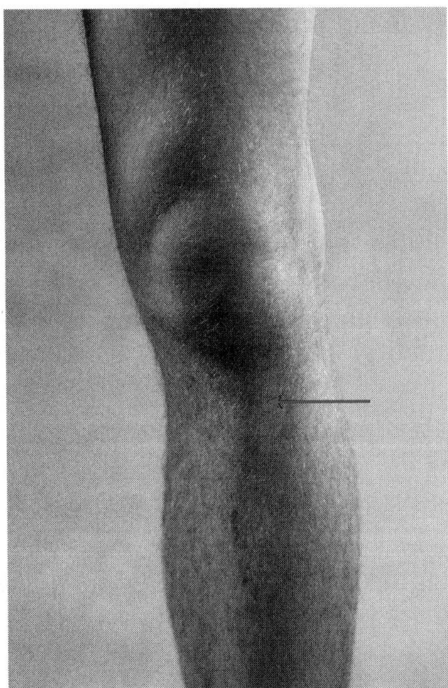

Figure 5-2: Don Smitson's point of pain.

1. Based on this scenario, what do you know about Mr. Smitson's injury?
   - *Male athlete*
   - *Cross-country runner*
   - *Chronic pain started 3 weeks ago*
   - *Pain only during and after practice*
   - *Mild edema near the tibial tuberosity*
   - *Anterior pain over the inferior pole of the patella*
   - *Pain occurs when quadriceps muscles are contracted*
   - *No deformity of patella and near tibial tuberosity*
2. To evaluate Mr. Smitson's injury effectively, you will need to gather additional information. What questions should you ask in addition to what is presented in this scenario?
   - *Is this injury a medical emergency?*
   - *Are there any preexisting injuries? If yes, what are they?*
   - *Are there any special tests that are important to perform? If yes, elaborate.*
   - *Are the results of the special tests positive or negative? What does each indicate?*
   - *Is there passive or active ROM in the knee?*
   - *What is the strength at the knee?*
   - *Did any type of fall happen to make the knee start hurting?*
   - *Does the knee feel unstable?*
   - *Is the patellar tendon thickened or have a change in temperature?*

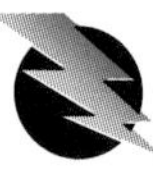

Brain Jolt

When palpating an inflamed tendon, it will feel thickened or wider when compared bilaterally.

3. Identify key terms and concepts, and then research each to broaden your knowledge of knee injuries.
   - What anatomical structures are involved?
     Tibial tuberosity
     Patella
     Tibia
     Femur
     Tibial plateau
     Inferior pole of the patella
   - What are the signs and symptoms of patellar tendonitis?
     Thickening of the patellar tendon
     Localized edema over the area
     Pain over the inferior pole of the patella
     Pain that occurs before, during, or after activity
     Increased temperature over the painful area
   - What are the signs and symptoms of Osgood-Schlatter disease?
     Edema over the tibial tuberosity
     Point tenderness over tibial tuberosity
     Pain with kneeling, jumping, or running
     Presence of deformity
4. Based on the information that you currently have and what was provided by your instructor, what are the possible differential diagnoses for Mr. Smitson's injury?
   Patellar tendonitis
   Osgood-Schlatter disease
   Avulsion of the patellar tendon from the tibial tuberosity

Why or why not?

For each assessment or diagnosis, write *why?* or *why not?* statements identifying why the information is correct or incorrect. Take details from your textbook, your own research, and data from Mr. Smitson's scenario to help you formulate an answer.

1. *Mr. Smitson has patellar tendonitis. Pain at the patella tendon and inferior pole of the patella, edema localized near the tibial tuberosity, and pain with activity, especially with contraction of the quadriceps, are symptoms that indicate patellar tendonitis.*
2. *Mr. Smitson does not have Osgood-Schlatter disease because there is no deformity or point tenderness at the tibial tuberosity.*
3. *Mr. Smitson does not have an avulsion because there is not moderate edema over the localized area, there is no deformity, and the pain is chronic.*

What do you think?

1. What is your assessment of Mr. Smitson's injury?
   Answer: *Patellar tendonitis*
2. Was your assessment of Mr. Smitson's injury correct?
   Answer: *Yes*
3. If not, explain what you did incorrectly and how you could have performed a better assessment.

Answer: ____________________

MODEL SCENARIO 3: JOSH MILLER

While playing soccer, Josh Miller dribbles the ball down the field, trips, and falls directly on his left knee. The playing surface is artificial turf, which allows for less impact absorption. Mr. Miller complains of pain directly over the top of the patella. He has localized point tenderness over the midportion of the patella. Mr. Miller did not feel or hear a pop or crack when landing on his left knee. Mild edema is already starting to form over the top of the patella when compared bilaterally (Fig. 5-3). The edema feels watery upon palpation, and Mr. Miller states that his knee feels tight when actively performing flexion and extension. He has no history of injury to his left knee. The tuning fork special test is negative.

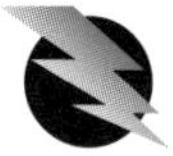

Brain Jolt

Always be sure to compare bilaterally when evaluating an injury.

1. Based on this scenario, what do you know about Mr. Miller's injury?
   - *Male athlete*
   - *Soccer player*
   - *Mechanism of injury (MOI) is falling directly on the knee*
   - *Acute injury*
   - *Hard injury surface*
   - *Localized pain and point tenderness over the patella*
   - *Mild edema that feels watery*
   - *No history of injuries*
   - *No popping or cracking sounds heard at the time of injury*
   - *Tuning fork special test negative*
2. To evaluate Mr. Miller's injury effectively, you will need to gather additional information. What questions should you ask in addition to what is presented in this scenario?
   - *Is this injury a medical emergency?*
   - *Are there any preexisting injuries? If yes, what are they?*
   - *Are there any special tests that are important to perform? If yes, elaborate.*
   - *Are the results of the special tests positive or negative? What does each result indicate?*
   - *Is there passive or active ROM in the knee?*
   - *What is the strength at the knee?*
   - *Does the knee feel unstable?*

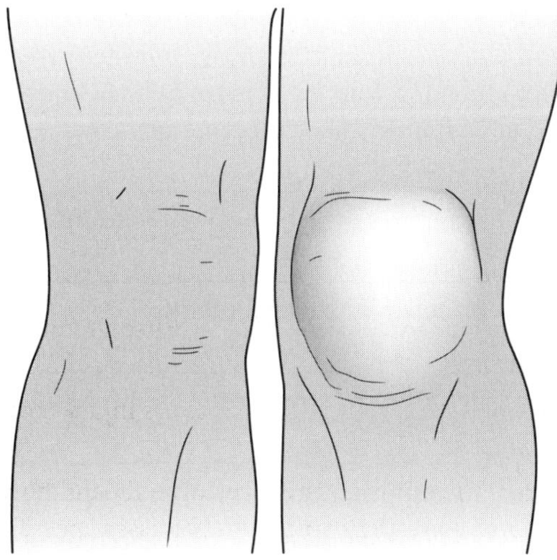

Figure 5-3: Josh Miller's edema.

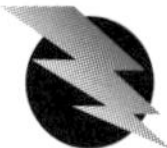

Brain Jolt

When this structure is inflamed, it typically has a watery feel. Learning to identify the different types of edema and how they feel during palpation will help you with the differential diagnosis.

3. Identify key terms and concepts, and then research each to broaden your knowledge of knee injuries.
   - What anatomical structures are involved?
     Patella
     Tibia
     Femur
     Patellar tendon
     Prepatellar bursa
     Suprapatellar bursa
     Infrapatellar bursa
     Pretibial bursa
   - *Define bilateral.*
     Directional term meaning "both sides"
   - What is intra-articular edema?
     Edema inside the joint space
   - What is extra-articular edema?
     Edema outside the joint that is palpable
   - What are the signs and symptoms of bursitis?
     Localized edema that is not intra-articular
     Redness
     Increased temperature over the painful area
     Edema that feels like fluid
   - What are the signs and symptoms of a patella fracture?
     Immediate edema
     Possible deformity
     Pain with movement
4. Based on the information that you currently have and what was provided by your instructor, what are the possible differential diagnoses for Mr. Miller's injury?
   Patellar bursitis
   Patella fracture

Why or why not?

For each assessment or diagnosis, write *why?* or *why not?* statements identifying why the information is correct or incorrect. Take details from your textbook, your own research, and data from Mr. Miller's scenario to help you formulate an answer.

1. *Mr. Miller has bursitis because the edema in the knee has a watery feel and is extra-articular.*
2. *Mr. Miller does not have a patellar fracture because of the type of edema that is present. In addition, movement of the patella is not painful and the tuning fork test result is negative, ruling out a fracture.*

What do you think?

1. What is your assessment of Mr. Miller's injury?
   Answer: *Patella bursitis*
2. Was your assessment of Mr. Miller's injury correct?
   Answer: *Yes*
3. If not, explain what you did incorrectly and how you could have performed a better assessment.
   Answer: __________

STUDENT SCENARIO 1: CALE HERRINGTON

Cale Herrington is a collegiate wrestler who is currently participating in a match. Mr. Herrington is seated behind his opponent with both his legs wrapped around the wrestler. When trying to break free, Mr. Herrington gets caught with his lower right leg being forced into a lateral varus and internally rotated position (Fig. 5-4). As Mr. Herrington's opponent falls to his right side, his opponent's body weight and elbow hits the medial side of Mr. Herrington's right knee, which is still in a varus and internally rotated position. On examination, Mr. Herrington is point tender over the lateral joint line and is partially bearing weight on his right leg when independently exiting the mat.

1. Based on this scenario, what do you know about Mr. Herrington's injury?
   - __________
   - __________
   - __________
   - __________

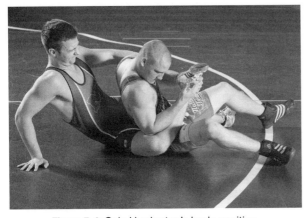

Figure 5-4: Cale Herrington's body position.

2. To evaluate Mr. Herrington's injury effectively, you will need to gather additional information. What questions should you ask in addition to what is presented in this scenario?
   - __________
   - __________
   - __________
   - __________

Brain Jolt
Pain is usually greatest with a grade 1 or grade 2 tear. A dull ache is normally described with a grade 3 tear.

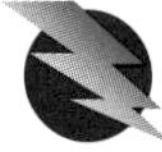

Brain Jolt
You can palpate this structure in the lateral joint line when the athlete has his legs in a figure-four position.

3. Identify key terms and concepts, and then research each to broaden your knowledge of knee injuries.
   - What anatomical structures are involved?
     Answer: __________
   - What structures are in the lateral joint line?
     Answer: __________
   - What is meant by internal rotation?
     Answer: __________
   - Describe the varus stress test.
     Answer: __________
   - Why is it important to have an understanding of different wrestling techniques?
     Answer: __________

4. Based on the information that you currently have and what was provided by your instructor, what are the possible differential diagnoses for Mr. Herrington's injury?

- ______________________________
- ______________________________
- ______________________________
- ______________________________

Why or why not?

For each assessment or diagnosis, write *why?* or *why not?* statements identifying why the information is correct or incorrect. Take details from your textbook, your own research, and data gathered from Mr. Herrington's scenario to help you formulate an answer.

1. ______________________________
2. ______________________________
3. ______________________________
4. ______________________________

What do you think?

1. What is your assessment of Mr. Herrington's injury?

   Answer: ______________________________
2. Was your assessment of Mr. Herrington's injury correct?

   Answer: ______________________________
3. If not, explain what you did incorrectly and how you could have performed a better assessment.

   Answer: ______________________________

STUDENT SCENARIO 2: OLIVIA JONES

While playing volleyball, Olivia Jones is jump-serving the ball and lands on the medial side of her foot, forcing her left knee into a valgus position. She is unable to continue with practice. Upon further assessment, Ms. Jones complains of pain deep inside her knee. She is unable to bear weight on her left leg without her left knee buckling. Ms. Jones lacks active full extension. During the assessment, Ms. Jones indicates that her knee is point tender along the medial joint line. Moderate to severe amounts of edema is noted (Fig. 5-5).

1. Based on this scenario, what do you know about Ms. Jones' injury?

- ______________________________
- ______________________________
- ______________________________
- ______________________________

2. To evaluate Ms. Jones' injury effectively, you will need to gather additional information. What questions should you ask in addition to what is presented in this scenario?

- ______________________________

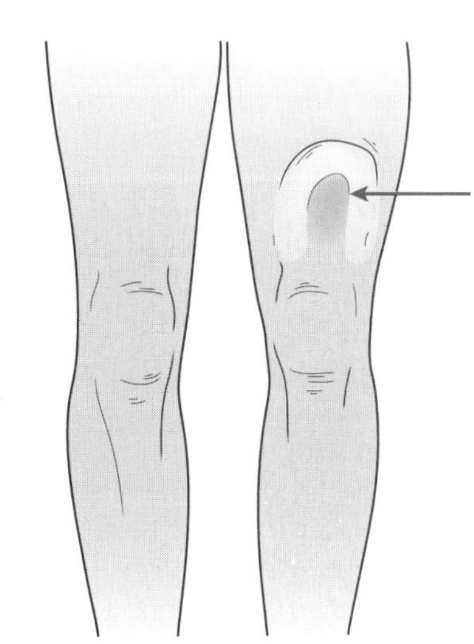

Figure 5-5: Olivia Jones' edema at the knee.

- ______________________________
- ______________________________
- ______________________________

Brain Jolt
The pattern of edema often associated with this injury is described as a "horseshoe pattern."

3. Identify key terms and concepts, and then research each to broaden your knowledge of knee injuries.
   - What anatomical structures are involved?

     Answer: ______________________________
   - Define *lateral*.

     Answer: ______________________________
   - Describe *valgus position*.

     Answer: ______________________________
   - What does *knee buckling* mean?

     Answer: ______________________________
   - What are the possible implications of a knee buckle?

     Answer: ______________________________
   - What is horseshoe-pattern edema?

     Answer: ______________________________
   - What are the indications of horseshoe-pattern edema?

     Answer: ______________________________
4. Based on the information that you currently have and what was provided by your instructor, what are the possible differential diagnoses for Ms. Jones' injury?
   - ______________________________
   - ______________________________
   - ______________________________
   - ______________________________

Why or why not?

For each assessment or diagnosis, write *why?* or *why not?* statements identifying why the information is correct or incorrect. Take details from your textbook, your own research, and data gathered from Ms. Jones' scenario to help you formulate an answer.

1. ______________________________
2. ______________________________
3. ______________________________
4. ______________________________

Conversation Buffer
When talking with an athlete after an injury, ensure that the athlete understands his or her injury and is focused on a positive and healthy recovery.

What do you think?

1. What is your assessment of Ms. Jones' injury?

   Answer: ______________________________
2. Was your assessment of Ms. Jones' injury correct?

   Answer: ______________________________
3. If not, explain what you did incorrectly and how you could have performed a better assessment.

   Answer: ______________________________

STUDENT SCENARIO 3: KELSEY MCELROY

Kelsey McElroy is a forward on the women's soccer team. She has no history of knee issues but has pronated feet, which are treated with physician-issued orthotics. Ms. McElroy also has genu valgum (Fig. 5-6a, 5-6b), which increases her Q angle. As she is running down the soccer field, Ms. McElroy firmly plants her foot on the ground and quickly changes direction to her right. She feels a pop over the top of her left knee, which makes her fall to the ground. Ms. McElroy states that she felt her patella shift when she pivoted, which was followed by excruciating pain. Your evaluation indicates mild to moderate edema and point tenderness around the patella.

1. Based on this scenario, what do you know about Ms. McElroy's injury?
   - ______________________________

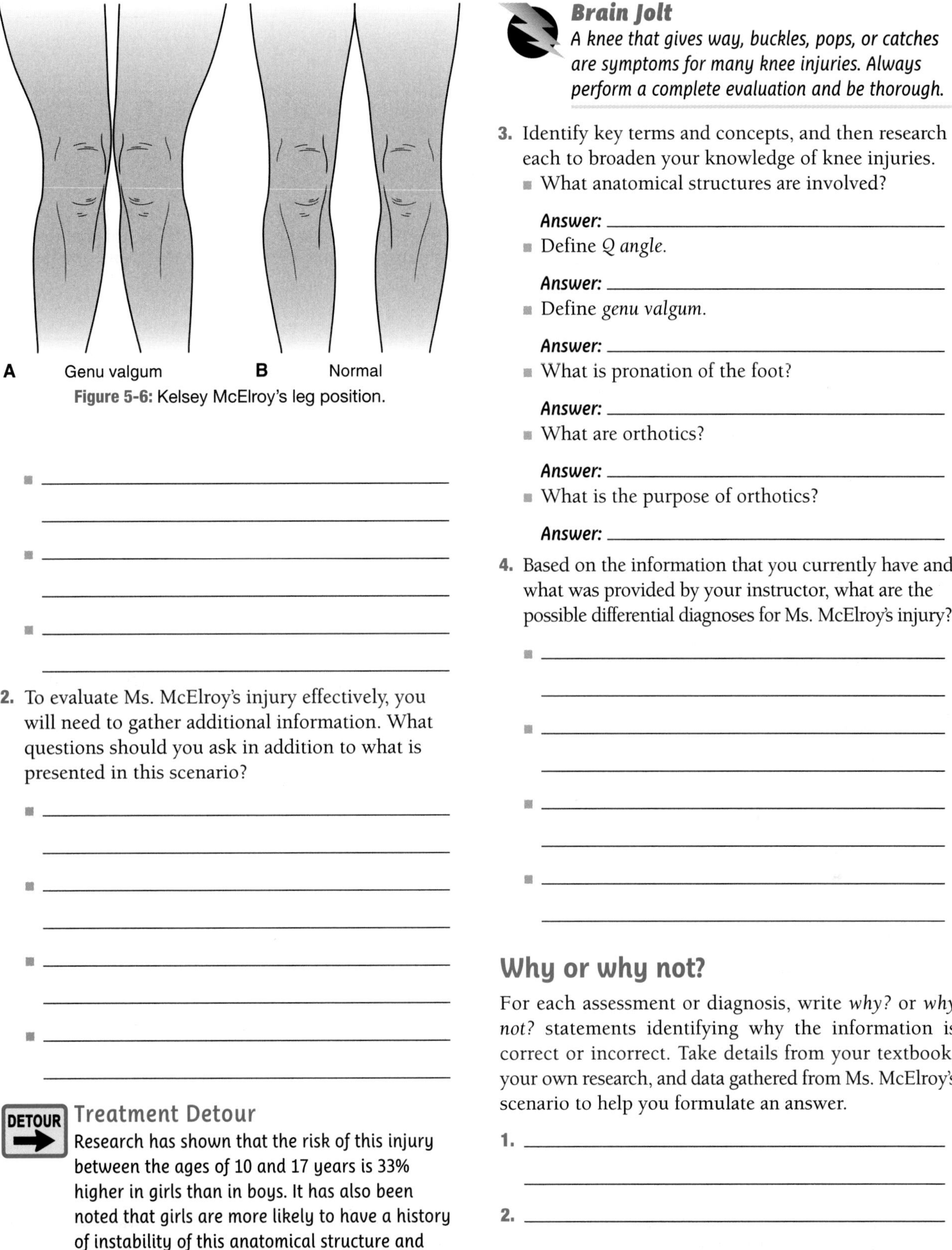

Figure 5-6: Kelsey McElroy's leg position.

- ______________________________
- ______________________________
- ______________________________

2. To evaluate Ms. McElroy's injury effectively, you will need to gather additional information. What questions should you ask in addition to what is presented in this scenario?
   - ______________________________
   - ______________________________
   - ______________________________
   - ______________________________

DETOUR **Treatment Detour**

Research has shown that the risk of this injury between the ages of 10 and 17 years is 33% higher in girls than in boys. It has also been noted that girls are more likely to have a history of instability of this anatomical structure and thus are at an even higher risk for this injury. The results of this study indicate that this injury most frequently occurred during low-risk or no-risk pivoting activities in women and attributed it to anatomical differences between males and females (Balcarek et al., 2010).

Brain Jolt

A knee that gives way, buckles, pops, or catches are symptoms for many knee injuries. Always perform a complete evaluation and be thorough.

3. Identify key terms and concepts, and then research each to broaden your knowledge of knee injuries.
   - What anatomical structures are involved?

     Answer: ______________________________
   - Define *Q angle.*

     Answer: ______________________________
   - Define *genu valgum.*

     Answer: ______________________________
   - What is pronation of the foot?

     Answer: ______________________________
   - What are orthotics?

     Answer: ______________________________
   - What is the purpose of orthotics?

     Answer: ______________________________
4. Based on the information that you currently have and what was provided by your instructor, what are the possible differential diagnoses for Ms. McElroy's injury?
   - ______________________________
   - ______________________________
   - ______________________________
   - ______________________________

Why or why not?

For each assessment or diagnosis, write *why?* or *why not?* statements identifying why the information is correct or incorrect. Take details from your textbook, your own research, and data gathered from Ms. McElroy's scenario to help you formulate an answer.

1. ______________________________
2. ______________________________
3. ______________________________
4. ______________________________

What do you think?

1. What is your assessment of Ms. McElroy's injury?

   Answer: ______________________

2. Was your assessment of Ms. McElroy's injury correct?

   Answer: ______________________

3. If not, explain what you did incorrectly and how you could have performed a better assessment.

   Answer: ______________________

STUDENT SCENARIO 4: KENNY WHITE

Kenny White is a senior on the men's basketball team. He gets a breakaway run and rushes to the basket to make a lay-up. As he lands, he feels a pop in his right knee and drops to the floor. Upon talking with Mr. White, he states that he thinks his knee "gave out" when landing. You noticed that Mr. White's right foot was slightly externally rotated when he landed (Fig. 5-7). When examining Mr. White's knee, you notice a rapid onset of edema over the anterior portion of the knee. Mr. White is unable to perform full weight-bearing on his right leg because of pain and instability in his knee. Mr. White has no history of knee injury.

1. Based on this scenario, what do you know about Mr. White's injury?
   - ______________________
   - ______________________
   - ______________________
   - ______________________

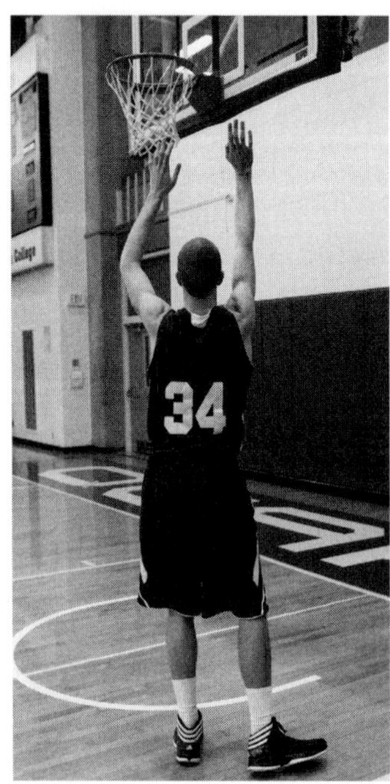

Figure 5-7: Kenny White's foot position.

2. To evaluate Mr. White's injury effectively, you will need to gather additional information. What questions should you ask in addition to what is presented in this scenario?
   - ______________________
   - ______________________
   - ______________________
   - ______________________

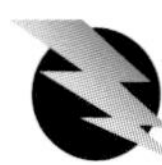

Brain Jolt

This structure can be related to a noncontact mechanism of injury. Female athletes are more prone to this injury because of wide Q angles.

3. Identify key terms and concepts, and then research each to broaden your knowledge of knee injuries.
   - What anatomical structures are involved?

     Answer: ______________________
   - What is meant by *rapid onset effusion*?

     Answer: ______________________
   - What can a pop or "giving out" feeling indicate?

     Answer: ______________________
   - Describe the different levels of weight-bearing.

     Answer: ______________________
   - How could this injury occur if there was no physical contact?

     Answer: ______________________

4. Based on the information that you currently have and what was provided by your instructor, what are the possible differential diagnoses for Mr. White's injury?

- ______________________________
- ______________________________
- ______________________________
- ______________________________

Why or why not?

For each assessment or diagnosis, write *why?* or *why not?* statements identifying why the information is correct or incorrect. Take details from your textbook, your own research, and data gathered from Mr. White's scenario to help you formulate an answer.

1. ______________________________
2. ______________________________
3. ______________________________
4. ______________________________

What do you think?

1. What is your assessment of Mr. White's injury?

   Answer: ______________________________

2. Was your assessment of Mr. White's injury correct?

   Answer: ______________________________

3. If not, explain what you did incorrectly and how you could have performed a better assessment.

   Answer: ______________________________

STUDENT SCENARIO 5: TYLER BREEN

Tyler Breen has been a catcher on a baseball team for many years. Mr. Breen noticed localized edema in his right knee a week ago. Besides his normal catcher's stance, and shifting from side to side to catch a ball, he has no additional mechanism that would lead to knee pain. Upon evaluation, Mr. Breen has mild edema over his medial joint line (Fig. 5-8), and he is unable to fully extend his right knee without it catching. Mr. Breen states that after a practice, he feels that his knee is "locked"; however, distraction of the right knee joint makes it feel better.

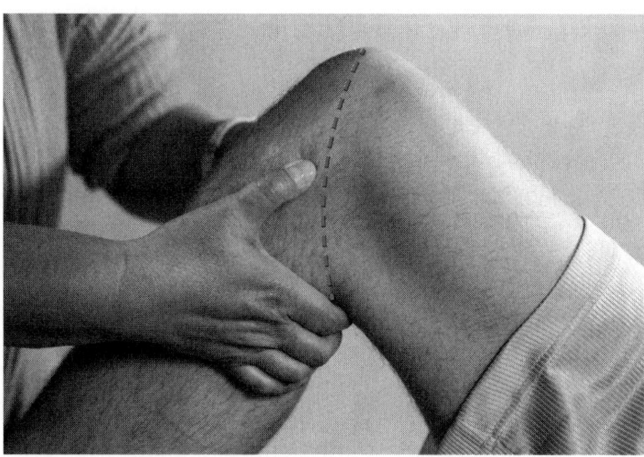

Figure 5-8: Tyler Breen's point of pain.

1. Based on this scenario, what do you know about Mr. Breen's injury?

- ______________________________
- ______________________________
- ______________________________
- ______________________________

2. To evaluate Mr. Breen's injury effectively, you will need to gather additional information. What questions should you ask yourself in addition to what is presented in this scenario?

- ______________________________
- ______________________________
- ______________________________

- ____________________

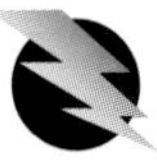

Brain Jolt

This medial structure is injured more often than the lateral structure because of its attachment to the capsule.

3. Identify key terms and concepts, and then research each to broaden your knowledge of knee injuries.
   - What anatomical structures are involved?

     Answer: ____________________
   - Define *distraction.*

     Answer: ____________________
   - Define *edema.*

     Answer: ____________________
   - What mechanical actions occur in the knee during extension and flexion?

     Answer: ____________________
   - What muscle "unlocks" the knee?

     Answer: ____________________
4. Based on the information that you currently have and what was provided by your instructor, what are the possible differential diagnoses for Mr. Breen's injury?
   - ____________________
   - ____________________
   - ____________________
   - ____________________

Why or why not?

For each assessment or diagnosis, write *why?* or *why not?* statements identifying why the information is correct or incorrect. Take details from your textbook, your own research, and data gathered from Mr. Breen's scenario to help you formulate an answer.

1. ____________________
2. ____________________
3. ____________________
4. ____________________

What do you think?

1. What is your assessment of Mr. Breen's injury?

   Answer: ____________________
2. Was your assessment of Mr. Breen's injury correct?

   Answer: ____________________
3. If not, explain what you did incorrectly and how you could have performed a better assessment.

   Answer: ____________________

STUDENT SCENARIO 6: ADAM SMITH

Adam Smith is an offensive lineman on the college football team. He is devoted to his weight room routine and is trying to increase and maintain his strength in his quadriceps and hamstrings. During the Saturday football game, a player falls into Mr. Smith, forcing his right knee inward and placing a valgus stress on the medial side of his knee (Fig. 5-9). During the moment of impact, Mr. Smith was standing with his right knee in a close-packed position. Mr. Smith complains of pain along his medial joint line and is unable to straighten his knee into full extension. Upon examination, Mr. Smith has instability when the right knee is slightly flexed. While you are obtaining his medical history, Mr. Smith states that he injured his right medial meniscus 2 years ago.

Conversation Buffer

When working with an athlete who lifts weights regularly and is devoted to a fitness plan, be sure to communicate with the athlete so that you are familiar with his or her fitness plan and style of weight lifts being performed. This knowledge can provide insight into the athlete's injury and allows you to address his or her future fitness plan.

1. Based on this scenario, what do you know about Mr. Smith's injury?
   - ____________________

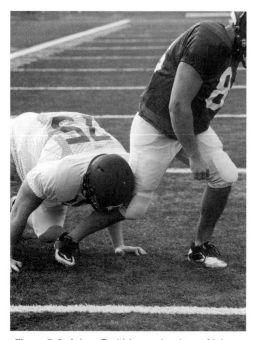

Figure 5-9: Adam Smith's mechanism of injury.

- ______________________________
- ______________________________
- ______________________________

2. To evaluate Mr. Smith's injury effectively, you will need to gather additional information. What questions should you ask in addition to what is presented in this scenario?

- ______________________________
- ______________________________
- ______________________________
- ______________________________

Brain Jolt

With this injury, there is minimal to absent edema. You will also notice more instability with 30 degrees of flexion versus full extension.

3. Identify key terms and concepts, and then research each to broaden your knowledge of knee injuries.
   - What anatomical structures are involved?

     Answer: ______________________________
   - *Define valgus.*

     Answer: ______________________________
   - Define *close-packed position.*

     Answer: ______________________________
   - Define *open-packed position.*

     Answer: ______________________________
   - What is the close-packed position for the knee joint?

     Answer: ______________________________
   - What is the open-packed position for the knee joint?

     Answer: ______________________________
   - What are the signs and symptoms of a meniscal injury?

     Answer: ______________________________
   - Why is it important to know the different techniques used by an offensive lineman during play?

     Answer: ______________________________
   - Why is it important to be familiar with the athlete's fitness plan?

     Answer: ______________________________

4. Based on the information that you currently have and what was provided by your instructor, what are the possible differential diagnoses for Mr. Smith's injury?

- ______________________________
- ______________________________
- ______________________________
- ______________________________

Why or why not?

For each assessment or diagnosis, write *why?* or *why not?* statements identifying why the information is correct or incorrect. Take details from your textbook, your own research, and data gathered from Mr. Smith's scenario to help you formulate an answer.

1. ______________________________
2. ______________________________
3. ______________________________

4. ______________________________

____

What do you think?

1. What is your assessment of Mr. Smith's injury?

   Answer: ______________________________

2. Was your assessment of Mr. Smith's injury correct?

   Answer: ______________________________

3. If not, explain what you did incorrectly and how you could have performed a better assessment.

   Answer: ______________________________

STUDENT SCENARIO 7: MIKE DRYER

Mike Dryer is a high school freshman and is the center on the football team. He experienced a 2-inch growth spurt this summer. Mr. Dryer complains of chronic knee pain, specifically over the front of his right patella and down to his right tibial tuberosity. Upon examining his right knee, you notice some deformity over the tibial tuberosity (Fig. 5-10a, 5-10b) and edema over the inferior pole of the patella and surrounding the tibial tuberosity. Mr. Dryer states that he has continual pain when jumping and running, and severe pain when kneeling on his right knee.

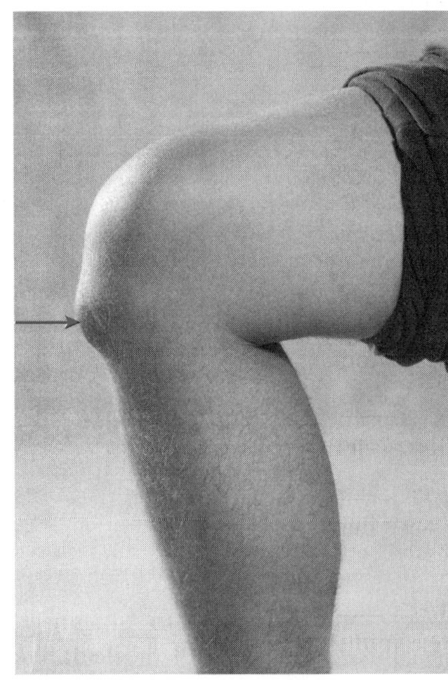

Figure 5-10a: Mike Dryer's knee.

1. Based on this scenario, what do you know about Mr. Dryer's injury?

   - ______________________________
   - ______________________________
   - ______________________________
   - ______________________________

Treatment Detour

This condition is most common in adolescence because the growth phase makes adolescents more susceptible to this type of injury. In girls, it most often occurs between the ages of 8 and 13 years, and in boys it occurs between the ages of 10 and 15 years. One study examined 956 adolescent students between the ages of 12 and 15 years enrolled in school in Brazil. The prevalence rate of this condition was 9.8% in this study. It was also concluded that regular practice of unsupervised sport activities in the pubertal phase and shortening of the rectus femoris were the main predispositions for this injury (Lucas de Lucena, 2011).

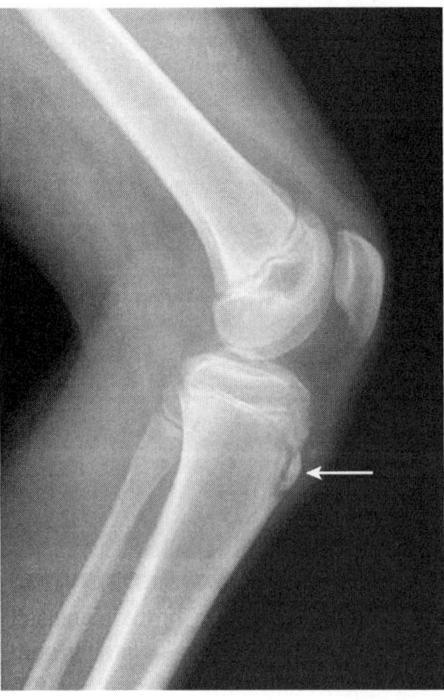

Figure 5-10b: X-ray of Mike Dryer's knee. (With permission from McKinnis, L. N. (2010). *Fundamentals of musculoskeletal imaging.* Philadelphia, PA: F.A. Davis, p. 398)

2. To evaluate Mr. Dryer's injury effectively, you will need to gather additional information. What

questions should you ask in addition to what is presented in this scenario?

- ______________________________
- ______________________________
- ______________________________
- ______________________________
- ______________________________
- ______________________________
- ______________________________

Brain Jolt

This condition is more common in boys and can be irritated by a substantial growth spurt, but it usually resolves itself by late adolescence.

3. Identify key terms and concepts, and then research each to broaden your knowledge of knee injuries.
   - What anatomical structures are involved?

     Answer: ______________________________
   - Define *edema.*

     Answer: ______________________________
   - Why is it important to know that the athlete has experienced a rapid growth spurt?

     Answer: ______________________________
   - Why is it important to know an athlete's age?

     Answer: ______________________________
   - Why might Mr. Dryer have increased pain with jumping, running, and kneeling?

     Answer: ______________________________
4. Based on the information that you currently have and what was provided by your instructor, what are the possible differential diagnoses for Mr. Dryer's injury?
   - ______________________________
   - ______________________________
   - ______________________________
   - ______________________________

Why or why not?

For each assessment or diagnosis, write *why?* or *why not?* statements identifying why the information is correct or incorrect. Take details from your textbook, your own research, and data gathered from Mr. Dryer's scenario to help you formulate an answer.

1. ______________________________
2. ______________________________
3. ______________________________
4. ______________________________

What do you think?

1. What is your assessment of Mr. Dryer's injury?

   Answer: ______________________________
2. Was your assessment of Mr. Dryer's injury correct?

   Answer: ______________________________
3. If not, explain what you did incorrectly and how you could have performed a better assessment.

   Answer: ______________________________

STUDENT SCENARIO 8: RACHAEL GORBON

Rachael Gorbon is a high school swimmer with a previous history of knee problems, including arthroscopic surgery to her right knee. Ms. Gorbon received rehab to her right knee for only five visits because of insurance limitations, after which she began a home exercise program. Ms. Gorbon quit her home exercise program after 2 weeks because she was not experiencing any more problems with her knee. However, Ms. Gorbon now notices anterior pain around the patella (Fig. 5-11). She states that she feels a nagging, uncomfortable pain while kicking in the pool. Ms. Gorbon also feels like her knee is weak when walking. When flexing her quadriceps, Ms. Gorbon experiences a grinding or grating feeling anteriorly over her patella.

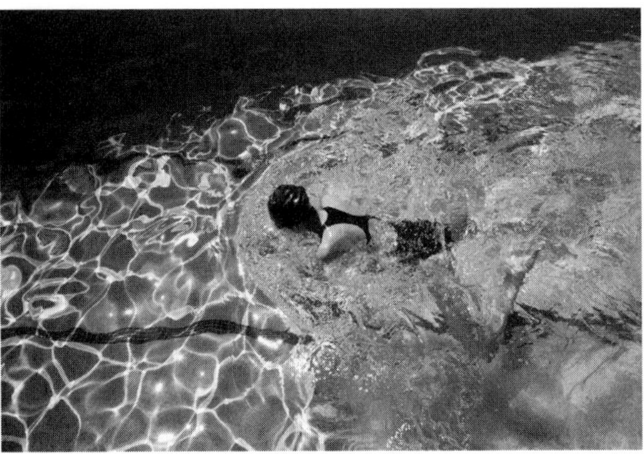

Figure 5-11: Rachael Gorbon's painful activity. (© Thinkstock)

1. Based on this scenario, what do you know about Ms. Gorbon's injury?
   - ______________________________
   - ______________________________
   - ______________________________
   - ______________________________

2. To evaluate Ms. Gorbon's injury effectively, you will need to gather additional information. What questions should you ask in addition to what is presented in this scenario?
   - ______________________________
   - ______________________________
   - ______________________________
   - ______________________________

Brain Jolt

When the knee is flexed passively and extended, there may be pain at the inferior pole of the patella. With this condition, there is normally atrophy with the involved vastus medialis oblique (VMO).

3. Identify key terms and concepts, and then research each to broaden your knowledge of knee injuries.
   - What anatomical structures are involved?

     Answer: ______________________________
   - Describe the characteristics of the medial meniscus.

     Answer: ______________________________
   - Describe the characteristics of the lateral meniscus.

     Answer: ______________________________
   - What are the main differences between the medial meniscus and lateral meniscus?

     Answer: ______________________________
   - What do the symptoms of grinding or grating indicate?

     Answer: ______________________________
   - Why is it important to know an athlete's surgical and rehabilitation history?

     Answer: ______________________________

4. Based on the information that you currently have and what was provided by your instructor, what are the possible differential diagnoses for Ms. Gorbon's injury?
   - ______________________________
   - ______________________________
   - ______________________________
   - ______________________________

Why or why not?

For each assessment or diagnosis, write *why?* or *why not?* statements identifying why the information is correct or incorrect. Take details from your textbook, your own research, and data gathered from Ms. Gorbon's scenario to help you formulate an answer.

1. ______________________________
2. ______________________________
3. ______________________________
4. ______________________________

What do you think?

1. What is your assessment of Ms. Gorbon's injury?

   Answer: ______________________________

2. Was your assessment of Ms. Gorbon's injury correct?

   Answer: ______

3. If not, explain what you did incorrectly and how you could have performed a better assessment.

   Answer: ______

STUDENT SCENARIO 9: MITCH ANDERSON

Mitch Anderson is a cross-country runner with a history of tight hamstrings. He stretches before practice, but does not do any stretching after his workouts. He often complains of a small pocket of edema that develops on his right medial tibia after running (Fig. 5-12). Mr. Anderson states that if he puts a knee sleeve on his right knee for support, the edema over the medial portion of the tibia often reabsorbs. Mr. Anderson has genu valgum. A weak vastus medialis with his right knee is noticed when testing his strength. Mr. Anderson notes a difference in the amount of edema on days that he runs on flat terrain versus sloped terrain.

1. Based on this scenario, what do you know about Mr. Anderson's injury?
   - ______
   - ______
   - ______
   - ______

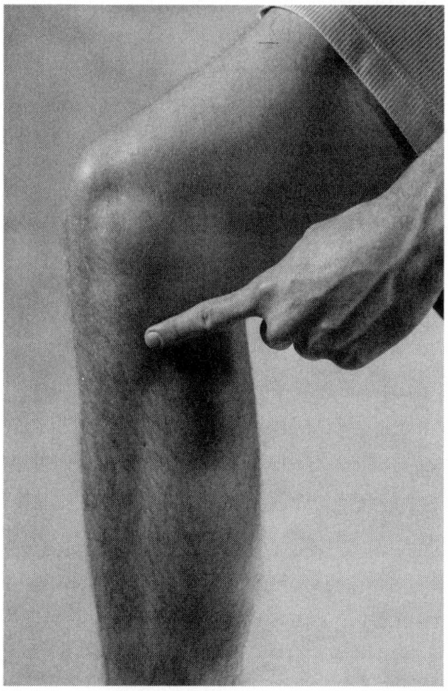

Figure 5-12: Mitch Anderson's area of pain.

2. To evaluate Mr. Anderson's injury effectively, you will need to gather additional information. What questions should you ask in addition to what is presented in this scenario?
   - ______
   - ______
   - ______
   - ______

Brain Jolt

This particular site can become irritated as a result of the insertion point of three muscles, often recalled with the phrase "Say Grace before tea."

3. Identify key terms and concepts, and then research each to broaden your knowledge of knee injuries.
   - What anatomical structures are involved?

     Answer: ______
   - What muscles compose the hamstring group?

     Answer: ______
   - What muscles insert medially near the knee?

     Answer: ______
   - Define *genu valgum.*

     Answer: ______
   - What is edema reabsorption?

     Answer: ______
   - What are the signs and symptoms of vastus medialis oblique weakness?

     Answer: ______

4. Based on the information that you currently have and what was provided by your instructor, what are the possible differential diagnoses for Mr. Anderson's injury?

- ____________________
- ____________________
- ____________________
- ____________________

Why or why not?

For each assessment or diagnosis, write *why?* or *why not?* statements identifying why the information is correct or incorrect. Take details from your textbook, your own research, and data gathered from Mr. Anderson's scenario to help you formulate an answer.

1. ____________________
2. ____________________
3. ____________________
4. ____________________

What do you think?

1. What is your assessment of Mr. Anderson's injury?

   Answer: ____________________

2. Was your assessment of Mr. Anderson's injury correct?

   Answer: ____________________

3. If not, explain what you did incorrectly and how you could have performed a better assessment.

   Answer: ____________________

STUDENT SCENARIO 10: EMILY ERTEL

Emily Ertel is a soccer, basketball, and softball player. Besides the strengthening program the coaches have her do, Ms. Ertel is not very assertive with improving her overall fitness. During her summer sports physical examination, she was told that she had tight hamstrings and quadriceps. Ms. Ertel also has decreased quadriceps strength, especially at her right VMO, and a small Q angle. Her right foot is pronated, which is creating additional stress on her right knee (Fig. 5-13). Upon palpation, mild point tenderness over the medial and lateral joint line is noted in her right knee.

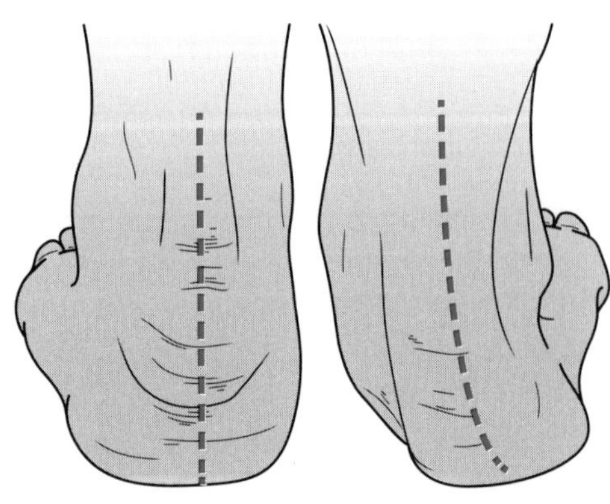

Figure 5-13: Emily Ertel's foot position.

1. Based on this scenario, what do you know about Ms. Ertel's injury?

- ____________________
- ____________________
- ____________________
- ____________________

2. To evaluate Ms. Ertel's injury effectively, you will need to gather additional information. What questions should you ask in addition to what is presented in this scenario?

- ____________________
- ____________________

- ______________________
  ____
- ______________________
  ____

Brain Jolt
The diagnosis for this injury can often be a catch-all name because of the lack of a specific mechanism and the lack of specific symptoms.

3. Identify key terms and concepts, and then research each to broaden your knowledge of knee injuries.
   - What anatomical structures are involved?

     Answer: ______________________
   - What is the vastus medialis oblique?

     Answer: ______________________
   - How does foot pronation affect the knee?

     Answer: ______________________
   - What are Q angle ratios?

     Answer: ______________________
   - How does an athletic trainer determine tightness in the hamstring or quadriceps muscles?

     Answer: ______________________
   - What information is covered in a sports physical examination?

     Answer: ______________________
4. Based on the information that you currently have and what was provided by your instructor, what are the possible differential diagnoses for Ms. Ertel's injury?
   - ______________________
     ____
   - ______________________
     ____
   - ______________________
     ____
   - ______________________
     ____

Why or why not?

For each assessment or diagnosis, write *why?* or *why not?* statements identifying why the information is correct or incorrect. Take details from your textbook, your own research, and data gathered from Ms. Ertel's scenario to help you formulate an answer.

1. ______________________
   ____
2. ______________________
   ____
3. ______________________
   ____
4. ______________________
   ____

What do you think?

1. What is your assessment of Ms. Ertel's injury?

   Answer: ______________________
2. Was your assessment of Ms. Ertel's injury correct?

   Answer: ______________________
3. If not, explain what you did incorrectly and how you could have performed a better assessment.

   Answer: ______________________

knowledge checklist

Table 5-1 offers a checklist that can be used by a peer, instructor, or preceptor to evaluate each part of a knee assessment. Use this checklist as a tool to ensure that the evaluation is complete and to assess your knowledge of the competencies that apply to this chapter.

TABLE 5-1 ■ Knee Assessment Competency Checklist

	Proficient *Can demonstrate and execute the skill properly*	**Proficient With Assistance** *Can demonstrate and execute the skill with minimal guidance or tips*	**Not Proficient** *Unable to demonstrate and execute the skill properly; need to be reevaluated at another time after further study and practice*
Athlete's Health History			
Medical history			
History of knee injury			
Type of sport and position played			
Mechanisms of Injury			
How did the injury occur?			
When does the pain occur?			
What makes the pain better or worse?			
Was the athlete's knee forced into an unusual direction?			
Was the athlete's foot planted?			
Were any pops, cracks, or snaps heard?			
Does the athlete experience pain going up or down stairs?			
How did the athlete's knee look at the time the injury occurred?			
Visual Observations			
Gait			
Edema			
Ecchymosis			
Deformity			
Knee symmetry (patellar alignment and muscle girth)			
Palpation			
Temperature change over the painful area; crepitus; deformity; intra-articular or extra-articular joint swelling; changes within the muscle fibers			
Quadriceps muscle group			
VMO			
Medial femoral condyle and epicondyle			
IT band			
Hamstring muscle group			
Popliteal fossa			
Gastrocnemius (medial and lateral head)			
Patella (including the bursa)			
Synovial plica			
Patellar tendon			
Tibial tuberosity (including the bursa)			
Tibial plateau (anterior edge)			

Continued

TABLE 5-1 ■ Knee Assessment Competency Checklist—cont'd

	Proficient	Proficient With Assistance	Not Proficient
Medial and lateral joint space			
MCL			
Pes anserine muscle group, tendons, and bursa			
LCL			
Gerdy's tubercle			
Fibular head			
ROM			
Passive or active			
Knee flexion			
Knee extension			
Strength			
Grade through manual muscle tests			
Knee flexion			
Knee extension			
Special Tests			
Anterior and posterior drawer test			
Lachman test			
Pivot shift test			
Jerk test			
Godfrey test			
Recurvatum test			
Valgus stress test (0 degrees flexion and 25–30 degrees flexion)			
Varus stress test (0 degrees flexion and 25–30 degrees flexion)			
Jerk test			
McMurray test			
Apley compression and distraction test			
Patellar apprehension test			
Clark test (patellar grind)			
Patellar compression test			
Neurological			
Q angle test			
L4–S2 nerve roots			
Achilles reflex			
Vascular			
Dorsal pedal pulse			
Posterior tibial pulse			
Popliteal pulse			
Capillary refill			
Final Assessment			
Sprain; strain; contusion; fracture, condition; severity			

*Be sure to always compare bilaterally.

IT, iliotibial; LCL, lateral collateral ligament; MCL, medial collateral ligament; ROM, range of motion; VMO, vastus medialis oblique.

REFERENCES

Balcarek, P., Jung, K., Ammon, J., Walde, T. A., Frosch, S., Schüttrumpf, J. P., . . . Frosch, K. H. (2010). Anatomy of lateral patellar instability, trochlear dysplasia and tibial tubercle-trochlear groove distance is more pronounced in women who dislocate the patella. *American Journal of Sports Medicine, 38*, 2320–2327.

Lucas de Lucena, G. (2011). Prevalence and associated factors of Osgood-Schlatter syndrome in a population-based sample of Brazilian adolescents. *American Journal of Sports Medicine, 39*, 415–420.

National Athletic Training Association. (2011). *Athletic training education competencies* (5th ed.). Retrieved from http://www.nata.org/sites/default/files/5th-Edition-Competencies-2011-PDF-Version.pdf

Prentice, W. (2010). *Arnheim's principles of athletic training: A competency-based approach* (14th ed.). New York, NY: McGraw-Hill.

Starkey, C., Brown, S. D., & Ryan, J. (2010). *Examination of orthopedic and athletic injuries* (3rd ed.). Philadelphia, PA: F.A. Davis.

Venes, D. (Ed.). (2009). *Taber's cyclopedic medical dictionary* (21st ed.). Philadelphia, PA: F.A. Davis.

chapter 6

Lower Extremity: The Hip, Thigh, and Lower Leg

chapter outline

athletic trainer's corner

Out there in the real world, one athletic trainer experienced the following:

As an athletic trainer, you are taught to be ready for any injury, but sometimes athletes get injuries that you never expect to see. This happened to me while working at a soccer camp over the summer.

During one of their scrimmages, a goalkeeper at the goal closest to me stepped to dive laterally to the right when her right leg became weak, causing her to fall. As I ran to her, I was trying to figure out what injury might cause her to collapse like that. I was assuming it would be a knee or ankle injury, but as I got closer to her, I could see her holding her thigh. When I asked her what happened, she said, "I tore my quad." This girl was 13 years old, and I was thinking that she might have strained the quadriceps muscle. A tear just did not seem possible. As I visually scanned her quadriceps muscle, I could see a large knot approximately three fourths of the way up her thigh. As I began to palpate her leg, I felt a large divot just inferior to the knot. At this point, I was shocked to realize she was correct, and then I was even more shocked when I started to think I would have to calm her down; however, she was already rather calm.

She stated that this had happened to her before and did not require surgery, but the prior injury did not feel like this before. I assisted her to the medical transport cart and we took her to the medical tent for further evaluation and treatment. We decided to pack her leg in ice and send her to the hospital. She went into surgery later that night. I never saw her again, but I received an e-mail a few weeks later saying that she was doing fine and was in rehabilitation to get back to playing.

Alex Geier, AT, ATC
Head Athletic Trainer, Ross High School
McCullough Hyde Memorial Hospital
Hamilton, Ohio

learning outcomes

After working through this chapter, you will be able to:

1. Verbalize the questions to use when obtaining a thorough medical history for an assessment.
2. Describe the principles of body movement at the hip, thigh, and lower leg and the various mechanisms of injury that affect the hip, thigh, and lower leg.
3. Compare and contrast the findings of various special tests and the role of diagnostic tests used during a hip, thigh, or lower leg evaluation.
4. Explain the medical terminology associated with the assessment of musculoskeletal injuries.
5. Verbalize the standard procedures used for a clinical evaluation of the hip, thigh, and lower leg, and interpret the findings for differential diagnoses.

MODEL SCENARIO 1: **REX HOTTINGER**

Rex Hottinger is a forward on his high school soccer team. He has a breakaway run toward the goal. As Mr. Hottinger runs toward the goal, the goalkeeper comes out of the goal box and advances toward Mr. Hottinger. As Mr. Hottinger slides, kicking the ball into the goal, the goalie collides with him. The goalkeeper's knee and body weight come down directly onto Mr. Hottinger's left quadriceps muscle. Mr. Hottinger has instant pain and temporary loss of quadriceps function. He is assisted off the field. Upon examination, Mr. Hottinger has acute mild edema and ecchymosis (Fig. 6-1). He has a lack of range of motion (ROM) with active knee flexion. At the end of the game, Mr. Hottinger is reevaluated and his quadriceps ROM has returned; however, he still has pain, and mild ecchymosis continues to be present at the area of trauma.

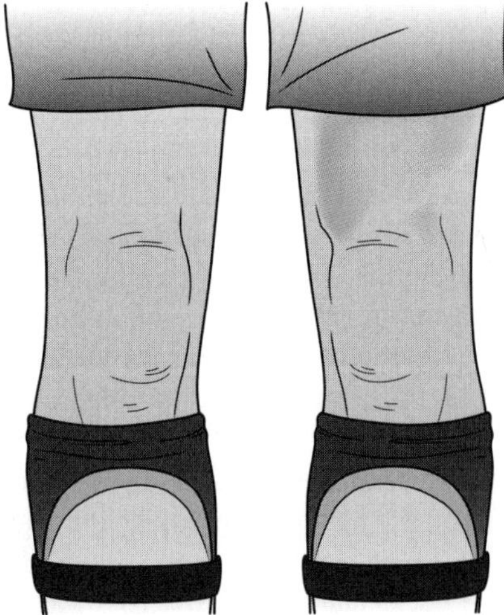

Figure 6-1: Rex Hottinger's thigh.

1. Based on this scenario, what do you know about Mr. Hottinger's injury?
   - *Male athlete*
   - *High school soccer player*
   - *Acute injury*
   - *Mechanism of injury: direct hit to the quadriceps muscle from an opponent's knee*
   - *Instant pain*
   - *Temporary loss of quadriceps function*
   - *Mild edema*
   - *Mild ecchymosis*
   - *Lack of ROM in knee flexion*
2. To evaluate Mr. Hottinger's injury effectively, you will need to gather additional information. What questions should you ask in addition to what is presented in this scenario?
   - *Is this injury a medical emergency?*
   - *Are there any preexisting injuries? If yes, what are they?*
   - *Are there any special tests that are important to perform? If yes, elaborate.*
   - *Are the results of the special tests positive or negative? What does each result indicate?*
   - *Are there gait irregularities?*
   - *Is there passive or active ROM at the knee and hip?*
   - *What is the strength at the knee and hip?*
   - *Are there deficits in the myotomes or dermatomes?*
3. Identify key terms and concepts, and then research each to broaden your knowledge of hip, thigh, and lower-leg injuries.
   - What anatomical structures are involved?

     Femur

     Quadriceps muscle group

- Define *edema.*
  Swelling; a localized or general condition when body tissues contain an excessive amount of fluid
- Define *ecchymosis.*
  A bruise; superficial bleeding under the skin
- What are myotomes?
  The motor component of a neurological screen
- What are dermatomes?
  The sensory component of a neurologic screen
- What does lack of ROM indicate?
  That there is possibly a difference in degree of active or passive motion at a specific joint; can also be a result of pain, edema in the area, or a muscle rupture
- What might a temporary loss of function indicate?
  That there has been trauma to the area and the muscle or nerve is involved

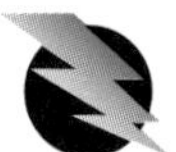

Brain Jolt

An acute injury of this nature needs to be iced immediately in knee flexion to help prevent the further loss of active ROM.

4. Based on the information that you currently have and what was provided by your instructor, what are the possible differential diagnoses for Mr. Hottinger's injury?
   Quadriceps contusion
   Femur fracture
   Quadriceps strain
   Myositis ossificans

Why or why not?

For each assessment or diagnosis, write *why?* or *why not?* statements identifying why the information is correct or incorrect. Take details from your textbook, your own research, and data from Mr. Hottinger's scenario to help you formulate an answer.

1. *Mr. Hottinger suffered a quadriceps contusion. The direct blow from the opponent's knee to Mr. Hottinger's quadriceps muscle caused trauma and ecchymosis.*
2. *Mr. Hottinger does not have a femur fracture because there is no deformity, and the results of the long-bone compression test are negative.*
3. *Mr. Hottinger does not have a quadriceps strain because there was no forceful, active ROM to tear the muscle fibers. Mr. Hottinger's active ROM returned by the end of the game.*
4. *Mr. Hottinger does not have myositis ossificans because it is a chronic condition that develops from repeated quadriceps injuries or improper treatment of a previous injury. In addition, myositis ossificans is a hard, calcified deformity within the muscle belly, which is not present in this injury.*

What do you think?

1. What is your assessment of Mr. Hottinger's injury?
   Answer: *Quadriceps contusion*
2. Was your assessment of Mr. Hottinger's injury correct?
   Answer: *Yes*
3. If not, explain what you did incorrectly and how you could have performed a better assessment.
   Answer: ____________________________________

MODEL SCENARIO 2: **DANIELLE MARTIN**

Danielle Martin is a gymnast who is training for the state competition. Throughout the regular season, Ms. Martin has experienced anterior tibial pain in her right leg. Ms. Martin states that she has seen a certified athletic trainer previously for her pain, and the pain has always subsided with treatment and rest. However, now the pain is more consistent and does not subside. The pain is present before and after activity and is greatest with the floor and vault routines. The anterior tibial pain is noticed only during the uneven bars event when she dismounts. Ms. Martin has localized pain at the middle shaft of the anterior right tibia (Fig. 6-2). She has no numbness or paraesthesia, and her strength is normal.

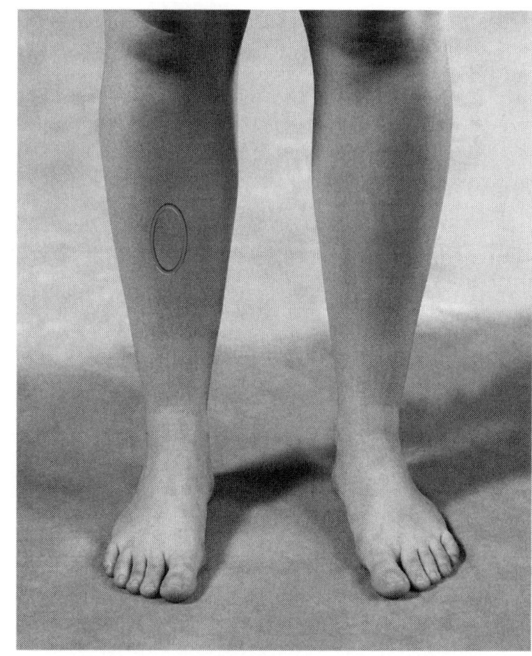

Figure 6-2: Danielle Martin's point of pain.

1. Based on this scenario, what do you know about Ms. Martin's injury?
   - *Female athlete*
   - *Gymnast*
   - *Chronic anterior shin pain*
   - *Normal strength*
   - *No numbness or paraesthesia*
   - *Pain beginning to localize*

- *Quicker onset of pain*
- *Most painful during floor and vault routines*
- *Constant pain that does not subside like it once did*

2. To evaluate Ms. Martin's injury effectively, you will need to gather additional information. What questions should you ask in addition to what is presented in this scenario?
   - *Is this injury a medical emergency?*
   - *Are there any preexisting injuries? If yes, what are they?*
   - *Are there any special tests that are important to perform? If yes, elaborate.*
   - *Are the results of the special tests positive or negative? What does each result indicate?*
   - *Are there gait irregularities?*
   - *Are there arch irregularities?*
   - *Is there passive or active ROM with dorsiflexion and plantar flexion?*
   - *What type of pain is it? For example, is the pain sharp, dull, or throbbing?*
3. Identify key terms and concepts, and then research each to broaden your knowledge of hip, thigh, and lower-leg injuries.
   - What anatomical structures are involved?
     Tibia
     Tibialis anterior muscle
   - Describe the different types of pain and what each indicates.
     Sharp pain indicates a fracture.
     Pins and needles or numbness indicates nerve pathology.
     Sharp and localized stinging indicates an acute injury.
     Aching or throbbing indicates a chronic or post injury (few days post injury).
     Radiating pain indicates pain dissipating away from the injured area along a nerve or along the length of a muscle.
   - Why might the onset of pain be quicker?
     The pain could have previously been muscular, but now it is either becoming chronic and the damage is worsening or becoming something more serious.
   - Why does Ms. Martin experience more pain during the floor and vault routines?
     The floor and vault are weight-bearing routines with increased impacts.
4. Based on the information that you currently have and what was provided by your instructor, what are the possible differential diagnoses for Ms. Martin's injury?
   Shin splints
   Tibial stress fracture
   Anterior exertional compartment syndrome

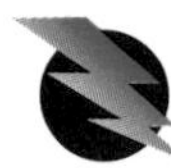

Brain Jolt

This injury is more accurately diagnosed with a radiograph.

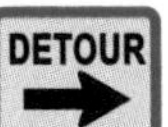

Treatment Detour

This injury occurs from repetitive activities and excessive load to this structure and is most common in the lower extremities. This injury is a possible assessment if an athlete has tenderness or edema over the involved anatomical structure after a change in training volume with limited rest periods. Women are thought to be at higher risk than males. In addition, poor nutrition and lifestyle habits, especially those with female athlete triad, increase the risk for this injury (Patel, Roth, & Kapil, 2011).

Why or why not?

For each assessment or diagnosis, write *why?* or *why not?* statements identifying why the information is correct or incorrect. Take details from your textbook, your own research, and data from Ms. Martin's scenario to help you formulate an answer.

1. *Ms. Martin does not have shin splints because the pain does not subside and is worse on the tibia, not the muscle. Treatment and rest may have helped with shin splints in the past, but the pain she is experiencing now is beyond this injury.*
2. *Ms. Martin has a tibial stress fracture because her pain is consistent and present during weight-bearing exercises, the tuning fork test is positive, and pain is localized to one area on the tibia.*
3. *Ms. Martin does not have anterior exertional compartment syndrome because she is not experiencing numbness or tingling and her strength in the dorsiflexion is normal.*

What do you think?

1. What is your assessment of Ms. Martin's injury?
   Answer: *Tibial stress fracture*
2. Was your assessment of Ms. Martin's injury correct?
   Answer: *Yes*
3. If not, explain what you did incorrectly and how you could have performed a better assessment.

   Answer: ______________________________

MODEL SCENARIO 3: **NICOLE TABOT**

Nicole Tabot is a cross-country runner. She comes to the athletic training room complaining of pain over her right tibia. She is treated with ice and calf stretching. A passive plantar flexion stretch, focusing on the tibialis anterior muscle, produces pain. While continuing with her season, Ms. Tabot comes to the athletic training room each day with the same symptoms. Three weeks before the end of the season, Ms. Tabot leaves practice because of the pressure she is experiencing from activity in her right tibia. She continues to complain of an anterior tightness and intense pain over her right tibia (Fig. 6-3). The pain subsides after a few hours, but she has residual soreness the next day. The results of a tap test are negative.

1. Based on this scenario, what do you know about Ms. Tabot's injury?
   - *Female athlete*
   - *Cross-country runner*
   - *Chronic mechanism of injury*
   - *Lower-leg anterior tightness and pain*
   - *Pain produced on passive stretching*
   - *Initial and intense pain subsides after activity*
   - *Has residual soreness the next day*
   - *Negative results of a tap test*
   - *Stretches and applies ice to the calf*
2. To evaluate Ms. Tabot's injury effectively, you will need to gather additional information. What questions should you ask in addition to what is presented in this scenario?
   - *Is this injury a medical emergency?*
   - *Are there any preexisting injuries? If yes, what are they?*
   - *Are there any special tests that are important to perform? If yes, elaborate.*
   - *Are the results of the special tests positive or negative? What does each result indicate?*
   - *Are there gait irregularities?*
   - *What type of pain is it? For example, is the pain sharp, dull, or throbbing?*
   - *Is there numbness or paraesthesia?*
   - *Is there point tenderness?*
   - *Is the tissue bony or soft?*
   - *Is there passive or active ROM in the dorsi and plantar flexion?*
   - *What is the strength at the ankle?*
3. Identify key terms and concepts, and then research each to broaden your knowledge of hip, thigh, and lower-leg injuries.
   - What anatomical structures are involved?

     Tibia

     Tibialis anterior muscle

     Anterior compartment of the lower leg

     Gastrocnemius
   - Define *plantar flexion.*

     Directional term of the foot: moving foot into extension in which the foot moves toward its bottom.
   - What is the tibialis anterior muscle?

     Muscle in the anterior compartment of the lower leg; a prime dorsiflexor
   - What does a negative tap test result indicate?

     No sign of a fracture
   - What is passive stretching?

     Movement performed by an athletic trainer or other person
   - Describe the different types of pain and what each indicates.

     Sharp pain indicates a fracture.

     Pins and needles or numbness indicates nerve pathology.

     Sharp and localized stinging indicates an acute injury.

     Aching or throbbing indicates a chronic or a post injury (few days post injury).

     Radiating pain indicates pain dissipating away from the injured area along a nerve or along the length of a muscle.
4. Based on the information that you currently have and what was provided by your instructor, what are

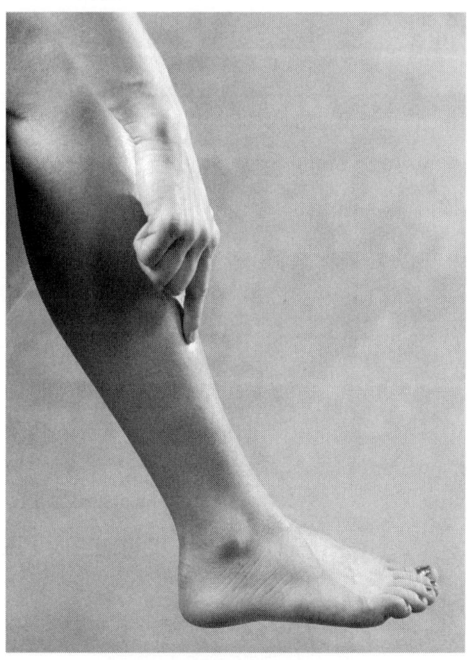

Figure 6-3: Nicole Tabot's area of pain.

the possible differential diagnoses for Ms. Tabot's injury?

Acute compartment syndrome
Tibialis anterior muscle strain
Tibia fracture
Chronic exertional compartment syndrome

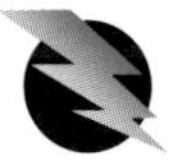

Brain Jolt
This injury can end the athlete's season, with either complete rest or surgery as two options of treatment.

Why or why not?

For each assessment or diagnosis, write *why?* or *why not?* statements identifying why the information is correct or incorrect. Take details from your textbook, your own research, and data from Ms. Tabot's scenario to help you formulate an answer.

1. *Ms. Tabot does not have acute compartment syndrome because it usually occurs secondary to a direct trauma, and her pain would not subside after activity if it was acute.*
2. *Ms. Tabot does not have a tibialis anterior muscle strain because her ROM and strength are normal, and there is no multiplicity of infection to indicate an acute strain.*
3. *Ms. Tabot does not have a tibia fracture because the results of the tap test are negative and there is no deformity.*
4. *Ms. Tabot has chronic exertional compartment syndrome because symptoms arise with activity and are consistent at a particular spot and pain diminishes when activity stops.*

What do you think?

1. What is your assessment of Ms. Tabot's injury?
   Answer: *Chronic exertional compartment syndrome*
2. Was your assessment correct for Ms. Tabot's injury?
   Answer: *Yes*
3. If not, explain what you did incorrectly and how you could have performed a better assessment.

   Answer: ________________

STUDENT SCENARIO 1: KEEGAN MARSHALL

Keegan Marshall is a senior lacrosse player for his high school. Mr. Marshall's team is facing off against the school archrival, which is making the game much more aggressive. He is proceeding down the field with the ball and is struck with a stick on his left side. The area of contact of the lacrosse stick is directly over the left iliac crest. Mr. Marshall feels a sharp pain, which causes limited active hip flexion. Mr. Marshall elicits an altered gait and has to be assisted off the field. Even after rest, Mr. Marshall continues to complain of pain and has difficulty with hip flexion and rotating his body to the left side. Ecchymosis and mild edema have developed over the left iliac crest (Fig. 6-4).

1. Based on this scenario, what do you know about Mr. Marshall's injury?
   - ________________
   - ________________
   - ________________
   - ________________
2. To evaluate Mr. Marshall's injury effectively, you will need to gather additional information. What questions should you ask in addition to what is presented in this scenario?
   - ________________
   - ________________

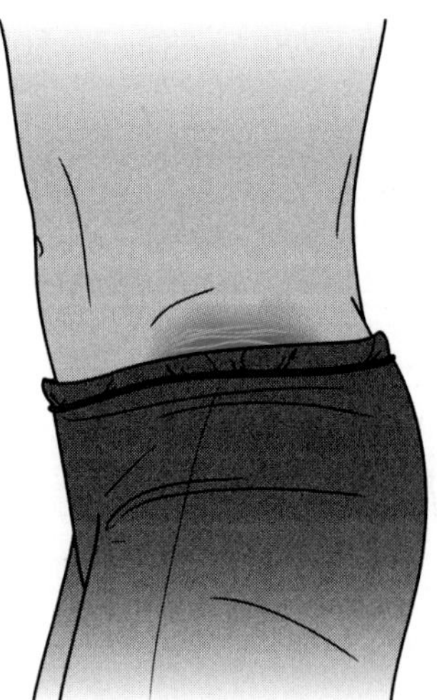

Figure 6-4: Keegan Marshall's hip.

- __________
- __________

3. Identify key terms and concepts, and then research each to broaden your knowledge of hip, thigh, and lower-leg injuries.
   - What anatomical structures are involved?

     Answer: __________
   - Define *ecchymosis*.

     Answer: __________
   - Define *edema*.

     Answer: __________
   - What is the iliac crest?

     Answer: __________
   - Why might a blow to the iliac crest limit hip flexion?

     Answer: __________
   - Why is it important to be familiar with lacrosse equipment?

     Answer: __________

> ***Brain Jolt***
> *Before this athlete can return to play, be sure to protect the contusion with additional padding.*

4. Based on the information that you currently have and what was provided by your instructor, what are the possible differential diagnoses for Mr. Marshall's injury?
   - __________
   - __________
   - __________
   - __________

Why or why not?

For each assessment or diagnosis, write *why?* or *why not?* statements identifying why the information is correct or incorrect. Take details from your textbook, your own research, and data from Mr. Marshall's scenario to help you formulate an answer.

1. __________
2. __________
3. __________
4. __________

What do you think?

1. What is your assessment of Mr. Marshall's injury?

   Answer: __________
2. Was your assessment correct for Mr. Marshall's injury?

   Answer: __________
3. If not, explain what you did incorrectly and how you could have performed a better assessment.

   Answer: __________

STUDENT SCENARIO 2: ERIC NOBLE

Eric Noble is a collegiate soccer player who has noticed a hard, bony deformity developing at the center of his left quadriceps muscle. After activity, the deformity is more defined if any type of contact occurs to that area. Mr. Noble allows 3 weeks to pass before he approaches the athletic trainer after practice. Mr. Noble is experiencing pain at the bony deformity. Upon evaluation, Mr. Noble has decreased ROM with knee flexion and extension and mild edema over the center of his left quadriceps muscle. There is localized point tenderness over the deformity. Mr. Noble stated he received a direct hit to the anterior portion of his quadriceps 1 month ago. Ecchymosis developed at the site of impact at that time (Fig. 6-5).

1. Based on this scenario, what do you know about Mr. Noble's injury?
   - __________
   - __________

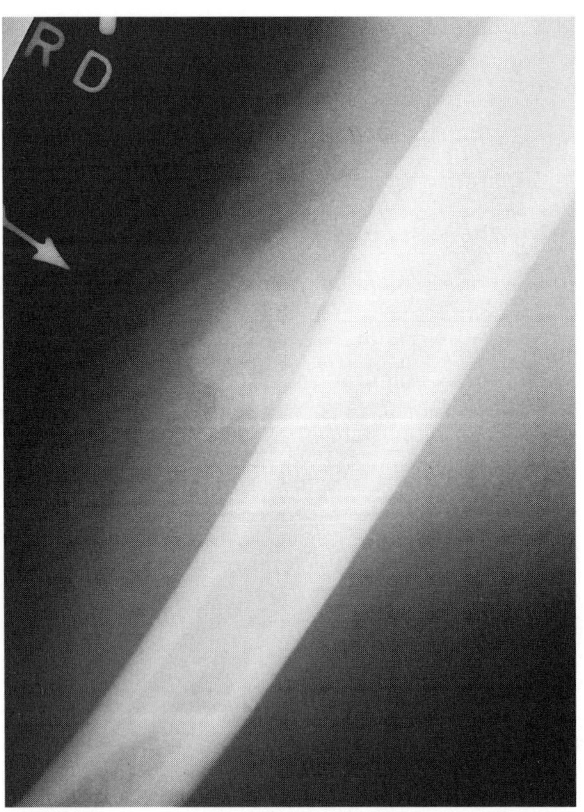

Figure 6-5: Eric Noble's radiograph. (With permission from Starkey, C., Brown, S. D., & Ryan, J. (2010). *Examination of orthopedic and athletic injuries.* Philadelphia, PA: F.A. Davis, p. 441)

- ____________________
- ____________________

2. To evaluate Mr. Noble's injury effectively, you will need to gather additional information. What questions should you ask in addition to what is presented in this scenario?
   - ____________________
   - ____________________
   - ____________________
   - ____________________
3. Identify key terms and concepts, and then research each to broaden your knowledge of hip, thigh, and lower-leg injuries.
   - What anatomical structures are involved?

     Answer: ____________________
   - Define *edema.*

     Answer: ____________________
   - Define *ecchymosis.*

     Answer: ____________________
   - Why does a bony deformity hinder knee flexion and extension?

     Answer: ____________________
   - What is the normal ROM for a knee flexion and extension?

     Answer: ____________________

Brain Jolt

This particular injury is treated with deep penetrating heat from an ultrasound machine or deep-tissue massage. These treatments help to dissipate the bony deformity that has developed.

4. Based on the information that you currently have and what was provided by your instructor, what are the possible differential diagnoses for Mr. Noble's injury?
   - ____________________
   - ____________________
   - ____________________
   - ____________________

Why or why not?

For each assessment or diagnosis, write *why?* or *why not?* statements identifying why the information is correct or incorrect. Take details from your textbook, your own research, and data from Mr. Noble's scenario to help you formulate an answer.

1. ____________________
2. ____________________
3. ____________________
4. ____________________

What do you think?

1. What is your assessment of Mr. Noble's injury?

   Answer: ____________________

2. Was your assessment correct for Mr. Noble's injury?

   Answer: ____________________

3. If not, explain what you did incorrectly and how you could have performed a better assessment.

   Answer: ____________________

STUDENT SCENARIO 3: SYMONE STANLEY

Symone Stanley is a recent college graduate. She is no longer involved with a collegiate sport, so she decides to join a coworker in training for a half marathon. Ms. Stanley was a softball player in college, and distance running is going to be new for her. The coworker is a former cross-country runner. The half marathon is 2 months away. Ms. Stanley wishes that she had obtained some new orthotics to address her foot pronation problem. Ms. Stanley quickly becomes accustomed to the training regimen and decides to add an additional 2 miles to her run today. She notices some anterior lower-leg pain after the run (Fig. 6-6). She ices her lower legs, but has increased soreness the next day. Ms. Stanley takes a few days of rest, and the pain subsides. The pain occurs again after her next run, this time only over the right lower leg. She continues with the same pattern for the next 3 weeks, until the week before the marathon. Now, everyday activity is painful.

1. Based on this scenario, what do you know about Ms. Stanley's injury?
   - ____________________
   - ____________________
   - ____________________
   - ____________________

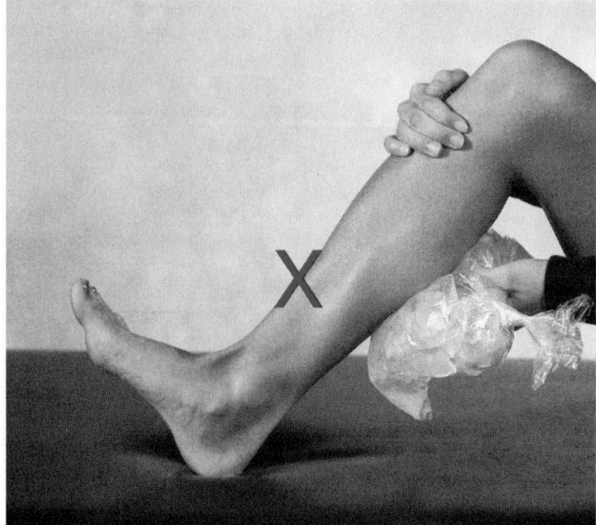

Figure 6-6: Symone Stanley's area of pain.

2. To evaluate Ms. Stanley's injury effectively, you will need to gather additional information. What questions should you ask in addition to what is presented in this scenario?
   - ____________________
   - ____________________
   - ____________________
   - ____________________

3. Identify key terms and concepts, and then research each to broaden your knowledge of hip, thigh, and lower-leg injuries.
   - What anatomical structures are involved?

   Answer: ____________________
   - How long is a half marathon?

   Answer: ____________________
   - What are reasonable mile increases for a beginning distance runner throughout training?

   Answer: ____________________
   - How do orthotics for foot pronation play a role in lower-leg pain?

   Answer: ____________________

4. Based on the information that you currently have and what was provided by your instructor, what are the possible differential diagnoses for Ms. Stanley's injury?
   - ____________________

- ______________________________
- ______________________________
- ______________________________

Brain Jolt

Chronic soreness and tenderness related to this injury can develop into hot spots if not properly treated and then progress into a more severe injury.

Why or why not?

For each assessment or diagnosis, write *why?* or *why not?* statements identifying why the information is correct or incorrect. Take details from your textbook, your own research, and data from Ms. Stanley's scenario to help you formulate an answer.

1. ______________________________
2. ______________________________
3. ______________________________
4. ______________________________

What do you think?

1. What is your assessment of Ms. Stanley's injury?

   Answer: ______________________________

2. Was your assessment correct for Ms. Stanley's injury?

   Answer: ______________________________

3. If not, please explain what you did incorrectly and how you could have performed a better assessment.

   Answer: ______________________________

STUDENT SCENARIO 4: TYLER ORTLIEB

Tyler Ortlieb is a senior forward on his high school soccer team. Mr. Ortlieb is dribbling the ball toward the goal and sees a player approaching from his right side. As he goes to take his shot on the goal with his right leg, the opponent slides in front of him. The opponent intends to kick the ball, but kicks Mr. Ortlieb's left shin. Mr. Ortlieb feels a crack and is then in a significant amount of pain. Mr. Ortlieb has a deformity and localized edema over the midtibial shaft and the midfibular shaft (Fig. 6-7). Mr. Ortlieb has complete lack of foot ROM, but still has a dorsal pedal pulse.

Brain Jolt

Ensure that any deformity is splinted properly for safe transport of the athlete.

1. Based on this scenario, what do you know about Mr. Ortlieb's injury?

   - ______________________________
   - ______________________________
   - ______________________________
   - ______________________________

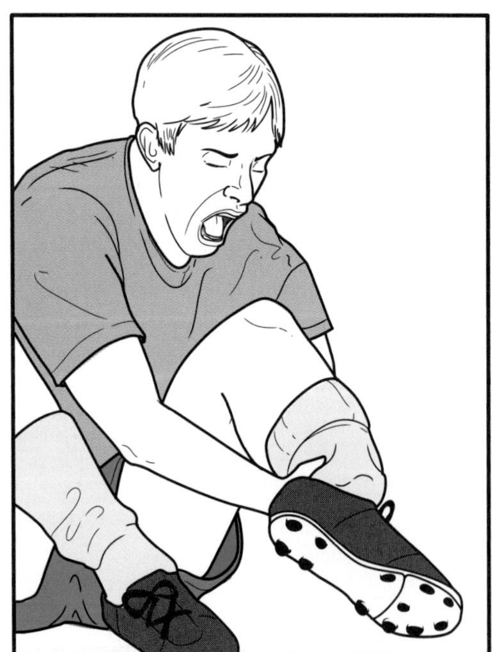

Figure 6-7: Tyler Ortlieb's leg.

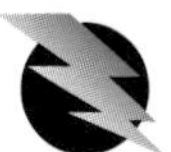

Brain Jolt
When an athlete has any type of deformity of the lower leg, always check the dorsal pedal pulse and capillary refill at the toes.

2. To evaluate Mr. Ortlieb's injury effectively, you will need to gather additional information. What questions should you ask in addition to what is presented in this scenario?
   - ______________________________
   - ______________________________
   - ______________________________
   - ______________________________

3. Identify key terms and concepts, and then research each to broaden your knowledge of hip, thigh, and lower-leg injuries.
   - What anatomical structures are involved?

     Answer: ______________________________
   - Define *plantar flexion.*

     Answer: ______________________________
   - What is a dorsal pedal pulse?

     Answer: ______________________________
   - Define *edema.*

     Answer: ______________________________
   - What is *capillary refill*?

     Answer: ______________________________
   - Why does Mr. Ortlieb have a complete lack of ROM in his foot?

     Answer: ______________________________

4. Based on the information that you currently have and what was provided by your instructor, what are the possible differential diagnoses for Mr. Ortlieb's injury?
   - ______________________________
   - ______________________________
   - ______________________________
   - ______________________________

Why or why not?

For each assessment or diagnosis, write *why?* or *why not?* statements identifying why the information is correct or incorrect. Take details from your textbook, your own research, and data from Mr. Ortlieb's scenario to help you formulate an answer.

1. ______________________________
2. ______________________________
3. ______________________________
4. ______________________________

What do you think?

1. What is your assessment of Mr. Ortlieb's injury?

   Answer: ______________________________
2. Was your assessment correct for Mr. Ortlieb's injury?

   Answer: ______________________________
3. If not, please explain what you did incorrectly and how you could have performed a better assessment.

   Answer: ______________________________

Conversation Buffer
When you see an athlete who has a severe injury with a gross deformity, you must be calm and reassuring. Athletes react differently to severe injuries, and it is important to calm them by telling them that they will be taken care of and that, although they have an injury, they will be just fine. Be sure not to gasp or make comments to startle your athlete or exacerbate his or her emotions. At this time, your athlete does not need the details of the deformity. Remember to always keep your athlete talking, maintain a light mood, and watch for symptoms of shock.

STUDENT SCENARIO 5: BROOKE MARROW

Brooke Marrow is a first baseman on her softball team. She has been experiencing anterior and medial hip tightness. Ms. Marrow comes to the athletic training room each day and has her hamstrings and iliotibial band stretched. Today at practice, a ball is thrown short in front of the first base. Ms. Marrow has to stretch to reach the ball. Her right foot is touching first base, and her left leg is lunged out in front of her (Fig. 6-8). After the play is over, Ms. Marrow notices some pain at her right hip and when she walks. Ms. Marrow is up next to bat and notices that she is unable to sprint to first base. She states that she has pain when flexing her hip. Ms. Marrow is removed from the game.

1. Based on this scenario, what do you know about Ms. Marrow's injury?
   - ______________________________
   - ______________________________
   - ______________________________
   - ______________________________

2. To evaluate Ms. Marrow's injury effectively, you will need to gather additional information. What questions should you ask in addition to what is presented in this scenario?
   - ______________________________
   - ______________________________
   - ______________________________
   - ______________________________

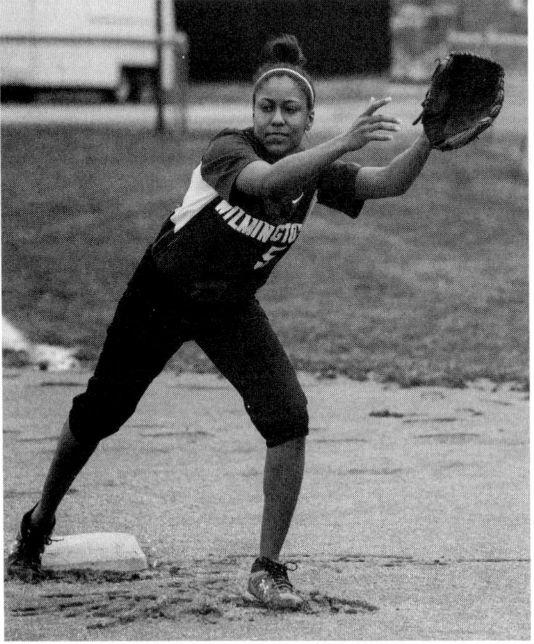

Figure 6-8: Brooke Marrow's body position.

3. Identify key terms and concepts, and then research each to broaden your knowledge of hip, thigh, and lower-leg injuries.
   - What anatomical structures are involved?

     Answer: ______________________________
   - What special tests will help you to determine hamstring, iliotibial band, and hip flexor tightness?

     Answer: ______________________________
   - With this injury, why would it hurt to walk?

     Answer: ______________________________
   - What anterior musculature could be causing some of Ms. Marrow's initial hip tightness?

     Answer: ______________________________
   - What medial musculature could be causing some of Ms. Marrow's initial hip tightness?

     Answer: ______________________________
   - Is having Ms. Marrow's hamstrings and iliotibial band stretched daily properly addressing her hip tightness? If no, explain.

     Answer: ______________________________

Brain Jolt

Be familiar with the two different types of hip spicas that can help with this type of injury and enable the athlete to return to play.

4. Based on the information that you currently have and what was provided by your instructor, what are the possible differential diagnoses for Ms. Marrow's injury?
   - ______________________________
   - ______________________________

- ______________________________
- ______________________________

3. ______________________________
4. ______________________________

Why or why not?

For each assessment or diagnosis, write *why?* or *why not?* statements identifying why the information is correct or incorrect. Take details from your textbook, your own research, and data from Ms. Marrow's scenario to help you formulate an answer.

1. ______________________________
2. ______________________________

What do you think?

1. What is your assessment of Ms. Marrow's injury?

   Answer: ______________________________

2. Was your assessment correct for Ms. Marrow's injury?

   Answer: ______________________________

3. If not, please explain what you did incorrectly and how you could have performed a better assessment.

   Answer: ______________________________

STUDENT SCENARIO 6: TIM GREEN

Tim Green is a football player who has sustained a lower-leg tibial fibular fracture. He is currently being transported to the hospital. He has a noticeable deformity in the midshaft of the right tibia and fibula. Localized edema has developed, and his dorsal pedal pulse, as seen in the example below (Fig. 6-9) has diminished. Mr. Green still has good capillary refill in his right toes. He has to have surgery to place a plate and two screws in his lower right leg to fix the spiral fracture. One day after surgery, while still in the hospital, he complains of increased pain in his lower leg. He notices a feeling of pressure that is extremely painful, and his dorsal pedal pulse has diminished again.

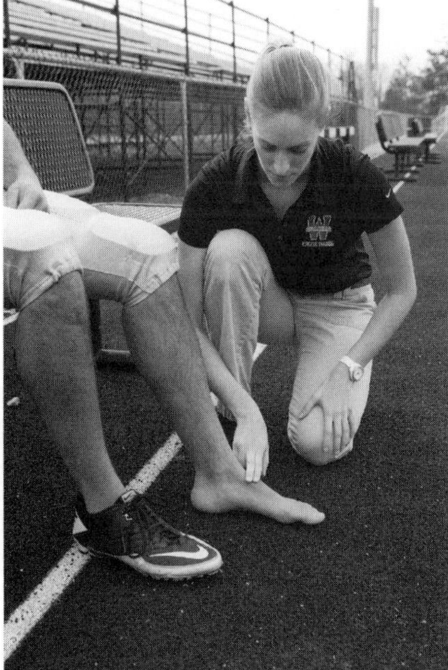

Figure 6-9: Tim Green's dorsal pedal pulse location.

1. Based on this scenario, what do you know about Mr. Green's injury?
   - ______________________________
   - ______________________________
   - ______________________________
   - ______________________________

2. To evaluate Mr. Green's injury effectively, you will need to gather additional information. What questions should you ask in addition to what is presented in this scenario?
   - ______________________________
   - ______________________________
   - ______________________________

- ______________________________

____

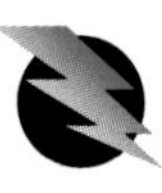

Brain Jolt

Surgery to the lower leg can produce residual swelling and cause these different sections to become inflamed and have increased pressure. This condition is a medical emergency.

3. Identify key terms and concepts, and then research each to broaden your knowledge of hip, thigh, and lower-leg injuries.
   - What anatomical structures are involved?

     Answer: ______________________________
   - Define *edema.*

     Answer: ______________________________
   - What is capillary refill?

     Answer: ______________________________
   - What is a spiral fracture?

     Answer: ______________________________
   - What is a dorsal pedal pulse?

     Answer: ______________________________
   - What are the surgical options for a tibial fibular fracture?

     Answer: ______________________________
   - What are the possible complications of surgery to correct a tibial fibular fracture?

     Answer: ______________________________
4. Based on the information that you currently have and what was provided by your instructor, what are the possible differential diagnoses for Mr. Green's injury?
   - ______________________________

     ____
   - ______________________________

     ____
   - ______________________________

     ____
   - ______________________________

     ____

Why or why not?

For each assessment or diagnosis, write *why?* or *why not?* statements identifying why the information is correct or incorrect. Take details from your textbook, your own research, and data from Mr. Green's scenario to help you formulate an answer.

1. ______________________________

   ____
2. ______________________________

   ____
3. ______________________________

   ____
4. ______________________________

   ____

What do you think?

1. What is your assessment of Mr. Green's injury?

   Answer: ______________________________
2. Was your assessment correct for Mr. Green's injury?

   Answer: ______________________________
3. If not, explain what you did incorrectly and how you could have performed a better assessment.

   Answer: ______________________________

STUDENT SCENARIO 7: MIKE WATSON

Mike Watson is a hockey player for his high school team and plays defense. During the game, he is skating backwards to defend against the offensive attacker. While he is attempting to quickly change directions for a body check, his push-off leg loses the inside edge on his skate, and he feels a sudden sharp pain along with a pulling sensation at his inner right thigh (Fig. 6-10). Once he regains his balance on the ice, he notices that he is unable to skate without pain and has an altered gait. Mr. Watson is quickly removed from the game and evaluated. On evaluation, he is point tender over the medial portion of the right quadriceps muscle and has limited strength and active ROM with adduction. There is no deformity or ecchymosis present.

1. Based on this scenario, what do you know about Mr. Watson's injury?
   - ______________________________

     ____
   - ______________________________

     ____

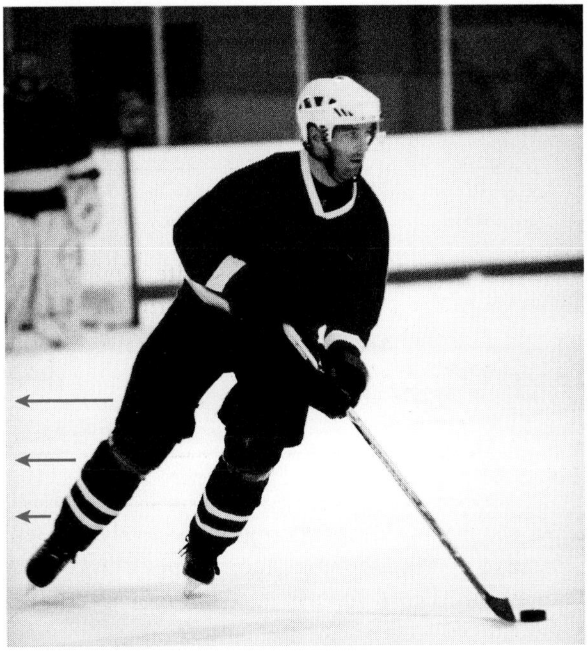

Figure 6-10: Mike Watson's mechanism of injury.
(© 2009 Jupiterimages © Thinkstock)

- ______________________________________
  ____
- ______________________________________
  ____

2. To evaluate Mr. Watson's injury effectively, you will need to gather additional information. What questions should you ask in addition to what is presented in this scenario?
   - ______________________________________
     ____
   - ______________________________________
     ____
   - ______________________________________
     ____
   - ______________________________________
     ____

3. Identify key terms and concepts, and then research each to broaden your knowledge of hip, thigh, and lower-leg injuries.
   - What anatomical structures are involved?

     Answer: ______________________________
   - Define *ecchymosis*.

     Answer: ______________________________
   - What does limited ROM indicate?

     Answer: ______________________________
   - What does limited strength indicate?

     Answer: ______________________________
   - What does a lack of deformity indicate?

     Answer: ______________________________
   - Why is it important to have an understanding of hockey terminology?

     Answer: ______________________________

4. Based on the information that you currently have and what was provided by your instructor, what are the possible differential diagnoses for Mr. Watson's injury?
   - ______________________________________
     ____
   - ______________________________________
     ____
   - ______________________________________
     ____
   - ______________________________________
     ____

Brain Jolt
Passive, active, and resistive strength tests should be performed, if tolerated, to determine exactly which muscle is injured.

Why or why not?

For each assessment or diagnosis, write *why?* or *why not?* statements identifying why the information is correct or incorrect. Take details from your textbook, your own research, and data from Mr. Watson's scenario to help you formulate an answer.

1. ______________________________________
   ____
2. ______________________________________
   ____
3. ______________________________________
   ____
4. ______________________________________
   ____

What do you think?

1. What is your assessment of Mr. Watson's injury?

   Answer: ____

2. Was your assessment correct for Mr. Watson's injury?

   Answer: ____

3. If not, explain what you did incorrectly and how you could have performed a better assessment.

   Answer: ____

STUDENT SCENARIO 8: BLAKE SHEPARD

Blake Shepard will soon be beginning his final year of high school. He has only 3 weeks left of summer break and has been enjoying his time off, spending today going out boating with his friends. Mr. Shepard has known how to water ski since he was 5 years old, and it is his turn for a trip around the lake. As he is water skiing behind the boat and approaching the first turn, he swings far out beside the boat. Mr. Shepard has to make his way back over the waves and loses his balance, causing him to wipe out and flip forward and onto his left side. He feels instant pain on his left side and is unable to move his left leg. While floating on his back, he notices a moderate deformity at his left quadriceps muscle. Mr. Shepard's friends have to drag him onto a makeshift board to get him to the shore. He notices that traction on the upper thigh (Fig. 6-11) helps to reduce some pain.

1. Based on this scenario, what do you know about Mr. Shepard's injury?
   - ____
   - ____
   - ____
   - ____

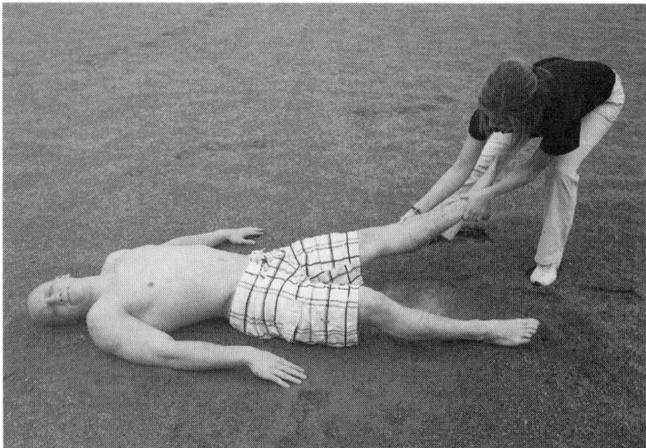

Figure 6-11: Blake Shepard's leg in traction.

2. To evaluate Mr. Shepard's injury effectively, you will need to gather additional information. What questions should you ask in addition to what is presented in this scenario?
   - ____
   - ____
   - ____
   - ____

3. Identify key terms and concepts, and then research each to broaden your knowledge of hip, thigh, and lower-leg injuries.
   - What anatomical structures are involved?

     Answer: ____
   - Define *traction.*

     Answer: ____
   - Why is Mr. Shepard unable to move his leg?

     Answer: ____
   - Why did Mr. Shepard's friends use a board to get him to shore?

     Answer: ____
   - Why does traction reduce Mr. Shepard's pain? Why is this information important in evaluating this injury?

     Answer: ____

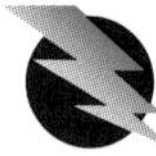

Brain Jolt

This injury is a medical emergency and requires traction to prevent further complications.

4. Based on the information that you currently have and what was provided by your instructor, what are

the possible differential diagnoses for Mr. Shepard's injury?

- ____________________
- ____________________
- ____________________
- ____________________

Why or why not?

For each assessment or diagnosis, write *why?* or *why not?* statements identifying why the information is correct or incorrect. Take details from your textbook, your own research, and data from Mr. Shepard's scenario to help you formulate an answer.

1. ____________________
2. ____________________
3. ____________________
4. ____________________

What do you think?

1. What is your assessment of Mr. Shepard's injury?

   Answer: ____________________

2. Was your assessment correct for Mr. Shepard's injury?

   Answer: ____________________

3. If not, explain what you did incorrectly and how you could have performed a better assessment.

   Answer: ____________________

STUDENT SCENARIO 9: MARK LINDEN

Mark Linden is a sprinter on the track and field team. He has a history of tight hamstrings, hamstring strains, and a functional leg-length discrepancy. In addition to his home exercise program for a stretching and strengthening of his hamstrings, Mr. Linden participated in the team practice yesterday, doing lunges and squats. He has noticed mild to moderate soreness in his hamstrings. After a hard practice yesterday, the coach decides to practice light and have each sprinter do 4 × 100-m race-pace sprints. Mr. Linden's stride does not feel normal; his right leg feels tight posteriorly, and his posture is uneven or unequal. As he completes his last 100 m, he feels a sharp pain and muscle weakness. He realizes that he is unable to fully extend his leg, and he drops to the track. On evaluation, a deformity is discovered on the posterior-lateral side of his leg (Fig. 6-12).

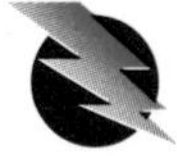

Brain Jolt

With any injury, remember the origins and insertions for the muscles that are around the involved area and palpate for incontinences in the muscle fibers.

1. Based on this scenario, what do you know about Mr. Linden's injury?

   - ____________________
   - ____________________

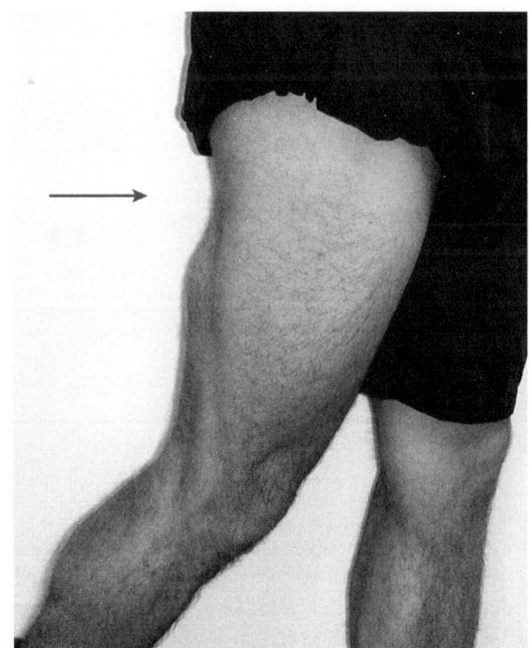

Figure 6-12: Mark Linden's posterior leg. (With permission from Starkey, C., Brown, S. D., & Ryan, J. (2010). *Examination of orthopedic and athletic injuries*. Philadelphia, PA: F. A. Davis, p. 423)

- ____________________
- ____________________

DETOUR

Treatment Detour

This type of injury is common and can range from mild to severe. An athlete is predisposed to this injury and a recurrence of injury if he or she has had prior injury and reduced flexibility. A systematic review of 18 research studies concluded that this injury has better subjective outcomes from patients, a greater rate of return to sport, and greater strength and endurance if treated surgically. Conservative treatment had low patient satisfaction, reduced strength, and lower rates of return to play (Harris, Griesser, & Best, 2011).

2. To evaluate Mr. Linden's injury effectively, you will need to gather additional information. What questions should you ask in addition to what is presented in this scenario?
   - ____________________
   - ____________________
   - ____________________
   - ____________________
3. Identify key terms and concepts, and then research each to broaden your knowledge of hip, thigh, and lower-leg injuries.
   - What anatomical structures are involved?

     Answer: ____________________
   - How is functional leg-length discrepancy determined?

     Answer: ____________________
   - What does functional leg-length discrepancy indicate?

     Answer: ____________________
   - How is hamstring tightness determined?

     Answer: ____________________
   - Is it normal to feel soreness in the hamstrings after performing lunges and squats?

     Answer: ____________________
   - Why is it important to have an understanding of track and field terminology?

     Answer: ____________________
   - Why might Mr. Linden's posture be unequal or uneven?

     Answer: ____________________
   - Unequal or uneven posture can lead to what condition?

     Answer: ____________________
   - What type of pain is associated with this injury, and what does this type indicate?

     Answer: ____________________
4. Based on the information that you currently have and what was provided by your instructor, what are the possible differential diagnoses for Mr. Linden's injury?
   - ____________________
   - ____________________
   - ____________________
   - ____________________

Why or why not?

For each assessment or diagnosis, write *why?* or *why not?* statements identifying why the information is correct or incorrect. Take details from your textbook, your own research, and data from Mr. Linden's scenario to help you formulate an answer.

1. ____________________
2. ____________________
3. ____________________
4. ____________________

What do you think?

1. What is your assessment of Mr. Linden's injury?

   Answer: ____________________
2. Was your assessment correct for Mr. Linden's injury?

   Answer: ____________________
3. If not, explain what you did incorrectly and how you could have performed a better assessment.

   Answer: ____________________

STUDENT SCENARIO 10: ANTHONY GOODRICH

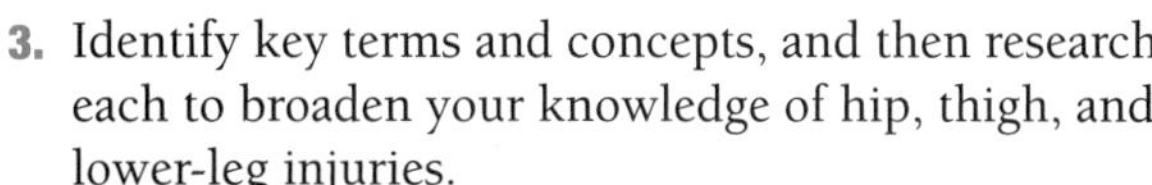

Anthony Goodrich is a cross-country runner. He has been complaining of left hip pain and tightness, and he feels the pain radiate down the left side of his left leg into the knee. He has noticed a tendon thickness occurring on the lateral side of his left knee. There is also localized point tenderness at Gerdy's tubercle (Fig. 6-13). The results of an Ober test are positive.

1. Based on this scenario, what do you know about Mr. Goodrich's injury?
   - ______________________________
   - ______________________________
   - ______________________________
   - ______________________________
2. To evaluate Mr. Goodrich's injury effectively, you will need to gather additional information. What questions should you ask in addition to what is presented in this scenario?
   - ______________________________
   - ______________________________
   - ______________________________
   - ______________________________

Figure 6-13: Anthony Goodrich's area of pain.

3. Identify key terms and concepts, and then research each to broaden your knowledge of hip, thigh, and lower-leg injuries.
   - What anatomical structures are involved?

     Answer: ______________________________
   - Explain the Ober test.

     Answer: ______________________________
   - What is radiating pain? What does it indicate?

     Answer: ______________________________
   - How is hip tightness determined?

     Answer: ______________________________
   - What does tendon thickness indicate?

     Answer: ______________________________
   - What inserts at Gerdy's tubercle?

     Answer: ______________________________
4. Based on the information that you currently have and what was provided by your instructor, what are the possible differential diagnoses for Mr. Goodrich's injury?
   - ______________________________
   - ______________________________
   - ______________________________
   - ______________________________

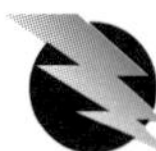

Brain Jolt

A foam roller will be an important tool to help the athlete's symptoms subside.

Why or why not?

For each assessment or diagnosis, write *why?* or *why not?* statements identifying why the information is correct or incorrect. Take details from your textbook, your own research, and data from Mr. Goodrich's scenario to help you formulate an answer.

1. ______________________________
2. ______________________________

3. ______________________________

____

4. ______________________________

____

What do you think?

1. What is your assessment of Mr. Goodrich's injury?

   Answer: ______________________________

2. Was your assessment correct for Mr. Goodrich's injury?

   Answer: ______________________________

3. If not, explain what you did incorrectly and how you could have performed a better assessment.

   Answer: ______________________________

Conversation Buffer

This injury can be nagging for runners. An aggressive treatment plan needs to include reducing the edema, initiating a stretching program, and evaluating hip-to-foot biomechanics. It is important to discuss the training plan with your athlete, because understanding this will help with treatment and may need to be modified if irritation persists.

knowledge checklist

Table 6-1 offers a checklist that can be used by a peer, instructor, or preceptor to evaluate each part of a hip, thigh, and lower-leg assessment. Use this checklist as a tool to ensure that the evaluation is complete and to assess your knowledge of the competencies that apply to this chapter.

TABLE 6-1 ■ Hip, Thigh, and Lower-Leg Assessment Competency Checklist

	Proficient *Can demonstrate and execute the skill properly*	**Proficient With Assistance** *Can demonstrate and execute the skill with minimal guidance or tips*	**Not Proficient** *Unable to demonstrate and execute the skill properly; need to be reevaluated at another time after further study and practice*
Athlete's Health History			
Medical history			
History of hip, thigh, or lower-leg injury			
Type of sport and position played			
Mechanisms of Injury			
How did the injury occur?			
When does pain occur?			
What makes the pain better or worse?			
Was the athlete's leg forced into an unusual direction?			
Is the athlete experiencing numbness or tingling?			
Were any pops, cracks, or snaps heard?			
Does the athlete experience pain going up or down stairs?			
How did the athlete's leg look at the time the injury(s) occurred?			
Visual Observations			
Gait			
Edema			
Ecchymosis			
Deformity			
Pelvic obliquity (ASIS, PSIS, and iliac crest alignment)			
Palpation			
Temperature change over the painful area; crepitus; deformity; intra-articular or extra-articular joint swelling; changes within the muscle fibers			
Iliac crest			
Greater trochanter and bursa			
Ischial tuberosity			
Posterior superior iliac spine			
Quadriceps muscle group			
Hamstring muscle group			
Tensor fasciae latae			
Iliotibial band			
Gluteus maximus			
Gluteus medius			
Adductor muscle group			
Sacroiliac joint			

Continued

TABLE 6-1 ■ Hip, Thigh, and Lower-Leg Assessment Competency Checklist—cont'd

	Proficient	Proficient With Assistance	Not Proficient
Sciatic nerve			
Muscles of the anterior compartment of the lower leg			
Range of Motion			
Passive or active			
Hip flexion			
Hip extension			
Hip abduction			
Hip adduction			
Hip internal rotation			
Hip external rotation			
Knee flexion			
Knee extension			
Strength			
Grade through manual muscle tests			
Hip flexion			
Hip extension			
Hip abduction			
Hip adduction			
Knee flexion			
Hip flexion			
Special Tests			
Hip scouring test or hip quadrant test			
Leg-length discrepancy (functional vs. anatomical)			
Q angle test			
Piriformis test			
Patrick test or FABER test			
Thomas test			
Ely test			
90/90 straight-leg raise test			
Ober test			
Trendelenburg test			
Long-bone compression test			
Tap-percussion-bump test			
Tuning fork test			
Squeeze or compression test			
Homan's sign			
Neurological			
Sciatic nerve			
Femoral nerve			
Vascular			
Dorsal pedal pulse			
Posterior tibial pulse			
Capillary refill			
Final Assessment			
Sprain; strain; contusion; fracture; condition; severity			

ASIS, anterior superior iliac spine; FABER, flexion abduction external rotation; IT, iliotibial; PSIS, posterior superior iliac spine.
*Be sure to always compare bilaterally.

REFERENCES

Harris, J. D., Griesser, M. J., & Best, T. M. (2011). Treatment of proximal hamstring ruptures—a systematic review. *International Journal of Sports Medicine, 32*, 490–495.

National Athletic Training Association. (2011). *Athletic training education competencies* (5th ed.). Retrieved from http://www.nata.org/sites/default/files/5th-Edition-Competencies-2011-PDF-Version.pdf

Patel, D. S., Roth, M., & Kapil, N. (2011). Stress fracture: Diagnosis, treatment, and prevention. *American Family Physician, 83*, 39–46.

Prentice, W. (2010). *Arnheim's principles of athletic training: A competency-based approach* (14th ed.). New York, NY: McGraw-Hill.

Starkey, C., Brown, S. D., & Ryan, J. (2010). *Examination of orthopedic and athletic injuries* (3rd ed.). Philadelphia, PA: F.A. Davis.

Venes, D. (Ed.) (2009). *Taber's cyclopedic medical dictionary* (21st ed.). Philadelphia, PA: F.A. Davis.

chapter 7

Upper Extremity: The Hand, Wrist, and Elbow

chapter outline

athletic trainer's corner

Out there in the real world, one athletic training student experienced the following:

One day, I was lifting furniture when I heard a loud "pop" sound in my left wrist. This is the same wrist I broke my freshman year in high school, and it still gives me frequent problems of sprains and instability. I tried flexing my wrist, but that caused a lot of pain. In addition, my lunate bone was subluxing. There was no edema or ecchymosis, but the pain and laxity of my carpal bones worried me. At the time, being an athletic training student, I knew that something was seriously wrong and I needed to undergo testing. The radiography results were negative, and I underwent magnetic resonance imaging (MRI). The MRI results indicated scapholunate dissociation. I had torn my scapholunate ligament, which holds the scaphoid and lunate together. This is the one ligament you do not want to tear because there currently is not much in terms of research or clinical guidelines on how to repair it. Two surgeons said that they could fix it, but I would lose 50% of my range of motion (ROM). With some research, I found a surgeon willing to perform a Brunelli procedure to repair my wrist. Although the Brunelli procedure is more extensive than other procedures, it was possible that I would not lose as much ROM with the Brunelli procedure. This was a risk I was willing to take. I'm glad I took the risk because I now have almost 100% ROM in my affected wrist.

Mitch Howard, AT, ATC
St. Louis, Missouri

learning outcomes

After working through this chapter, you will be able to:

1. Verbalize the questions to use when obtaining a thorough medical history for an assessment.
2. Describe the principles of body movement at the hand, wrist, and elbow and the various mechanisms of injury that affect the hand, wrist, and elbow.
3. Compare and contrast the findings of various special tests and the role of diagnostic tests used during a hand, wrist, and elbow evaluation.
4. Explain the medical terminology associated with the assessment of musculoskeletal injuries.
5. Verbalize the standard procedures used for a clinical evaluation of the hand, wrist, and elbow and interpret the findings for differential diagnoses.

MODEL SCENARIO 1: STEVE LOFTUS

Steve Loftus is a linebacker for his college football team. As he attempts to block his opponent during practice, he grabs the opponent's shoulder pads, and his right index finger gets caught in his opponent's jersey. His finger is forced into extension at the same time he is trying to flex his fingers and hold his opponent. After the play, Mr. Loftus walks off the field to be evaluated and tells the athletic trainer he felt a pop when trying to hold onto his opponent. He has good ROM in his first, third, fourth, and fifth phalanges and complains only of pain with flexion of his right index finger. There is no apparent edema or deformity. On further evaluation, the athletic trainer notices that Mr. Loftus is unable to flex his right index finger at the distal interphalangeal (DIP) joint when the proximal interphalangeal (PIP) joint is stabilized (Fig. 7-1).

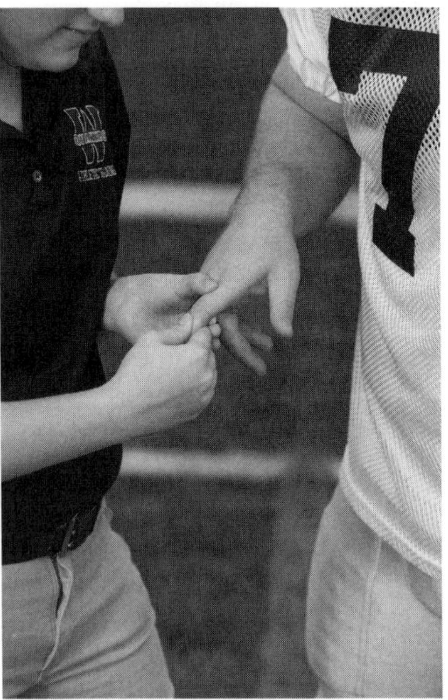

Figure 7-1: Steve Loftus' Finger

1. Based on the previous scenario, what do you know about Mr. Loftus' injury?
   - *Male athlete*
   - *Collegiate linebacker*
   - *Mechanism of injury: grabbing an opponent*
   - *Injured right index finger*
   - *No deformity*
   - *No edema*
   - *Felt a pop when grabbing an opponent*
   - *Pain with flexion of right index finger*
   - *Unable to flex DIP joint of index finger when the PIP is stabilized*

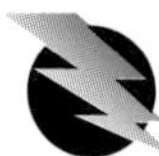

Brain Jolt

The athletic trainer must splint this injury immediately in extension, and then refer the athlete to a physician to avoid further complications.

Conversation Buffer

You will want to explain to the athlete the importance of maintaining extension of the injured finger when removing or changing the splint for any reason. The athlete needs to understand that allowing this injury to return to flexion can increase the recovery period and lead to other complications. Explaining this concept will increase the athlete's compliance with proper treatment.

2. To evaluate Mr. Loftus' injury effectively, you will need to gather additional information. What questions should you ask in addition to what is presented in this scenario?
   - *Is this injury a medical emergency?*
   - *Are there any preexisting injuries? If yes, what are they?*
   - *Are there any special tests that are important to perform? If yes, elaborate.*
   - *Are the results of the special tests positive or negative? What does each result indicate?*

- *Does the athlete have any numbness or tingling?*
- *Are there any changes in temperature of the affected area?*
- *Is ecchymosis present?*

3. Identify key terms and concepts, and then research each to broaden your knowledge of hand, wrist, and elbow injuries.
   - What anatomical structures might be involved in Mr. Loftus' injury?
     Flexor digitorum profundus (FDP)
     Flexor digitorum superficialis (FDS)
     Distal interphalangeal joint
     PIP
     Interphalangeal (IP) ligaments
   - Define *edema.*
     Swelling; a localized or general condition that causes body tissues to contain an excessive amount of fluid
   - Where are the muscle insertions for the FDP?
     The muscle insertions for the FDP are at the base of the middle phalanges of digits 2 through 5.
   - Where are the muscle insertions for the FDS?
     The muscle insertions for the FDS are at the sides of the middle phalanges of digits 2 through 5.
   - What does the abbreviation *PIP* stand for?
     Proximal interphalangeal joint
   - What does the abbreviation *DIP* stand for?
     Distal interphalangeal joint
   - What is affected if Mr. Loftus is unable to flex his finger at the DIP joint?
     The FDP muscle flexes the finger at the DIP joint; if the FDP muscle is avulsed, he is unable to actively flex at the DIP joint.
   - What does a popping sensation indicate?
     A popping sensation can indicate a ruptured muscle or an avulsion of a muscle tendon.

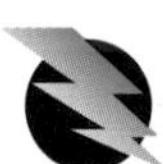

Brain Jolt

A helpful way to remember the insertion of the FDS versus FDP is to think that FDS "splits and inserts on the sides of the middle phalanges." The "s" in "splits" and "sides" correlates to the "s" in FDS.

4. Based on the information that you currently have and what was provided by your instructor, what are the possible differential diagnoses for Mr. Loftus' injury?
   Boutonniere deformity
   Mallet finger
   Jersey finger
   Finger flexor strain

Why or why not?

For each assessment or diagnosis, write *why?* or *why not?* statements identifying why the information is correct or incorrect. Take details from your textbook, your own research, and data from Mr. Loftus' scenario to help you formulate an answer.

1. *Mr. Loftus does not have a boutonniere deformity because there is no significant deformity present. In addition, his PIP joint is in extension, which is not possible with this deformity because the central extensor tendon is ruptured.*
2. *Mr. Loftus does not have a mallet finger because he is able to extend the DIP joint of his index finger, which is not possible with a mallet finger because the extensor digitorum longus is avulsed.*
3. *Mr. Loftus has a jersey finger because his PIP joint can flex and extend, but the DIP joint of his index finger cannot flex, showing that the FDP tendon is avulsed.*
4. *Mr. Loftus does not have a finger flexor strain because a strain is typically associated with limited range of motion (ROM), and Mr. Loftus has no ROM.*

What do you think?

1. What is your assessment of Mr. Loftus' injury?
   Answer: *Jersey finger, an avulsion of the FDP tendon*
2. Was your assessment of Mr. Loftus' injury correct?
   Answer: *Yes*
3. If not, explain what you did incorrectly and how you could have performed a better assessment.

   Answer: ____________________

MODEL SCENARIO 2: JUDY SIMS

Judy Sims is a gymnast who comes to the athletic training room complaining of wrist pain. She states that she is able to continue practicing, but by the end of practice her right wrist is extremely painful. Her wrist proves most painful during extension. She has a small soft mass on the dorsal side of her wrist over the distal row of the carpal bones (Fig. 7-2). Besides the mass, there is no edema or ecchymosis. The mass is slightly movable and is point tender. Ms. Sims states that the mass appeared

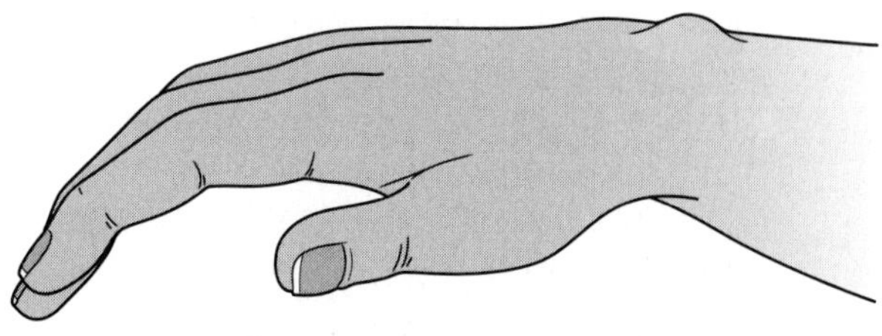

Figure 7-2: Judy Sims' wrist.

3 weeks ago, but it was asymptomatic until a few days ago. Her wrist strength and ROM are good in all directions.

1. Based on the previous scenario, what do you know about Ms. Sims' injury?
   - *Female athlete*
   - *Gymnast*
   - *Pain in right wrist*
   - *Pain began a few days ago*
   - *Able to finish practice but wrist is painful*
   - *Small soft mass on dorsal side of right wrist over distal row of carpal bones*
   - *No edema*
   - *No ecchymosis*
   - *Slightly movable mass*
   - *Point tender over mass*
   - *Mass present for 3 weeks, but asymptomatic until a few days ago*
   - *Good ROM and strength in all directions*
2. To evaluate Ms. Sims' injury effectively, you will need to gather additional information. What questions should you ask in addition to what is presented in this scenario?
   - *Is this a medical emergency?*
   - *Are there any preexisting injuries? If yes, what are they?*
   - *Are there any special tests that are important to perform? If yes, elaborate.*
   - *Are the results of the special tests positive or negative? What does each indicate?*
   - *Does Ms. Sims' mass ever change in size?*
   - *Has Ms. Sims had a similar mass anywhere else?*
3. Identify key terms and concepts, and then research each to broaden your knowledge of hand, wrist, and elbow injuries.
   - What anatomical structures might be involved in Ms. Sims' injury?
     Carpal bones
     Radius
     Ulna
   - Define *asymptomatic.*
     Having no symptoms, meaning there is no pain or functional limitations
   - Define *edema.*
     Swelling; a localized or general condition that causes body tissues to contain an excessive amount of fluid
   - Define *ecchymosis.*
     A bruise; superficial bleeding under the skin
   - Why would the mass be soft and slightly movable?
     The mass could be a collection of fluid within the tendinous sheath or joint capsule, which causes it to be movable.
   - If Ms. Sims' strength and ROM are good, why is her wrist most painful in extension?
     When the wrist is in extension, especially with added weight such as a handstand or other gymnastics moves, the compression of the wrist bones pinches the mass. This repetitive pinching inflames the mass and causes pain.
   - What are all of the directions for ROM of the wrist?
     Flexion
     Extension
     Ulnar deviation
     Radial deviation
     Supination
     Pronation
4. Based on the information that you currently have and what was provided by your instructor, what are the possible differential diagnoses for Ms. Sims' injury?
   Sprained wrist
   Wrist ganglion cyst
   Bursitis

Why or why not?

For each assessment or diagnosis, write *why?* or *why not?* statements identifying why the information is correct or incorrect. Take details from your textbook, your own research, and data from Ms. Sims' scenario to help you formulate an answer.

1. *Ms. Sims does not have a sprained wrist because her ROM and strength are good. A sprain would produce less localized edema and would cause a temperature change of the affected area.*
2. *Ms. Sims has a wrist ganglion cyst because there is a small movable mass with no temperature change of the affected area.*
3. *Ms. Sims does not have bursitis because there is not a bursa to be inflamed in the affected location.*

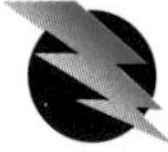

Brain Jolt
After proper diagnosis, this condition is easily treated and is typically harmless.

What do you think?

1. What is your assessment of Ms. Sims' injury?
   Answer: *Wrist ganglion cyst*
2. Was your assessment of Ms. Sims' injury correct?
   Answer: *Yes*
3. If not, explain what you did incorrectly and how you could have performed a better assessment.

   Answer: ____________________

MODEL SCENARIO 3: **BRUCE LOGAN**

Bruce Logan is a collegiate wrestler who competes in the 175-lb weight class. The day before a match, he is wrestling a fellow teammate and subsequently is brought down to the mat where he lands on the tip of his left elbow. He complains of pain with elbow extension. Within 1 hour, he begins experiencing localized point tenderness and moderate edema over his left olecranon process (Fig. 7-3). The results of a forearm compression test are positive, and Mr. Logan is referred for radiography, the results of which are negative. As Mr. Logan's pain decreases, the edema continues to increase. Heat is produced over the injured area.

1. Based on the previous scenario, what do you know about Mr. Logan's injury?
   - *Male athlete*
   - *Collegiate wrestler*
   - *Mechanism of injury: acute from a direct hit to the elbow*
   - *Localized point tenderness over the olecranon process*
   - *Moderate edema over the olecranon process*
   - *Positive forearm compression test*
   - *Negative radiograph results*
   - *Pain with elbow extension*
   - *Acute temperature changes of the affected area*
2. To evaluate Mr. Logan's injury effectively, you will need to gather additional information. What questions should you ask in addition to what is presented in this scenario?
   - *Is this injury a medical emergency?*
   - *Are there any preexisting injuries? If yes, what are they?*
   - *Are there any special tests that are important to perform? If yes, elaborate.*
   - *Are the results of the special tests positive or negative? What does each result indicate?*
   - *Does the athlete experience any numbness or tingling?*
   - *Are deformities present?*
   - *What are the elbow and shoulder carrying positions?*
   - *What is the ROM and strength at the elbow?*

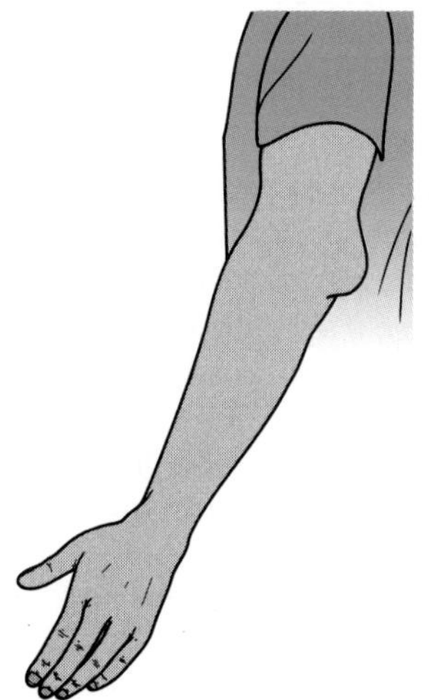

Figure 7-3: Bruce Logan's elbow.

3. Identify key terms and concepts, and then research each to broaden your knowledge of hand, wrist, and elbow injuries.
   - What anatomical structures might be involved in Mr. Logan's injury?
     Elbow extensors
     Ulna
     Olecranon process
     Olecranon bursae
     Humerus
     Medial and lateral epicondyles
     Radius
   - Define *edema.*
     Swelling; a localized or general condition that causes body tissues to contain an excessive amount of fluid
   - What does a positive compression test indicate?
     A positive compression test indicates a possible fracture, but a radiograph is needed to confirm the diagnosis of fracture.
   - Why is there temperature change with this particular acute injury?
     There is increased temperature change because the edema present is a result of the inflamed bursa from an acute mechanism of injury.

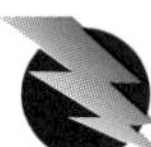

Brain Jolt
When an Ace bandage with a pad is placed directly over the edema, the edema tends to dissipate quickly. When the bandage is removed, the edema can reappear in the same localized area.

4. Based on the information that you currently have and what was provided by your instructor, what are the possible differential diagnoses for Mr. Logan's injury?
   Olecranon fracture
   Olecranon bursitis
   Radius fracture
   Medial epicondylitis

Why or why not?

For each assessment or diagnosis, write *why?* or *why not?* statements identifying why the information is correct or incorrect. Take details from your textbook, your own research, and data from Mr. Logan's scenario to help you formulate an answer.

1. *Mr. Logan does not have an olecranon fracture because the radiographs did not confirm this. When localized point tenderness and positive compression test results*

are present, radiographs are needed to rule out a fracture.

2. *Mr. Logan has olecranon bursitis because the subcutaneous olecranon bursae is easily injured from a direct hit to the olecranon process. The edema from this injury is localized with a temperature change over the affected area from the acute injury.*
3. *Mr. Logan does not have a radius fracture because the radiographs did not confirm a diagnosis of fracture, and he is not point tender over the radius. His pain is over the olecranon process, which is part of the ulna.*
4. *Mr. Logan does not have medial epicondylitis because this condition is a chronic over-use injury that is typically not the result of a direct hit, such as Mr. Logan's mechanism of injury. Medial epicondylitis is usually a result of repetitive forceful flexion of the wrist and valgus stress on the medial side of the elbow.*

What do you think?

1. What is your assessment of Mr. Logan's injury?
   Answer: *Olecranon bursitis*
2. Was your assessment of Mr. Logan's injury correct?
   Answer: *Yes*
3. If not, explain what you did incorrectly and how you could have performed a better assessment.

   Answer: ____________________

STUDENT SCENARIO 1: JEAN WINTERROAD

Jean Winterroad is a collegiate softball pitcher who is ranked number one in her conference. She continually exhibits forced left wrist flexion after she releases the softball during pitches. Her coach has instructed her to correct her mechanics, but she continues to go back to her old habit. After a weekend of two games per day, Ms. Winterroad complains that her wrist is sore and painful over the anterior (palmar) surface of her left hand (Fig. 7-4). She states that she has noticed decreased strength in her left thumb. Jean Winterroad has paraesthesia radiating into her left third phalange, and edema is present over the palmar surface of her left wrist.

1. Based on the previous scenario, what do you know about Ms. Winterroad's injury?
   - ____________________
   - ____________________
   - ____________________
   - ____________________

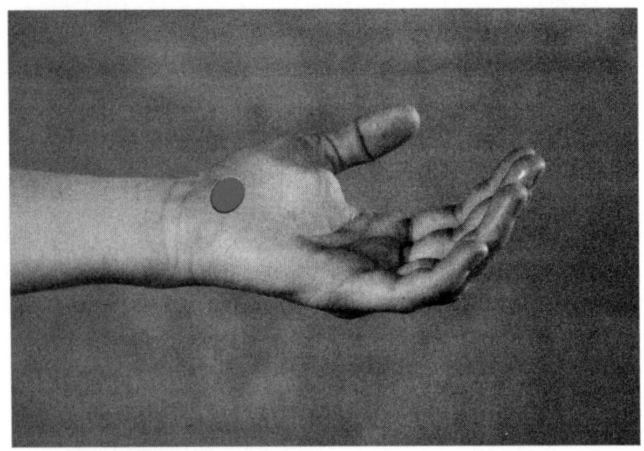

Figure 7-4: Jean Winterroad's area of pain.

2. To evaluate Ms. Winterroad's injury effectively, you will need to gather additional information. What questions should you ask in addition to what is presented in this scenario?
   - ____________________
   - ____________________
   - ____________________
   - ____________________

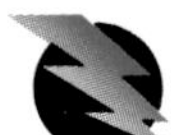

Brain Jolt

Computer programmers are not the only people who suffer from this condition. Wrist flexor tendonitis is typically the initial diagnosis; however, if left untreated, flexor tendonitis can develop into this condition.

3. Identify key terms and concepts, and then research each to broaden your knowledge of hand, wrist, and elbow injuries.
   - What anatomical structures might be involved in Ms. Winterroad's injury?

   Answer: ____________________

- Define *edema*.

  Answer: ______

- Define *paraesthesia*.

  Answer: ______

- Why is there paraesthesia in Ms. Winterroad's left third phalange?

  Answer: ______

- Why might there be decreased strength in Ms. Winterroad's thumb?

  Answer: ______

- Why is it important for the athletic trainer to become familiar with a softball pitcher's throwing mechanics?

  Answer: ______

DETOUR **Treatment Detour**

A research study was conducted to establish the most accurate combination of special tests to diagnose a compression injury of the median nerve. The results reported that a hand elevation test followed by the Phalen test were the best predictors for this wrist injury. Therefore, when an injury of this type is suspected, it is important to perform the hand elevation test and then the Phalen test to implement the most clinically accurate practices (Amirfeyz et al., 2011).

4. Based on the information that you currently have and what was provided by your instructor, what are the possible differential diagnoses for Ms. Winterroad's injury?

- ______
- ______
- ______
- ______

Why or why not?

For each assessment or diagnosis, write *why?* or *why not?* statements identifying why the information is correct or incorrect. Take details from your textbook, your own research, and data from Ms. Winterroad's scenario to help you formulate an answer.

1. ______
2. ______
3. ______
4. ______

What do you think?

1. What is your assessment of Ms. Winterroad's injury?

   Answer: ______

2. Was your assessment of Ms. Winterroad's injury correct?

   Answer: ______

3. If not, explain what you did incorrectly and how you could have performed a better assessment.

   Answer: ______

STUDENT SCENARIO 2: HOLLY CAIN

Holly Cain is home from college for the holiday break. After the break, her spring tennis season will begin. The tennis coach has the team doing conditioning exercises, but no hitting until the team returns from break. While Ms. Cain is home, it snows 3 to 4 inches, so she helps her dad shovel snow for 2 hours. The next morning, she has pain on the lateral side of her right elbow (Fig. 7-5), which is her dominant side. By the end of the day, Ms. Cain calls her school's certified athletic trainer to ask what she needs to do for treatment. She describes her symptoms, which are pain with active wrist extension, pain with full extension of the elbow, pain in the forearm, and edema over the lateral epicondyle. She is instructed to apply ice to the injury for 20 minutes, take an anti-inflammatory medication, and then wrap the area with an Ace bandage. She is scheduled to be evaluated when she returns back to campus.

1. Based on the previous scenario, what do you know about Ms. Cain's injury?

- ______
- ______

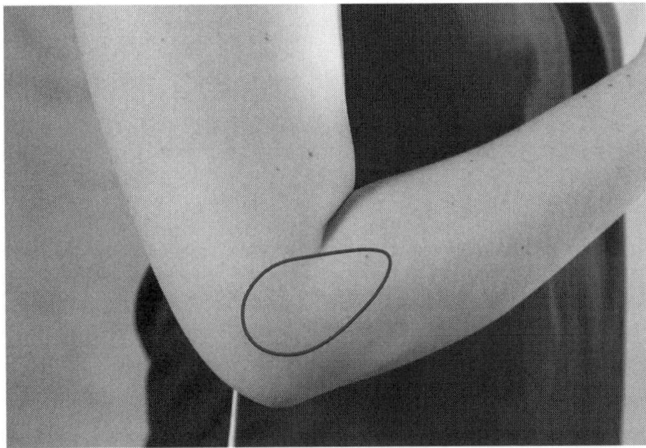

Figure 7-5: Holly Cain's area of pain.

- ______________________________
- ______________________________

2. To effectively evaluate Ms. Cain's injury, you will need to gather additional information. What questions should you ask in addition to what is presented in this scenario?

- ______________________________
- ______________________________
- ______________________________
- ______________________________

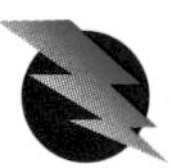

Brain Jolt

This injury can become a nagging injury if the athlete does not stay proactive in icing the area after practice and until the symptoms are under control. This injury also benefits from the use of a neoprene sleeve or strap placed over the area that reduces tension during practice.

3. Identify key terms and concepts, and then research each to broaden your knowledge of hand, wrist, and elbow injuries.

- What anatomical structures might be involved in Ms. Cain's injury?

  Answer: ______________________________
- Explain active wrist extension.

  Answer: ______________________________
- Define *edema.*

  Answer: ______________________________
- Why does Ms. Cain experience pain with wrist and elbow extension?

  Answer: ______________________________
- How is pain with extension related to the lateral epicondyle?

  Answer: ______________________________
- Why does the athletic trainer tell Ms. Cain to ice the area and then wrap it using an Ace bandage?

  Answer: ______________________________
- Why is an anti-inflammatory medication suggested to Ms. Cain?

  Answer: ______________________________
- Why is it important to know that Ms. Cain was shoveling snow before the injury occurred in relation to Ms. Cain's pain?

  Answer: ______________________________

4. Based on the information that you currently have and what was provided by your instructor, what are the possible differential diagnoses for Ms. Cain's injury?

- ______________________________
- ______________________________
- ______________________________
- ______________________________

Why or why not?

For each assessment or diagnosis, write *why?* or *why not?* statements identifying why the information is correct or incorrect. Take details from your textbook, your own research, and data from Ms. Cain's scenario to help you formulate an answer.

1. ______________________________

2. ______________________________

3. ______________________________

4. ______________________________

What do you think?

1. What is your assessment of Ms. Cain's injury?

   Answer: ______________________

2. Was your assessment of Ms. Cain's injury correct?

   Answer: ______________________

3. If not, explain what you did incorrectly and how you could have performed a better assessment.

   Answer: ______________________

STUDENT SCENARIO 3: PATRICK HOWELL

Patrick Howell is a sprinter and hurdler on a collegiate track and field team. Mr. Howell was sick before the track meet, but is no longer running a fever and is cleared by the campus physician to participate. Mr. Howell's coach places him in only two events, a sprint and a hurdle event. Before the hurdle event, he notices some fatigue. As Mr. Howell approaches his first hurdle, he realizes his legs and body feel heavy. As he jumps over the second hurdle, his trail leg catches the hurdle and he falls to the track. Most of Mr. Howell's body weight comes down onto his right wrist, forcing it into extension. His right wrist is painful, and moderate edema immediately appears over the dorsal side of the carpal bones. Mr. Howell has point tenderness on the radial side of his wrist and in the anatomical snuff box (Fig. 7-6). Radiographs do not indicate a fracture.

1. Based on the previous scenario, what do you know about Mr. Howell's injury?
   - ______________________
   - ______________________
   - ______________________
   - ______________________

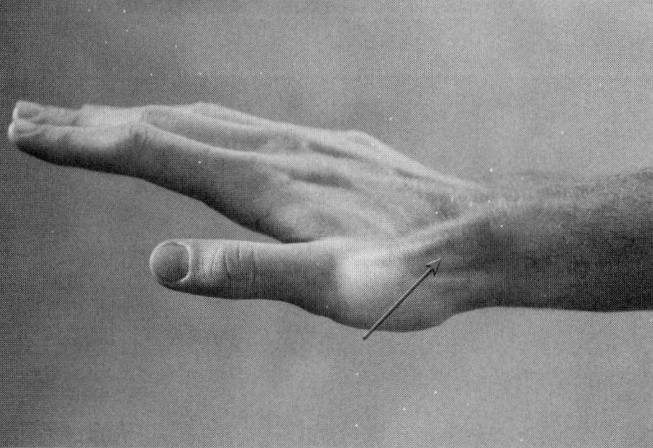

Figure 7-6: Patrick Howell's point of tenderness.

2. To evaluate Mr. Howell's injury effectively, you will need to gather additional information. What questions should you ask in addition to what is presented in this scenario?
   - ______________________
   - ______________________
   - ______________________
   - ______________________

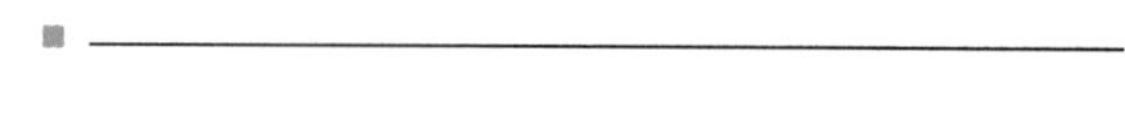

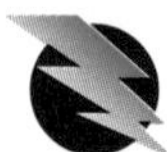

Brain Jolt
The structure in the anatomical snuff box has a low blood supply that leaves it vulnerable to necrosis and degenerative changes.

3. Identify key terms and concepts, and then research each to broaden your knowledge of hand, wrist, and elbow injuries.
   - What anatomical structures might be involved in Mr. Howell's injury?

     Answer: ______________________
   - Define *edema.*

     Answer: ______________________
   - Explain the location of the anatomical snuff box.

     Answer: ______________________
   - Define *carpal bones.*

     Answer: ______________________
   - Identify and name each carpal bone.

     Answer: ______________________
   - What is the radial side of the wrist?

     Answer: ______________________

- What does an athletic trainer palpate in the anatomical snuff box?

  Answer: ______________________

- Is there any reason to monitor Mr. Howell for a fracture even though his radiographs were negative?

  Answer: ______________________

4. Based on the information that you currently have and what was provided by your instructor, what are the possible differential diagnoses for Mr. Howell's injury?

   - ______________________
   - ______________________
   - ______________________
   - ______________________

Why or why not?

For each assessment or diagnosis, write *why?* or *why not?* statements identifying why the information is correct or incorrect. Take details from your textbook, your own research, and data from Mr. Howell's scenario to help you formulate an answer.

1. ______________________
2. ______________________
3. ______________________
4. ______________________

Treatment Detour

DETOUR

This injury, which accounts for 60% of wrist injuries, is common in active individuals. It is frequently missed or misdiagnosed, which can lead to complications. As a result, any athlete who is injured by falling on an outstretched hand should be evaluated for this particular wrist injury. Beyond a physical examination, the evaluation must include radiographs of all views of the wrist. If the radiographs are inconclusive, further diagnostic testing is warranted. It is important to remember that a diagnosis of this wrist injury is challenging, but following a good evaluation and frequent follow-up evaluations, the athlete has a low risk of complications (Tysver & Jawa, 2010).

Conversation Buffer

With this injury, there is sometimes a long waiting period before the athlete returns to play without major signs or symptoms of the injury. Some athletes do not understand that complications can arise if this injury is not treated properly. Therefore, the athletic trainer should explain the injury to the athlete with the rationale for suspending play temporarily.

What do you think?

1. What is your assessment of Mr. Howell's injury?

   Answer: ______________________

2. Was your assessment of Mr. Howell's injury correct?

   Answer: ______________________

3. If not, explain what you did incorrectly and how you could have performed a better assessment.

   Answer: ______________________

STUDENT SCENARIO 4: BEN OSTERBRACH

Ben Osterbrach is a collegiate golfer who competes in the conference finals at a course where he has been playing 18 holes every day for the last 3 days. It is important to note that Mr. Osterbrach is right handed, has improper mechanics with his golf swing, and has a history of medial epicondylitis. On the second day, Mr. Osterbrach feels occasional numbness in his left elbow that radiates down the anterior medial side of his left forearm. Today, the last day of finals, Mr. Osterbrach begins to experience soreness on the ulnar side of his elbow. When recreating his golf swing (Fig. 7-7), he feels a stress on the left elbow when releasing the right hand too early. Toward the end of the finals, Mr. Osterbrach takes a swing and feels a pop over his left elbow on the ulnar side.

1. Based on the previous scenario, what do you know about Mr. Osterbrach's injury?

   - ______________________

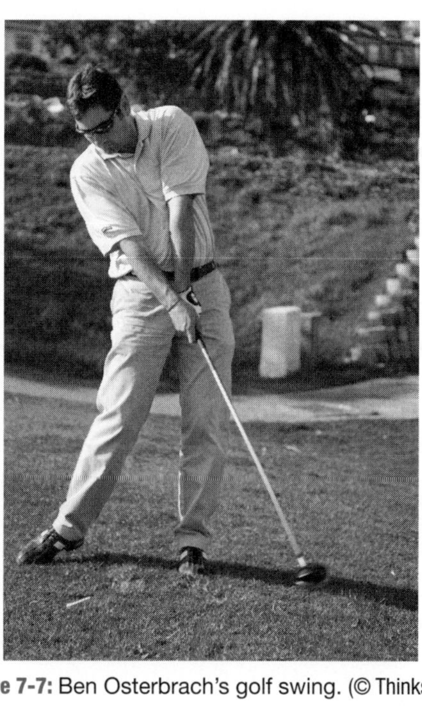

Figure 7-7: Ben Osterbrach's golf swing. (© Thinkstock)

- ______________________________
- ______________________________
- ______________________________

2. To evaluate Mr. Osterbrach's injury effectively, you will need to gather additional information. What questions should you ask in addition to what is presented in this scenario?
   - ______________________________
   - ______________________________
   - ______________________________
   - ______________________________

3. Identify key terms and concepts, and then research each to broaden your knowledge of hand, wrist, and elbow injuries.
   - What anatomical structures might be involved in Mr. Osterbrach's injury?

     Answer: ______________________________
   - Define *epicondylitis*.

     Answer: ______________________________
   - What are the signs and symptoms of epicondylitis?

     Answer: ______________________________
   - What can radiating numbness indicate?

     Answer: ______________________________
   - When Mr. Osterbrach feels stress on the ulnar side of his elbow, what structures may be stressed?

     Answer: ______________________________
   - What does a popping sensation indicate?

     Answer: ______________________________
   - Why is it important to know that Mr. Osterbrach is right side dominant?

     Answer: ______________________________

4. Based on the information that you currently have and what was provided by your instructor, what are the possible differential diagnoses for Mr. Osterbrach's injury?
   - ______________________________
   - ______________________________
   - ______________________________
   - ______________________________

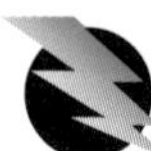

Brain Jolt

It is important to know the athlete's medical history because this provides insight into the current injury. It is also helpful to know whether the athlete is currently rehabilitating an injury, because this can lead to muscle imbalances that can increase the athlete's risk of further injury.

Why or why not?

For each assessment or diagnosis, write *why?* or *why not?* statements identifying why the information is correct or incorrect. Take details from your textbook, your own research, and data from Mr. Osterbrach's scenario to help you formulate an answer.

1. ______________________________
2. ______________________________
3. ______________________________

4. ______________________________

____

What do you think?

1. What is your assessment of Mr. Osterbrach's injury?

   Answer: ______________________________

2. Was your assessment of Mr. Osterbrach's injury correct?

   Answer: ______________________________

3. If not, explain what you did incorrectly and how you could have performed a better assessment.

   Answer: ______________________________

STUDENT SCENARIO 5: LUCY DOYLE

Lucy Doyle is a certified athletic trainer who is helping with athletic coverage at a high school lacrosse game. It rained earlier today, but ceased by game time. Ms. Doyle is called onto the field for an injured player and loses her footing on the wet grass. She braces for the fall with her left arm. As her left hand hits the ground, she feels the weight of her body shift more toward the radial side of her thumb. Her wrist forces itself into hyperextension as her weight moves proximal to the wrist and thumb, and she experiences a cracking sensation followed by extreme pain. There is a deformity of her distal forearm near the wrist (Fig. 7-8). A splint is applied, and she is transported for radiography.

1. Based on the previous scenario, what do you know about Ms. Doyle's injury?
   - ______________________________
   - ______________________________
   - ______________________________
   - ______________________________

2. To evaluate Ms. Doyle's injury effectively, you will need to gather additional information. What questions should you ask in addition to what is presented in this scenario?
   - ______________________________
   - ______________________________
   - ______________________________
   - ______________________________

Figure 7-8: Lucy Doyle's wrist.

3. Identify key terms and concepts, and then research each to broaden your knowledge of hand, wrist, and elbow injuries.
   - What anatomical structures might be involved in Ms. Doyle's injury?

     Answer: ______________________________
   - Define *radial side.*

     Answer: ______________________________
   - Define *proximal.*

     Answer: ______________________________
   - Define *distal.*

     Answer: ______________________________
   - Define *wrist hyperextension.*

     Answer: ______________________________
   - What can a cracking sensation indicate?

     Answer: ______________________________
   - How should the deformity in this scenario be splinted?

     Answer: ______________________________
   - Why is a radiograph the diagnostic test of choice for this injury?

     Answer: ______________________________

Brain Jolt
This injury gets its name because of the unique shape it forms on a radiograph.

4. Based on the information that you currently have and what was provided by your instructor, what are the possible differential diagnoses for Ms. Doyle's injury?
   - ______________________________

- ______________________________
- ______________________________
- ______________________________

2. ______________________________
3. ______________________________
4. ______________________________

Why or why not?

For each assessment or diagnosis, write *why?* or *why not?* statements identifying why the information is correct or incorrect. Take details from your textbook, your own research, and data from Ms. Doyle's scenario to help you formulate an answer.

1. ______________________________

What do you think?

1. What is your assessment of Ms. Doyle's injury?

   Answer: ______________________________
2. Was your assessment of Ms. Doyle's injury correct?

   Answer: ______________________________
3. If not, explain what you did incorrectly and how you could have performed a better assessment.

   Answer: ______________________________

STUDENT SCENARIO 6: CASEY MADISON

Casey Madison plays the position of center on his college football team. He is always catching his fingers between helmets, and other players step on his toes. As Mr. Madison tries to move past a defensive lineman, his first phalange on his right hand is smashed between two helmets. He experiences instant pain and a moderate amount of edema over the DIP and PIP joints. After the game, he is able to move the joints, but with pain. Mr. Madison notices ecchymosis developing underneath the first phalange nail bed and around the DIP joint (Fig. 7-9). When the pain subsides, there is an increase in pressure at the tip of his first phalange.

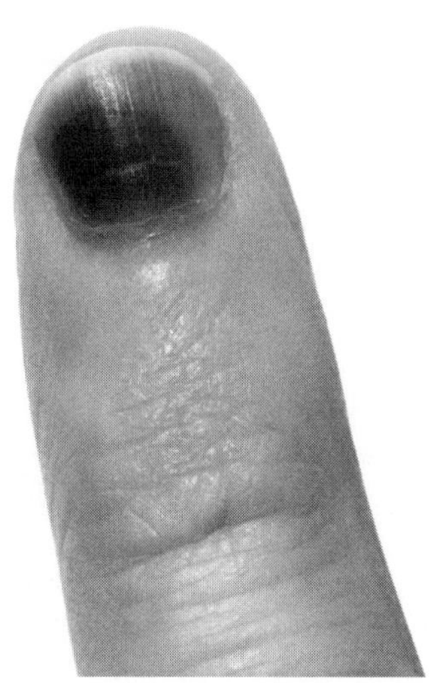

Figure 7-9: Casey Madison's finger. (© Thinkstock)

1. Based on the previous scenario, what do you know about Mr. Madison's injury?
   - ______________________________
   - ______________________________
   - ______________________________
   - ______________________________
2. To evaluate Mr. Madison's injury effectively, you will need to gather additional information. What questions should you ask in addition to what is presented in this scenario?
   - ______________________________
   - ______________________________
   - ______________________________
   - ______________________________

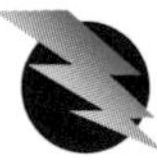

Brain Jolt
With this injury, it is common to relieve pressure by creating a hole in the nail bed.

3. Identify key terms and concepts, and then research each to broaden your knowledge of hand, wrist, and elbow injuries.
   - What anatomical structures might be involved in Mr. Madison's injury?

     Answer: ________________
   - Define *ecchymosis.*

     Answer: ________________
   - Define *edema.*

     Answer: ________________
   - Define *phalange.*

     Answer: ________________
   - What does the abbreviation *DIP* stand for?

     Answer: ________________
   - Why does Mr. Madison feel increased pressure on the tip of his first phalange?

     Answer: ________________
   - Why would a hole in the nail bed relieve pain from this injury?

     Answer: ________________
4. Based on the information that you currently have and what was provided by your instructor, what are the possible differential diagnoses for Mr. Madison's injury?
   - ________________
   - ________________
   - ________________
   - ________________

Why or why not?

For each assessment or diagnosis, write *why?* or *why not?* statements identifying why the information is correct or incorrect. Take details from your textbook, your own research, and data from Mr. Madison's scenario to help you formulate an answer.

1. ________________
2. ________________
3. ________________
4. ________________

What do you think?

1. What is your assessment of Mr. Madison's injury?

   Answer: ________________
2. Was your assessment of Mr. Madison's injury correct?

   Answer: ________________
3. If not, explain what you did incorrectly and how you could have performed a better assessment.

   Answer: ________________

STUDENT SCENARIO 7: CURTIS EDES

Today is Curtis Edes' big day at the state wrestling finals for the 145-lb weight class. He has wrestled his opponent before and is confident that he will win the match. Unfortunately, Mr. Edes' opponent pins him in the second period. Mr. Edes is furious and proceeds to the locker room, where he punches the wall with his right hand in anger. He has instant pain at the metacarpophalangeal (MCP) joints. His fifth MCP joint is point tender, and mild edema develops over his third, fourth, and fifth MCP joints. He notices a deformity on the dorsal side of his hand (Fig. 7-10), and is taken to the hospital for radiography.

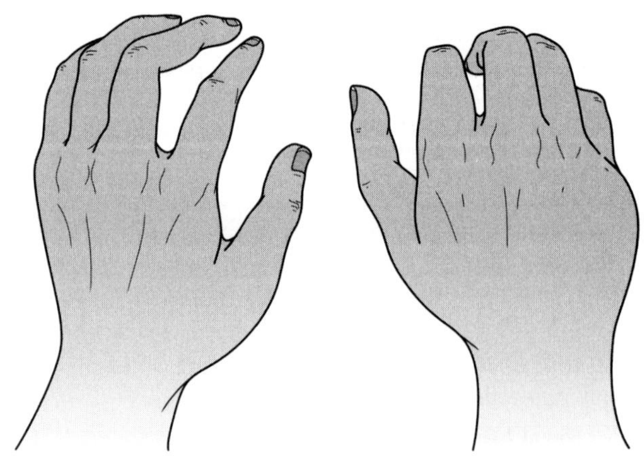

Figure 7-10: Curtis Edes' hand.

1. Based on the previous scenario, what do you know about Mr. Edes' injury?
   - ______________________________
   - ______________________________
   - ______________________________
   - ______________________________

2. To effectively evaluate Mr. Edes' injury, you will need to gather additional information. What questions should you ask in addition to what is presented in this scenario?
   - ______________________________
   - ______________________________
   - ______________________________
   - ______________________________

Brain Jolt

This injury frequently goes untreated because athletes are embarrassed to admit that they hurt themselves out of anger by punching something. If left untreated, the deformity can cause degenerative problems later in life.

3. Identify key terms and concepts, and then research each to broaden your knowledge of hand, wrist, and elbow injuries.
   - What anatomical structures might be involved in Mr. Edes' injury?

     Answer: ______________________________
   - What does the abbreviation *MCP* stand for?

     Answer: ______________________________
   - What is the dorsal side of the hand?

     Answer: ______________________________
   - What should the athletic trainer assess when the athlete has a deformity in the hand?

     Answer: ______________________________
   - Why is radiography the diagnostic test of choice for this injury?

     Answer: ______________________________

4. Based on the information that you currently have and what was provided by your instructor, what are the possible differential diagnoses for Mr. Edes' injury?
   - ______________________________
   - ______________________________
   - ______________________________
   - ______________________________

Why or why not?

For each assessment or diagnosis, write *why?* or *why not?* statements identifying why the information is correct or incorrect. Take details from your textbook, your own research, and data from Mr. Edes' scenario to help you formulate an answer.

1. ______________________________
2. ______________________________
3. ______________________________
4. ______________________________

What do you think?

1. What is your assessment of Mr. Edes' injury?

   Answer: ______________________________
2. Was your assessment of Mr. Edes' injury correct?

   Answer: ______________________________
3. If not, explain what you did incorrectly and how you could have performed a better assessment.

   Answer: ______________________________

STUDENT SCENARIO 8: CRYSTAL CREECH

Crystal Creech is a freshman goalkeeper for her high school soccer team who is learning how to cover the goal more effectively when a shot is being made. Ms. Creech blocks a corner shot on the goal and tries to catch it with both hands, but catches the ball with only her right hand. The ball hits the anterior or palm side of her right hand while forcing her right thumb into excessive abduction. She has pain and point tenderness over her first MCP joint and is not able to continue playing in the game. She did not feel a pop or crack sensation. Because she has a positive valgus test result at the MCP joint of the thumb (Fig. 7-11), she is splinted and referred to an orthopedic physician.

1. Based on the previous scenario, what do you know about Ms. Creech's injury?

- ______________________________
- ______________________________
- ______________________________
- ______________________________

2. To evaluate Ms. Creech's injury effectively, you will need to gather additional information. What questions should you ask in addition to what is presented in this scenario?

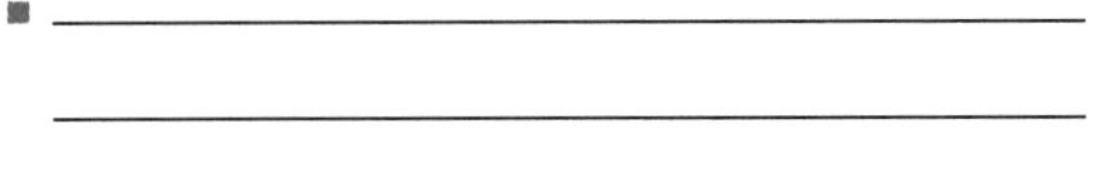

- ______________________________
- ______________________________
- ______________________________
- ______________________________

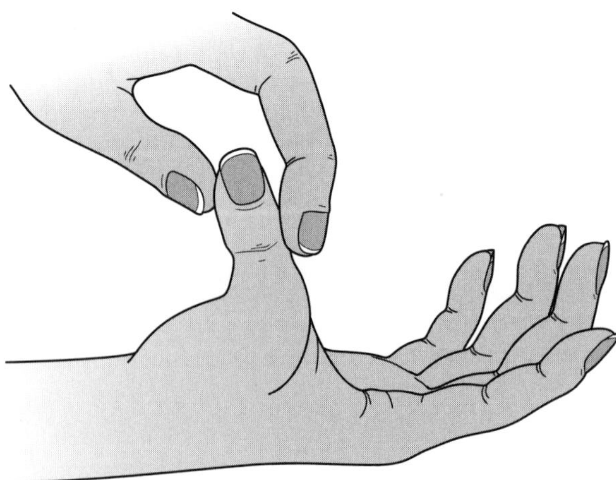

Figure 7-11: Crystal Creech's thumb.

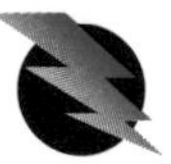

Brain Jolt

This injury is often referred to as skier's thumb or gamekeeper's thumb.

3. Identify key terms and concepts, and then research each to broaden your knowledge of hand, wrist, and elbow injuries.

- What anatomical structures might be involved in Ms. Creech's injury?

  Answer: ______________________________
- Define *thumb abduction.*

  Answer: ______________________________
- What does the abbreviation *MCP* stand for?

  Answer: ______________________________
- What is the valgus stress test of the thumb? What does it test?

  Answer: ______________________________
- How should Ms. Creech's injury be splinted?

  Answer: ______________________________
- When is it appropriate to refer an athlete to a physician, and what does this process entail?

  Answer: ______________________________

4. Based on the information that you currently have and what was provided by your instructor, what are the possible differential diagnoses for Ms. Creech's injury?

- ______________________________
- ______________________________
- ______________________________
- ______________________________

Why or why not?

For each assessment or diagnosis, write *why?* or *why not?* statements identifying why the information is correct or incorrect. Take details from your textbook, your

own research, and data from Ms. Creech's scenario to help you formulate an answer.

1. ______________________________________

____

2. ______________________________________

____

3. ______________________________________

____

4. ______________________________________

____

What do you think?

1. What is your assessment of Ms. Creech's injury?

   Answer: ______________________________

2. Was your assessment of Ms. Creech's injury correct?

   Answer: ______________________________

3. If not, explain what you did incorrectly and how you could have performed a better assessment.

   Answer: ______________________________

STUDENT SCENARIO 9: **SARAH JOHNSON**

Sarah Johnson is a field hockey player finishing her final season with the high school team before she plays in college next year. Ms. Johnson has a history of slashing (striking) players on the forearm to free the ball from her opponents. Her team is winning 3 to 2 with 1 minute left in the game. The opponent guarding Ms. Johnson has been a victim of her aggressive forearm striking in the past. As Ms. Johnson proceeds to perform a forward pass with her left arm that is holding her stick, her opponent purposely strikes her over the radius and ulna bones. Ms. Johnson feels excruciating pain. Evaluation reveals a complete loss of function and ROM in her left hand and wrist. Deformity is present (Fig. 7-12), and by the time Ms. Johnson is assisted off the field, she experiences localized edema at the midshaft of her radius and ulna bones.

Brain Jolt

It is important to handle an acute deformity correctly to ensure the athlete's safety. If the athlete cannot be moved safely, then the athlete should not be moved at all.

Figure 7-12: Sarah Johnson's arm.

1. Based on the previous scenario, what do you know about Ms. Johnson's injury?
   - ______________________________________
   - ______________________________________
   - ______________________________________
   - ______________________________________
2. To evaluate Ms. Johnson's injury effectively, you will need to gather additional information. What questions should you ask in addition to what is presented in this scenario?
   - ______________________________________
   - ______________________________________
   - ______________________________________
   - ______________________________________
3. Identify key terms and concepts, and then research each to broaden your knowledge of hand, wrist, and elbow injuries.
   - What anatomical structures might be involved in Ms. Johnson's injury?

     Answer: ______________________________

- Define *edema*.

Answer: ________________

- What types of deformities are possible with this injury?

Answer: ________________

- What might Ms. Johnson's increasing pain indicate?

Answer: ________________

- Why did Ms. Johnson experience complete loss of function and ROM?

Answer: ________________

- Ms. Johnson has a noticeable deformity. What measures should be taken to assist her off the field correctly and safely?

Answer: ________________

4. Based on the information that you currently have and what was provided by your instructor, what are the possible differential diagnoses for Ms. Johnson's injury?

- ________________
- ________________
- ________________
- ________________

Why or why not?

For each assessment or diagnosis, write *why?* or *why not?* statements identifying why the information is correct or incorrect. Take details from your textbook, your own research, and data from Ms. Johnson's scenario to help you formulate an answer.

1. ________________
2. ________________
3. ________________
4. ________________

What do you think?

1. What is your assessment of Ms. Johnson's injury?

   Answer: ________________

2. Was your assessment of Ms. Johnson's injury correct?

   Answer: ________________

3. If not, explain what you did incorrectly and how you could have performed a better assessment.

   Answer: ________________

STUDENT SCENARIO 10: MEG LUTTRELL

Meg Luttrell has been a gymnast for 10 years. She is skilled at each event, but the floor exercise is her favorite. She is learning how to do a running front tuck, which will eventually be added to her floor routine. To feel comfortable, she first performs the front tuck on a trampoline and large mat. She completes a few attempts successfully, but on her last try she has too much momentum and lands at the edge of the mat. She falls forward and puts her hands to the floor. She rotates her feet around as her left hand remains stationary on the floor. Because her hand is stationary, her left elbow is forced to torque or pivot abnormally. Ms. Luttrell feels a pop and a crack sensation and experiences immediate pain and deformity (Fig. 7-13). Ms. Luttrell has diminished sensation distal to the injury, and her pulse is faint in her left wrist. Her arm is stabilized above and below the joint while the paramedics are called. A vacuum splint is placed, and she is transported to the hospital.

Conversation Buffer

This injury typically has an obvious deformity. It is important to have someone maintain crowd control to avoid the surprising gasps from bystanders. It is also important to keep the athlete calm, because athletes may go into shock sometimes with a deformity of this nature.

1. Based on the previous scenario, what do you know about Ms. Luttrell's injury?

- ________________
- ________________
- ________________

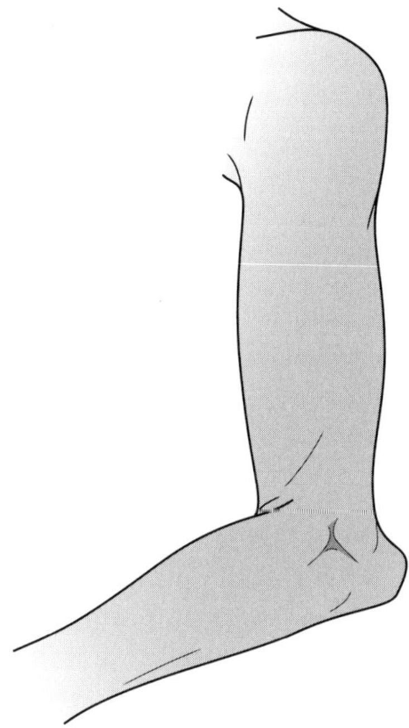

Figure 7-13: Meg Luttrell's elbow.

- ______________________________

____

2. To evaluate Ms. Luttrell's injury effectively, you will need to gather additional information. What questions should you ask in addition to what is presented in this scenario?
   - ______________________________
   - ______________________________
   - ______________________________
   - ______________________________

3. Identify key terms and concepts, and then research each to broaden your knowledge of hand, wrist, and elbow injuries.
   - What anatomical structures might be involved in Ms. Luttrell's injury?

     Answer: ______________________________
   - Define *distal.*

     Answer: ______________________________
   - What is a *vacuum splint*?

     Answer: ______________________________
   - What may a popping sensation indicate?

     Answer: ______________________________
   - What can a cracking sensation indicate?

     Answer: ______________________________
   - Why does Ms. Luttrell have diminished sensation distal to the injury?

     Answer: ______________________________
   - Why does Ms. Luttrell's pulse in her left wrist feel faint?

     Answer: ______________________________
   - Why is Ms. Luttrell's arm stabilized above and below the affected joint?

     Answer: ______________________________
   - Why are the paramedics called?

     Answer: ______________________________

4. Based on the information that you currently have and what was provided by your instructor, what are the possible differential diagnoses for Ms. Luttrell's injury?
   - ______________________________
   - ______________________________
   - ______________________________
   - ______________________________

Brain Jolt
This elbow position is referred to as a gunstock deformity.

Why or why not?

For each assessment or diagnosis, write *why?* or *why not?* statements identifying why the information is correct or incorrect. Take details from your textbook, your own research, and data from Ms. Luttrell's scenario to help you formulate an answer.

1. ______________________________
2. ______________________________
3. ______________________________
4. ______________________________

What do you think?

1. What is your assessment of Ms. Luttrell's injury?

   Answer: ______________________________

2. Was your assessment of Ms. Luttrell's injury correct?

   Answer: ______________________________

3. If not, explain what you did incorrectly and how you could have performed a better assessment.

   Answer: ______________________________

knowledge checklist

Table 7-1 offers a checklist that can be used by a peer, instructor, or preceptor to evaluate each part of a hand, wrist, or elbow assessment. Use this checklist as a tool to ensure that the evaluation is complete and to assess your knowledge of the competencies that apply to this chapter.

TABLE 7-1 ■ Hand, Wrist, and Elbow Assessment Competency Checklist

	Proficient *Can demonstrate and execute the skill properly*	**Proficient With Assistance** *Can demonstrate and execute the skill with minimal guidance or tips*	**Not Proficient** *Unable to demonstrate and execute the skill properly; need to be reevaluated at another time after further study and practice*
Athlete's Health History			
Medical history			
History of hand, wrist, or elbow injury			
Type of sport and position played			
When did the injury occur?			
Mechanisms of Injury			
How did the injury occur?			
When does the pain occur?			
What makes the pain better or worse?			
Was the athlete's hand, wrist, or elbow forced into an unusual position?			
Does the athlete experience numbness or tingling?			
Were any pops, cracks, or snaps felt or heard?			
How did the athlete's hand, wrist, or elbow look at the time the injury occurred?			
Visual Observations			
Arm carry			
Edema			
Ecchymosis			
Deformity			
Palpation			
Temperature change over the painful area, crepitus, deformity, intra-articular or extra-articular joint swelling, changes within the muscle fibers			
Medial epicondyle of the humerus			
Lateral epicondyle of the humerus			
Cubital fossa			
Olecranon process and bursa			
Radius			
Ulna			
Radial head			
Ulnar collateral ligament			
Radial collateral ligament			
Annular ligament			

Continued

TABLE 7-1 ■ Hand, Wrist, and Elbow Assessment Competency Checklist—cont'd

	Proficient	Proficient With Assistance	Not Proficient
Elbow flexor muscle group			
Elbow extensor muscle group			
Supination muscle group			
Pronator muscle group			
Wrist extensor muscle group			
Wrist flexor muscle group			
Radial styloid process			
Ulnar styloid process			
Lister's tubercle			
Eight (8) carpal bones			
Hook of the hamate			
Anatomical snuff box			
Metacarpals (1–5)			
Thenar eminence			
Hypothenar eminence			
MCP joint collateral ligaments			
IP joint collateral ligaments			
Five (5) phalanges (IP, DIP, PIP, MCP)			
ROM			
Passive or active			
Elbow flexion			
Elbow extension			
Supination			
Pronation			
Wrist extension			
Wrist flexion			
Ulnar deviation			
Radial deviation			
Finger flexion			
Finger extension			
Finger abduction			
Finger adduction			
Opposition			
Reposition			
Thumb flexion			
Thumb extension			
Thumb abduction			
Thumb adduction			
Strength			
Grade through manual muscle tests			
Elbow flexion			
Elbow extension			
Supination			
Pronation			
Wrist flexion			
Wrist extension			
Ulnar deviation			
Radial deviation			
Finger flexion			
Finger extension			

TABLE 7-1 ■ Hand, Wrist, and Elbow Assessment Competency Checklist—cont'd

	Proficient	Proficient With Assistance	Not Proficient
Finger abduction			
Finger adduction			
Opposition			
Reposition			
Thumb flexion			
Thumb extension			
Thumb abduction			
Thumb adduction			
Special Tests			
Compression test			
Tap, percussion, bump test			
Varus stress test (metacarpophalangeal, interphalangeal, and elbow joints)			
Valgus stress test (metacarpophalangeal, interphalangeal, and elbow joints)			
Tinel sign			
Hyperextension test			
Pinch grip test			
Finkelstein test			
Phalen test			
Hand elevation test			
Intercarpal glide test			
IP joint stress test			
MCP joint stress test			
Murphy sign			
Neurological			
Median nerve			
Ulnar nerve			
Radial nerve			
Biceps reflex			
Triceps reflex			
Brachioradialis reflex			
Vascular			
Radial pulse			
Capillary refill			
Final Assessment			
Sprain, strain, contusion, fracture, condition, severity			

IP, Interphalangeal; DIP, Distal Interphalangeal; PIP, Proximal Interphalangeal; MCP, Metacarpophalangeal.
*Be sure to always compare bilaterally.

REFERENCES

Amirfeyz, R., Clark, D., Parsons, B., Melotti, R., Bhatia, R., Leslie, I., & Bannister, G. (2011). Clinical tests for carpal tunnel syndrome in contemporary practice. *Archives of Orthopaedic and Trauma Surgery, 131*, 471–474.

National Athletic Training Association. (2011). *Athletic training education competencies* (5th ed.). Retrieved from http://www.nata.org/sites/default/files/5th-Edition-Competencies-2011-PDF-Version.pdf

Prentice, W. (2010). *Arnheim's principles of athletic training: A competency-based approach* (14th ed.). New York, NY: McGraw-Hill.

Starkey, C., Brown, S. D., & Ryan, J. (2010). *Examination of orthopedic and athletic injuries* (3rd ed.). Philadelphia, PA: F.A. Davis.

Tysver, T., & Jawa, A. (2010). Scaphoid fractures. *Clinical orthopaedics and related research, 468*, 2553–2555.

Venes, D. (Ed.). (2009). *Taber's cyclopedic medical dictionary* (21st ed.). Philadelphia, PA: F.A. Davis.

chapter 8

Upper Extremity: The Shoulder

chapter outline

athletic trainer's corner

Out there in the real world, one athletic trainer experienced the following:

During a surprisingly warm Saturday morning in early October I was covering a junior varsity football game. One of the running backs was sprinting down the sideline when he was tackled. He landed on the tip of his shoulder, briefly paused, and then slowly rose to his feet. He was cradling his right arm as he walked toward the sideline. As I began evaluating him, I considered possible involvement of the acromioclavicular joint or a fractured clavicle. With the help of a couple of varsity players milling on the sideline, we removed the injured athlete's shoulder pads and immediately saw an anterior dislocation of the sternoclavicular joint. I placed his arm in a sling, applied ice, and sent him to the emergency room with his parents. It was a quick reminder that you cannot assume that a typical injury has occurred based on an initial assessment. I was thankful the athlete did not experience a posterior dislocation.

Kari Terrell, MSEd, AT, ATC
Highland District Hospital
East Clinton High School
Hillsboro, Ohio

learning outcomes

After working through this chapter, you will be able to:

1. Verbalize the questions to use when obtaining a thorough medical history for an assessment.
2. Describe the principles of body movement at the shoulder and the various mechanisms of injury that affect the shoulder.
3. Compare and contrast the findings of various special tests and the role of diagnostic tests used during a shoulder evaluation.
4. Explain the medical terminology associated with the assessment of musculoskeletal injuries.
5. Verbalize the standard procedures used for a clinical evaluation of the shoulder and interpret the findings for differential diagnoses.

MODEL SCENARIO 1: JOANN HARTMAN

JoAnn Hartman is playing soccer in a weekend tournament in her hometown. She is an aggressive forward who is one of the top scorers on her team. Ms. Hartman receives the ball from a teammate and is on a fast breakaway to the goal. As she gets inside the goal box, a defender slide tackles her just before the goalkeeper gets the ball, and Ms. Hartman collides with the defender and the goalie. She hears a cracking sound and experiences immediate pain. As she leaves the field in a panic, she supports her left arm with her right hand, keeps her left arm next to her body, and rotates her head to the right side. Upon evaluation, there is a visible deformity (Fig. 8-1), no apparent edema, no ecchymosis, and mild paraesthesia in her upper left arm. Ms. Hartman has normal capillary refill on the affected side. Ms. Hartman has pain with palpation to the shoulder and clavicle and has pain with any shoulder range of motion.

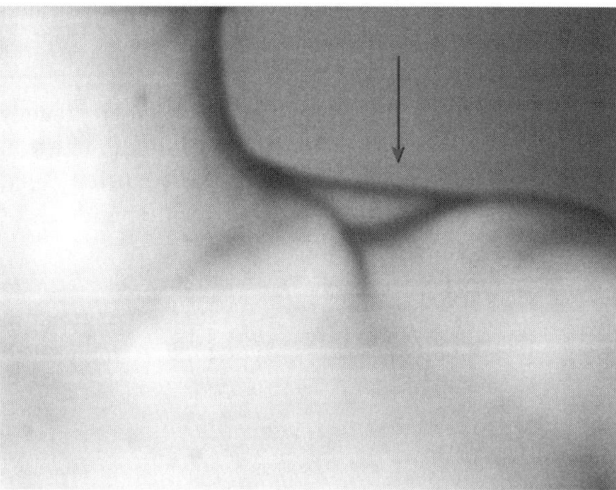

Figure 8-1: JoAnn Hartman's left shoulder. (From Starkey, C., Brown, S. D., & Ryan, J. (2010). *Examination of orthopedic and athletic injuries.* Philadelphia, PA: F.A. Davis, p. 632)

1. Based on this scenario, what do you know about Ms. Hartman's injury?
   - *Female athlete*
   - *Soccer player*
   - *Mechanism of injury: collision with two people, a possible direct hit*
   - *Pain with palpation of the shoulder and clavicle*
   - *Pain with any shoulder range of motion*
   - *Deformity present*
   - *No edema*
   - *No ecchymosis*
   - *Mild paraesthesia in the upper arm*
   - *Good capillary refill*
   - *Supports the left arm to her body with her right arm*
   - *Head is rotated to her right side*
   - *Heard a cracking sound*

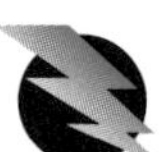

Brain Jolt
Immediately after the injury, a sling and possibly a swath are needed to take weight off the affected area.

2. To evaluate Ms. Hartman's injury effectively, you will need to gather additional information. What questions should you ask in addition to what is presented in this scenario?
   - *Is this injury a medical emergency?*
   - *Are there any preexisting injuries? If yes, what are they?*
   - *Are there any special tests that are important to perform? If yes, elaborate.*
   - *Are the results of the special tests positive or negative? What does each result indicate?*
   - *Does the athlete have any numbness?*

- *Where is Ms. Hartman's deformity located?*
- *What structures are affected by the deformity?*
- *Is there pain with range of motion of the elbow or wrist?*

3. Identify key terms and concepts, and then research each to broaden your knowledge of shoulder injuries.

- What anatomical structures might be involved in Ms. Hartman's injury?
  Clavicle
  Humerus
  Acromioclavicular (AC) joint
  Scapula
  Sternoclavicular (SC) joint
- Define *edema.*
  Swelling; a localized or general condition that causes body tissues to contain an excessive amount of fluid
- Define *ecchymosis.*
  A bruise; superficial bleeding under the skin
- Define *paraesthesia.*
  A tingling or a prickling sensation associated with an injury
- What is a capillary refill test? What does it test? What does a positive result indicate?
  The capillary refill test provides information on the quantity and quality of blood flow to the extremities. It is performed on the nail bed of the fingers and toes. The test is positive for a compromised artery when there is a markedly slow or absent return of the nail's natural color.
- Why are Ms. Hartman's carrying position and posture important to note?
  Ms. Hartman supports her left arm with her right arm. She keeps her arm close to her body, and her head is rotated to the right side. This position and posture usually indicate a clavicle fracture.
- Why would Ms. Hartman experience mild paraesthesia in her upper arm?
  Ms. Hartman could experience a tingling sensation, or paraesthesia, if the nerves in her arm are injured or if the nerves are temporarily symptomatic as a result of the trauma.
- What can a cracking sound indicate?
  A cracking sound can indicate a fracture.

4. Based on the information that you currently have and what was provided by your instructor, what are the possible differential diagnoses for Ms. Hartman's injury?
Clavicle fracture
Humeral fracture
AC separation
Shoulder dislocation

Why or why not?

For each assessment or diagnosis, write *why?* or *why not?* statements identifying why the information is correct or incorrect. Take details from your textbook, your own research, and data from Ms. Hartman's scenario to help you formulate an answer.

1. *Ms. Hartman has a clavicle fracture because her posture is typical with this injury, she heard a cracking sound, and deformity is present on the distal one-third of the clavicle. Ms. Hartman experiences pain with shoulder range of motion, which is directly related to her clavicular movement. She also has pain with palpation of the clavicle.*
2. *Ms. Hartman does not have a humeral fracture because she is point tender over the clavicle. The visible deformity is over the clavicle, not the humerus.*
3. *Ms. Hartman does not have an AC separation because the deformity is over the shaft of the clavicle and is not isolated to the AC joint. A deformity involving an AC separation appears as a raised clavicle at the AC joint (a step deformity), and not as a break in the shaft of the clavicle as with Ms. Hartman's injury.*
4. *Ms. Hartman does not have a shoulder dislocation because there is no displacement of the humeral head, and the deformity involves the clavicle.*

What do you think?

1. What is your assessment of Ms. Hartman's injury?
   Answer: *Clavicle fracture*
2. Was your assessment of Ms. Hartman's injury correct?
   Answer: *Yes*
3. If not, explain what you did incorrectly and how you could have performed a better assessment.

   Answer: ________________________________

MODEL SCENARIO 2: CHRIS PATTERSON

Chris Patterson is a freshman football player for a college team that is in the beginning of its season. To determine a baseline of each athlete's strength, the coaches have each player perform maximum weight lifts for different exercises. Mr. Patterson wants to be a starting player this season and is eager to prove that he has been training over the summer. After a few warm-up repetitions on the bench press, he is ready to lift his maximum weight. With a spotter standing by, Mr. Patterson attempts to lower the weight to his chest, but when he starts to raise the weight, he feels a pop in his chest and immediately drops the weight on his sternum and pectoral region. The spotter helps to free him from the weight, but Mr. Patterson is in immense pain. He cannot horizontally adduct his right arm and has intense pain while attempting active adduction and shoulder flexion of his right arm. On evaluation, Mr. Patterson has a deformity near his axilla and pectoral region area on his right side (Fig. 8-2).

1. Based on this scenario, what do you know about Mr. Patterson's injury?
   - *Male athlete*
   - *Football player*
   - *Mechanism of injury: maximum weight lift on the bench press*
   - *Heard a popping sound*
   - *No horizontal adduction of the right shoulder*
   - *Intense pain with right shoulder flexion and adduction*
   - *Deformity on the right side of chest, near the axilla*
2. To evaluate Mr. Patterson's injury effectively, you will need to gather additional information. What questions should you ask in addition to what is presented in this scenario?
   - *Is this injury a medical emergency?*
   - *Are there any preexisting injuries? If yes, what are they?*

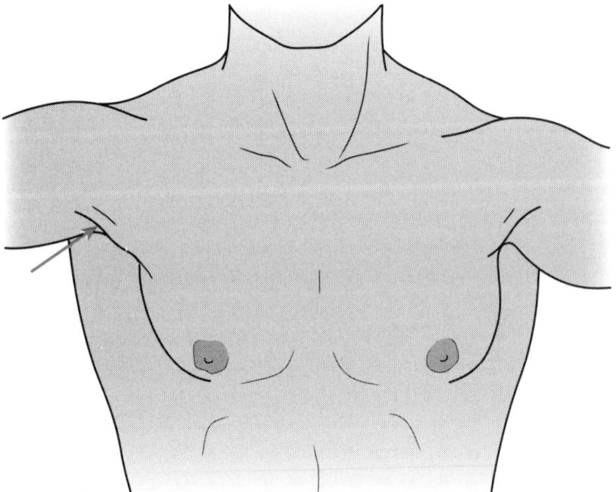

Figure 8-2: Chris Patterson's deformity.

   - *Are there any special tests that are important to perform? If yes, elaborate.*
   - *Are the results of the special tests positive or negative? What does each result indicate?*
   - *Is there any issue with his heart or lungs from the injury that might signal a serious injury?*
   - *Does the athlete have any numbness or tingling?*
   - *Is there pain with passive shoulder movements?*
   - *Is there a deformity near the glenohumeral (GH) joint?*
   - *Is edema present?*
   - *Is ecchymosis present?*
   - *Is there a palpable divot in the muscle fibers?*
   - *What is Mr. Patterson's range of motion (ROM) at the shoulder and elbow in all motions?*
3. Identify key terms and concepts, and then research each to broaden your knowledge of shoulder injuries.
   - What anatomical structures might be involved in Mr. Patterson's injury?

     Humerus
     Scapula
     Clavicle
     Pectoralis major
     Pectoralis minor
     Anterior and middle deltoid
     Biceps brachii
   - Define *horizontal adduction.*

     A directional term for movement toward the median plane of the body with the shoulder at a 90-degree angle
   - Define *axilla.*

     The armpit or underarm
   - Define *adduction.*

     A directional term for movement toward the median of the body
   - What can a popping sound indicate?

     A popping sound could indicate a muscle or ligament rupture.
   - What might a deformity in the chest indicate?

     A deformity in the chest could indicate muscle recoil after a rupture. In this case, there is a divot in the muscle fibers near the deformity.
4. Based on the information that you currently have and what was provided by your instructor, what are the possible differential diagnoses for Mr. Patterson's injury?

   Shoulder dislocation
   Pectoralis major rupture
   Coracobrachialis rupture

Why or why not?

For each assessment or diagnosis, write *why?* or *why not?* statements identifying why the information is correct or incorrect. Take details from your textbook, your

own research, and data from Mr. Patterson's scenario to help you formulate an answer.

1. *Mr. Patterson does not have a shoulder dislocation because he has a deformity on his chest, which is not near the GH joint. In addition, he has pain or lack of function only with horizontal adduction, adduction, and shoulder flexion. In a shoulder dislocation, there is no active or passive range of motion, because with a ball-in-socket joint the humeral head must be in the glenoid fossa to have motion.*
2. *Mr. Patterson has a pectoralis major rupture because he has pain and lack of function with horizontal adduction, adduction, and shoulder flexion. There is a deformity on the right side of the chest, near his axilla. Most likely, the muscle has recoiled to the muscle's origin site.*
3. *Mr. Patterson does not have a coracobrachialis rupture because there is no pain or loss of function in horizontal adduction with a coracobrachialis rupture. In addition, the deformity would appear on the arm, not the axilla and chest.*

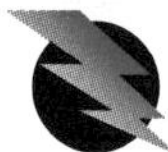

Brain Jolt

This type of injury typically occurs at the insertion point or the most movable part instead of the origin.

What do you think?

1. What is your assessment of Mr. Patterson's injury?
   Answer: *Pectoralis major rupture*
2. Was your assessment of Mr. Patterson's injury correct?
   Answer: *Yes*
3. If not, please explain what you did incorrectly and how you could have performed a better assessment.

   Answer: ____________________

MODEL SCENARIO 3: **RYAN MOORE**

Ryan Moore is a member of a collegiate swim team, and freestyle is his best stroke. The team is midway through the season, which means they are swimming a high volume each week. It is common for the team to swim 6,000 meters or more during a practice. Mr. Moore notices soreness in his shoulders after practice, but the soreness in the right shoulder does not diminish over time. Mr. Moore feels a pop when he actively takes the GH joint through full ROM. The pop sensation is painful and occurs anteriorly to the coracoid process. He has point tenderness over the coracoacromial space (Fig. 8-3). On evaluation, he has excessive passive external rotation, but limited internal rotation of the GH joint. He experiences pain with the Hawkins-Kennedy test.

1. Based on this scenario, what do you know about Mr. Moore's injury?
   - *Male athlete*
   - *Collegiate freestyle swimmer*

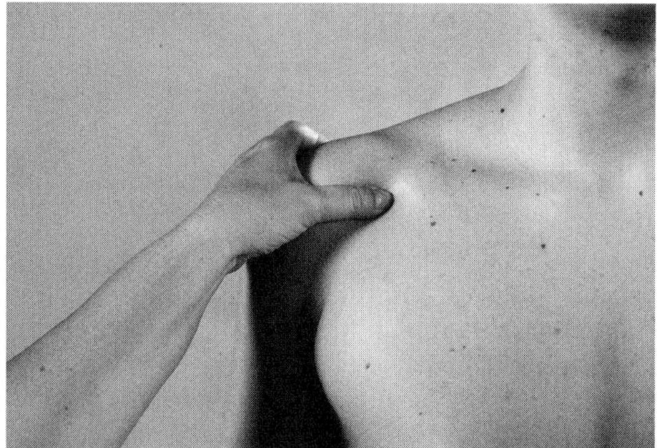

Figure 8-3: Ryan Moore's point tenderness.

   - *Mechanism of injury: chronic midseason soreness*
   - *Both shoulders sore after practice; right shoulder stays sore continuously*
   - *Popping sound heard with full active GH joint ROM*
   - *Point tender over the coracoacromial space*
   - *Excessive passive external shoulder rotation*
   - *Limited passive internal shoulder rotation*
   - *Positive Hawkins-Kennedy test result*
2. To evaluate Mr. Moore's injury effectively, you will need to gather additional information. What questions should you ask in addition to what is presented in this scenario?
   - *Is this injury a medical emergency?*
   - *Are there any preexisting injuries? If yes, what are they?*
   - *Are there any special tests that are important to perform? If yes, elaborate.*
   - *Are the results of the special tests positive or negative? What does each result indicate?*
   - *Does the athlete experience any numbness or paraesthesia?*
   - *Is edema present?*
   - *Is ecchymosis present?*
   - *What is Mr. Moore's shoulder carrying position?*
   - *What is Mr. Moore's strength and ROM at the GH joint in all motions?*
3. Identify key terms and concepts, and then research each to broaden your knowledge of shoulder injuries.
   - What anatomical structures might be involved in Mr. Moore's injury?
     Acromion process
     Clavicle

Coracoid process
Humerus
Biceps brachii tendon
GH joint
AC joint
Rotator cuff (RTC)
Biceps brachii
Subacromial bursae

- Why does Mr. Moore experience a pop sensation with full GH joint ROM?
  The thickened muscle tendons move and hit the arch with extreme ROM.
- What is done in a Hawkins-Kennedy test; what does it test; and what does a positive result indicate?
  The Hawkins-Kennedy test is done with the GH joint abducted to 90 degrees and the humerus internally rotated. It tests for RTC impingement. In a positive test result, the athlete has pain with motion, especially at the end ROM. This result indicates that the RTC, mainly the supraspinatus or the long head of the biceps brachii tendon, is impinged between the greater tuberosity and the inferior side of the acromion process.
- What is passive external rotation at the GH joint?
  This motion is performed by the athletic trainer. The GH joint is rotated laterally with the elbow joint flexed at a 90-degree angle.
- What is passive internal rotation at the GH joint?
  This motion is performed by the athletic trainer. The GH joint is rotated medially with the elbow joint flexed at a 90-degree angle.

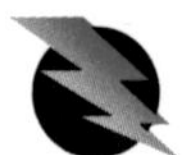

Brain Jolt
This condition can result from anatomical variation of the coracoacromial arch, muscle weakness, muscle fatigue, and restricted GH ROM.

4. Based on the information that you currently have and what was provided by your instructor, what are the possible differential diagnoses for Mr. Moore's injury?
   Glenoid labrum tear
   Shoulder impingement
   Bicipital tendonitis
   Shoulder subluxation

Why or why not?

For each assessment or diagnosis, write *why?* or *why not?* statements identifying why the information is correct or incorrect. Take details from your textbook, your own research, and data from Mr. Moore's scenario to help you formulate an answer.

1. *Mr. Moore does not have a glenoid labrum tear. Normally, a glenoid labrum tear is secondary to a dislocation or subluxation. A glenoid labrum tear does not cause a positive Hawkins-Kennedy test result.*
2. *Mr. Moore has shoulder impingement. The coracoacromial arch or space is where the supraspinatus, subacromial bursa, and the long head of the biceps brachii tendon are located. Repetitive ROM, primarily overhead activities, causes compression to the space, which causes irritation and inflammation to the involved structures. This situation leads to edema and thickening of the tendons, which decreases the space and impinges the anatomical structures involved. All these components produce a positive Hawkins-Kennedy test result.*
3. *Mr. Moore does not have bicipital tendonitis. The popping sound and point tenderness are not located over the bicipital groove where the bicep tendon is located.*
4. *Mr. Moore does not have shoulder subluxation. With shoulder subluxation, there is a feeling of instability when performing any ROM. If he had shoulder subluxation, he also would not be able to perform horizontal or overhead exercises without pain and would exhibit decreased strength.*

What do you think?

1. What is your assessment of Mr. Moore's injury?
   Answer: *Shoulder impingement*
2. Was your assessment correct for Mr. Moore's injury?
   Answer: *Yes*
3. If not, explain what you did incorrectly and how you could have performed a better assessment.

   Answer: ______________________________

STUDENT SCENARIO 1: COLTON BEAN

Colton Bean is an offensive lineman who plays left tackle on a football team. He has a history of right shoulder weakness and weak internal and external rotation of the right shoulder. He has been on a home exercise program to help increase his strength. He is participating in a blocking drill and is up against a fellow player who outweighs him by 75 lb. It is a three-person play, and as the running back runs by Mr. Bean with the ball, the defensive player tries to maneuver his way by Mr. Bean and attempts to tackle the running back. Mr. Bean is engaged with the defensive player and protects the running back when he is pushed backwards. As the defensive player makes a move to Mr. Bean's inside, Mr. Bean shifts, pushing force to the right side of his body, which puts him in a compromising position. As Mr. Bean reaches out to stop the defensive player, his right shoulder joint is externally rotated with slight horizontal abduction. Mr. Bean feels a popping and tearing sensation and intense pain. He notices a deformity at his deltoid muscle and anterior surface of his shoulder (Fig. 8-4).

Treatment Detour

A traumatic shoulder injury is often a result of a posterior force placed on an abducted and externally rotated shoulder. This injury occurs in other joints and in different directions, but it occurs most often in the shoulder, accounting for 94% to 98% of all of these types of shoulder injuries. When evaluating an athlete who experiences this mechanism of injury, be sure to palpate for this shoulder injury first, and then test the shoulder's ROM (Sims & Spina, 2009).

1. Based on this scenario, what do you know about Mr. Bean's injury?
   - ______________________________
   - ______________________________
   - ______________________________
   - ______________________________

2. To evaluate Mr. Bean's injury effectively, you will need to gather additional information. What questions should you ask in addition to what is presented in this scenario?
   - ______________________________
   - ______________________________
   - ______________________________
   - ______________________________

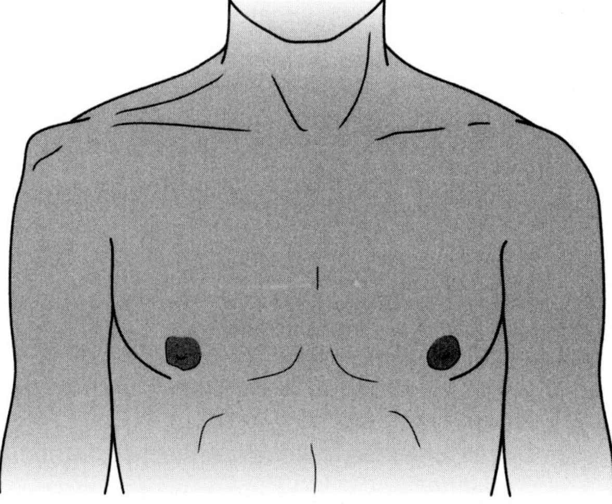

Figure 8-4: Colton Bean's shoulder.

Brain Jolt

After this injury is treated, a Bankart or Hill-Sachs lesion is identified as a complication of the trauma that could slow down the recovery process.

3. Identify key terms and concepts, and then research each to broaden your knowledge of shoulder injuries.
   - What anatomical structures might be involved in Mr. Bean's injury?

     Answer: ______________________________
   - Define *horizontal abduction*.

     Answer: ______________________________
   - Define *external rotation*.

     Answer: ______________________________
   - Where is the deltoid muscle located?

     Answer: ______________________________
   - What can a pop or tearing sensation indicate?

     Answer: ______________________________
   - Shoulder weakness can lead to what conditions?

     Answer: ______________________________
   - What are the possible explanations for Mr. Bean's deformity?

     Answer: ______________________________

4. Based on the information that you currently have and what was provided by your instructor, what are the possible differential diagnoses for Mr. Bean's injury?
   - ______________________________
   - ______________________________
   - ______________________________
   - ______________________________

Why or why not?

For each assessment or diagnosis, write *why?* or *why not?* statements identifying why the information is correct or incorrect. Take details from your textbook, your own research, and data from Mr. Bean's scenario to help you formulate an answer.

1. ______________________________

   ____

2. ______________________________

   ____

3. ______________________________

   ____

4. ______________________________

   ____

What do you think?

1. What is your assessment of Mr. Bean's injury?

   Answer: ______________________________

2. Was your assessment correct for Mr. Bean's injury?

   Answer: ______________________________

3. If not, explain what you did incorrectly and how you could have performed a better assessment.

   Answer: ______________________________

STUDENT SCENARIO 2: WILL ISAAC

Will Isaac is the starting running back on a college football team that is in a highly competitive conference. He is extremely talented, but the team has a weak offensive line as a result of senior graduations. Because of the highly competitive conference and the weak offensive line, Mr. Isaac takes numerous hard hits during every game. Before practice, Mr. Isaac sees the athletic trainer and complains of pain in his right shoulder and numbness in his right arm and hand. He states that in the middle of practice and games, his arm and hand begin to go numb. When this happens, he says that it feels like his gloves get tighter. Outside of football, Mr. Isaac says that the numbness in his arm and hand happen when he is sleeping and when he drives 3 hours home during school breaks. His strength and ROM at his shoulder and elbow are normal; however, he says that before his arm and hand go numb, he feels like his grip strength is weak. On evaluation, his grip strength is normal. The result of the Roos test is positive (Fig. 8-5).

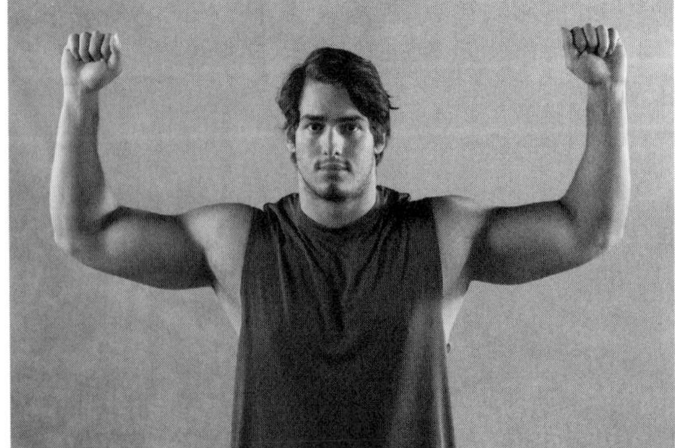

Figure 8-5: Will Isaac's test position for Roos test.

1. Based on this scenario, what do you know about Mr. Isaac's injury?

   - ______________________________

     ____
   - ______________________________

     ____
   - ______________________________

     ____
   - ______________________________

     ____

2. To evaluate Mr. Isaac's injury effectively, you will need to gather additional information. What questions should you ask in addition to what is presented in this scenario?

   - ______________________________

     ____
   - ______________________________

     ____
   - ______________________________

     ____
   - ______________________________

     ____

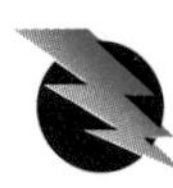

Brain Jolt

With this injury, a few anatomical structures are affected, including an artery, vein, and nerve; this results in the symptoms of this condition.

Treatment Detour

The proper assessment for this elusive, often debilitating condition is challenging because of the low accuracy rates of clinical tests and a wide range of anatomical etiology. Try to narrow down and identify the precise neurovascular structure that is involved, and refer the athlete for diagnostic tests (Nichols, 2009).

3. Identify key terms and concepts, and then research each to broaden your knowledge of shoulder injuries.
   - What anatomical structures might be involved in Mr. Isaac's injury?

     Answer: ______
   - What could be causing the numbness in Mr. Isaac's arm and hand?

     Answer: ______
   - What could be causing Mr. Isaac's gloves to feel tighter?

     Answer: ______
   - What could cause Mr. Isaac's grip strength to decrease?

     Answer: ______
   - How do repetitive hard hits have a role in this injury?

     Answer: ______
   - Why would Mr. Isaac have symptoms after waking from sleep?

     Answer: ______
   - Why would Mr. Isaac have symptoms after driving for long periods of time?

     Answer: ______
   - What is the Roos test? What does it test? What does a positive result indicate?

     Answer: ______
4. Based on the information that you currently have and what was provided by your instructor, what are the possible differential diagnoses for Mr. Isaac's injury?
   - ______
   - ______
   - ______
   - ______

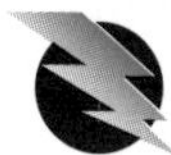

Brain Jolt

With this injury, athletes often complain of having symptoms outside of sports. Athletes often notice more symptoms while performing activities of daily living.

Why or why not?

For each assessment or diagnosis, write *why?* or *why not?* statements identifying why the information is correct or incorrect. Take details from your textbook, your own research, and data from Mr. Isaac's scenario to help you formulate an answer.

1. ______
2. ______
3. ______
4. ______

What do you think?

1. What is your assessment of Mr. Isaac's injury?

   Answer: ______
2. Was your assessment correct for Mr. Isaac's injury?

   Answer: ______
3. If not, explain what you did incorrectly and how you could have performed a better assessment.

   Answer: ______

STUDENT SCENARIO 3: ANDREW SAWYER

Andrew Sawyer is a pitcher on a baseball team. He has anterior pain in the right shoulder, which is his pitching arm. He has localized pain and edema around the bicipital groove and anterior deltoid. He states that while pitching 2 days ago he felt a popping sensation. Since then, he feels discomfort with active ROM and is unable to pitch without pain. He also comments that he feels as though he cannot throw as hard as usual. Upon evaluation, Mr. Sawyer has pain and discomfort with active forward flexion, horizontal adduction, and external rotation of his right shoulder. An O'Brien test result is positive (Fig. 8-6), and an anterior apprehension test result is negative.

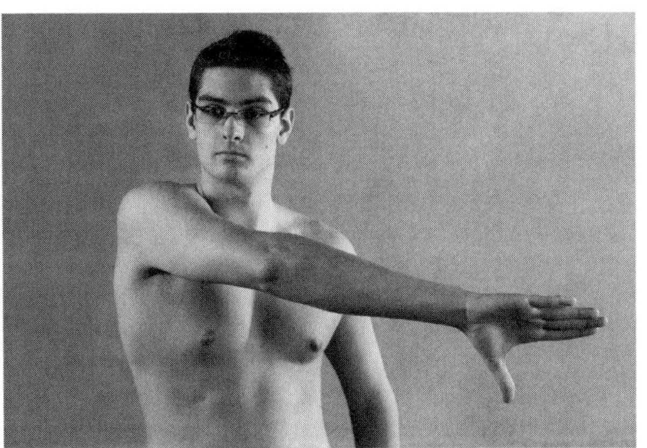

Figure 8-6: Andrew Sawyer's O'Brien test.

1. Based on this scenario, what do you know about Mr. Sawyer's injury?
   - ______________________________
   - ______________________________
   - ______________________________
   - ______________________________

2. To evaluate Mr. Sawyer's injury effectively, you will need to gather additional information. What questions should you ask in addition to what is presented in this scenario?
   - ______________________________
   - ______________________________
   - ______________________________
   - ______________________________

Brain Jolt

Similar to the knee, athletes with this injury may report experiencing a catching sensation.

3. Identify key terms and concepts, and then research each to broaden your knowledge of shoulder injuries.
   - What anatomical structures might be involved in Mr. Sawyer's injury?

     Answer: ______________________________
   - Define *edema.*

     Answer: ______________________________
   - Define *shoulder forward flexion.*

     Answer: ______________________________
   - Define *horizontal adduction.*

     Answer: ______________________________
   - Define *external rotation.*

     Answer: ______________________________
   - Where is the bicipital groove located? What lies within the groove?

     Answer: ______________________________
   - What is an O'Brien test? What does it test? What does a positive result indicate?

     Answer: ______________________________
   - What is an anterior apprehension test? What does it test? What does a positive result indicate?

     Answer: ______________________________

4. Based on the information that you currently have and what was provided by your instructor, what are the possible differential diagnoses for Mr. Sawyer's injury?
   - ______________________________
   - ______________________________
   - ______________________________
   - ______________________________

Why or why not?

For each assessment or diagnosis, write *why?* or *why not?* statements identifying why the information is correct or incorrect. Take details from your textbook, your own research, and data from Mr. Sawyer's scenario to help you formulate an answer.

1. ______________________________
2. ______________________________
3. ______________________________
4. ______________________________

What do you think?

1. What is your assessment of Mr. Sawyer's injury?

   Answer: ______

2. Was your assessment correct for Mr. Sawyer's injury?

   Answer: ______

3. If not, explain what you did incorrectly and how you could have performed a better assessment.

   Answer: ______

STUDENT SCENARIO 4: JAKE DAVIS

Jake Davis is a wide receiver on a football team. He has a history of AC joint sprains in his left shoulder. The previous sprains have been grade 1 with no deformity and have required a sling for 1 to 2 days. Mr. Davis is running a new route when a player comes from his right side and tackles him. He falls directly on his left shoulder and immediately feels pain and experiences loss of full ROM of his left shoulder. He states there is no burning sensation, but that his shoulder feels unstable. A piano key sign test result is positive, and radiographs show some deformity with the clavicle near the AC joint (Fig. 8-7).

1. Based on this scenario, what do you know about Mr. Davis' injury?
   - ______
   - ______
   - ______
   - ______

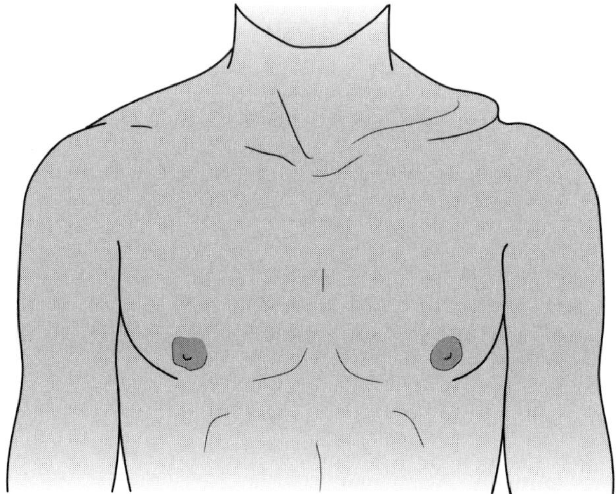

Figure 8-7: Jake Davis' shoulder.

2. To evaluate Mr. Davis' injury effectively, you will need to gather additional information. What questions should you ask in addition to what is presented in this scenario?
   - ______
   - ______
   - ______
   - ______

3. Identify key terms and concepts, and then research each to broaden your knowledge of shoulder injuries.
   - What anatomical structures might be involved in Mr. Davis' injury?

     Answer: ______
   - Where is the AC joint located?

     Answer: ______
   - What is a grade 1 AC sprain?

     Answer: ______
   - Why does Mr. Davis have full loss of movement in his shoulder?

     Answer: ______
   - Why does Mr. Davis' shoulder feel unstable?

     Answer: ______
   - What is the piano key sign test? What does it test? What does a positive result indicate?

     Answer: ______

4. Based on the information that you currently have and what was provided by your instructor, what are the possible differential diagnoses for Mr. Davis' injury?
   - ______

- ____________________
- ____________________
- ____________________

Brain Jolt

With this injury, aggressive rehabilitation should be followed to increase strength, flexibility, and ROM of the joint. Additional protective equipment should be worn over the joint when participating in sports.

Conversation Buffer

This injury has varying degrees of severity. Be sure to talk with the athlete and coach so that they understand that recovery time and return to play is determined by the severity of the injury.

Why or why not?

For each assessment or diagnosis, write *why?* or *why not?* statements identifying why the information is correct or incorrect. Take details from your textbook, your own research, and data from Mr. Davis' scenario to help you formulate an answer.

1. ____________________
2. ____________________
3. ____________________
4. ____________________

What do you think?

1. What is your assessment of Mr. Davis' injury?

   Answer: ____________________
2. Was your assessment correct for Mr. Davis' injury?

   Answer: ____________________
3. If not, explain what you did incorrectly and how you could have performed a better assessment.

   Answer: ____________________

STUDENT SCENARIO 5: PAIGE GREEN

Paige Green comes to the athletic training room with a complaint of left arm pain. She is a swimmer who is currently starting the tapering phase of her season. She states that her left shoulder is normally sore after practice, but she has recently noticed the pain radiating down into her arm. On evaluation, she has localized edema over the anterior surface of her deltoid and down into her bicep muscle, no point tenderness over the coracoacromial ligament, and mild point tenderness over the bicipital groove (Fig. 8-8). She has a positive speed's test, a 5/5 strength test result, and active resistive horizontal abduction.

1. Based on this scenario, what do you know about Ms. Green's injury?
   - ____________________
   - ____________________
   - ____________________
   - ____________________
2. To evaluate Ms. Green's injury effectively, you will need to gather additional information. What questions should you ask in addition to what is presented in this scenario?
   - ____________________
   - ____________________
   - ____________________
   - ____________________
3. Identify key terms and concepts, and then research each to broaden your knowledge of shoulder injuries.
   - What anatomical structures might be involved in Ms. Green's injury?

     Answer: ____________________
   - Define *edema.*

     Answer: ____________________

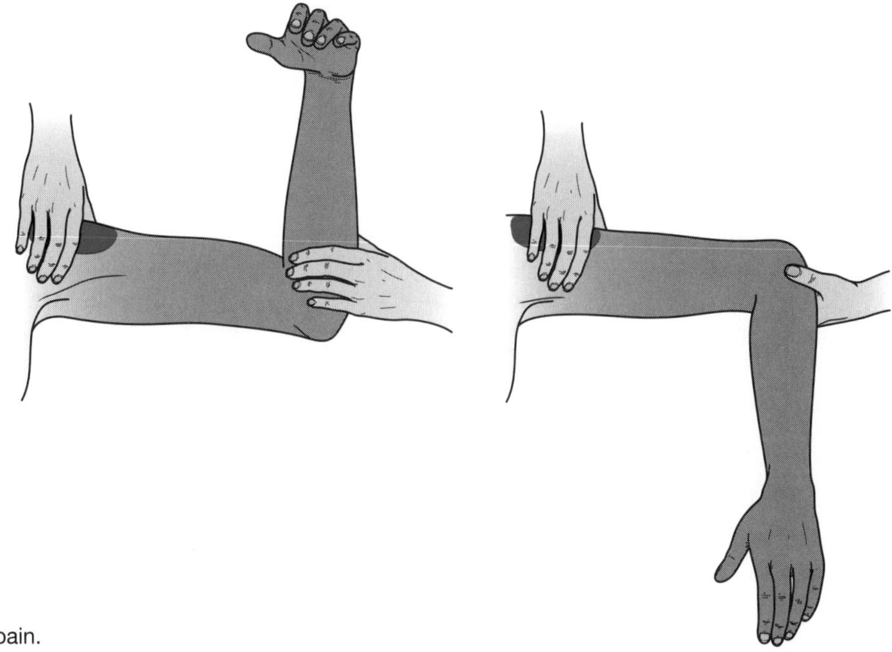

Figure 8-8: Paige Green's point of pain.

- Define *horizontal abduction.*

  Answer: ___

- Explain a tapering phase in swimming.

  Answer: ___

- Where is the coracoacromial ligament located?

  Answer: ___

- What might the pain radiating down Ms. Green's arm indicate?

  Answer: ___

- What is a speed's test, what does it test, and what does a positive result indicate?

  Answer: ___

- What does a positive 5/5 strength test result indicate?

  Answer: ___

- What are the other grades for strength?

  Answer: ___

Brain Jolt

Athletes who participate in overhead activities often develop this injury from overuse of this muscle, which is found in a special groove.

4. Based on the information that you currently have and what was provided by your instructor, what are the possible differential diagnoses for Ms. Green's injury?

- ___
- ___
- ___
- ___

Why or why not?

For each assessment or diagnosis, write *why?* or *why not?* statements identifying why the information is correct or incorrect. Take details from your textbook, your own research, and data from Ms. Green's scenario to help you formulate an answer.

1. ___

2. ___

3. ___

4. ___

What do you think?

1. What is your assessment of Ms. Green's injury?

Answer: ___

2. Was your assessment correct for Ms. Green's injury?

Answer: ___

3. If not, explain what you did incorrectly and how you could have performed a better assessment.

Answer: ___

STUDENT SCENARIO 6: AMY MCCLELLAN

Amy McClellan is a volleyball player who plays front row. This position has Ms. McClellan frequently blocking at the net and hitting from the outside. The teammate who normally substitutes for Ms. McClellan is sick, so she has played the entire game. At the end of the third match, she states that her right shoulder is sore with active ROM. Any overhead ROM or horizontal abduction greater than 90 degrees is painful. Ms. McClellan states she has pain near the deltoid muscle and has developed edema on her anterior shoulder. She has no history of problems with her shoulder, and an empty can test result is positive (Fig. 8-9).

1. Based on this scenario, what do you know about Ms. McClellan's injury?

- ____________________
- ____________________
- ____________________
- ____________________

2. To evaluate Ms. McClellan's injury effectively, you will need to gather additional information. What questions should you ask in addition to what is presented in this scenario?

- ____________________
- ____________________
- ____________________
- ____________________

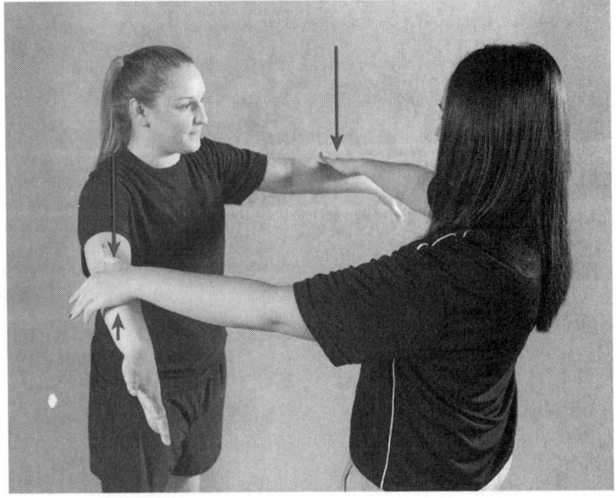

Figure 8-9: Amy McClellan's empty can test.

Brain Jolt

This muscle group is often remembered by the acronym SITS.

Conversation Buffer

Proper treatment of this injury is vital for an athlete to avoid future injury. Although this injury might not seem severe to the athlete, it is important to discuss the injury with the athlete and help him or her understand that this injury leads to weakness. It could also lead to further recurrent injuries if not treated and rehabilitated correctly.

3. Identify key terms and concepts, and then research each to broaden your knowledge of shoulder injuries.

- What anatomical structures might be involved in Ms. McClellan's injury?

  Answer: ____________________
- Define *edema.*

  Answer: ____________________
- Define *horizontal abduction.*

  Answer: ____________________
- Where is the deltoid muscle located?

  Answer: ____________________
- Why does Ms. McClellan have increased pain with ROM greater than 90 degrees?

  Answer: ____________________
- What is the empty can test? What does it test? What does a positive result indicate?

  Answer: ____________________

4. Based on the information that you currently have and what was provided by your instructor, what are the possible differential diagnoses for Ms. McClellan's injury?

- ____________________
- ____________________
- ____________________

- ______________________________

  ____

Why or why not?

For each assessment or diagnosis, write *why?* or *why not?* statements identifying why the information is correct or incorrect. Take details from your textbook, your own research, and data from Ms. McClellan's scenario to help you formulate an answer.

1. ______________________________

   ____

2. ______________________________

   ____

3. ______________________________

   ____

4. ______________________________

   ____

What do you think?

1. What is your assessment of Ms. McClellan's injury?

   Answer: ______________________________

2. Was your assessment correct for Ms. McClellan's injury?

   Answer: ______________________________

3. If not, explain what you did incorrectly and how you could have performed a better assessment.

   Answer: ______________________________

STUDENT SCENARIO 7: BILLY MALAKITE

Billy Malakite is a wrestler who has discomfort in his right arm and believes that he is unable to finish the match while pinning the opponent down. Each time he flexes his elbow and retracts his scapula, he notices a considerable strength difference in his right shoulder. Mr. Malakite states he has some shoulder irritation and pain around his ribs from a previous match in which an opponent tried to roll him onto his back. When that happened, his right arm was in full shoulder extension and horizontal abduction. The opponent extended Mr. Malakite's right arm back past his head, which put an extreme pull on his upper right rib cage. He has no history of shoulder or rib injuries. When performing a wall push-up, a deformity of a posterior structure is present (Fig. 8-10).

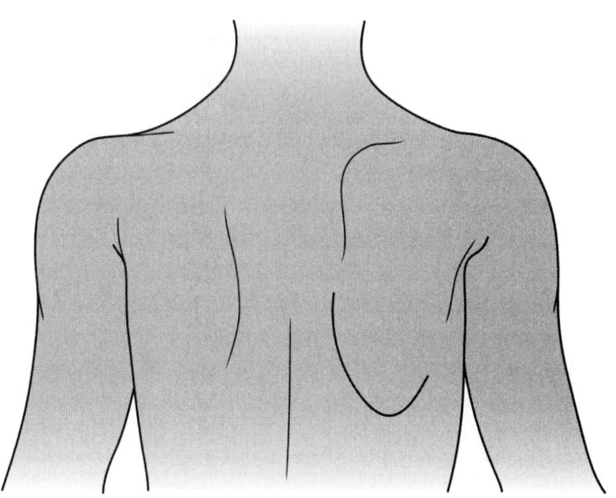

Figure 8-10: Billy Malakite's deformity.

1. Based on this scenario, what do you know about Mr. Malakite's injury?

   - ______________________________

     ____

   - ______________________________

     ____

   - ______________________________

     ____

   - ______________________________

     ____

2. To evaluate Mr. Malakite's injury effectively, you will need to gather additional information. What questions should you ask in addition to what is presented in this scenario?

   - ______________________________

     ____

   - ______________________________

     ____

   - ______________________________

     ____

   - ______________________________

     ____

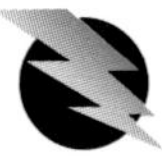

Brain Jolt

With this condition, a posterior structure of the body can appear to "fly" when performing a wall push-up. Note whether the issue appears bilaterally. This condition can be a result of nerve damage or muscular involvement.

3. Identify key terms and concepts, and then research each to broaden your knowledge of shoulder injuries.
   - What anatomical structures might be involved in Mr. Malakite's injury?

     Answer: ____________
   - Define *retract.*

     Answer: ____________
   - Define *shoulder extension.*

     Answer: ____________
   - Define *horizontal abduction.*

     Answer: ____________
   - Why does Mr. Malakite feel a pull in the upper rib cage when his right arm is extended back past his head?

     Answer: ____________
4. Based on the information that you currently have and what was provided by your instructor, what are the possible differential diagnoses for Mr. Malakite's injury?
   - ____________
   - ____________
   - ____________
   - ____________

Why or why not?

For each assessment or diagnosis, write *why?* or *why not?* statements identifying why the information is correct or incorrect. Take details from your textbook, your own research, and data from Mr. Malakite's scenario to help you formulate an answer.

1. ____________
2. ____________
3. ____________
4. ____________

What do you think?

1. What is your assessment of Mr. Malakite's injury?

   Answer: ____________
2. Was your assessment correct for Mr. Malakite's injury?

   Answer: ____________
3. If not, explain what you did incorrectly and how you could have performed a better assessment.

   Answer: ____________

STUDENT SCENARIO 8: EVA CANTY

Eva Canty throws shot put for her college track team. She states that when she throws or does a bench press, her left shoulder feels loose, as though it will "pop out." She does not remember a specific incident where she hurt her shoulder, but the feeling is occurring more frequently and appears to be progressing. On evaluation, she has positive GH joint play inferiorly, anteriorly, and posteriorly. The active range of motion (AROM) of her shoulder in all directions is good except she has excessive horizontal external rotation (Fig. 8-11) bilaterally. When nearing the end ranges of motion, she states that her shoulder feels like it could "pop out."

1. Based on this scenario, what do you know about Ms. Canty's injury?
   - ____________
   - ____________
   - ____________
   - ____________

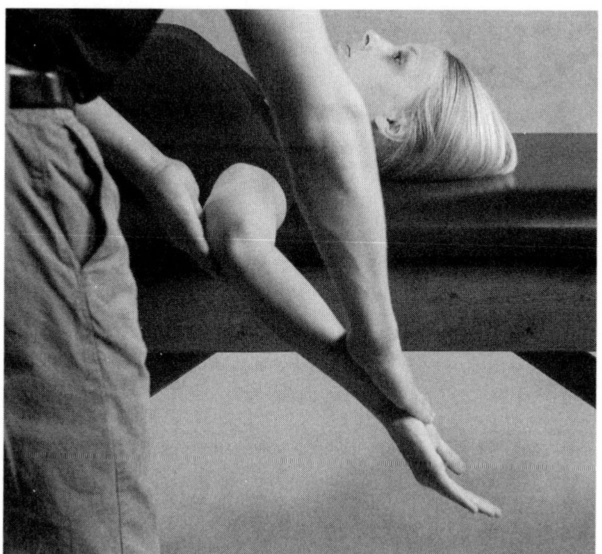

Figure 8-11: Eva Canty's horizontal external rotation.

2. To evaluate Ms. Canty's injury effectively, you will need to gather additional information. What questions should you ask in addition to what is presented in this scenario?
   - ______________________________
   - ______________________________
   - ______________________________
   - ______________________________

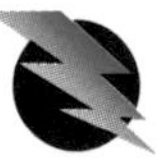

Brain Jolt

Strengthening the muscles of the shoulder joint and shoulder girdle can sometimes help this injury, but surgery is required to help permanently resolve the problem.

3. Identify key terms and concepts, and then research each to broaden your knowledge of shoulder injuries.
   - What anatomical structures might be involved in Ms. Canty's injury?

     Answer: ______________________________
   - Define *anterior.*

     Answer: ______________________________
   - Define *inferior.*

     Answer: ______________________________
   - Define *posterior.*

     Answer: ______________________________
   - Define *bilateral.*

     Answer: ______________________________
   - What is GH joint play? What does it test? What does a positive result indicate?

     Answer: ______________________________
   - Ms. Canty's shoulder feels loose, as though it will "pop out." What might this indicate?

     Answer: ______________________________
   - What might the feeling of the shoulder popping out at the end ROM indicate?

     Answer: ______________________________
   - Why is it important to note that Ms. Canty has excessive horizontal external rotation bilaterally?

     Answer: ______________________________
4. Based on the information that you currently have and what was provided by your instructor, what are the possible differential diagnoses for Ms. Canty's injury?
   - ______________________________
   - ______________________________
   - ______________________________
   - ______________________________

Why or why not?

For each assessment or diagnosis, write *why?* or *why not?* statements identifying why the information is correct or incorrect. Take details from your textbook, your own research, and data from Ms. Canty's scenario to help you formulate an answer.

1. ______________________________
2. ______________________________
3. ______________________________
4. ______________________________

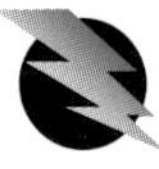

Brain Jolt

With this injury, be sure to check the bilateral laxity of other joints. This information could provide helpful insight to any additional problems the athlete may experience.

What do you think?

1. What is your assessment of Ms. Canty's injury?

   Answer: ______

2. Was your assessment correct for Ms. Canty's injury?

   Answer: ______

3. If not, explain what you did incorrectly and how you could have performed a better assessment.

   Answer: ______

STUDENT SCENARIO 9: COURTNEY TRUMAN

Courtney Truman is the goalkeeper on her school soccer team. She is defending against a shot on goal when she falls onto the tip of her left shoulder, hitting her acromion. She notices discomfort in her shoulder, but she experiences more persistent pain in her clavicle. She does not mention anything about her injury until the game is over. After the game, she has pain with active horizontal abduction and is unable to perform horizontal adduction without intense pain at the clavicle. She also has localized edema and a slight deformity over the left sternoclavicular (SC) joint when compared bilaterally (Fig. 8-12).

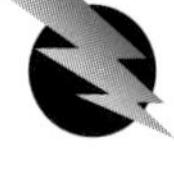

Brain Jolt

This injury is uncommon, but once this area is injured, it behaves like a sprained ankle and recurs easily.

1. Based on this scenario, what do you know about Ms. Truman's injury?
   - ______
   - ______
   - ______
   - ______

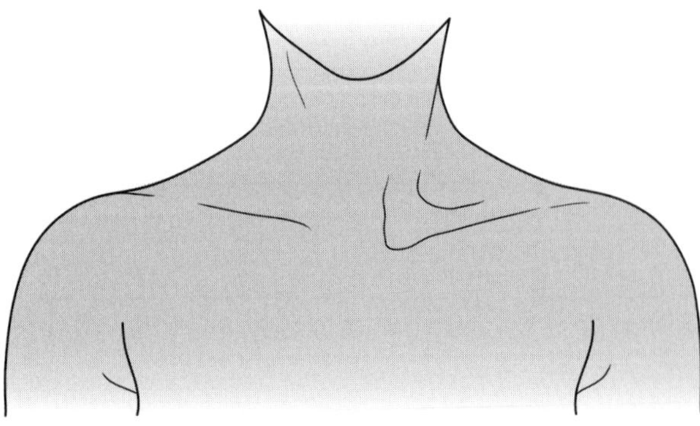

Figure 8-12: Courtney Truman's SC joint.

2. To evaluate Ms. Truman's injury effectively, you will need to gather additional information. What questions should you ask in addition to what is presented in this scenario?
   - ______
   - ______
   - ______
   - ______

3. Identify key terms and concepts, and then research each to broaden your knowledge of shoulder injuries.
   - What anatomical structures might be involved in Ms. Truman's injury?

     Answer: ______
   - Define *horizontal abduction.*

     Answer: ______
   - Define *deformity.*

     Answer: ______
   - Define *horizontal adduction.*

     Answer: ______
   - Define *edema.*

     Answer: ______
   - Define *bilateral.*

     Answer: ______
   - Where is the SC joint located?

     Answer: ______

- Why does Ms. Truman experience pain in the clavicle with movement?

  Answer: ______

4. Based on the information that you currently have and what was provided by your instructor, what are the possible differential diagnoses for Ms. Truman's injury?

   - ______
   - ______
   - ______
   - ______

Why or why not?

For each assessment or diagnosis, write *why?* or *why not?* statements identifying why the information is correct or incorrect. Take details from your textbook, your own research, and data from Ms. Truman's scenario to help you formulate an answer.

1. ______
2. ______
3. ______
4. ______

What do you think?

1. What is your assessment of Ms. Truman's injury?

   Answer: ______

2. Was your assessment correct for Ms. Truman's injury?

   Answer: ______

3. If not, explain what you did incorrectly and how you could have performed a better assessment.

   Answer: ______

STUDENT SCENARIO 10: MCKENZIE HUFF

McKenzie Huff is a pole-vaulter on her high school track team. It rained just before practice, causing the track's surface to be slippery. On her last jump, as Ms. Huff is forced up and over the bar, her pole slips on the stopper, causing her body to shift in a different direction when traveling over the bar. She is angled on her right side and, without thinking, extends her right arm out to catch her fall onto the mat. She feels a pop and crack sensation in her upper arm. There is intense pain and immediate development of effusion at her humerus and around the deltoid region (Fig. 8-13). She is unable to extend her arm and has a diminished radial pulse. Her arm is stabilized, and the paramedics are called.

1. Based on this scenario, what do you know about Ms. Huff's injury?

   - ______
   - ______
   - ______
   - ______

2. To evaluate Ms. Huff's injury effectively, you will need to gather additional information. What questions should you ask in addition to what is presented in this scenario?

   - ______
   - ______
   - ______
   - ______

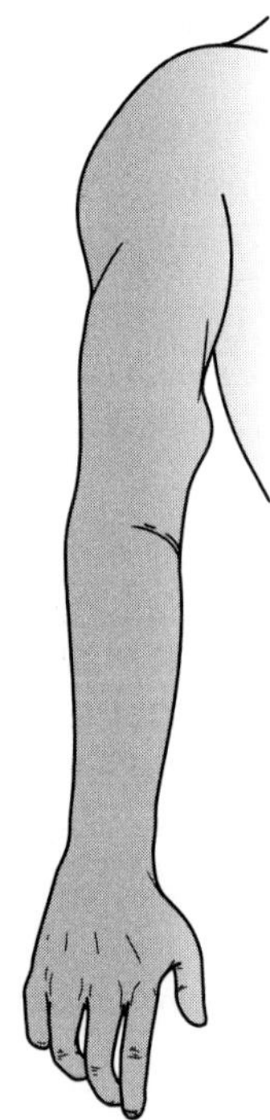

Figure 8-13: McKenzie Huff's humerus fracture.

3. Identify key terms and concepts, and then research each to broaden your knowledge of shoulder injuries.
   - What anatomical structures might be involved in Ms. Huff's injury?

     Answer: ______________________
   - Define *effusion.*

     Answer: ______________________
   - What might a pop and crack sensation indicate?

     Answer: ______________________
   - Where is the radial pulse located?

     Answer: ______________________
   - What does a diminished radial pulse indicate?

     Answer: ______________________
   - Why is Ms. Huff unable to extend her arm? What could this indicate?

     Answer: ______________________
   - Why are the emergency paramedics called?

     Answer: ______________________
   - Why is it important to become familiar with pole-vaulting?

     Answer: ______________________
4. Based on the information that you currently have and what was provided by your instructor, what are the possible differential diagnoses for Ms. Huff's injury?
   - ______________________
   - ______________________
   - ______________________
   - ______________________

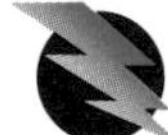

Brain Jolt

Always remember the importance that the epiphyseal plate has on an athlete's growth and development.

Why or why not?

For each assessment or diagnosis, write *why?* or *why not?* statements identifying why the information is correct or incorrect. Take details from your textbook, your own research, and data from Ms. Huff's scenario to help you formulate an answer.

1. ______________________
2. ______________________
3. ______________________
4. ______________________

What do you think?

1. What is your assessment of Ms. Huff's injury?

   Answer: ______________________
2. Was your assessment correct for Ms. Huff's injury?

   Answer: ______________________
3. If not, explain what you did incorrectly and how you could have performed a better assessment.

   Answer: ______________________

Conversation Buffer

Sometimes the drive to improve and win impedes a coach's vision of proper training conditions for the athletes. Remember to educate coaches about proper safety, and point out the potential risks weather can pose to a sporting event.

knowledge checklist

Table 8-1 offers a checklist that can be used by a peer, instructor, or preceptor to evaluate each part of a shoulder assessment. Use this checklist as a tool to ensure that the evaluation is complete and to assess your knowledge of the competencies that apply to this chapter.

TABLE 8-1 ■ Shoulder Assessment Competency Checklist

	Proficient *Can demonstrate and execute the skill properly*	**Proficient With Assistance** *Can demonstrate and execute the skill with minimal guidance or tips*	**Not Proficient** *Unable to demonstrate and execute the skill properly; need to be reevaluated at another time after further study and practice*
Athlete's Health History			
Medical history			
History of shoulder injury			
Type of sport and position played			
When did the injury occur?			
Mechanisms of Injury			
How did the injury occur?			
When does the pain occur?			
What makes the pain better or worse?			
Was the athlete's arm or shoulder forced into an unusual position?			
Is the athlete experiencing numbness or tingling?			
Were any pops, cracks, or snaps felt or heard?			
How did the athlete's arm and shoulder look at the time the injury occurred?			
Visual Observations			
Arm carry			
Edema			
Ecchymosis			
Deformity			
Head position			
Palpation			
Temperature change over the painful area, crepitus, deformity, intra-articular or extra-articular joint swelling, changes within the muscle fibers			
Jugular notch			
Sternoclavicular joint			
Clavicle			
Acromion process			
Acromioclavicular joint			
Coracoid process			
Humeral head			
Great tuberosity of the humerus			
Lesser tuberosity of the humerus			
Bicipital groove			
Humerus			
Pectoralis major			
Pectoralis minor			
Coracobrachialis			

Continued

TABLE 8-1 ■ Shoulder Assessment Competency Checklist—cont'd

	Proficient	Proficient With Assistance	Not Proficient
Deltoid			
Spine of scapula			
Superior angle of scapula			
Inferior angle of scapula			
Rotator cuff			
Teres major			
Rhomboids			
Levator scapulae			
Trapezius			
Latissimus dorsi			
Triceps brachii			
Range of Motion			
Passive or active			
Flexion			
Extension			
Abduction			
Horizontal abduction			
Adduction			
Horizontal adduction			
Internal rotation			
Horizontal internal rotation			
External rotation			
Horizontal external rotation			
Scapular retraction			
Scapular protraction			
Scapular elevation			
Scapular depression			
Scapular upward rotation			
Scapular downward rotation			
Strength			
Grade through manual muscle tests			
Flexion			
Extension			
Abduction			
Horizontal abduction			
Adduction			
Horizontal adduction			
Internal rotation			
Horizontal internal rotation			
External rotation			
Horizontal external rotation			
Scapular retraction			
Scapular protraction			
Scapular elevation			
Scapular depression			
Scapular upward rotation			
Scapular downward rotation			

TABLE 8-1 ■ Shoulder Assessment Competency Checklist—cont'd

	Proficient	Proficient With Assistance	Not Proficient
Special Tests			
Apley scratch test			
Empty can (Jobe) test			
Hawkins-Kennedy test			
Sulcus sign			
Speed's test			
Drop arm test			
Yergason test			
Neer test			
Clunk test			
Anterior apprehension test/crank test			
Posterior apprehension test/crank test			
GH translation/joint play anterior, inferior, posterior			
Sternoclavicular joint stress test			
Piano key sign			
Compression-rotation (grind) test			
Adson test			
Allen test			
O'Brien test			
Roos test			
Neurological			
Brachial plexus			
Biceps reflex			
Triceps reflex			
Brachioradialis reflex			
Vascular			
Radial pulse			
Brachial pulse			
Capillary refill			
Final Assessment			
Sprain, strain, contusion, fracture, condition, severity			

*Be sure to always compare bilaterally.

REFERENCES

National Athletic Training Association. (2011). *Athletic training education competencies* (5th ed.). Retrieved from http://www.nata.org/sites/default/files/5th-Edition-Competencies-2011-PDF-Version.pdf

Nichols, A. (2009). Diagnosis and management of thoracic outlet syndrome. *Current Sports Medicine Reports, 8*, 240–249.

Prentice, W. (2010). *Arnheim's principles of athletic training: A competency-based approach* (14th ed.). New York, NY: McGraw-Hill.

Sims, K., & Spina, A. (2009). Traumatic anterior shoulder dislocation: A case study of nonoperative management in mixed martial arts athlete. *The Journal of the Canadian Chiropractic Association, 53*, 261–271.

Starkey, C., Brown, S. D., & Ryan, J. (2010). Examination of orthopedic and athletic injuries (3rd ed.). Philadelphia, PA: F.A. Davis.

Venes, D. (Ed.). (2009). *Taber's cyclopedic medical dictionary* (21st ed.). Philadelphia, PA: F.A. Davis.

chapter 9

The Head, Neck, and Trunk

chapter outline

athletic trainer's corner

Out there in the real world, one athletic trainer experienced the following:

Late in the afternoon in mid-January at the finals of a middle school wrestling invitational, a 128-lb wrestler's headgear slipped down around his neck. The official stopped the match and called for an injury time out. While evaluating the young wrestler, I noticed that he was having difficulty catching his breath and he said that he was "a little dizzy." Being the typical athlete, he was furious with me when I defaulted him in the finals, because he was sure that he could continue with the match. After monitoring him briefly, his signs and symptoms did not improve. When he tried to take a drink of sports drink, I could hear a clicking sound and he could not swallow. Immediately, I notified the athlete's parents and coaches that he needed to be taken to the emergency department. After radiographic imaging, a fracture of the hyoid bone was diagnosed, which is an injury normally seen only with hangings and strangulation cases. Luckily, the young man's condition was stabilized and he was sent to a children's hospital, where he was monitored and treated. His season was finished, but he was allowed to return to wrestling the next season.

Mindy Smith, MS, AT, ATC, PTA
Drayer Physical Therapy Institute
Head Athletic Trainer, Wilmington High School
Physical Therapy Assistant
Wilmington, Ohio

learning outcomes

After working through this chapter, you will be able to:

1. Verbalize the questions to use when obtaining a thorough medical history for an assessment.
2. Describe the principles of body movement at the head, neck, and trunk and the various mechanisms of injury that affect the head, neck, and trunk.
3. Compare and contrast the findings of various special tests and the role of diagnostic tests used during a head, neck, and trunk evaluation.
4. Explain the medical terminology associated with the assessment of musculoskeletal injuries.
5. Verbalize the standard procedures used for a clinical evaluation of the head, neck, and trunk and interpret the findings for differential diagnoses

MODEL SCENARIO 1: **DEBRA ROSS**

Debra Ross is a soccer player who is playing midfield and confronts another female player for a head ball. The two girls collide in midair while fighting for a line-driven ball from the defensive sweeper. Ms. Ross makes contact with the ball, but with poor form. As a result, the ball hits her head more anteriorly and forces her neck to go farther into extension (Fig. 9-1). She finishes the first half of the game, which has approximately 7 minutes left to play; however, at halftime she complains of neck pain and stiffness while performing active neck range of motion (ROM). She is point tender, bilaterally, on the lateral sides of the neck. Her passive ROM is good, but she has limited active ROM motion with flexion, extension, and rotation of the neck with pain.

1. Based on this scenario, what do you know about Ms. Ross' injury?
   - *Female athlete*
   - *Soccer player*
   - *Mechanism of injury: forced neck extension from a poorly headed soccer ball*
   - *Neck pain and stiffness*
   - *Point tender bilaterally on the lateral side of the neck*
   - *Good PROM in all directions*
   - *Limited active ROM in flexion, extension, and rotation of the neck with pain*

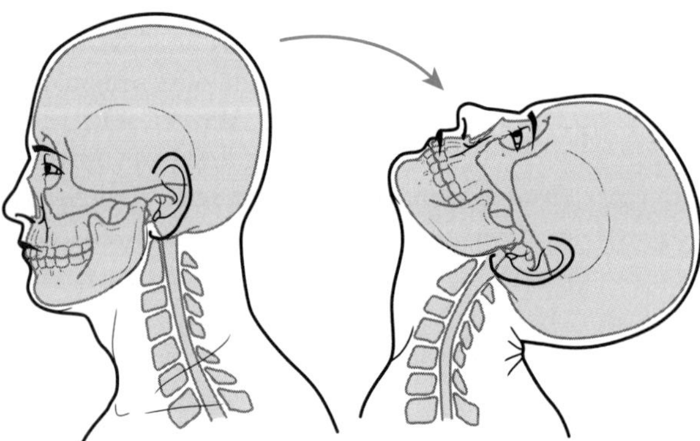

Figure 9-1: Debra Ross' neck motion.

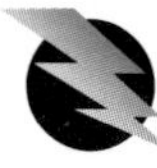

Brain Jolt

This muscle is commonly referred to as the whiplash muscle.

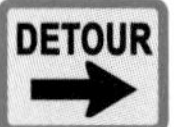

Treatment Detour

Whiplash is usually triggered by an accident, motor vehicle or sport related, involving an acceleration-deceleration mechanism. The goal for an evaluation is to determine nervous system involvement and rule out fractures. Research shows that magnetic resonance imaging is not useful in diagnosing whiplash unless significant neurologic symptoms are present or a fracture is suggested. Therefore, when whiplash is suggested, performing a full range of clinical evaluations is important to pinpoint the source of the pain. Hopefully this evaluation provides sufficient information to determine whether further interventions are needed (van Suijlekom et al., 2010).

2. To evaluate Ms. Ross' injury, you will need to gather additional information. What questions should you ask in addition to what is presented in this scenario?
   - *Is this injury a medical emergency?*
   - *Are there any preexisting injuries? If yes, what are they?*
   - *Are there any special tests that are important to perform? If yes, elaborate.*
   - *Are the results of the special tests positive or negative? What does each result indicate?*
   - *Does the athlete have any numbness or tingling?*
   - *Is edema present?*
   - *Is ecchymosis present?*
   - *Does the athlete have pain at the vertebral column?*

- *Does the athlete have pain along the spinous processes?*
- *Does the athlete have any symptoms of a concussion?*

3. Identify key terms and concepts, and then research each to broaden your knowledge of head, neck, and trunk injuries.
   - What anatomical structures might be involved in Ms. Ross' injury?
     Sternocleidomastoid
     Cervical vertebrae
     Cranium
   - Define *bilateral*.
     Affecting two or both sides
   - What are the symptoms of a concussion?
     Symptoms of a concussion include headache, dizziness, blurred vision, nausea, tinnitus, impaired coordination, impaired balance, impaired memory, nystagmus, photophobia, and tinnitus.
   - What is proper form for a head ball in soccer?
     A person should be centered in front of the ball, make contact with the ball just proximal to the center of the head, and use the neck muscles to change the direction of the soccer ball. Allowing the ball to hit anteriorly on the forehead can result in injury.
   - What is the meaning of the abbreviation *PROM*?
     Passive range of motion
   - Why is Ms. Ross point tender bilaterally on the lateral side of the neck?
     Ms. Ross is point tender because that is where the sternocleidomastoid (SCM) runs on both sides. This muscle flexes the neck when contracted bilaterally and rotates and laterally flexes the neck when used unilaterally.
   - Why is Ms. Ross' PROM good?
     There typically is no pain when a muscle is moved passively because the evaluator is moving the neck; therefore, there is no muscle contraction to cause pain.
   - Why would there be a possible injury to a neck flexor when the head was forced into extension?
     When there is an unexpected forced action, the muscle contracts to limit the motion; this is a protection mechanism.
4. Based on the information that you currently have and what was provided by your instructor, what are the possible differential diagnoses for Ms. Ross' injury?
   Cervical fracture
   SCM strain
   Concussion

Why or why not?

For each assessment or diagnosis, write *why?* or *why not?* statements identifying why the information is correct or incorrect. Take details from your textbook, your own research, and data from Ms. Ross' scenario to help you formulate an answer.

1. *Ms. Ross does not have a cervical fracture because she does not report any tenderness on the cervical vertebrae. The cervical compression test and the Spurling test are both negative for a fracture.*
2. *Ms. Ross has a SCM strain because she is point tender over the muscle bilaterally. She has pain with neck extension from the stretching of the SCM and pain with flexion and rotation, which is the main action of this muscle. The mechanism of injury of forced extension elicits a muscle contraction leading to a strained muscle.*
3. *Ms. Ross does not have a concussion because she does not exhibit any concussion symptoms.*

What do you think?

1. What is your assessment of Ms. Ross' injury?
   Answer: *SCM strain or whiplash*
2. Was your assessment of Ms. Ross' injury correct?
   Answer: *Yes*
3. If not, please explain what you did incorrectly and how you could have performed a better assessment.

   Answer: ________________________________

MODEL SCENARIO 2: BECKY HONISCH

Becky Honisch, a basketball player, is playing in the conference championship game. The score is close, and the game is getting aggressive. The ball is tipped by Ms. Honisch's teammate; in hopes of keeping it inbounds, Ms. Honisch dives toward the ball (Fig. 9-2). In the process of flipping the ball back inbounds, she hits the back of her head on the court. Ms. Honisch hesitates a bit before getting up, but runs a few more plays before asking to be "subbed out." The athletic trainer uses the sideline concussion assessment tool (SCAT) to evaluate Ms. Honisch. She reports a mild headache and mild photophobia, and she states that she was a bit dizzy while on the court but is currently no longer dizzy. She has no nystagmus or nausea, and her balance, coordination, and memory are normal. At her 15-minute recheck, her symptoms are improving and she has developed no new symptoms. At her 30-minute recheck, all symptoms are gone. Upon reevaluation the next day, she remains asymptomatic.

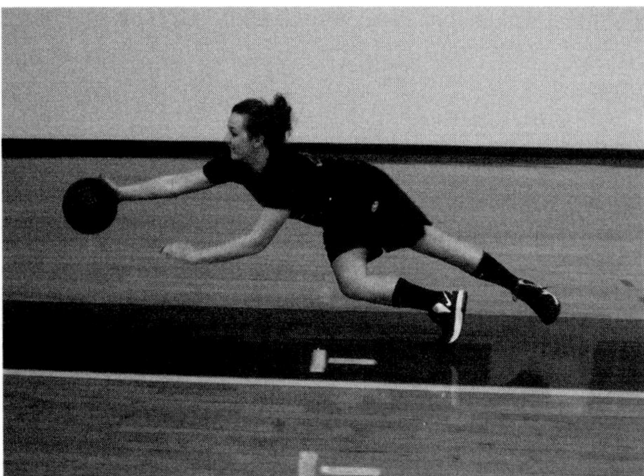

Figure 9-2: Becky Honisch's dive.

1. Based on this scenario, what do you know about Ms. Honisch's injury?
   - *Female athlete*
   - *Basketball player*
   - *Mechanism of injury: diving for the ball and hitting the back of the head on the court*
   - *Mild headache*
   - *Mild photophobia*
   - *Dizzy while on the court but is not currently*
   - *No nystagmus*
   - *No nausea*
   - *Normal balance, coordination, and memory*
   - *Symptoms are improving after 15 min, and are gone after 30 min*
2. To evaluate Ms. Honisch's injury effectively, you will need to gather additional information. What questions should you ask in addition to what is presented in this scenario?
   - *Is this injury a medical emergency?*
   - *Are there any preexisting injuries? If yes, what are they?*
   - *Are there any special tests that are important to perform? If yes, elaborate.*
   - *Are the results of the special tests positive or negative? What does each indicate?*
   - *Does the athlete have any numbness or tingling?*
   - *Is tinnitus present?*
   - *Are the pupils equal and reactive?*
   - *Are the cranial nerves normal?*
   - *Is there any point tenderness on the skull?*
   - *Is crepitus or blood present?*
3. Identify key terms and concepts, and then research each to broaden your knowledge of head, neck, and trunk injuries.
   - What anatomical structures might be involved in Ms. Honisch's injury?
     Cranium, skull
     Brain
     Cranial nerves
   - What are the signs and symptoms of a concussion?
     Symptoms of a concussion include headache, dizziness, blurred vision, nausea, tinnitus, impaired coordination, impaired balance, impaired memory, nystagmus, photophobia, and tinnitus.
   - Define *photophobia.*
     Unusual sensitivity to light
   - Define *nystagmus.*
     Abnormal eye tracking; eye tends to skip when tracking
   - Have Ms. Honisch's balance, coordination, and memory been tested?
     Yes, using a SCAT for a quantitative score.
   - Why was Ms. Honisch rechecked after 15 min and then again after 30 min?
     It is important to recheck concussion symptoms every 15 min to ensure that the athlete does not develop new symptoms, or to ensure the current symptoms do not become worse. If symptoms worsen, they could be a sign of an epidural or subdural hematoma.

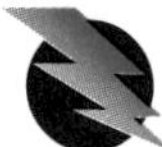

Brain Jolt

Because of the importance of rechecking concussion symptoms to rule out more serious injuries, it is best not to allow the athlete to take any pain medication that could mask new symptoms until you are certain that concussion symptoms are not present.

4. Based on the information that you currently have and what was provided by your instructor, what are the possible differential diagnoses for Ms. Honisch's injury?
   Concussion
   Subdural hematoma
   Skull fracture

Why or why not?

For each assessment or diagnosis, write *why?* or *why not?* statements identifying why the information is correct or incorrect. Take details from your textbook, your own research, and data from Ms. Honisch's scenario to help you formulate an answer.

1. *Ms. Honisch has a concussion because she has a few mild symptoms, such as headache, photophobia, and dizziness, which according to the Zurich Statement are all symptoms of a concussion. Her SCAT score for a concussion is good, and her symptoms improved after 15 min and subsided within 30 min.*
2. *Ms. Honisch does not have a subdural hematoma because her symptoms improved; her symptoms never lingered or became more severe.*
3. *Ms. Honisch does not have a skull fracture because she does not have any deformity or crepitus on her skull.*

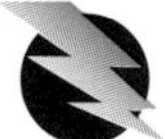

Brain Jolt

Remember, every athlete reacts differently to a concussion. Conducting proper tests is important, and having baseline tests available for all your athletes is helpful to compare to the current evaluation.

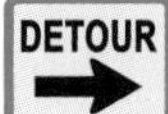

Treatment Detour

In a prospective study over 11 years, concussion data were collected at 25 high schools in a large public school system. The findings showed that concussions have an incidence rate of 0.24 per 1,000 athletes. Boys' sports account for 75% of all concussions, and football has the highest incidence rate, accounting for half of these concussions. However, girls' soccer has the most concussions for a girls' sport, and the second highest incidence rate for all the sports studied. The study found that the concussion incidence rate increased 15.5% annually, and it increased in all sports. Therefore, proper training on the detection, treatment, and prevention of concussions is important. Education should not be limited to sports that are thought to have traditionally high concussion risks, because concussions occur in all sports (Lincoln et al., 2011).

What do you think?

1. What is your assessment of Ms. Honisch's injury?
   Answer: *Concussion*
2. Was your assessment of Ms. Honisch's injury correct?
   Answer: *Yes*
3. If not, explain what you did incorrectly and how you could have performed a better assessment.
   Answer: ______________________________

MODEL SCENARIO 3: KEITH ALBRIGHT

Keith Albright participates in kickboxing. Through many years of hard work, he has become highly accomplished at his art. He has been preparing hard for an upcoming competition against a fellow classmate because he knows that the fight will be challenging. Two minutes into the competition, Mr. Albright is caught off guard when his opponent uses an illegal direct kick to the anterior portion of his chest and ribs (Fig. 9-3). He has a sharp pain with inspiration and has localized point tenderness over the anterior middle section of his sixth and seventh ribs. With palpation, crepitus is felt over the sixth and seventh ribs. He is referred for radiography.

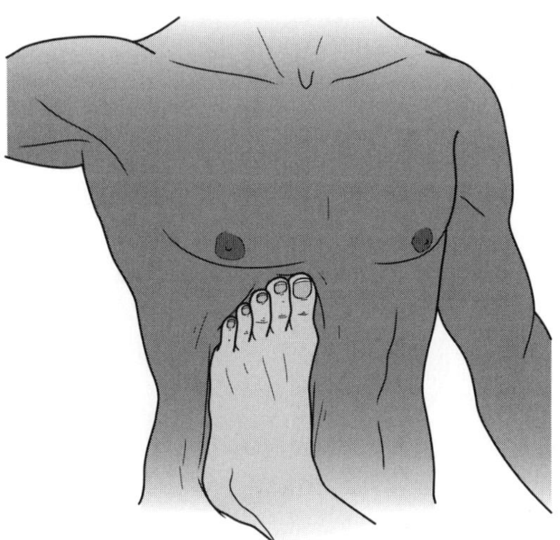

Figure 9-3: Keith Albright's mechanism of injury.

1. Based on this scenario, what do you know about Mr. Albright's injury?
   - *Male athlete*
   - *Kickboxer*
   - *Mechanism of injury: kick to the anterior chest and ribs*
   - *Sharp pain with inspiration*
   - *Localized point tenderness at ribs 6 and 7*
   - *Crepitus with palpation*
   - *Referred for radiography*
2. To evaluate Mr. Albright's injury effectively, you will need to gather additional information. What questions should you ask in addition to what is presented in this scenario?
   - *Is this injury a medical emergency?*
   - *Are there any preexisting injuries? If yes, what are they?*
   - *Are there any special tests that are important to perform? If yes, elaborate.*
   - *Are the results of the special tests positive or negative? What does each result indicate?*
   - *Does the athlete have any numbness or tingling?*
   - *Is edema present?*
   - *Is ecchymosis present?*
   - *Are there any deformities?*
   - *Is shortness of breath present?*

3. Identify key terms and concepts, and then research each to broaden your knowledge of head, neck, and trunk injuries.
   - What anatomical structures might be involved in Mr. Albright's injury?
     Ribs
     Lungs
     Sternum
     Xiphoid process
     Costal cartilage
   - Define *crepitus*.
     A crackling or rattling sound made by a body part
   - Define *inspiration*.
     Inhalation; drawing air into the lungs
   - Define *anterior*.
     In front of or on the abdominal side of the body
   - What might Mr. Albright be at risk for with a direct hit to the anterior chest?
     A sternum fracture or rib fracture; consequently, a possible punctured lung

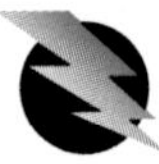

Brain Jolt

With a direct blow to ribs 1 through 9, the ribs can be pushed posteriorly, possibly causing damage to the lungs, which is a life-threatening emergency.

4. Based on the information that you currently have and what was provided by your instructor, what are the possible differential diagnoses for Mr. Albright's injury?
   Rib contusion
   Costochondral separation
   Rib fracture
   Sternum fracture

Why or why not?

For each assessment or diagnosis, write *why?* or *why not?* statements identifying why the information is correct or incorrect. Take details from your textbook, your own research, and data from Mr. Albright's scenario to help you formulate an answer.

1. *Mr. Albright does not have a rib contusion because no pain is experienced on both expiration and inspiration. He also has some crepitus over ribs 6 and 7, which is a sign of an instability or a possible fracture.*
2. *Mr. Albright does not have a costochondral separation because the pain is not localized at the costal cartilage junction. His pain is more localized over the middle portion of the bone.*
3. *Mr. Albright has a rib fracture. A direct or an indirect blow causes rib fractures. The kick Mr. Albright received was a direct blow to the anterior surfaces of ribs 6 and 7. Mr. Albright has a sign of crepitus, which is normally associated with instability of a bone and a positive rib compression test.*
4. *Mr. Albright does not have a sternum fracture because of the location of his symptoms.*

What do you think?

1. What is your assessment of Mr. Albright's injury?
   Answer: *Rib fracture*
2. Was your assessment of Mr. Albright's injury correct?
   Answer: *Yes*
3. If not, please explain what you did incorrectly and how you could have performed a better assessment.

   Answer: ____________________

STUDENT SCENARIO 1: JONATHAN MCKAY

Jonathan McKay is a sweeper on his soccer team. His opponent has a breakaway ball, and Mr. McKay moves to his right to guard the player. The opponent takes a line drive shot on goal. Mr. McKay thinks that he can perform a head ball, clearing the ball, before it gets to the goal. As Mr. McKay jumps up, he loses his footing and the ball hits him directly over the left eye. He is assisted off the field as a result of the diplopia that he is experiencing. He is developing edema and ecchymosis around the eye and zygomatic bone (Fig. 9-4). He has trouble with upwardly rotating the eye and has a history of concussions.

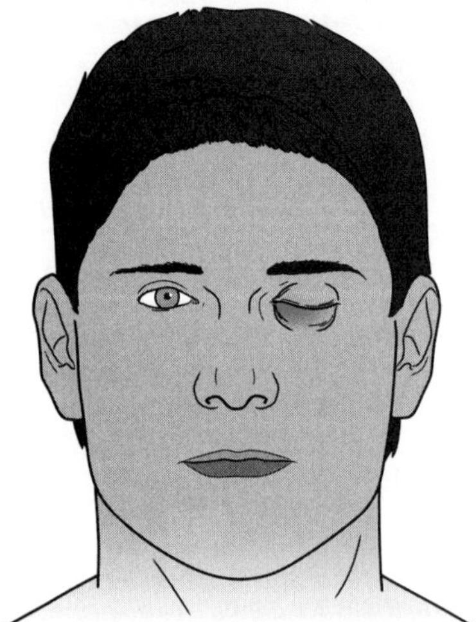

Figure 9-4: Jonathan McKay's eye.

1. Based on this scenario, what do you know about Mr. McKay's injury?
   - ____________________
     ____

- ______________________________
- ______________________________
- ______________________________

2. To evaluate Mr. McKay's injury effectively, you will need to gather additional information. What questions should you ask in addition to what is presented in this scenario?
   - ______________________________
   - ______________________________
   - ______________________________
   - ______________________________

Brain Jolt
This eye injury is often referred to as the trap door injury *or a* blowout injury.

3. Identify key terms and concepts, and then research each to broaden your knowledge of head, neck, and trunk injuries.
   - What anatomical structures might be involved in Mr. McKay's injury?

     Answer: ______________________________
   - Define *diplopia.*

     Answer: ______________________________
   - Define *edema.*

     Answer: ______________________________
   - Define *ecchymosis.*

     Answer: ______________________________
   - Define *concussion.*

     Answer: ______________________________
   - What are the signs and symptoms of a concussion?

     Answer: ______________________________
   - Where are the zygomatic bones located?

     Answer: ______________________________
   - Why is a history of concussions important to this athlete and scenario?

     Answer: ______________________________
   - Why does Mr. McKay have trouble with upward rotation of the eye? What does this indicate?

     Answer: ______________________________

4. Based on the information that you currently have and what was provided by your instructor, what are the possible differential diagnoses for Mr. McKay's injury?
   - ______________________________
   - ______________________________
   - ______________________________
   - ______________________________

Why or why not?

For each assessment or diagnosis, write *why?* or *why not?* statements identifying why the information is correct or incorrect. Take details from your textbook, your own research, and data from Mr. McKay's scenario to help you formulate an answer.

1. ______________________________
2. ______________________________
3. ______________________________
4. ______________________________

Conversation Buffer
Any eye injury should be treated with extreme caution. With this particular injury, the athlete should follow specific guidelines to ensure the best outcome. The injured eye needs to be lightly covered, avoiding any pressure to the area, and the athlete needs to be transported immediately to a hospital in the recumbent position. Explain to your athlete that these guidelines are strict; ignoring them places the athlete at further risk for vision loss.

What do you think?

1. What is your assessment of Mr. McKay's injury?

   Answer: ______________________________
2. Was your assessment correct for Mr. McKay's injury?

   Answer: ______________________________
3. If not, explain what you did incorrectly and how you could have performed a better assessment.

   Answer: ______________________________

STUDENT SCENARIO 2: DIRK BRUSH

Dirk Brush is a running back on his college football team. He is a fast, explosive player who frequently powers through tackles and offensive holes. Mr. Brush is handed the ball and sees a hole to the right of the center on the opposing team. He charges through and is sandwiched hard from his left and right sides by defensive players. He is slow to get up and seems disoriented, and he is removed from the game for evaluation. He states that he has vertigo and a headache, but he believes that he never lost consciousness. He is held out for the remainder of the game and is evaluated 15 min later. The same symptoms remain, but now he has nausea, blurred vision, and a dilated pupil on the left side (Fig. 9-5); his condition seems to be deteriorating. He is transported immediately to the hospital for additional testing.

1. Based on this scenario, what do you know about Mr. Brush's injury?

- ____________________
- ____________________
- ____________________
- ____________________

2. To evaluate Mr. Brush's injury effectively, you will need to gather additional information. What questions should you ask in addition to what is presented in this scenario?

- ____________________
- ____________________
- ____________________
- ____________________

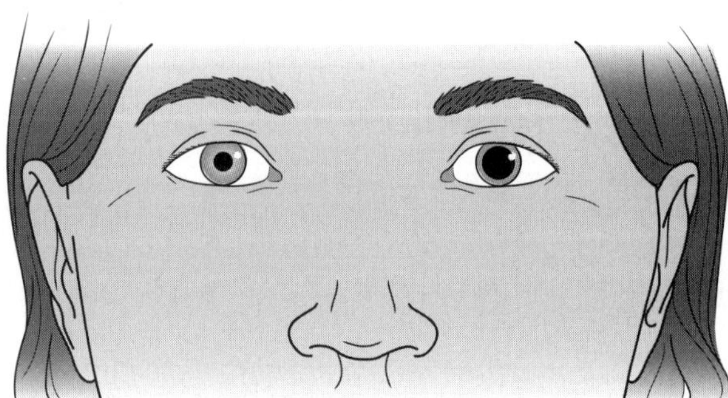

Figure 9-5: Dirk Brush's eye.

Brain Jolt

Head injuries that worsen or do not improve need to be treated as medical emergencies. Being conservative is always best. When in doubt, transport by ambulance.

3. Identify key terms and concepts, and then research each to broaden your knowledge of head, neck, and trunk injuries.

- What anatomical structures might be involved in Mr. Brush's injury?

  Answer: ____________________
- Define *vertigo.*

  Answer: ____________________
- Define *edema.*

  Answer: ____________________
- Define *ecchymosis.*

  Answer: ____________________
- What are the signs and symptoms of a concussion?

  Answer: ____________________
- Why is Mr. Brush's deterioration and new symptoms a concern?

  Answer: ____________________
- Why is only one of Mr. Brush's pupils dilated?

  Answer: ____________________
- Why is blurred vision important to note?

  Answer: ____________________
- Why is Mr. Brush prevented from participating in the game?

  Answer: ____________________
- Why is Mr. Brush transported to a hospital immediately?

  Answer: ____________________

4. Based on the information that you currently have and what was provided by your instructor, what are the possible differential diagnoses for Mr. Brush's injury?

- ____________________
- ____________________

- ______________________________
- ______________________________

Why or why not?

For each assessment or diagnosis, write *why?* or *why not?* statements identifying why the information is correct or incorrect. Take details from your textbook, your own research, and data from Mr. Brush's scenario to help you formulate an answer.

1. ______________________________
2. ______________________________
3. ______________________________
4. ______________________________

What do you think?

1. What is your assessment of Mr. Brush's injury?

   Answer: ______________________________

2. Was your assessment correct for Mr. Brush's injury?

   Answer: ______________________________

3. If not, explain what you did incorrectly and how you could have performed a better assessment.

   Answer: ______________________________

STUDENT SCENARIO 3: JEREMY CLAY

Jeremy Clay is a freshman defensive lineman on his college football team. He is participating in a drill that focuses on getting low and tackling the offensive player. His first two attempts are unsuccessful. On his third attempt, he powers out of his stance and begins to lower his left shoulder. He slips when he powers out of the drill, causing his form to change. His head lowers from the proper "head up" technique for hitting, and he hits the opponent with the top of his head (Fig. 9-6). This impact produces an axial loading to the vertebral column, and he drops to the ground and is motionless. He has immediate cervical pain and remains conscious. His head is immediately stabilized, and then Mr. Clay is assessed by the athletic trainer. He is experiencing numbness and paraesthesia in his limbs and has point tenderness over cervical vertebrae 5 and 6. He is placed on a spine board, fitted with a cervical spine collar, and transported by an ambulance to the nearest hospital.

1. Based on this scenario, what do you know about Mr. Clay's injury?
   - ______________________________
   - ______________________________
   - ______________________________
   - ______________________________
2. To evaluate Mr. Clay's injury effectively, you will need to gather additional information. What questions should you ask in addition to what is presented in this scenario?
   - ______________________________

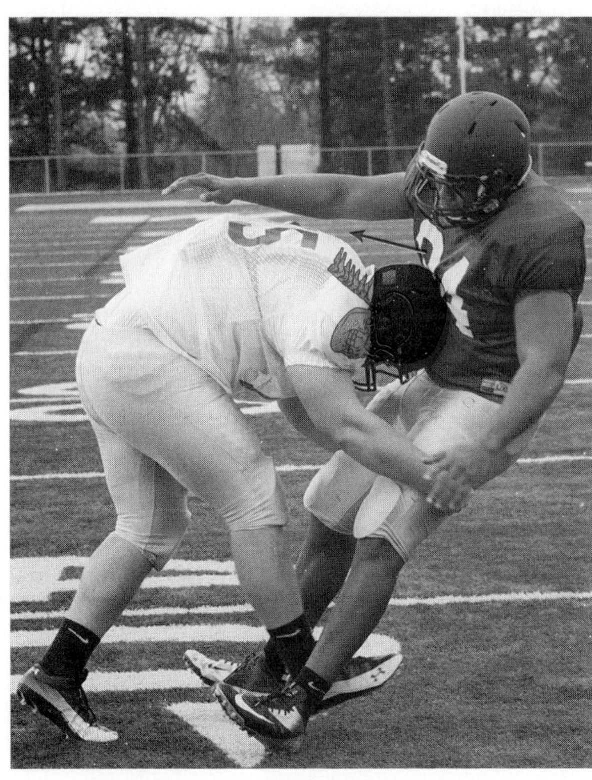

Figure 9-6: Jeremy Clay hitting his opponent.

- ________________________________
- ________________________________
- ________________________________

Conversation Buffer

In football, good technique is essential to reducing the risk of injury. Talking with athletes about proper technique when hitting or tackling an opponent is important. Athletes need to keep their heads up so that they can always see their opponents. Putting the head down creates a risk for serious neck injuries that can change the athlete's life forever.

3. Identify key terms and concepts, and then research each to broaden your knowledge of head, neck, and trunk injuries.
   - What anatomical structures might be involved in Mr. Clay's injury?

     Answer: ____________________
   - Define *axial loading*.

     Answer: ____________________
   - Define *vertebral column*.

     Answer: ____________________
   - Where is the vertebral column located?

     Answer: ____________________
   - Where are cervical vertebrae 1 through 7 located?

     Answer: ____________________
   - What might the symptoms of numbness and paraesthesia indicate?

     Answer: ____________________
   - Why is Mr. Clay stabilized immediately?

     Answer: ____________________
   - Describe the proper technique for fitting a cervical spine collar and using a back board.

     Answer: ____________________
   - Why is it important to become familiar with the proper form for hitting and tackling in football?

     Answer: ____________________

4. Based on the information that you currently have and what was provided by your instructor, what are the possible differential diagnoses for Mr. Clay's injury?
   - ________________________________
   - ________________________________
   - ________________________________
   - ________________________________

Why or why not?

For each assessment or diagnosis, write *why?* or *why not?* statements identifying why the information is correct or incorrect. Take details from your textbook, your own research, and data from Mr. Clay's scenario to help you formulate an answer.

1. ________________________________
2. ________________________________
3. ________________________________
4. ________________________________

What do you think?

1. What is your assessment of Mr. Clay's injury?

   Answer: ____________________
2. Was your assessment correct for Mr. Clay's injury?

   Answer: ____________________
3. If not, explain what you did incorrectly and how you could have performed a better assessment.

   Answer: ____________________

STUDENT SCENARIO 4: DAWN OTT

Dawn Ott is playing in a softball game. The game is tied, and she is ready to steal third base. The catcher fumbles the ball, and the third base coach signals for her to steal third base; however, the third base coach underestimates the amount of time needed to get to third base, resulting in a close play. To try to arrive at the base safely, she dives for the bag, overshooting it and hitting her stomach sharply on the base (Fig. 9-7). She rolls in pain

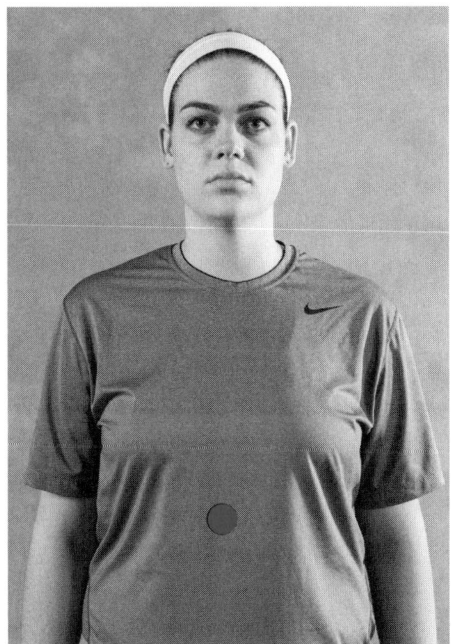

Figure 9-7: Dawn Ott's point of impact.

while holding her abdomen. She is unable to talk and is violently gasping for air. After a few seconds, she finally calms down and is able to reassure the athletic trainer that she has no other pain and is feeling better.

1. Based on this scenario, what do you know about Ms. Ott's injury?
   - ______________________________
   - ______________________________
   - ______________________________
   - ______________________________
2. To evaluate Ms. Ott's injury effectively, you will need to gather additional information. What questions should you ask in addition to what is presented in this scenario?
   - ______________________________
   - ______________________________
   - ______________________________
   - ______________________________
3. Identify key terms and concepts, and then research each to broaden your knowledge of head, neck, and trunk injuries.
   - What anatomical structures might be involved in Ms. Ott's injury?

     Answer: ______________________________
   - Why was Ms. Ott grasping her abdomen?

     Answer: ______________________________
   - Why was Ms. Ott gasping for air?

     Answer: ______________________________
   - Is there a possibility of an airway obstruction?

     Answer: ______________________________
   - Why could Ms. Ott not speak?

     Answer: ______________________________
   - Why did the injury subside without any additional signs of injury?

     Answer: ______________________________
4. Based on the information that you currently have and what was provided by your instructor, what are the possible differential diagnoses for Ms. Ott's injury?
   - ______________________________
   - ______________________________
   - ______________________________
   - ______________________________

Brain Jolt

Athletes tend to be scared and prone to panic because of this injury. To help the athlete, use a firm and confident voice, press your hand firmly on the athlete's abdomen, and instruct the athlete to push his or her stomach into your hand while taking a deep breath. This activity helps the symptoms subside quicker.

Why or why not?

For each assessment or diagnosis, write *why?* or *why not?* statements identifying why the information is correct or incorrect. Take details from your textbook, your own research, and data from Ms. Ott's scenario to help you formulate an answer.

1. ______________________________
2. ______________________________

3. ______________________________

____

4. ______________________________

____

What do you think?

1. What is your assessment of Ms. Ott's injury?

   Answer: ______________________

2. Was your assessment correct for Ms. Ott's injury?

   Answer: ______________________

3. If not, explain what you did incorrectly and how you could have performed a better assessment.

   Answer: ______________________

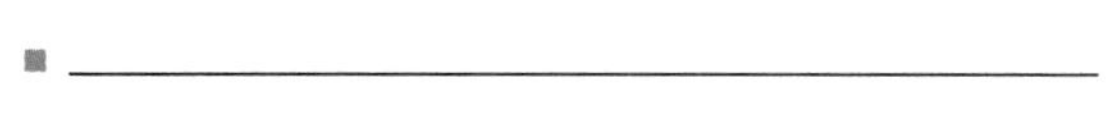

STUDENT SCENARIO 5: DOMINIC TURNER

Dominic Turner is a basketball player who is known to be aggressive on the court. As a loose ball occurs, Mr. Turner reaches forward for the ball and is elbowed on the lateral side of his nose by an opponent. He experiences immediate pain and epistaxis. The first objective of care is to control the epistaxis. Once this is under control, the injury is further assessed, and some mild deformity of his nose is noted (Fig. 9-8). Mild edema develops, and he has trouble breathing through the left nostril, which is the side that received the direct blow. He is referred for radiography.

1. Based on this scenario, what do you know about Mr. Turner's injury?
   - ______________________________
   - ______________________________
   - ______________________________
   - ______________________________

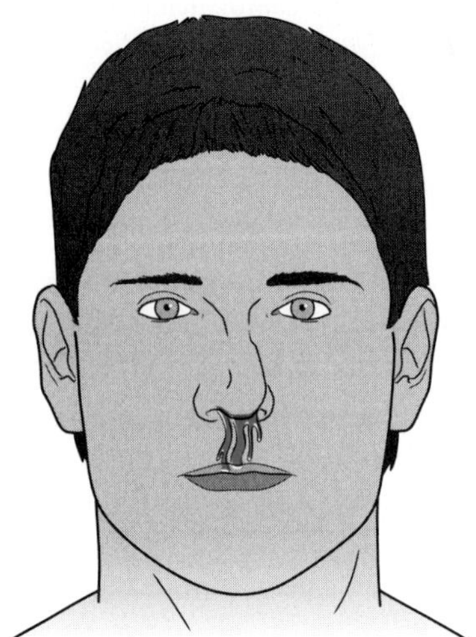

Figure 9-8: Dominic Turner's nose.

2. To evaluate Mr. Turner's injury effectively, you will need to gather additional information. What questions should you ask in addition to what is presented in this scenario?
   - ______________________________
   - ______________________________
   - ______________________________
   - ______________________________

3. Identify key terms and concepts, and then research each to broaden your knowledge of head, neck, and trunk injuries.
   - What anatomical structures might be involved in Mr. Turner's injury?

     Answer: ______________________
   - Define *epistaxis.*

     Answer: ______________________
   - Define *edema.*

     Answer: ______________________
   - Why is radiography the diagnostic test of choice in this scenario?

     Answer: ______________________
   - How are deformities determined? What key aspects should be evaluated when determining deformity?

     Answer: ______________________
   - Why is Mr. Turner having difficulty breathing from the left nostril? What might this indicate?

     Answer: ______________________

Brain Jolt

Raccoon eyes are common with this injury.

4. Based on the information that you currently have and what was provided by your instructor, what are the possible differential diagnoses for Mr. Turner's injury?

- ______________________________
- ______________________________
- ______________________________
- ______________________________

Why or why not?

For each assessment or diagnosis, write *why?* or *why not?* statements identifying why the information is correct or incorrect. Take details from your textbook, your own research, and data from Mr. Turner's scenario to help you formulate an answer.

1. ______________________________
2. ______________________________
3. ______________________________
4. ______________________________

What do you think?

1. What is your assessment of Mr. Turner's injury?

   Answer: ______________________________

2. Was your assessment correct for Mr. Turner's injury?

   Answer: ______________________________

3. If not, explain what you did incorrectly and how you could have performed a better assessment.

   Answer: ______________________________

STUDENT SCENARIO 6: BILL FABIAN

Bill Fabian is an offensive lineman on his college football team. He has been having trouble with a weak left deltoid muscle, but he has not mentioned anything to a medical staff member for fear of being removed from participation. In the past four games, however, he has twice experienced some numbness and paraesthesia in his shoulder over the deltoid region that sometimes travels down to his fingers but lasts for only a few minutes. The results of a brachial plexus traction test are positive (Fig. 9-9). He also has a history of a herniated cervical disc at the C4 level and has normal neck active range of motion.

1. Based on this scenario, what do you know about Mr. Fabian's injury?

- ______________________________
- ______________________________
- ______________________________
- ______________________________

2. To evaluate Mr. Fabian's injury effectively, you will need to gather additional information. What

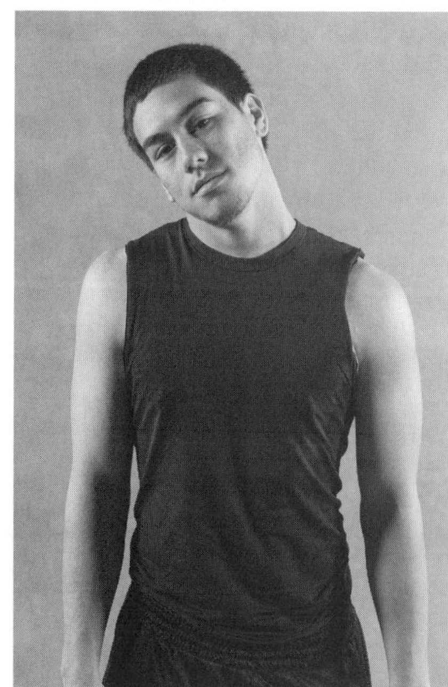

Figure 9-9: Bill Fabian's motion to reproduce pain.

questions should you ask in addition to what is presented in this scenario?

- ____________________
- ____________________
- ____________________
- ____________________

Brain Jolt
Seeing a player coming off the field with a "dead arm" is normal with this injury.

3. Identify key terms and concepts, and then research each to broaden your knowledge of head, neck, and trunk injuries.
   - What anatomical structures might be involved in Mr. Fabian's injury?

     Answer: ____________________
   - Define the brachial plexus traction test, how to perform the test, and what a positive test indicates.

     Answer: ____________________
   - Why can shoulder depression reproduce symptoms?

     Answer: ____________________
   - Define *herniated cervical disc.*

     Answer: ____________________
   - What are the signs and symptoms of a herniated cervical disc?

     Answer: ____________________
   - Where is the deltoid muscle located?

     Answer: ____________________
   - What might the symptoms of numbness and paraesthesia indicate?

     Answer: ____________________
   - Why would the numbness and paraesthesia travel to Mr. Fabian's fingers?

     Answer: ____________________
   - Why does Mr. Fabian's numbness and paraesthesia last only a few minutes?

     Answer: ____________________
4. Based on the information that you currently have and what was provided by your instructor, what are the possible differential diagnoses for Mr. Fabian's injury?
   - ____________________
   - ____________________
   - ____________________
   - ____________________

Why or why not?

For each assessment or diagnosis, write *why?* or *why not?* statements identifying why the information is correct or incorrect. Take details from your textbook, your own research, and data from Mr. Fabian's scenario to help you formulate an answer.

1. ____________________
2. ____________________
3. ____________________
4. ____________________

What do you think?

1. What is your assessment of Mr. Fabian's injury?

   Answer: ____________________
2. Was your assessment correct for Mr. Fabian's injury?

   Answer: ____________________
3. If not, explain what you did incorrectly and how you could have performed a better assessment.

   Answer: ____________________

STUDENT SCENARIO 7: LAURIA YEARY

Lauria Yeary is home for summer vacation and is dog-sitting for a friend. When she reaches down to pick up the dog bowl, the small dog jumps up, causing both of their mouths to collide. She was talking when this collision happened, causing her mouth to be open. She experiences immediate pain and blood in her mouth, feeling as though something dislodged when the collision occurred. Ms. Yeary inspects the dog and sees no injuries. She inspects her mouth and notices that blood is gushing from her front lower gum and tooth socket; she notices a gap (Fig. 9-10).

1. Based on this scenario, what do you know about Ms. Yeary's injury?
   - ____________________________
   - ____________________________
   - ____________________________
   - ____________________________

2. To evaluate Ms. Yeary's injury effectively, you will need to gather additional information. What questions should you ask in addition to what is presented in this scenario?
   - ____________________________
   - ____________________________
   - ____________________________
   - ____________________________

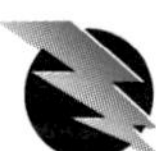

Brain Jolt

A glass of milk is one way to preserve this structure.

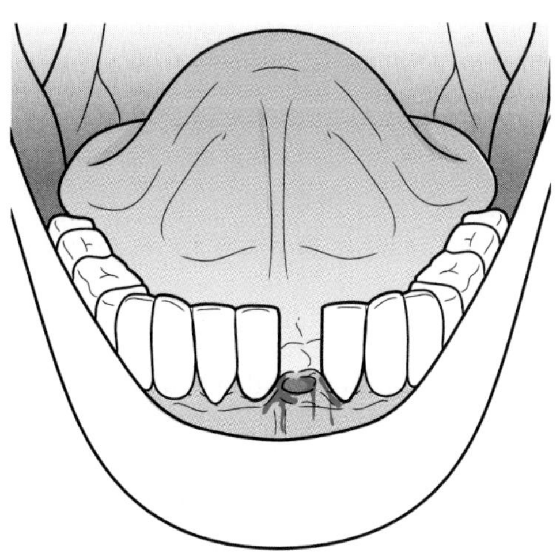

Figure 9-10: Lauria Yeary's mouth.

3. Identify key terms and concepts, and then research each to broaden your knowledge of head, neck, and trunk injuries.
   - What anatomical structures might be involved in Ms. Yeary's injury?

     Answer: ____________________
   - In this scenario, is it important to seek a dentist immediately?

     Answer: ____________________
   - Save-a-tooth (dental product) and milk are the best options to preserve a tooth, but if these are not available, how should the tooth be stored?

     Answer: ____________________
   - What determines whether the tooth can or should be replaced on site?

     Answer: ____________________

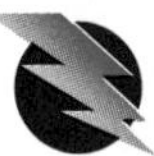

Brain Jolt

Time is of the essence in this injury. Do not delay calling a dentist.

4. Based on the information that you currently have and what was provided by your instructor, what are the possible differential diagnoses for Ms. Yeary's injury?
   - ____________________________
   - ____________________________
   - ____________________________
   - ____________________________

Why or why not?

For each assessment or diagnosis, write *why?* or *why not?* statements identifying why the information is correct or incorrect. Take details from your textbook, your own research, and data from Ms. Yeary's scenario to help you formulate an answer.

1. ____________________________
2. ____________________________
3. ____________________________
4. ____________________________

What do you think?

1. What is your assessment of Ms. Yeary's injury?

   Answer: ______________________________

2. Was your assessment correct for Ms. Yeary's injury?

   Answer: ______________________________

3. If not, explain what you did incorrectly and how you could have performed a better assessment.

   Answer: ______________________________

STUDENT SCENARIO 8: NATHAN BROWN

Nathan Brown is wrestling on the floor with his brother when his brother compresses Mr. Brown's right side of his head down to the floor. This pressure causes Mr. Brown's right ear to become irritated. He does not seem to experience any hearing loss, but he notices that the auricle of his ear has significant edema (Fig. 9-11). Although a hematoma develops, he does not seem to experience any pain with the injury. Mr. Brown is a wrestler for his school's team and the season has just ended.

1. Based on this scenario, what do you know about Mr. Brown's injury?

   - ______________________________
   - ______________________________
   - ______________________________
   - ______________________________

2. To evaluate Mr. Brown's injury effectively, you will need to gather additional information. What questions should you ask in addition to what is presented in this scenario?

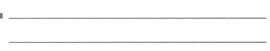

   - ______________________________
   - ______________________________
   - ______________________________
   - ______________________________

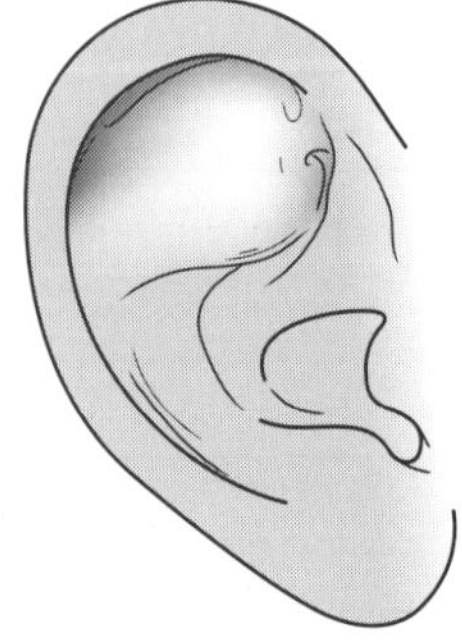

Figure 9-11: Nathan Brown's ear.

Brain Jolt

This injury is common with wrestlers and can be prevented by wearing proper headgear.

3. Identify key terms and concepts, and then research each to broaden your knowledge of head, neck, and trunk injuries.
   - What anatomical structures might be involved in Mr. Brown's injury?

     Answer: ______________________________
   - Define *compression.*

     Answer: ______________________________
   - Define *hematoma.*

     Answer: ______________________________
   - Define *edema.*

     Answer: ______________________________
   - Define *auricle.*

     Answer: ______________________________
   - Where is the auricle located?

     Answer: ______________________________
   - Why is there no pain associated with this injury?

     Answer: ______________________________
   - Is the fact that Mr. Brown is a wrestler important to the evaluation?

     Answer: ______________________________

4. Based on the information that you currently have and what was provided by your instructor, what are the possible differential diagnoses for Mr. Brown's injury?

   - ______________________________

- ______________________________
- ______________________________
- ______________________________

2. ______________________________
3. ______________________________
4. ______________________________

Why or why not?

For each assessment or diagnosis, write *why?* or *why not?* statements identifying why the information is correct or incorrect. Take details from your textbook, your own research, and data from Mr. Brown's scenario to help you formulate an answer.

1. ______________________________

What do you think?

1. What is your assessment of Mr. Brown's injury?

   Answer: ______________________________

2. Was your assessment correct for Mr. Brown's injury?

   Answer: ______________________________

3. If not, explain what you did incorrectly and how you could have performed a better assessment.

   Answer: ______________________________

STUDENT SCENARIO 9: ALEXIS CHILDREY

Alexis Childrey is a cheerleader, and her team is learning new stunts for their halftime routine. Ms. Childrey's role as a base is to catch her teammate after she is tossed in the air for a stunt. When her teammate is on the descent, the teammate loses her confidence and her arms are no longer tight against her body. As Alexis Childrey catches the teammate, the teammate's elbow strikes Ms. Childrey in the lateral side of the mandible near the ear. Ms. Childrey experiences immediate pain and a lack of movement in her jaw. She panics because she cannot close her mouth and is having difficulty communicating her pain. A deformity is obvious (Fig. 9-12).

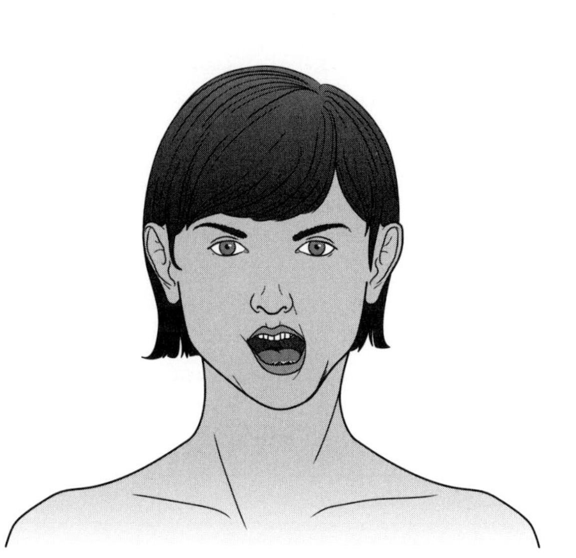

Figure 9-12: Alexis Childrey's jaw.

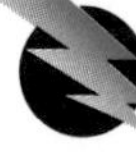

Brain Jolt

With this injury, an athlete can be immobilized with a Philadelphia collar as long as it does not create further pain. The athlete should be referred immediately to a dentist or physician.

1. Based on this scenario, what do you know about Ms. Childrey's injury?
   - ______________________________
   - ______________________________
   - ______________________________
   - ______________________________

2. To evaluate Ms. Childrey's injury effectively, you will need to gather additional information. What questions should you ask in addition to what is presented in this scenario?
   - ______________________________
   - ______________________________
   - ______________________________

- ______________________________

3. Identify key terms and concepts, and then research each to broaden your knowledge of head, neck, and trunk injuries.
   - What anatomical structures might be involved in Ms. Childrey's injury?

     Answer: ______________________________
   - What is a Philadelphia collar?

     Answer: ______________________________
   - Why is Ms. Childrey unable to close her mouth?

     Answer: ______________________________
   - Why is Ms. Childrey having trouble communicating?

     Answer: ______________________________
   - What might Ms. Childrey's deformity indicate? What other injury should be ruled out?

     Answer: ______________________________
4. Based on the information that you currently have and what was provided by your instructor, what are the possible differential diagnoses for Ms. Childrey's injury?
   - ______________________________
   - ______________________________
   - ______________________________

- ______________________________

Why or why not?

For each assessment or diagnosis, write *why?* or *why not?* statements identifying why the information is correct or incorrect. Take details from your textbook, your own research, and data from Ms. Childrey's scenario to help you formulate an answer.

1. ______________________________
2. ______________________________
3. ______________________________
4. ______________________________

What do you think?

1. What is your assessment of Ms. Childrey's injury?

   Answer: ______________________________
2. Was your assessment correct for Ms. Childrey's injury?

   Answer: ______________________________
3. If not, explain what you did incorrectly and how you could have performed a better assessment.

   Answer: ______________________________

STUDENT SCENARIO 10: MARY ANNE NORTON

Mary Anne Norton is a basketball player on the women's team. She is 6 feet, 3 inches tall and, because of her height, is a post player. She is well-known for her rebounding skills and stats. Ms. Norton is passed a breakaway ball. She dribbles to the hoop, slightly flexes her abdominals, and then extends to shoot the ball into the basket. Her momentum throws her off balance, and she is too close to the basket to get the shot off, which causes her to overextend her upper body back toward the basket (Fig. 9-13). She experiences immediate pain in her anterior torso and is removed from the game. On evaluation, she states that she has a history of an inguinal hernia. She had been experiencing some abdominal soreness since the last basketball game and notices the pain when she extends or rotates her body. The pain is similar to a stretching or a tearing feeling that occurs superior and laterally to her umbilicus. A lower abdominal rebound test is negative.

1. Based on this scenario, what do you know about Ms. Norton's injury?
   - ______________________________
   - ______________________________
   - ______________________________
   - ______________________________

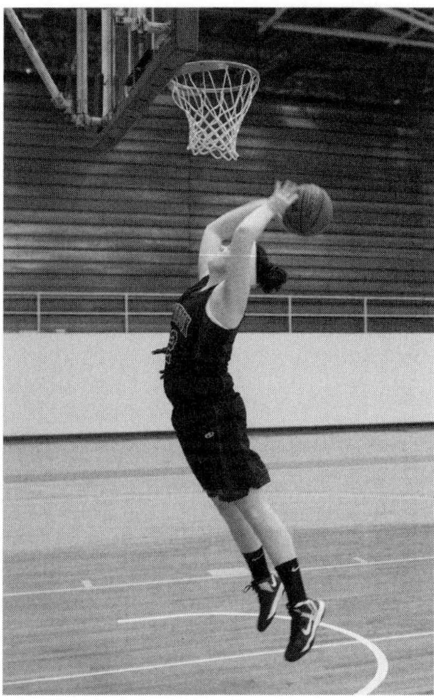

Figure 9-13: Mary Anne Norton's mechanism of injury.

2. To evaluate Ms. Norton's injury effectively, you will need to gather additional information. What questions should you ask yourself in addition to what is presented in this scenario?
   - ______________________________
   - ______________________________
   - ______________________________
   - ______________________________

3. Identify key terms and concepts, and then research each to broaden your knowledge of head, neck, and trunk injuries.
   - What anatomical structures might be involved in Ms. Norton's injury?

     Answer: ______________________________
   - Define *superior.*

     Answer: ______________________________
   - Define *lateral.*

     Answer: ______________________________
   - Define *inguinal hernia.*

     Answer: ______________________________
   - What are the signs and symptoms of an inguinal hernia?

     Answer: ______________________________
   - Define *umbilicus.*

     Answer: ______________________________
   - Where is the umbilicus located?

     Answer: ______________________________
   - What are the muscles of the abdomen?

     Answer: ______________________________
   - What is a rebound test? What does it test? What does a positive result indicate?

     Answer: ______________________________

4. Based on the information that you currently have and what was provided by your instructor, what are the possible differential diagnoses for Ms. Norton's injury?
   - ______________________________
   - ______________________________
   - ______________________________
   - ______________________________

Brain Jolt

The torso has four core parts. This injury involves a structure involved within the "six-pack" muscle.

Why or why not?

For each assessment or diagnosis, write *why?* or *why not?* statements identifying why the information is correct or incorrect. Take details from your textbook, your own research, and data from Ms. Norton's scenario to help you formulate an answer.

1. ______________________________
2. ______________________________
3. ______________________________
4. ______________________________

What do you think?

1. What is your assessment of Ms. Norton's injury?

   Answer: ______________________________

2. Was your assessment correct for Ms. Norton's injury?

   Answer: ______________________________

3. If not, explain what you did incorrectly and how you could have performed a better assessment.

   Answer: ______________________________

knowledge checklist

Table 9-1 offers a checklist that can be used by a peer, instructor, or preceptor to evaluate each part of a head, neck, or trunk assessment. Use this checklist as a tool to ensure that the evaluation is complete and to assess your knowledge of the competencies that apply to this chapter.

TABLE 9-1 ■ Head, Neck, and Trunk Assessment Competency Checklist

	Proficient *Can demonstrate and execute the skill properly*	**Proficient With Assistance** *Can demonstrate and execute the skill with minimal guidance or tips*	**Not Proficient** *Unable to demonstrate and execute the skill properly; need to be reevaluated at another time after further study and practice*
Athlete's Health History			
Medical history			
History of head, neck, or trunk injury			
Type of sport and position played			
When did the injury occur?			
Mechanisms of Injury			
How did the injury occur?			
When does the pain occur?			
What makes the pain better or worse?			
Was the athlete's head, neck, or trunk forced into an unusual position?			
Is the athlete experiencing numbness or tingling?			
Were any pops, cracks, or snaps felt or heard?			
Did loss of consciousness occur? (Refer to full concussion assessment)			
Visual Observations			
Level of shoulders			
Edema			
Ecchymosis			
Deformity/misalignment			
Palpation			
Temperature change over the painful area, crepitus, deformity, intra-articular or extra-articular joint swelling, changes within the muscle fibers			
Hyoid			
Sternocleidomastoid			
Scalenes			
Carotid artery			
Lymph nodes			
Transverse processes			
Spinous processes			
Trapezius			
Levator scapulae			
Skull			
Nasal bone			
Nasal cartilage			
Maxilla			

Continued

TABLE 9-1 ■ Head, Neck, and Trunk Assessment Competency Checklist—cont'd

	Proficient	Proficient With Assistance	Not Proficient
Temporomandibular joint			
External ear			
Teeth			
Mandible			
Orbital rim			
Frontal bone			
Zygomatic bone			
Sternum			
Xiphoid process			
Costal cartilage			
Ribs			
Rectus abdominis			
Internal oblique			
External oblique			
Range of Motion			
Passive or active			
Flexion of neck			
Extension of neck			
Lateral rotation of neck			
Lateral flexion of neck			
Flexion of trunk			
Extension of trunk			
Lateral flexion of trunk			
Rotation of trunk			
Temporomandibular joint motion			
Eye movement			
Strength			
Grade through manual muscle tests			
Flexion of neck			
Extension of neck			
Lateral rotation of neck			
Lateral flexion of neck			
Flexion of trunk			
Extension of trunk			
Lateral flexion of trunk			
Rotation of trunk			
Special Tests			
Spring test			
Cervical compression test			
Spurling test			
Cervical distraction test			
Vertebral artery test			
Valsalva maneuver			
Shoulder abduction test			
Brachial plexus traction test			
Concussion (refer to standardized concussion assessment)			
Rib compression test			

TABLE 9-1 ■ Head, Neck, and Trunk Assessment Competency Checklist—cont'd

	Proficient	Proficient With Assistance	Not Proficient
Neurological			
Cranial nerve assessment			
Brachial plexus (upper quarter)			
Lumbar plexus (lower quarter)			
Babinski test			
Vascular			
Radial pulse			
Brachial pulse			
Carotid pulse			
Dorsal pedal pulse			
Capillary refill			
Final Assessment			
Sprain, strain, contusion, fracture, condition, severity			

*Be sure to always compare bilaterally.

REFERENCES

Lincoln, A. E., Caswell, S. V., Almquist, J. L., Dunn, R. E., Norris, J. B., & Hinton R. Y. (2011). Trends in concussion incidence in high school sports. *The American Journal of Sports Medicine, 39*, 958–963.

National Athletic Training Association. (2011). *Athletic training education competencies* (5th ed.). Retrieved from http://www.nata.org/sites/default/files/5th-Edition-Competencies-2011-PDF-Version.pdf

Prentice, W. (2010). *Arnheim's principles of athletic training: A competency-based approach* (14th ed.). New York, NY: McGraw-Hill.

Starkey, C., Brown, S. D., & Ryan, J. (2010). *Examination of orthopedic and athletic injuries* (3rd ed.). Philadelphia, PA: F.A. Davis.

Van Suijlekom, H., et al. (2010). Whiplash-associated disorders. *Pain Practice, 10*, 131–136.

Venes, D. (Ed.) (2009). *Taber's cyclopedic medical dictionary* (21st ed.). Philadelphia, PA: F.A. Davis.

chapter 10

Lower Back, Sacroiliac Joint, and Pelvis

chapter outline

athletic trainer's corner

Out there in the real world, one athletic trainer experienced the following:

During my junior year of college, I cared for an athlete who complained of back pain. He believed he had done more than simply pull a muscle at cheerleading practice, where he performed many repetitive motions into lumbar extension. My initial reaction to this injury was to simply assume he had a muscle strain. I examined him, but he was too sore to allow a full evaluation. I gave him some exercises to help stretch the lumbar musculature and relax the area where he was having pain. Several days later, the athlete returned and stated that he had pain radiating down one of his legs but only with certain motions. At this point, I knew that the exercises were clearly not the solution to his back pain. I informed the team physician of the athlete's symptoms; he referred the athlete for imaging. The results of the examination revealed that the athlete had a spondylolisthesis that required immediate attention. This situation taught me that back pain in athletes is not a condition to dismiss lightly. The athlete could have something more serious underneath the spasms and muscle soreness.

Becky Honisch, PT, AT, ATC, DPT
Brownsburg, Indiana

learning outcomes

After working through this chapter, you will be able to:

1. Verbalize the questions to use when obtaining a thorough medical history for an assessment.
2. Describe the principles of body movement at the lower back, sacroiliac joint, and pelvis and the various mechanisms of injury that affect the lower back, sacroiliac joint, and pelvis.
3. Compare and contrast the findings of various special tests and the role of diagnostic tests used during a lower back, sacroiliac joint, or pelvis evaluation.
4. Explain medical terminology associated with assessment of musculoskeletal injuries.
5. Verbalize the standard procedures used for a clinical evaluation of the lower back, sacroiliac joint, and pelvis and interpret the findings for differential diagnoses.

MODEL SCENARIO 1: **PAULA SAUNDER**

Paula Saunder is a member of the volleyball team who plays all positions except the back row. Ms. Saunder has a history of tight hamstrings and weak core muscles that cause her to experience low back pain after practice. She has pain as a result of outside hitting that requires repetitive back hyperextension. She comes to the athletic training room with a complaint of low back discomfort, but she also is experiencing numbness and paraesthesia in her legs bilaterally. She has localized point tenderness over the lumbar (L5–S1) vertebrae and has a step deformity of the vertebrae at the L5–S1 level (Fig. 10-1). Special tests indicate a positive spring test of the low back at vertebrae L5–S1 and a negative straight-leg raise test result.

1. Based on this scenario, what do you know about Ms. Saunder's injury?
   - *Female athlete*
   - *Volleyball player*
   - *Mechanism of injury: chronic low back condition*
   - *Pain occurring after practice when focusing on outside hitting with repetitive hyperextension*
   - *Tight hamstrings and a weak core*
   - *Bilateral numbness and paraesthesia in the legs*
   - *Point tenderness over L5–S1*
   - *Step deformity at L5–S1*
   - *Positive spring test*
   - *Negative straight-leg test result*

Figure 10-1: Paula Saunder's deformity.

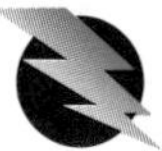

Brain Jolt
When an individual has this injury, he or she often has a history of spondylolysis. This patient's injury is an advanced version of spondylolysis, one precedes the other. Both of these conditions are verified by radiography.

2. To evaluate Ms. Saunder's injury effectively, you will need to gather additional information. What questions should you ask in addition to what is presented in this scenario?
   - *Is this injury a medical emergency?*
   - *Are there any preexisting injuries? If yes, what are they?*
   - *Are there any special tests that are important to perform? If yes, elaborate.*
   - *Are the results of the special tests positive or negative? What does each indicate?*
   - *What is the athlete's strength at the trunk and hips?*
   - *What is the athlete's range of motion (ROM) in the trunk and hips?*
   - *What is the athlete's gait pattern?*
   - *Is edema present?*
   - *Is ecchymosis present?*
3. Identify key terms and concepts, and then research each to broaden your knowledge of lower back, sacroiliac joint, and pelvic injuries.
   - What anatomical structures might be involved in Ms. Saunder's injury?
     Pelvis
     Lumbar vertebrae
     Sacroiliac joint

- Define *bilateral*.
  Affecting two or both sides
- What is the spring test?
  During a spring test, the evaluator applies a downward force with the palm of his or her hand over the vertebra, looking for any type of excessive movement between the vertebrae anteriorly and posteriorly.
- What is a straight-leg raise test? What are its different angles of testing?
  In the straight-leg raise test, the athlete lies supine and the evaluator passively raises the affected leg. This test is performed to determine whether the athlete has sacroiliac (SI) joint problems, sciatic nerve issues, or lumbar spine problems. If pain is felt when the leg is raised 0 to 30 degrees, it indicates an inflamed nerve or hip involvement. If pain is felt when the leg is raised 30 to 60 degrees, it indicates a sciatic nerve issue. If pain is felt when the leg is raised 70 to 90 degrees, it indicates an SI joint problem. Pain below 70 degrees indicates disc involvement.
- What does a step deformity mean in relation to the vertebrae?
  A step deformity is often referred to when talking about spondylolisthesis. It describes how the deformity feels when palpating the lower lumbar vertebrae from the anterior slippage of the vertebrae. Spondylolisthesis normally occurs between L5 to S1.
- Why does Ms. Saunder have bilateral numbness and paraesthesia?
  There is compression on the nerve root from the anterior misalignment of the vertebrae.

4. Based on the information that you currently have and what was provided by your instructor, what are the possible differential diagnoses for Ms. Saunder's injury?
   Lumbar strain
   Sciatica
   Spondylolisthesis
   Spondylolysis

Why or why not?

For each assessment or diagnosis, write *why?* or *why not?* statements identifying why the information is correct or incorrect. Take details from your textbook, your own research, and data from Ms. Saunder's scenario to help you formulate an answer.

1. *Ms. Saunder does not have a lumbar strain because she has localized point tenderness at vertebrae L5–S1, and step deformity is felt with palpation at the L5–S1 level. A lumbar strain has more generalized soreness and no deformity.*
2. *Ms. Saunder does not have sciatica because her numbness and paraesthesia occurs in both legs, and she does not have any point tenderness over her gluteus maximus and posterior superior iliac spine (PSIS) region on one or both legs. In addition, her straight-leg raise test results are negative.*
3. *Ms. Saunder has spondylolisthesis because she has a step deformity that is felt at vertebrae L5–S1, and numbness and paraesthesia that occurs in both legs as a result of the compression on the nerve from misalignment.*
4. *Ms. Saunder does not have spondylolysis because no step deformity is present with this type of injury. With spondylolysis, a radiographic examination reveals a fracture of the pars interarticularis between the superior and inferior facets of the vertebrae but no misalignment or slippage. This condition is commonly known as the Scotty dog view.*

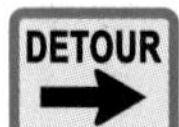

Treatment Detour

Ninety-three gymnasts were a part of a study that examined the prevalence rate and risk factors for spondylolisthesis. Of this sample, 6.5% of participants were found to have this condition. The results show that gender and height were not determinant factors for this condition. Those who had the condition were heavier, had been practicing gymnastics for more years and more hours per week, and had been competing at a high level. This information can help you to develop prevention and strengthening programs for these athletes with one or more of these risk factors to keep them healthy and competing in their sport (Toueg et al., 2010).

What do you think?

1. What is your assessment of Ms. Saunder's injury?
   Answer: *Spondylolisthesis*
2. Was your assessment of Ms. Saunder's injury correct?
   Answer: *Yes*
3. If not, explain what you did incorrectly and how you could have performed a better assessment.

Answer: ______________________

MODEL SCENARIO 2: HANNAH YOCKEY

Hannah Yockey is on the equestrian team at her college. Her horse has been having problems jumping the barriers for competition. Yesterday in practice, Ms. Yockey's horse halted right before a jump and threw Ms. Yockey. She hit the ground hard and landed on her buttocks (Fig. 10-2). She was extremely sore initially; however, after gathering herself from the fall, she seemed alright, although she felt a bit "banged up." Hannah Yockey stopped training her horse for the day and went home. Her pain level increased during the night, rendering her unable to sit down without intense discomfort to her buttocks. Leaning to one side when sitting was more comfortable, but lying prone was the most comfortable position. She has good strength and ROM at the hip with no history of injury.

1. Based on this scenario, what do you know about Ms. Yockey's injury?
   - *Female athlete*
   - *Equestrian*
   - *Mechanism of injury: thrown from a horse, landed on the buttocks*
   - *Unable to sit without intense pain*
   - *Tolerable to lean to one side when sitting*
   - *Most comfortable when lying prone*
   - *Good strength and ROM at the hip*
   - *No history of injuries*
2. To evaluate Ms. Yockey's injury effectively, you will need to gather additional information. What questions should you ask in addition to what is presented in this scenario?
   - *Is this injury a medical emergency?*
   - *Are there any preexisting injuries? If yes, what are they?*
   - *Are there any special tests that are important to perform? If yes, elaborate.*
   - *Are the results of the special tests positive or negative? What does each result indicate?*
   - *Does the athlete have any numbness or paraesthesia?*
   - *Is ecchymosis present?*
   - *Does the athlete exhibit any changes in gait pattern?*
   - *Where is the athlete most point tender?*
   - *Are radiographs available?*
   - *Are the athlete's os coxae misaligned?*
   - *Does the athlete have any leg-length discrepancies?*
   - *Are there any changes in bladder or bowel function?*
3. Identify key terms and concepts, and then research each to broaden your knowledge of lower back, sacroiliac joint, and pelvic injuries.
   - What anatomical structures might be involved in Ms. Yockey's injury?
     Gluteus maximus
     Gluteus minimus
     Gluteus medius
     Right and left os coxae
     Sacrum
     Coccyx
   - Define *prone.*
     Directional term meaning "lying on one's stomach"
   - Why would Ms. Yockey experience intense pain when sitting?
     When Ms. Yockey hit the ground, she may have bruised or fractured the bony anatomy in the buttocks.
   - When sitting, Ms. Yockey experiences less pain when she leans to one side. What might this indicate?
     Although Ms. Yockey may have bruised or fractured the bony anatomy in the buttocks, having less pain when leaning to one side can indicate that the ischium or the os coxae are not involved, because these bones bear weight when leaning and would be painful under a weight load.

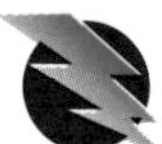

Brain Jolt
Not much treatment is available for this injury. Rest and inactivity typically heal the injury.

4. Based on the information that you currently have and what was provided by your instructor, what are the possible differential diagnoses for Ms. Yockey's injury?
   Contusion to gluteus maximus
   Misalignment of os coxae
   Fractured coccyx

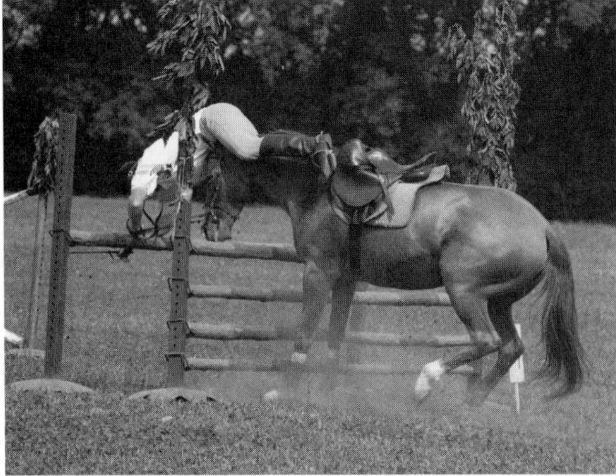

Figure 10-2: Hannah Yockey's fall. (© Thinkstock)

Why or why not?

For each assessment or diagnosis, write *why?* or *why not?* statements identifying why the information is correct or incorrect. Take details from your textbook, your own research, and data from Ms. Yockey's scenario to help you formulate an answer.

1. *Ms. Yockey does not have a contused gluteus maximus because leaning to one side to sit, which places direct pressure on the muscle, is less painful. In addition, strength and ROM at the hip are good.*
2. *Ms. Yockey does not have a misalignment of the os coxae because she does not have a leg-length discrepancy. Her anterior superior iliac spine (ASIS) and posterior iliac spine (PSIS) align and she has good ROM.*
3. *Ms. Yockey has a fractured coccyx because she experiences the most pain when sitting. She is most point tender over the coccyx, and the radiography results were positive for a fractured coccyx.*

What do you think?

1. What is your assessment of Ms. Yockey's injury?
   Answer: *Fractured coccyx*
2. Was your assessment of Ms. Yockey's injury correct?
   Answer: *Yes*
3. If not, explain what you did incorrectly and how you could have performed a better assessment.

   Answer: ________________________________

MODEL SCENARIO 3: HANK GELLER

Hank Geller is a pole-vaulter who is experiencing back and upper-leg pain. He states that the pain has been present for approximately 2 weeks but is increasing. Mr. Geller states that the pain is the worst in the leg compared with his back, and it is increasingly painful when he sneezes and lifts weights. On evaluation, he has positive Milgram test and slump test results (Fig. 10-3). Mr. Geller's lower extremity dermatomes and myotomes are normal.

1. Based on this scenario, what do you know about Mr. Geller's injury?
   - *Male athlete*
   - *Pole-vaulter*
   - *Back pain and upper-leg pain*
   - *Pain for 2 weeks that is becoming increasingly worse*
   - *Increased pain when sneezing and lifting weights*
   - *Positive Milgram test result*
   - *Positive slump test result*
   - *Normal lower extremity dermatomes and myotomes*

Figure 10-3: Hank Geller's slump test.

2. To evaluate Mr. Geller's injury effectively, you will need to gather additional information. What questions should you ask in addition to what is presented in this scenario?
   - *Is this injury a medical emergency?*
   - *Are there any preexisting injuries? If yes, what are they?*
   - *Are there any special tests that are important to perform? If yes, elaborate.*
   - *Are the results of the special tests positive or negative? What does each result indicate?*
   - *Is the athlete's strength and ROM in the trunk and legs good?*
   - *Are reflexes in the lower extremities normal?*
   - *Is edema present?*
   - *Are there any changes in bowel or bladder function?*
   - *Is there any point tenderness in the muscles of the buttocks?*

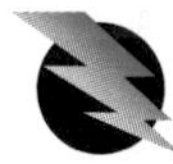

Brain Jolt
A herniated intervertebral disc, spinal stenosis, or distal nerve entrapment correlates with and causes this injury.

3. Identify key terms and concepts, and then research each to broaden your knowledge of lower back, sacroiliac joint, and pelvic injuries.
   - What anatomical structures might be involved in Mr. Geller's injury?
     Lumbar vertebrae
     Vertebral disc
     Pelvis
     Gluteus maximus
     Hamstrings

- Define *dermatomes.*
  The sensory component of a neurologic screen
- Define *myotomes.*
  The motor component of a neurologic screen
- Define *herniated intervertebral disc.*
  A displacement of the nucleus pulposus of a ruptured intervertebral disc
- Define *spinal stenosis.*
  A narrowing of the spinal canal caused by degenerative or traumatic changes
- Define *distal nerve entrapment.*
  Compression of a nerve or nerves that can cause nerve damage
- What is the Milgram test? What does a positive result indicate?
  During a Milgram test, the patient lies supine and is instructed to perform a bilateral straight-leg raise to the height of 2 to 6 inches. The athlete is then instructed to hold the position for 30 seconds. A positive result means that the athlete is unable to hold the position, cannot lift his or her leg, or experiences pain when performing the activity. A positive result indicates an increased intrathecal or extrathecal pressure, which causes pressure on a lumbar nerve root.
- What is the slump test and what does a positive result indicate?
  During a slump test, the athlete sits over the edge of a table and performs the following in sequence: (1) athlete slumps forward and rounds the shoulders, keeping the cervical spine in neutral; pressure is then applied; (2) athlete flexes the cervical spine by bringing his or her chin to the chest; (3) athlete actively extends the knee; (4) athlete's ankle is actively dorsiflexed; (5) athlete repeats these steps bilaterally. The result is positive if sciatic pain or any neurologic symptoms are reproduced. A positive result indicates impingement of the spinal cord or nerve roots.
- Why does Mr. Geller experience increased pain with sneezing and lifting weights?
  When sneezing or lifting weights, there is an increase in intrathecal pressure on the lumbar nerve root.

4. Based on the information that you currently have and what was provided by your instructor, what are the possible differential diagnoses for Mr. Geller's injury?
   Cauda equina syndrome
   Piriformis muscle spasm
   Facet joint dysfunction
   Nerve root impingement

Why or why not?

For each assessment or diagnosis, write *why?* or *why not?* statements identifying why the information is correct or incorrect. Take details from your textbook, your own research, and data from Mr. Geller's scenario to help you formulate an answer.

1. *Mr. Geller does not have cauda equina syndrome. Although he has leg pain, his deep tendon reflexes are not absent, and no changes in bladder or bowel function have occurred.*
2. *Mr. Geller does not have a piriformis muscle spasm. His strength is good, and he has lower back pain. A spasm could pinch the sciatic nerve and produce neurologic symptoms, but no tenderness is felt in the muscle.*
3. *Mr. Geller does not have facet joint dysfunction. Most of his pain is felt in the legs versus the back. The quadrant test result is negative.*
4. *Mr. Geller has lumbar nerve root impingement. He has a positive Milgram test and slump test and positive Valsalva maneuver results. Most of his pain is in his legs versus his back.*

What do you think?

1. What is your assessment of Mr. Geller's injury?
   Answer: *Nerve root impingement*
2. Was your assessment of Mr. Geller's injury correct?
   Answer: *Yes*
3. If not, explain what you did incorrectly and how you could have performed a better assessment.
   Answer: ____________________

STUDENT SCENARIO 1: KYLIE ASHBACHER

Kylie Ashbacher is a cross-country runner who has been experiencing some low back pain since she started running this season. As the mileage increases, the pain increases across her lower back. She finds that when she runs on uneven ground, she gets some relief. It always seems to be her right side that is sore after each practice. On evaluation, Ms. Ashbacher states that she had a prior injury when she was in the fifth grade; she jumped out of a tree and fractured her left tibia at the epiphyseal plate. Although she has not had any restrictions or problems with that leg since the break healed, she does have some weakness with her hip abductors on her right side. When Ms. Ashbacher walks, a dip or drop with her pelvis is noted on her left side (Fig. 10-4).

1. Based on this scenario, what do you know about Ms. Ashbacher's injury?
   - ____________________
     ____

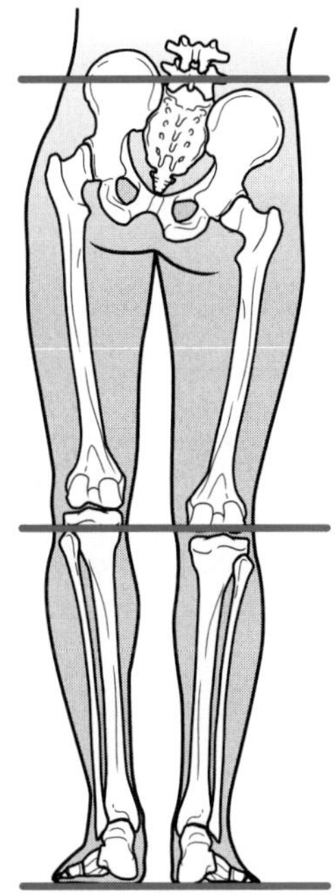

Figure 10-4: Kylie Ashbacher's pelvic orientation.

- ______________________________
- ______________________________
- ______________________________

2. To evaluate Ms. Ashbacher's injury effectively, you will need to gather additional information. What questions should you ask in addition to what is presented in this scenario?

- ______________________________
- ______________________________
- ______________________________
- ______________________________

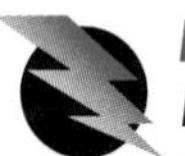

Brain Jolt

If some hip imbalance is noted, first determine whether the discrepancy is true or apparent. A misaligned pelvis can be the result of other anatomical or functional issues.

3. Identify key terms and concepts, and then research each to broaden your knowledge of lower back, sacroiliac joint, and pelvic injuries.

- What anatomical structures might be involved in Ms. Ashbacher's injury?

  Answer: ______________________________
- Define *epiphyseal plate.*

  Answer: ______________________________
- What are hip abductors? What muscles are included in this group?

  Answer: ______________________________
- Why might Ms. Ashbacher's pelvis dip or drop on the left side?

  Answer: ______________________________
- Why does Ms. Ashbacher seem to feel pain relief on uneven ground?

  Answer: ______________________________
- Why do Ms. Ashbacher's previous injuries have a role in this injury?

  Answer: ______________________________

4. Based on the information that you currently have and what was provided by your instructor, what are the possible differential diagnoses for Ms. Ashbacher's injury?

- ______________________________
- ______________________________
- ______________________________
- ______________________________

Why or why not?

For each assessment or diagnosis, write *why?* or *why not?* statements identifying why the information is correct or incorrect. Take details from your textbook, your own research, and data from Ms. Ashbacher's scenario to help you formulate an answer.

1. ______________________________

2. ______________________________

3. ______________________________

4. ______________________________

____

What do you think?

1. What is your assessment of Ms. Ashbacher's injury?

Answer: ______________________________

2. Was your assessment of Ms. Ashbacher's injury correct?

Answer: ______________________________

3. If not, explain what you did incorrectly and how you could have performed a better assessment.

Answer: ______________________________

STUDENT SCENARIO 2: KINO RAMSEY

Kino Ramsey is a catcher on his college baseball team. He has a history of tight hip flexors, but otherwise no other previous injury. He has completed the preseason training and spring break tournament and is now complaining of low back pain. He does not experience any numbness or paraesthesia, but the pain is starting to hinder his performance in the catcher's stance. On evaluation, Mr. Ramsey has weakness in his hamstrings and a positive Thomas test result. He also has a noticeable lordotic curve (Fig. 10-5).

1. Based on this scenario, what do you know about Mr. Ramsey's injury?

- ______________________________
- ______________________________
- ______________________________
- ______________________________

2. To evaluate Mr. Ramsey's injury effectively, you will need to gather additional information. What questions should you ask in addition to what is presented in this scenario?

- ______________________________
- ______________________________
- ______________________________
- ______________________________

Figure 10-5: Kino Ramsey's posture.

Brain Jolt

Back pain does not always originate in the back. Remember to look at the entire picture and the whole athlete to determine what could be causing the problem.

3. Identify key terms and concepts, and then research each to broaden your knowledge of lower back, sacroiliac joint, and pelvic injuries.

- What anatomical structures might be involved in Mr. Ramsey's injury?

  Answer: ______________________________
- Define *lordotic curve*.

  Answer: ______________________________
- What causes a lordotic curve?

  Answer: ______________________________
- Explain other vertebral curvatures.

  Answer: ______________________________
- How does hip flexor tightness play a role in lower back pain?

  Answer: ______________________________
- How is a manual muscle test for the hamstrings conducted?

  Answer: ______________________________
- What is the Thomas test? What does a positive result indicate?

  Answer: ______________________________

4. Based on the information that you currently have and what was provided by your instructor, what are the possible differential diagnoses for Mr. Ramsey's injury?
   - ______
   - ______
   - ______
   - ______

Why or why not?

For each assessment or diagnosis, write *why?* or *why not?* statements identifying why the information is correct or incorrect. Take details from your textbook, your own research, and data from Mr. Ramsey's scenario to help you formulate an answer.

1. ______
2. ______
3. ______
4. ______

What do you think?

1. What is your assessment of Mr. Ramsey's injury?

   Answer: ______
2. Was your assessment of Mr. Ramsey's injury correct?

   Answer: ______
3. If not, explain what you did incorrectly and how you could have performed a better assessment.

   Answer: ______

STUDENT SCENARIO 3: JAMES HERALD

James Herald is a football player. He joins the team in the weight room to work on his legs and low back exercises. Mr. Herald is working on his form with the deadlift technique. He has a tendency to lock his knees when bending over to grab the bar to begin the lift. Keeping his legs straight while lifting the bar places added stress on his low back, and he feels an uncomfortable stretching at his low back during his lift. During evaluation, uneven PSISs are observed. His right PSIS is higher than the left (Fig. 10-6), and his right ASIS is lower than the left. He has point tenderness directly over the sacrum and near the right PSIS, in addition to pain with trunk flexion and extension and positive SI compression and distraction test results.

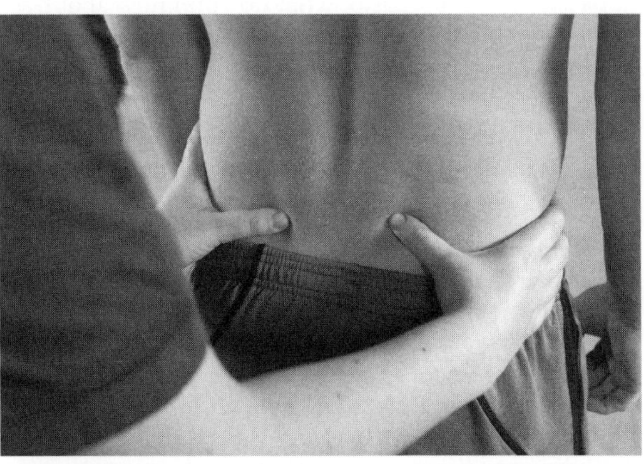

Figure 10-6: James Herald's posterior superior iliac spine.

1. Based on this scenario, what do you know about Mr. Herald's injury?
   - ______
   - ______
   - ______
   - ______
2. To evaluate Mr. Herald's injury effectively, you will need to gather additional information. What questions should you ask in addition to what is presented in this scenario?
   - ______
   - ______
   - ______
   - ______

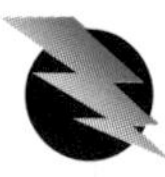

Brain Jolt
When there is pelvic asymmetry, the side that is painful is usually the involved side.

3. Identify key terms and concepts, and then research each to broaden your knowledge of lower back, sacroiliac joint, and pelvic injuries.
   - What anatomical structures might be involved in Mr. Herald's injury?

     Answer: ______
   - How is the athlete's PSIS level determined? What does it indicate if one is higher than the other?

     Answer: ______
   - How is the athlete's ASIS level determined? What does it indicate if one is lower than the other?

     Answer: ______
   - What is the SI compression test? What does a positive result indicate?

     Answer: ______
   - What is the SI distraction test? What does a positive result indicate?

     Answer: ______
   - Why is it important for the athletic trainer to be familiar with proper deadlift technique?

     Answer: ______
4. Based on the information that you currently have and what was provided by your instructor, what are the possible differential diagnoses for Mr. Herald's injury?
   - ______
   - ______
   - ______
   - ______

Why or why not?

For each assessment or diagnosis, write *why?* or *why not?* statements identifying why the information is correct or incorrect. Take details from your textbook, your own research, and data from Mr. Herald's scenario to help you formulate an answer.

1. ______
2. ______
3. ______
4. ______

What do you think?

1. What is your assessment of Mr. Herald's injury?

   Answer: ______
2. Was your assessment of Mr. Herald's injury correct?

   Answer: ______
3. If not, explain what you did incorrectly and how you could have performed a better assessment.

   Answer: ______

STUDENT SCENARIO 4: CURTIS SEXTON

Curtis Sexton is a track runner who participates in the hurdle events by running the 50- and 300-yard hurdles. His coach has him focus on strengthening his hip abductors and hip external rotator muscles in the hope that these exercises will help him to clear the hurdles with ease. He notices a pain in his right hip, which is in the leg that extends horizontally and abducts over the hurdle. Initially, the pain feels similar to soreness from weight room exercises. Now, he notices pain when walking and when seated. Occasionally, he has some numbness that radiates down the back of his leg and into his foot. He states that the numbness is worse when his gluteus maximus feels tight and spasms. He is point tender in the middle of his right gluteus maximus (Fig. 10-7), and there is no history of a lower back injury.

1. Based on this scenario, what do you know about Mr. Sexton's injury?
   - ______
   - ______
   - ______
   - ______

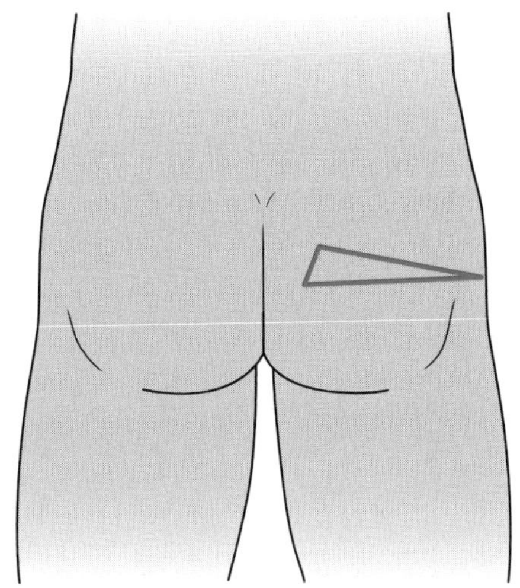

Figure 10-7: Curtis Sexton's point of tenderness.

2. To evaluate Mr. Sexton's injury effectively, you will need to gather additional information. What questions should you ask in addition to what is presented in this scenario?
   - ______________________________
   - ______________________________
   - ______________________________
   - ______________________________

3. Identify key terms and concepts, and then research each to broaden your knowledge of lower back, sacroiliac joint, and pelvic injuries.
   - What anatomical structures might be involved in Mr. Sexton's injury?

     Answer: ______________________________
   - Define *muscle spasm.*

     Answer: ______________________________
   - What are hip abductors? What muscles are included in this group?

     Answer: ______________________________
   - What are external rotators? What muscles are included in this group?

     Answer: ______________________________
   - Why would Mr. Sexton's pain progress to pain with walking and sitting?

     Answer: ______________________________
   - Why does Mr. Sexton's numbness get worse with muscle tightness and spasms?

     Answer: ______________________________
   - Why is it important for athletic trainers to be familiar with the proper hurdle form?

     Answer: ______________________________

4. Based on the information that you currently have and what was provided by your instructor, what are the possible differential diagnoses for Mr. Sexton's injury?
   - ______________________________
   - ______________________________
   - ______________________________
   - ______________________________

Brain Jolt

In some individuals, the sciatic nerve runs through this structure and can produce symptoms. The nerve is not always the root of the problem.

Why or why not?

For each assessment or diagnosis, write *why?* or *why not?* statements identifying why the information is correct or incorrect. Take details from your textbook, your own research, and data from Mr. Sexton's scenario to help you formulate an answer.

1. ______________________________
2. ______________________________
3. ______________________________
4. ______________________________

What do you think?

1. What is your assessment of Mr. Sexton's injury?

   Answer: ______________________________
2. Was your assessment of Mr. Sexton's injury correct?

   Answer: ______________________________
3. If not, explain what you did incorrectly and how you could have performed a better assessment.

   Answer: ______________________________

STUDENT SCENARIO 5: SHERRI MASON

Sherri Mason is a personal trainer who trains for bodybuilding competitions. She is frequently plagued with recurrent hamstring problems and is trying to resolve them before she has to stop training because of pain. Ms. Mason states that the last time she strained her hamstring was 3 months earlier. On evaluation, her hamstring strength is fair with no pain on her right leg, but the hamstring is atrophied when compared bilaterally (Fig. 10-8). The athletic trainer is trying to find the origin of the recurrent issues. On further evaluation, Ms. Mason has a positive Trendelenburg test result, and she experiences pain with hip extension with a bent knee.

1. Based on this scenario, what do you know about Ms. Mason's injury?
   - ______________________________
   - ______________________________
   - ______________________________
   - ______________________________

2. To evaluate Ms. Mason's injury effectively, you will need to gather additional information. What questions should you ask in addition to what is presented in this scenario?
   - ______________________________
   - ______________________________
   - ______________________________
   - ______________________________

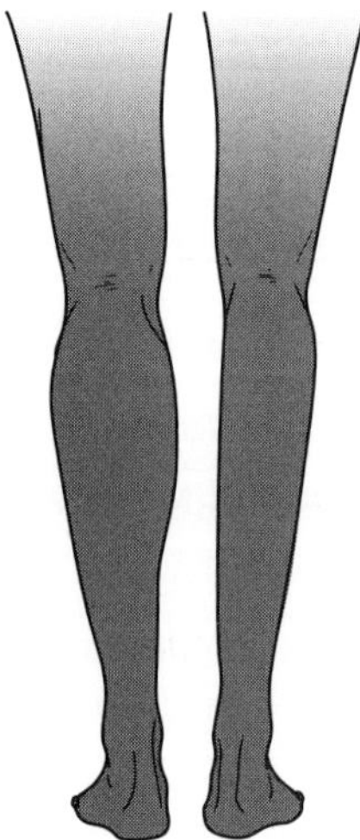

Figure 10-8: Sherri Mason's atrophy.

3. Identify key terms and concepts, and then research each to broaden your knowledge of lower back, sacroiliac joint, and pelvic injuries.
   - What anatomical structures might be involved in Ms. Mason's injury?

     Answer: ______________________________
   - Define *atrophy*.

     Answer: ______________________________
   - Define *bilaterally*.

     Answer: ______________________________
   - How is strength graded?

     Answer: ______________________________
   - Why would Ms. Mason experience pain with hip extension with the knee bent?

     Answer: ______________________________
   - What is the Trendelenburg test? What does a positive result indicate?

     Answer: ______________________________

Brain Jolt

Athletes can be fit and have well-defined muscles; however, sometimes they forget to train the smaller muscles. Remember to check these small but important muscles when evaluating your athletes.

4. Based on the information that you currently have and what was provided by your instructor, what are the possible differential diagnoses for Ms. Mason's injury?
   - ______________________________
   - ______________________________
   - ______________________________
   - ______________________________

Why or why not?

For each assessment or diagnosis, write *why?* or *why not?* statements identifying why the information is correct or incorrect. Take details from your textbook, your own research, and data from Ms. Mason's scenario to help you formulate an answer.

1. ______________________________

2. ______________________________

3. ______________________________

4. ______________________________

What do you think?

1. What is your assessment of Ms. Mason's injury?

   Answer: ______________________________

2. Was your assessment of Ms. Mason's injury correct?

   Answer: ______________________________

3. If not, explain what you did incorrectly and how you could have performed a better assessment.

   Answer: ______________________________

STUDENT SCENARIO 6: KAY GINTER

Kay Ginter has been a gymnast for 13 years, starting when she was 5 years old. She is excited to be reaching her goal of being on a collegiate gymnastics team, and her body has adapted to the many stresses exerted on it over the years. After her freshman year, Ms. Ginter continues to have low back pain that seems to fan out over her lower back. The pain is always worse in the morning, which prohibits her from fully standing straight as a result of a feeling of muscle weakness. She has a positive well straight-leg raise test result (Fig. 10-9) and has pain that radiates into both gluteus maximus muscles when performing a prone press-up.

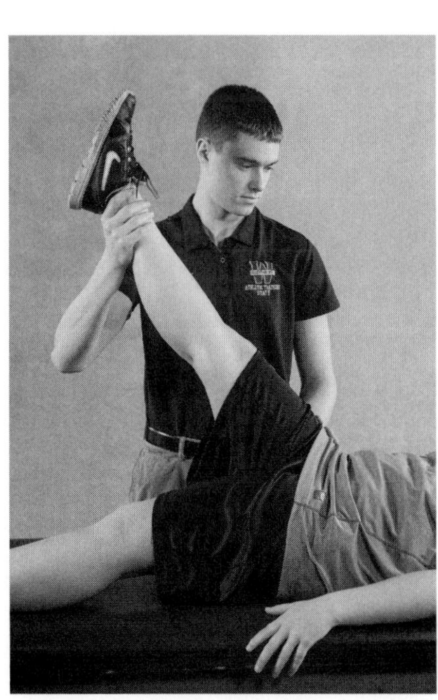

Figure 10-9: Kay Ginter's well straight-leg raise test.

1. Based on this scenario, what do you know about Ms. Ginter's injury?

   - ______________________________
   - ______________________________
   - ______________________________
   - ______________________________

2. To evaluate Ms. Ginter's injury effectively, you will need to gather additional information. What questions should you ask in addition to what is presented in this scenario?

   - ______________________________
   - ______________________________
   - ______________________________
   - ______________________________

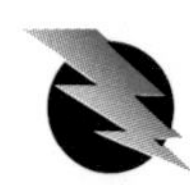

Brain Jolt

This injury causes back pain upon sneezing.

Treatment Detour

This injury is a common cause of lower extremity radicular pain. Research has shown that patients with this condition can relieve their symptoms without surgery. However, this study looks into the subsequent recurrence of symptoms in those patients who resolve this injury nonsurgically. Twenty-five percent of individuals who had resolved symptoms for at least 1 month had recurrence of symptoms within 1 year. Radicular pain is most likely to return in patients who took longer to have resolving symptoms from the initial episode (Suri, Rainville, Hunter, Li, & Katz, 2012).

3. Identify key terms and concepts, and then research each to broaden your knowledge of lower back, sacroiliac joint, and pelvic injuries.
   - What anatomical structures might be involved in Ms. Ginter's injury?

     Answer: ________________
   - Explain the term *prone press-up.*

     Answer: ________________
   - Define *radiating pain.*

     Answer: ________________
   - Why does Ms. Ginter experience radiating pain with a prone press-up?

     Answer: ________________
   - Why is Ms. Ginter's pain worse in the morning?

     Answer: ________________
   - What is the well straight-leg raise test? What does a positive result indicate?

     Answer: ________________
4. Based on the information that you currently have and what was provided by your instructor, what are the possible differential diagnoses for Ms. Ginter's injury?
   - ________________
   - ________________
   - ________________
   - ________________

Why or why not?

For each assessment or diagnosis, write *why?* or *why not?* statements identifying why the information is correct or incorrect. Take details from your textbook, your own research, and data from Ms. Ginter's scenario to help you formulate an answer.

1. ________________
2. ________________
3. ________________
4. ________________

What do you think?

1. What is your assessment of Ms. Ginter's injury?

   Answer: ________________
2. Was your assessment of Ms. Ginter's injury correct?

   Answer: ________________
3. If not, explain what you did incorrectly and how you could have performed a better assessment.

   Answer: ________________

STUDENT SCENARIO 7: BRETT GREGORY

Brett Gregory is a football offensive lineman who experiences low back aching and discomfort after practice. He also finds that sitting in a certain position for longer than 5 min causes mild low back discomfort. He participates in a blocking drill at practice when he notices that his back feels weak. During the last drill, he is forced into extreme hyperextension that causes moderate low back pain. On evaluation, he reproduces the pain when performing the single-leg (stork) stance test (Fig. 10-10).

1. Based on this scenario, what do you know about Mr. Gregory's injury?
   - ________________
   - ________________
   - ________________

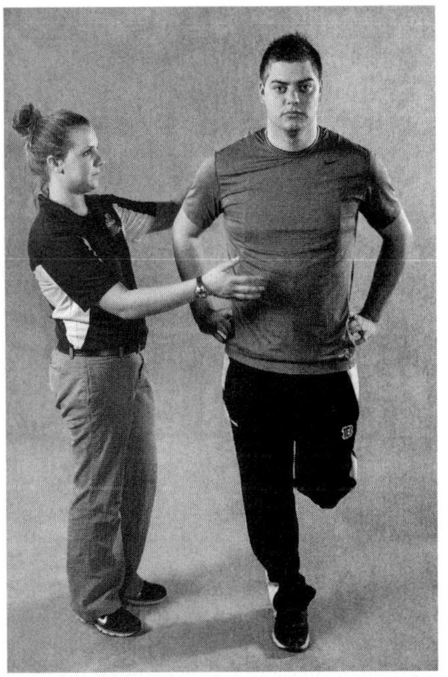

Figure 10-10: Brett Gregory's single-leg stance test.

- ______________________________
  ____

2. To evaluate Mr. Gregory's injury effectively, you will need to gather additional information. What questions should you ask in addition to what is presented in this scenario?
   - ______________________________
     ____
   - ______________________________
     ____
   - ______________________________
     ____
   - ______________________________
     ____

Brain Jolt

The Scotty dog sign will verify this injury.

3. Identify key terms and concepts, and then research each to broaden your knowledge of lower back, sacroiliac joint, and pelvic injuries.
   - What anatomical structures might be involved in Mr. Gregory's injury?

     Answer: ______________________________
   - Define *hyperextension.*

     Answer: ______________________________
   - Why would Mr. Gregory experience increasing pain when sitting for extended periods?

     Answer: ______________________________
   - What might a feeling of weakness indicate?

     Answer: ______________________________
   - What is the single-leg stance test? What does a positive result indicate?

     Answer: ______________________________

Brain Jolt

Misdiagnosis of this injury can lead to a more serious injury. Do not delay referral to a physician.

4. Based on the information that you currently have and what was provided by your instructor, what are the possible differential diagnoses for Mr. Gregory's injury?
   - ______________________________
     ____
   - ______________________________
     ____
   - ______________________________
     ____
   - ______________________________
     ____

Why or why not?

For each assessment or diagnosis, write *why?* or *why not?* statements identifying why the information is correct or incorrect. Take details from your textbook, your own research, and data from Mr. Gregory's scenario to help you formulate an answer.

1. ______________________________
   ____
2. ______________________________
   ____
3. ______________________________
   ____
4. ______________________________
   ____

What do you think?

1. What is your assessment of Mr. Gregory's injury?

   Answer: ______________________________
2. Was your assessment of Mr. Gregory's injury correct?

   Answer: ______________________________
3. If not, explain what you did incorrectly and how you could have performed a better assessment.

   Answer: ______________________________

STUDENT SCENARIO 8: AMBER NELSON

Amber Nelson is a collegiate swimmer. She has a history of low back problems that develop mid-season from performing the butterfly stroke. Ms. Nelson comes to the athletic training room stating that her low back started hurting again 2 weeks ago. On evaluation, she has point tenderness over the left PSIS adjacent to the S2 spinous process. She has additional pain when seated rather than standing and has experienced radiating pain over the left gluteus maximus and into the left upper hamstring. She is unable to perform active back extension without low back pain. A straight-leg raise test result is positive at 30 to 60 degrees with foot dorsiflexion (Fig. 10-11).

1. Based on this scenario, what do you know about Ms. Nelson's injury?
   - ______________________________
   - ______________________________
   - ______________________________
   - ______________________________

2. To evaluate Ms. Nelson's injury effectively, you will need to gather additional information. What questions should you ask in addition to what is presented in this scenario?
   - ______________________________
   - ______________________________
   - ______________________________
   - ______________________________

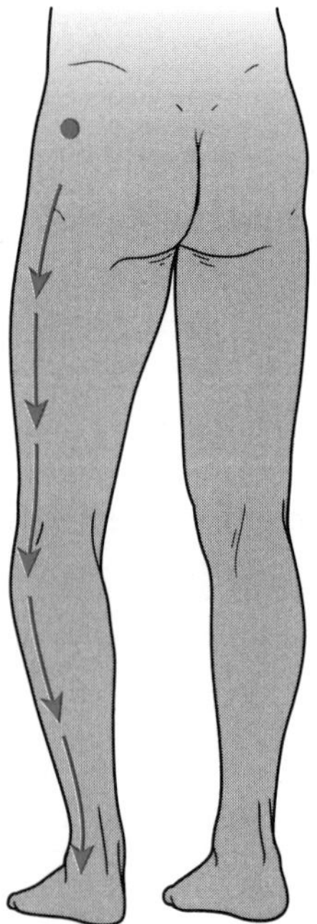

Figure 10-11: Amber Nelson's area of pain.

Brain Jolt

Do not forget to apply pressure over and into the popliteal fossa when straightening the leg in the straight-leg raise test.

3. Identify key terms and concepts, and then research each to broaden your knowledge of lower back, sacroiliac joint, and pelvic injuries.
   - What anatomical structures might be involved in Ms. Nelson's injury?

     Answer: ______________________________
   - Define *radiating pain.*

     Answer: ______________________________
   - Why would Ms. Nelson have more pain when seated versus standing?

     Answer: ______________________________
   - What might radiating pain in the gluteus maximus and hamstrings indicate?

     Answer: ______________________________
   - Why is it important for athletic trainers to be familiar with the butterfly stroke?

     Answer: ______________________________
   - What is a straight-leg raise test? What are the different positions? Why are 30 to 60 degrees important? What does a positive result indicate?

     Answer: ______________________________

4. Based on the information that you currently have and what was provided by your instructor, what are the possible differential diagnoses for Ms. Nelson's injury?
   - ______________________________
   - ______________________________
   - ______________________________
   - ______________________________

Why or why not?

For each assessment or diagnosis, write *why?* or *why not?* statements identifying why the information is correct or incorrect. Take details from your textbook, your own research, and data from Ms. Nelson's scenario to help you formulate an answer.

1. ______________________________

____

2. ______________________________

____

3. ______________________________

____

4. ______________________________

____

What do you think?

1. What is your assessment of Ms. Nelson's injury?

   Answer: ______________________________

2. Was your assessment of Ms. Nelson's injury correct?

   Answer: ______________________________

3. If not, explain what you did incorrectly and how you could have performed a better assessment.

   Answer: ______________________________

STUDENT SCENARIO 9: DARYL HUBER

Daryl Huber is a forward on the men's soccer team. He has recently missed each shot on goal that he has taken, kicking the ball either directly to the goalie or wide of the goal. His coach is having him practice only shots on goal for the entire 2-hour practice. Because he plays on the right side of the goal, he is kicking with his right leg. He begins his practice by hitting each shot into the goal. As practice continues, he notices that he is developing a soreness located around the groin area on his right leg. Each time he brings the leg across the body or adducts the hip, he feels this discomfort (Fig. 10-12). He attributes soreness to the long practices of performing only one drill and dismisses the discomfort. One week passes, and Mr. Huber decides that he should tell the certified athletic trainer that the pain in his groin has gotten worse. On evaluation, Mr. Huber displays point tenderness over his lower abdominal area. He is already predisposed to any type of lower abdominal injury as a result of his weak core strength that was tested earlier in the season.

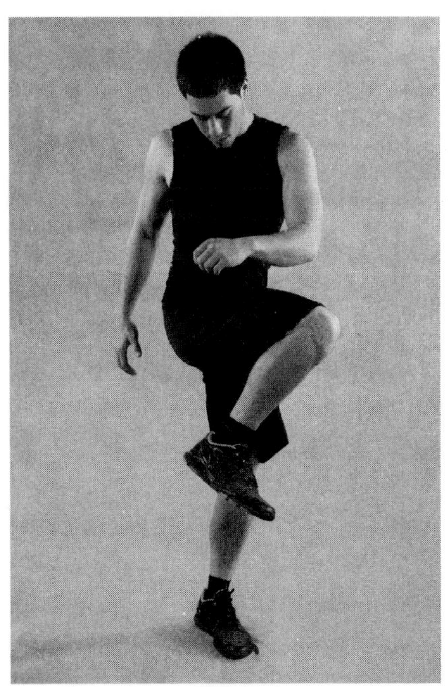

Figure 10-12: Daryl Huber's pain-causing action.

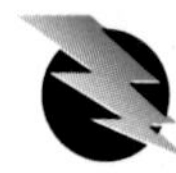

Brain Jolt

If misdiagnosed, this injury can be prolonged and disabling for an athlete.

1. Based on this scenario, what do you know about Mr. Huber's injury?

   - ______________________________

     ____
   - ______________________________

     ____
   - ______________________________

     ____
   - ______________________________

     ____

2. To evaluate Mr. Huber's injury effectively, you will need to gather additional information. What questions should you ask in addition to what is presented in this scenario?

   - ______________________________

     ____
   - ______________________________

     ____

- ____
- ____

3. Identify key terms and concepts, and then research each to broaden your knowledge of lower back, sacroiliac joint, and pelvic injuries.
   - What anatomical structures might be involved in Mr. Huber's injury?

     Answer: ______________________________

   - Define *predisposed.*

     Answer: ______________________________

   - Define *adduction of the hip.*

     Answer: ______________________________

   - What is core strength? Why is this important in athletic training evaluations?

     Answer: ______________________________

   - What might pain in the groin and with adduction indicate?

     Answer: ______________________________

4. Based on the information that you currently have and what was provided by your instructor, what are the possible differential diagnoses for Mr. Huber's injury?
   - ____
   - ____
   - ____
   - ____

Conversation Buffer

As the evaluator, you might need to ask the athlete personal questions and palpate personal or intimate areas of the body. Inform the athlete of which body area needs to be examined. Doing so can help the athlete feel more comfortable and alleviate any uncertainties regarding your actions. Have a witness available, especially if the athlete is of the opposite sex.

Why or why not?

For each assessment or diagnosis, write *why?* or *why not?* statements identifying why the information is correct or incorrect. Take details from your textbook, your own research, and data from Mr. Huber's scenario to help you formulate an answer.

1. ____
2. ____
3. ____
4. ____

What do you think?

1. What is your assessment of Mr. Huber's injury?

   Answer: ______________________________

2. Was your assessment of Mr. Huber's injury correct?

   Answer: ______________________________

3. If not, explain what you did incorrectly and how you could have performed a better assessment.

   Answer: ______________________________

STUDENT SCENARIO 10: ROD THOMPSON

Rod Thompson is a certified athletic trainer at a Division III college. He is 45 years old and enjoys going to the gym 3 days a week to perform cardiovascular exercises. The college athletic training room has just recently received their supplies for the year, and Mr. Thompson knows that he will need to lift many boxes as a result. At the end of the day, he notices soreness in his lower back even though he has no history of injury. He attributes the soreness to lifting and rotating his lower back while moving the supplies. When he wakes up the following morning, he experiences moderate pain, soreness, and point tenderness over the L1–L5 transverse processes (Fig. 10-13). There is no radiating pain, numbness, or paraesthesia in his lower extremities.

1. Based on this scenario, what do you know about Mr. Thompson's injury?
   - ____
   - ____

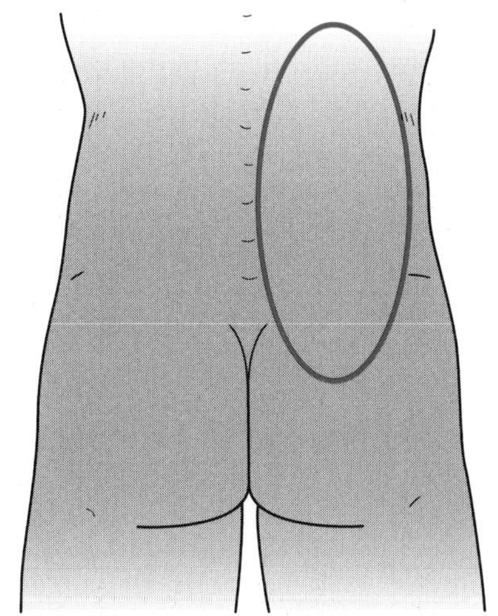

Figure 10-13: Rod Thompson's point of pain.

- ______________________________
- ______________________________

2. To evaluate Mr. Thompson's injury effectively, you will need to gather additional information. What questions should you ask in addition to what is presented in this scenario?
   - ______________________________
   - ______________________________
   - ______________________________
   - ______________________________

3. Identify key terms and concepts, and then research each to broaden your knowledge of lower back, sacroiliac joint, and pelvic injuries.
   - What anatomical structures might be involved in Mr. Thompson's injury?

     Answer: ______________________________
   - Define *cardiovascular exercise.*

     Answer: ______________________________
   - Define *lumbar rotation.*

     Answer: ______________________________
   - Define *lower extremity.*

     Answer: ______________________________
   - Define *radiating pain.*

     Answer: ______________________________
   - Where are the L1–L5 vertebrae located?

     Answer: ______________________________
   - If Mr. Thompson experiences numbness or paraesthesia, what could this indicate?

     Answer: ______________________________
   - Why would Mr. Thompson's pain become worse the following day?

     Answer: ______________________________

4. Based on the information that you currently have and what was provided by your instructor, what are the possible differential diagnoses for Mr. Thompson's injury?
   - ______________________________
   - ______________________________
   - ______________________________
   - ______________________________

Brain Jolt

At any age, core strength is the key to a healthy back.

Brain Jolt

Proper lifting techniques are crucial to protecting the back.

Why or why not?

For each assessment or diagnosis, write *why?* or *why not?* statements identifying why the information is correct or incorrect. Take details from your textbook, your own research, and data from Mr. Thompson's scenario to help you formulate an answer.

1. ______________________________
2. ______________________________
3. ______________________________
4. ______________________________

What do you think?

1. What is your assessment of Mr. Thompson's injury?

   Answer: ______

2. Was your assessment of Mr. Thompson's injury correct?

   Answer: ______

3. If not, explain what you did incorrectly and how you could have performed a better assessment.

   Answer: ______

knowledge checklist

Table 10-1 offers a checklist that can be used by a peer, instructor, or preceptor to evaluate each part of a lower back, sacroiliac joint, and pelvis assessment. Use this checklist as a tool to ensure that the evaluation is complete and to assess your knowledge of the competencies that apply to this chapter.

TABLE 10-1 ■ Lower Back, Sacroiliac Joint, and Pelvis Assessment Competency Checklist

	Proficient *Can demonstrate and execute the skill properly*	**Proficient With Assistance** *Can demonstrate and execute the skill with minimal guidance or tips*	**Not Proficient** *Unable to demonstrate and execute the skill properly; need to be reevaluated at another time after further study and practice*
Athlete's Health History			
Medical history			
History of injury to low back, sacroiliac joint, or pelvis injuries			
Type of sport and position played			
When did the injury occur?			
Any changes in bladder or bowel function?			
Mechanisms of Injury			
How did the injury occur?			
When does the pain occur?			
What makes the pain better or worse?			
Is there a position that makes the pain subside?			
Does the athlete experience numbness or tingling?			
Were any pops, cracks, or snaps felt or heard?			
Was a leg or the trunk forced into an unusual position?			
When did the pain begin?			
Visual Observations			
Posture			
Edema			
Ecchymosis			
Deformity, misalignment			
Gait pattern			
Palpation			
Temperature change over the painful area, crepitus, deformity, intra-articular or extra-articular joint swelling, changes within the muscle fibers			
Spinous processes			
Iliac crests			
Posterior superior iliac spine			
Gluteals			
Ischial tuberosity			
Greater trochanter			
Sciatic nerve			
Pubic symphysis			

Continued

TABLE 10-1 ■ Lower Back, Sacroiliac Joint, and Pelvis Assessment Competency Checklist—cont'd

	Proficient	Proficient With Assistance	Not Proficient
Range of Motion			
Passive or active			
Trunk flexion			
Trunk extension			
Trunk rotation			
Trunk lateral flexion			
Hip flexion			
Hip extension			
Hip adduction			
Hip abduction			
Strength			
Grade through manual muscle tests			
Trunk flexion			
Trunk extension			
Trunk rotation			
Trunk lateral flexion			
Hip flexion			
Hip extension			
Hip adduction			
Hip abduction			
Special Tests			
Spring test			
Valsalva maneuver			
Milgram test			
Kernig–Brudzinski test			
Straight-leg raise test			
Well straight-leg raise test			
Slump test			
Quadrant test			
Femoral nerve stretch test			
Trendelenburg test			
Bowstring test			
Thomas test			
Single leg stance test			
SI compression/distraction test			
Leg Length Measurements			
Neurological			
Lumbar plexus (lower quarter)			
Vascular			
Dorsal pedal pulse			
Capillary refill			
Final Assessment			
Sprain, strain, contusion, fracture, condition, severity			

*Be sure to always compare bilaterally.

REFERENCES

National Athletic Training Association. (2011). *Athletic training education competencies* (5th ed.). Retrieved from http://www.nata.org/sites/default/files/5th-Edition-Competencies-2011-PDF-Version.pdf

Prentice, W. (2010). *Arnheim's principles of athletic training: A competency-based approach* (14th ed.). New York, NY: McGraw-Hill.

Starkey, C., Brown, S. D., & Ryan, J. (2010). *Examination of orthopedic and athletic injuries* (3rd ed.). Philadelphia, PA: F.A. Davis.

Suri, P. S., Rainville, J., Hunter, D. J., Li, L., & Katz, J. N. (2012). Recurrence of radicular pain or back pain after nonsurgical treatment of symptomatic lumbar disk herniation. *Archive of Physical Medicine and Rehabilitation, 93*, 690–695.

Toueg, C .W., et al. (2010). Prevalence of spondylolisthesis in a population of gymnasts. *Studies in Health Technology and Informatics, 158*, 132–137.

Venes, D. (Ed.). (2009). *Taber's cyclopedic medical dictionary* (21st ed.). Philadelphia, PA: F.A. Davis.

part three

Rehabilitation and Therapeutic Exercise

chapter 11

Lower Extremity: The Ankle and Foot

chapter outline

athletic trainer's corner

Here is what one athletic training student experienced while rehabilitating an athlete's injury:

One of the most memorable rehabilitation programs I implemented was for a football player with a syndesmotic ankle sprain. The injury occurred during a preseason scrimmage and resulted in mild ecchymosis and edema to the athlete's ankle. Although it seemed that the athlete would heal quickly, he struggled to regain his strength and proprioception throughout the next week of rehabilitation. We worked together to prepare him for a scrimmage the following week, but he was not ready, which was discouraging for both of us. We did not give up though, and throughout the next week he worked even harder to regain the strength he had lost. Finally, he was able to play in the first game of the season. He was thankful for everything I had done for him, and I was proud of the effort he put forth. Even when you do everything right, I learned that rehabilitation still takes time. For an athletic trainer, this makes an athlete's return to play even more rewarding. I will always remember this special rehabilitation experience.

Erin Dettwiler, AT, ATC
Dayton Sports Medicine Institute
Dayton Dunbar High School
Dayton, Ohio

learning outcomes

After working through this chapter, you will be able to:

1. Describe seven different goals of rehabilitation and the importance each plays in the overall rehabilitation protocol.
2. Verbalize indications for performing ankle and foot rehabilitative techniques.
3. Discuss modifications and progressions that are used during a rehabilitation program for the ankle and foot.
4. Discuss outcome measures used to identify activity levels and return-to-play guidelines for all ankle and foot injuries.
5. Explain what modality choice is proper for rehabilitation by using indications and contraindications and the principles and theory related to the physiological response of the intervention.

introduction

In the profession of athletic training, you are inevitably exposed to many injuries as a result of athletic or recreational activities. Throughout this chapter, many examples of conditions and injuries are presented, and you are asked to design a rehabilitation program to help these patients recover and resume their active lifestyles. These activities will help you to fine-tune your rehabilitation skills and develop new and beneficial rehabilitation plans. Before you begin a rehabilitation plan, be sure that you completely understand the injury—that is, how it occurred and what body part has been injured. By implementing all the information you have learned in the classroom, you can determine the best exercises and modalities to use in your program.

As you work through the exercises in this chapter, remember the phases of healing (Table 11-1), which describe the inflammatory, proliferation, and maturation responses that occur with ankle and foot injuries.

TABLE 11-1 ■ Phases of Healing

Phase	Stages of Inflammation	Duration
Phase 1: Inflammatory response	Acute	0–14 days after injury
	Subacute	14–31 days after injury
	Chronic	14–31 days after injury
Phase 2: Repair, regeneration (proliferation)		72 hours to 4–6 weeks after injury
Phase 3: Remodeling, maturation		Can begin at 3 weeks to 1 year or more after injury

The brain jolts in this chapter are tips to help you bridge the gap from the actual diagnosis to the treatment plan. Each brain jolt leads you toward information that can assist you during the rehabilitation process. You might discover repetitive information that reinforces important information and aids learning.

MODEL SCENARIO 1: WADE WILHELM

Wade Wilhelm is a 10-year-old multisport athlete. He plays football, basketball, and baseball. He is beginning his baseball season and notices pain on his posterior calcaneus only when he is participating. He is taken to his pediatrician and examined. On evaluation, he has a bony prominence that has developed over the posterior side of the calcaneus and localized edema that has developed just below the insertion point of the Achilles tendon. In addition, he has a decreased passive range of motion (ROM) and strength with dorsiflexion. Sever disease is diagnosed (Fig. 11-1).

1. Based on this scenario, what do you know about Mr. Wilhelm's injury?
   - *Male athlete*
   - *Ten years old*
   - *Mechanism of injury: chronic*
   - *Active in sports*

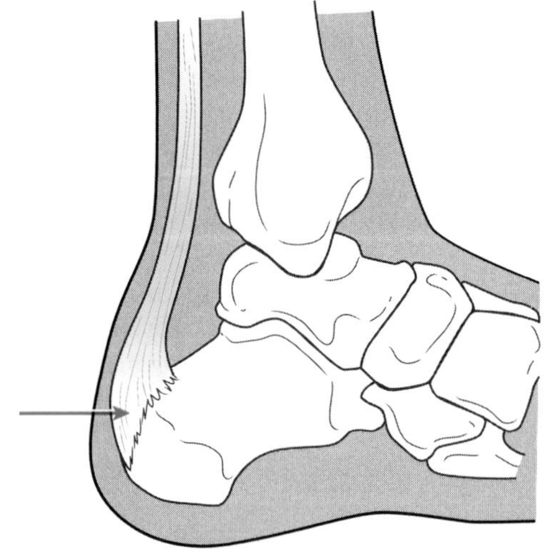

Figure 11-1: Wade Wilhelm's calcaneus.

- *Pain at posterior calcaneus only with participation in sports*
- *Bony prominence over posterior calcaneus*
- *Localized edema below the Achilles tendon*
- *Decreased passive ROM*

2. To rehabilitate Mr. Wilhelm's injury effectively, you will need to gather additional information. What questions should you ask in addition to what is presented in this scenario?
   - *Are there any preexisting injuries? If yes, what are they?*
   - *How long has the athlete experienced this pain?*
   - *What is the athlete's pain level and type of pain felt?*
   - *What is the strength at the ankle other than dorsiflexion?*
   - *What is the ROM at the ankle?*
   - *Does the athlete have any numbness or paraesthesia?*
   - *Is the edema localized in the bursa?*
3. Identify key terms and concepts, and then research each to broaden your knowledge about the rehabilitation of ankle and foot injuries.
   - What anatomical structures might be involved in Mr. Wilhelm's injury?
     Calcaneus
     Achilles tendon
     Muscles superficial to posterior compartment of the lower leg
   - What is Sever disease?
     Sever disease is a traction injury at the apophysis of the calcaneus where the Achilles tendon attaches. This disease primarily affects young, active children.
   - In which phase of healing is this injury?
     This injury occurs at the inflammatory response phase.
   - Define *edema.*
     Swelling; a localized or general condition that causes body tissues to contain an excessive amount of fluid
   - Define *pediatrician.*
     A physician who specializes in infant-to-adolescent internal medicine or care
   - Define *bony prominence.*
     A tuberosity or growth that develops on a bone
   - What is the insertion point of the Achilles tendon?
     The calcaneus is the insertion point of the Achilles tendon.
4. Based on the information that you currently have and what was provided by your instructor, how will you begin Mr. Wilhelm's rehabilitation?
   The initial part of the evaluation is conducted with a physical examination. Based on the results of this evaluation, start by applying ice to the area. Because the surface area is small, an ice cup can be used for 7 to 10 minutes. If Mr. Wilhelm's parents are concerned about his pain, recommend that they talk with their pediatrician about proper medications that can be used. He can also try to increase flexibility by using a foam roller over his gastrocnemius. A heel lift can also be used to reduce pain. He should be placed on limited playing status until the pain and inflammation subside.

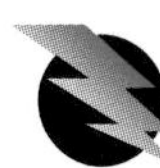

Brain Jolt

Documentation while rehabilitating an athlete is a crucial component of athletic training. Documenting the athlete's progression is necessary to encourage continuous athlete evaluations; this ensures the most effective rehabilitation and helps you protect yourself in the event of a lawsuit.

Why or why not?

How will Mr. Wilhelm's rehabilitation progress? For the *why?* portion of each exercise, explain why you chose a particular exercise or activity as part of your program. Describe which rehabilitation goals the exercise or activity covers, and describe the key indicators for progression. For the *why not?* portion of each exercise, explain why other rehabilitation exercises or activities were not chosen and what to avoid during rehabilitation for this injury. Gather details from the textbook, your own research, and data from Mr. Wilhelm's scenario to help formulate your answer.

Why?

- ***Foam roller.*** *This activity helps with the rehabilitation goal of increasing ROM and can be progressed to towel stretches and an inclined board once the athlete has healed and the pain levels decrease.*
- ***Towel curls with toes.*** *This activity is used for the rehabilitation goal of increasing strength and to strengthen the intrinsic muscles of the foot. This activity also helps to increase strength and can progress by adding a weight at the end of the towel once the athlete performs the activity with ease.*
- ***Seated calf raises.*** *This activity is used for the rehabilitation goal of increasing strength and to strengthen the superficial posterior compartment. It also helps to achieve the goal of increasing strength and can progress to weight-bearing double-leg raises, followed by weight-bearing single-leg raises, once the seated exercises are no longer a challenge for the athlete.*
- ***Resistance band exercises.*** *This activity is used for the rehabilitation goal of increasing strength and to strengthen the ankle. This exercise can be progressed by using different colored bands that provide increased resistance, following each manufacturer's guidelines for resistance color. Increase repetitions and number of sets once the athlete performs the exercises with ease.*
- ***Ice cup.****This modality delivers concentrated cryotherapy to an area. It also helps with the rehabilitation goal of decreasing pain, edema, and inflammation.*

Why not?

- *Other exercises were not implemented because typical strengthening exercises do not address ROM in the ankle.*
- *Avoid any exercise or resistance technique that is too strenuous or places excessive stress or tension on the Achilles tendon, because this can further damage the structures involved.*

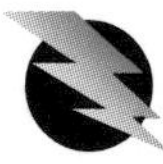

Brain Jolt
Raising the heel often provides relief in Sever disease.

What do you think?

1. Based on your rehabilitation protocol, discuss the indicators for a limited or full return to play with the athlete. Include a rough timeline for return to play, if applicable, which is affected by the athlete's compliance with the rehabilitation program.
   - ***Limited return to play.*** *The athlete can return to play with limited participation if he or she: (1) has only mild pain but is generally pain free with most activities; (2) has no active edema; (3) is able to perform sport-specific activities without pain or a limp; or (4) has good strength, ROM, and proprioception.*
   - ***Full return to play.*** *The athlete can attain full return-to-play status if he performs sport-specific activities without any symptoms and achieves a muscle strength grade of 5/5 with comparable strength bilaterally, full ROM, and normal proprioception.*
2. Are modifications or required protective equipment needed to return to play?
   - *A heel lift can be used to help with this condition.*

MODEL SCENARIO 2: JANET PLATT

Janet Platt is a college soccer player who has a history of foot injuries. Since the soccer season began 1 month ago, Ms. Platt has noticed pain on the right side of the posterior calcaneus. Moderate localized edema has developed, representing with a watery feel, upon palpation but no visible blister. The area is more inflamed after Ms. Platt wears her soccer cleats during practice. She decides to ask the certified athletic trainer (ATC) to examine her foot. Retrocalcaneal bursitis is diagnosed (Fig. 11-2).

1. Based on this scenario, what do you know about Ms. Platt's injury?
   - *Female athlete*
   - *Soccer player*
   - *Previous foot injuries*
   - *Mechanism of injury: chronic*
   - *Pain over right posterior calcaneus*
   - *Edema that feels watery and increases with soccer play*
   - *No visible blister evident*
2. To rehabilitate Ms. Platt's injury effectively, you will need to gather additional information. What questions should you ask in addition to what is presented in this scenario?
   - *Are there any preexisting injuries? If yes, what are they?*
   - *How long has the athlete experienced this pain?*
   - *What is the athlete's pain level and type of pain felt?*
   - *What is the strength in the foot and ankle?*
   - *What is the ROM in the foot and ankle?*
   - *Does the athlete have any numbness or paraesthesia?*
   - *Is the Achilles tendon thickened?*

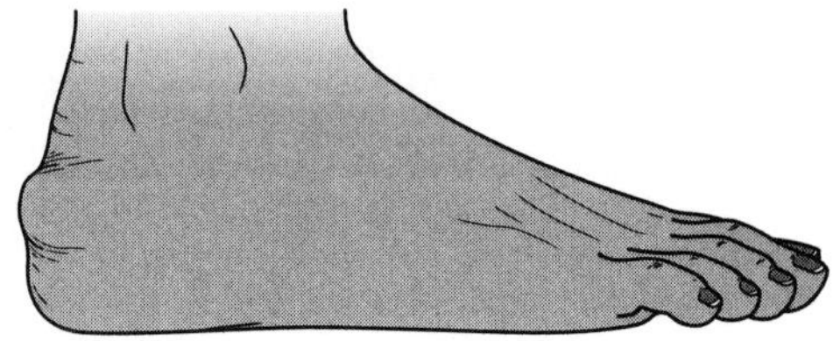

Figure 11-2: Janet Platt's heel.

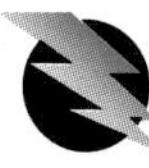

Brain Jolt
The "pump bump" can become easily inflamed and painful. Adding an extra layer between the area and the shoe can reduce the pain and friction and enhance recovery.

3. Identify key terms and concepts, and then research each to broaden your knowledge about the rehabilitation of ankle and foot injuries.
   - What anatomical structures might be involved in Ms. Platt's injury?
     Calcaneus
     Achilles tendon
     Retrocalcaneal bursa
   - What is retrocalcaneal bursitis?
     An inflammation of the bursa that lies over the calcaneus and sits between the calcaneus and the Achilles tendon
   - In which phase of healing is this injury?
     This injury occurs at the inflammatory response phase.
   - Define *edema.*
     Swelling; a localized or general condition that causes body tissues to contain an excessive amount of fluid

- What does watery edema indicate?
  When a bursa becomes inflamed, fluid collects but has the feeling of a watery substance.

4. Based on the information that you currently have and the information that was provided by your instructor, how will you begin Ms. Platt's rehabilitation?
   Retrocalcaneal bursitis is an inflammation of the bursa that is located between the Achilles tendon and the calcaneus. It becomes inflamed because of pressure and the friction that a rigid shoe heel can cause. Focus on decreasing the edema on the calcaneus with a compression pad and elastic wrap. Next, begin a stretching program with the superficial posterior compartment followed by the Achilles tendon. Discuss using an anti-inflammatory medication and instruct the athlete to follow the PRICE (prevention, rest, ice, compression, and elevation) regimen at home. Inspect the athlete's shoes and recommend a new pair if needed.

Why or why not?

How will Ms. Platt's rehabilitation progress? For the *why?* portion of each exercise, explain why you chose a particular exercise or activity as part of your program, describe which rehabilitation goals the exercise or activity covers, and describe the key indicators for progression. For the *why not?* portion of each exercise, explain why other rehabilitation exercises or activities were not chosen and what to avoid during rehabilitation for this injury. Gather details from the textbook, your own research, and data from Ms. Platt's scenario to help formulate your answer.

Why?

- ***Towel stretching.*** *This activity is not intense enough to cause further injury. This activity also helps with the rehabilitation goal of increasing ROM, and it can be progressed to an incline board once the athlete no longer benefits from towel stretching and pain levels decrease.*
- ***Adjust compression wrap.*** *Remove the compression pad after the edema decreases and add only an elastic wrap to decrease the edema further.*
- ***Pulsed ultrasound.*** *If edema fails to decrease with PRICE, then a pulsed ultrasound modality can help disperse the edema.*
- ***Resistance band exercises.*** *This activity is used for the rehabilitation goal of increasing strength and to strengthen the ankle. This exercise can be progressed by using different colored bands following each manufacturer's guidelines for resistance color. Increase repetitions and number of sets once the athlete performs the exercises with ease.*

Why not?

- *Avoid direct friction to the area, as well as any activity that increases the bursitis edema, such as thermal modalities, while still in the inflammatory stage of healing.*

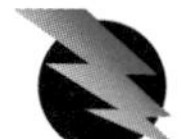

Brain Jolt
To limit the risk of tendonitis, remember to increase repetitions and number of sets before increasing resistance.

What do you think?

1. Based on your rehabilitation protocol, discuss the indicators for a limited or full return to play with the athlete. Include a rough timeline for return to play, if applicable, which is affected by the athlete's compliance with the rehabilitation program.
   - ***Limited or full return to play.*** *Retrocalcaneal bursitis is an injury that causes discomfort. The bursitis does not normally decrease the athlete's strength or ROM. As long as he or she is able to participate without compensation and the bursitis continues to subside, the athlete is not normally kept out of competition.*
2. Are modifications or required protective equipment needed to return to play?
   - *Verifying that the athlete's soccer cleats and recreation shoes fit properly prevents unnecessary friction on the posterior heel.*

STUDENT SCENARIO 1: **HALEY ROE**

Haley Roe is a volleyball player. Two days ago, she sustained a syndesmotic ankle sprain (Fig. 11-3). She fell onto another player's foot while forcefully dorsiflexing her right foot, and she is now experiencing pain with eversion. She is unable to bear weight on her right foot, and appears to have moderate edema and ecchymosis. She has a positive Kleiger test result and, based on the Ottawa ankle rules, she is referred to the team doctor for a radiography. Ms. Roe has been unable to bear weight and is wearing an elastic wrap with compression pad. In addition, PRICE has been added to her rehabilitation program. She just returned to play 1 week ago after being out for 2 months because of a grade 2 lateral ankle sprain to the anterior talofibular ligament.

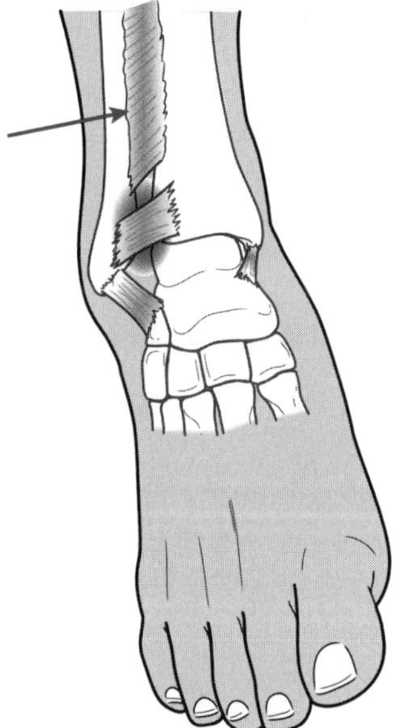

Figure 11-3: Haley Roe's ankle.

1. Based on this scenario, what do you know about Ms. Roe's injury?

- ______________________
- ______________________
- ______________________
- ______________________

2. To rehabilitate Ms. Roe's injury effectively, you will need to gather additional information. What questions should you ask in addition to what is presented in this scenario?

- ______________________
- ______________________
- ______________________
- ______________________

Brain Jolt

Syndesmotic ankle sprains take longer to heal than inversion and eversion ankle sprains. If healing does not progress, this injury can be repaired surgically.

Conversation Buffer

The rate of healing and the timeline for return to play varies significantly and is often unpredictable. Be cautious about your predictions concerning the return to play of an injured athlete when speaking with the coach or athlete. As a result of this unpredictability, you could unintentionally provide false expectations that might set up the coach and athlete for disappointment in the long run. Assess the individual's progress on a daily basis to better determine recovery time.

Treatment Detour

Ankle injuries are the most common injury sustained by athletes; however, syndesmotic sprains account for 10% to 20% of all ankle sprains and are the most frustrating and problematic sprains. This section focuses on the management of these injuries, which tend to have a delay in recovery and significant pain associated with them. Athletes who sustain these "high" ankle sprains are usually unable to walk after the injury because of fibular movement during gait, specifically during the stance phase. Complete immobilization in a cast or boot and partial or non-weight-bearing is best for a good progression through the healing process and ultimately a quicker recovery (Williams, Jones, & Amendola, 2007).

3. Identify key terms and concepts, and then research each to broaden your knowledge about the rehabilitation of ankle and foot injuries.

- What anatomical structures might be involved in Ms. Roe's injury?

  Answer: ______________________
- In which phase of healing is this injury?

  Answer: ______________________
- Define the term *syndesmotic ankle sprain.*

  Answer: ______________________
- Define *edema.*

  Answer: ______________________
- Define *ecchymosis.*

  Answer: ______________________
- Define *dorsiflexion.*

  Answer: ______________________
- Define *eversion.*

  Answer: ______________________
- What are the Ottawa ankle rules?

  Answer: ______________________
- Does Ms. Roe's previous injury play a role in her current injury?

  Answer: ______________________

- Why is Ms. Roe's injury considered a non–weight-bearing injury?

  Answer: ______

- What is the Kleiger test? What does it test? What does a positive result indicate?

  Answer: ______

4. Based on the information that you currently have and what was provided by your instructor, how will you begin Ms. Roe's rehabilitation?

- ______
- ______
- ______
- ______

Why or why not?

How will Ms. Roe's rehabilitation progress? For the *why?* portion of each exercise, explain why you chose a particular exercise or activity as part of your program. Describe which rehabilitation goals the exercise or activity covers, and describe the key indicators for progression. For the *why not?* portion of each exercise, explain why other rehabilitation exercises or activities were not chosen and what to avoid during rehabilitation for this injury. Gather details from the textbook, your own research, and data from Ms. Roe's scenario to help formulate your answer.

Why?

- ______
- ______
- ______
- ______

Why not?

- ______
- ______

What do you think?

1. Based on your rehabilitation protocol, discuss the indicators for a limited return or full return to play. Include a rough timeline for return to play, if applicable, which is affected by the athlete's compliance with the rehabilitation program.

- ______
- ______
- ______
- ______

2. Are modifications or required protective equipment needed to return to play?

- ______
- ______

STUDENT SCENARIO 2: SAM AMBROSS

Sam Ambross has been experiencing a significant amount of pain on the plantar surface of his right foot near his calcaneus while running (Fig. 11-4). He is evaluated by the ATC, who diagnoses plantar fasciitis. He is placed on a limited participation status with his cross-country team. He has no history of injury, and the ATC suggests that Mr. Ambross consult a podiatrist for a soft, nonrigid orthotic. In addition, he should consider using a soft heel cup.

1. Based on this scenario, what do you know about Mr. Ambross' injury?

- ______
- ______

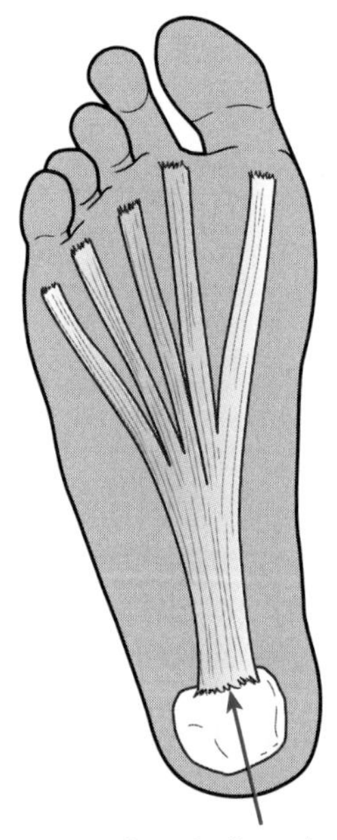

Figure 11-4: Sam Ambross' pain.

- ______________________________
- ______________________________

2. To rehabilitate Mr. Ambross' injury effectively, you will need to gather additional information. What questions should you ask in addition to what is presented in this scenario?
   - ______________________________
   - ______________________________
   - ______________________________
   - ______________________________

3. Identify key terms and concepts, and then research each to broaden your knowledge about the rehabilitation of ankle and foot injuries.
   - What anatomical structures might be involved in Mr. Ambross' injury?

     Answer: ______________________________
   - In which phase of healing is this injury?

     Answer: ______________________________
   - Define the term *plantar fasciitis*.

     Answer: ______________________________
   - Define *plantar surface*.

     Answer: ______________________________
   - Define *podiatrist*.

     Answer: ______________________________
   - Define *orthotics*.

     Answer: ______________________________
   - Why are soft, nonrigid orthotics recommended for Mr. Ambross?

     Answer: ______________________________
   - Why is a soft heel cup recommended for Mr. Ambross?

     Answer: ______________________________

4. Based on the information that you currently have and what was provided by your instructor, how will you begin Mr. Ambross' rehabilitation?
   - ______________________________
   - ______________________________
   - ______________________________
   - ______________________________

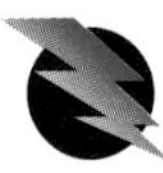

Brain Jolt

With plantar fasciitis, sometimes the patient is placed in a night splint to maintain flexibility and the ROM gains that were achieved in rehabilitation.

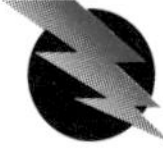

Brain Jolt

When treating this injury, remember to treat the "big picture." Consider what anatomical structure extends into the plantar fascia. Treating the flexor muscle of the main stabilizing phalange of the foot can also help.

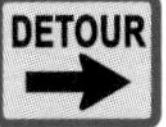

Treatment Detour

Plantar fasciitis is said to be the most common cause of heel pain, affecting 10% of the population. Instrument-assisted, soft-tissue mobilization with the Graston technique is often helpful in treating this condition, as well as other conditions involving soft tissue. The technique has been shown to reduce recovery time, decrease pain, and increase ROM by breaking up adhesions and regaining flexibility. In a study of 10 people reporting heel pain, each was treated with the Graston technique a maximum of eight times over a 3- to 8-week period, one to two times per week. They also participated in a home stretching plan three times daily. Seventy percent of the group showed improvements in pain and disability. When treating athletes, the Graston technique is an option if conventional measures are not successful (Looney, Srokose, Fernández-de-las-Peñas, & Cleland, 2011).

Why or why not?

How will Mr. Ambross' rehabilitation progress? For the *why?* portion of each exercise, explain why you chose a particular exercise or activity as part of your program. Describe which rehabilitation goals the exercise or activity covers, and describe the key indicators for progression. For the *why not?* portion of each exercise, explain why other rehabilitation exercises or activities were not chosen and what to avoid during rehabilitation for this injury. Gather details from the textbook, your own research, and data from Mr. Ambross' scenario to help formulate your answer.

Why?

- ______________________________
  ____
- ______________________________
  ____
- ______________________________
  ____
- ______________________________
  ____

Why not?

- ______________________________
  ____

What do you think?

1. Based on your rehabilitation protocol, discuss the indicators for a limited or full return to play. Include a rough timeline for return to play, if applicable, which is affected by the athlete's compliance with the rehabilitation program.
   - ______________________________
     ____
   - ______________________________
     ____
   - ______________________________
     ____
   - ______________________________
     ____
2. Are modifications or personal protective equipment needed to return to play?
   - ______________________________
     ____

STUDENT SCENARIO 3: CHRIS HOWARD

Chris Howard is a member of his college's track and field team. His main event is the long jump. Mr. Howard has been visiting the ATC for discomfort under his right first metatarsal that occurs when he pushes off the ground (Fig. 11-5). A negative radiographic examination rules out a sesamoid bone fracture, but sesamoiditis is diagnosed. Mr. Howard is placed on limited participation to allow the edema to decrease, but his repeated jumping causes his great toe to hyperextend repetitively, creating increased pressure and weight-bearing on the sesamoid bones. This overuse causes inflammation of the area.

1. Based on this scenario, what do you know about Mr. Howard's injury?
   - ______________________________
     ____
   - ______________________________
     ____

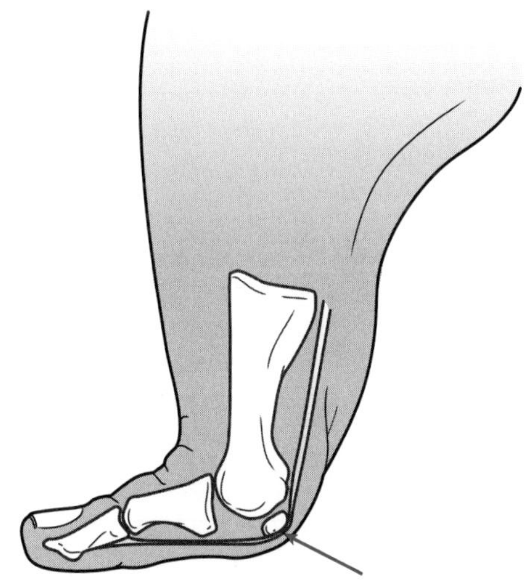

Figure 11-5: Chris Howard's position when painful.

- __________
- __________

2. To rehabilitate Mr. Howard's injury effectively, you will need to gather additional information. What questions should you ask in addition to what is presented in this scenario?
   - __________
   - __________
   - __________
   - __________
3. Identify key terms and concepts, and then research each to broaden your knowledge about ankle and foot injuries.
   - What anatomical structures might be involved in Mr. Howard's injury?

     Answer: __________
   - In which phase of healing is this injury?

     Answer: __________
   - Define *great toe.*

     Answer: __________
   - Define *sesamoid.*

     Answer: __________
   - What is the anatomical role of the sesamoid bones?

     Answer: __________

Brain Jolt
When treating sesamoiditis, a donut pad is one tool that can be used to relieve pressure on the metatarsal head.

4. Based on the information that you currently have and what was provided by your instructor, how will you begin Mr. Howard's rehabilitation?
   - __________
   - __________
   - __________
   - __________

Why or why not?

How will Mr. Howard's rehabilitation progress? For the *why?* portion of each exercise, explain why you chose a particular exercise or activity as part of your program. Describe which rehabilitation goals the exercise or activity covers, and describe the key indicators for progression. For the *why not?* portion of each exercise, explain why other rehabilitation exercises or activities were not chosen and what to avoid during rehabilitation for this injury. Gather details from the textbook, your own research, and data from Mr. Howard's scenario to help formulate your answer.

Why?

- __________
- __________
- __________
- __________

Why not?

- __________
- __________

What do you think?

1. Based on your rehabilitation protocol, discuss the indicators for a limited or full return to play. Include a rough timeline for return to play, if applicable, which is affected by the athlete's compliance with the rehabilitation program.
   - __________
   - __________
   - __________
   - __________

2. Are modifications or personal protective equipment needed to return to play?

- ______________________________

- ______________________________

STUDENT SCENARIO 4: **LUKE MADISON**

Luke Madison plays center on the football team. Because of his position, he has a history of other players stepping on his feet. After Saturday's football game, Mr. Madison notices a great deal of pain in his right foot (Fig. 11-6). On Monday, the ATC evaluates his foot and refers him to the team doctor, hoping that the doctor will order radiographs. The ATC believes that a Jones fracture is possible. Mr. Madison's signs and symptoms include localized edema and point tenderness over the proximal fifth metatarsal, and he is unable to walk without a limp. Mr. Madison has a positive tap and compression test result over the fifth metatarsal. Radiography is positive for a Jones fracture, and he is issued crutches.

1. Based on this scenario, what do you know about Mr. Madison's injury?

- ______________________________

- ______________________________

- ______________________________

- ______________________________

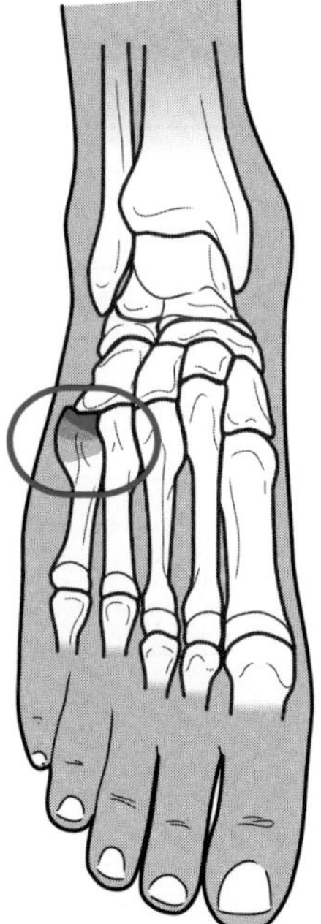

Figure 11-6: Luke Madison's area of pain.

2. To rehabilitate Mr. Madison's injury effectively, you will need to gather additional information. What questions should you ask in addition to what is presented in this scenario?

- ______________________________

- ______________________________

- ______________________________

- ______________________________

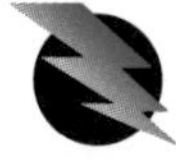

Brain Jolt

A nonunion fracture is a fracture that fails to unite and heal properly. It is diagnosed when 9 months have passed without healing from the time of injury.

Conversation Buffer

Whenever options for the treatment of injuries vary from traditional forms or from the "gold standard," ensure that the athlete and the parents understand the pros and cons of the recommended treatment. Consult current research studies to support or refute a given treatment to allow the athlete and parents to make their own judgments. If the information is unclear, encourage a second opinion from physicians to ensure that the right treatment is chosen for the athlete.

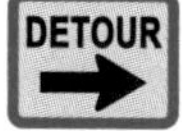

Treatment Detour

Jones fractures have a history of delayed union or nonunion following fracture to the styloid process of the fifth metatarsal. This is thought to be a result of vascular insufficiency. To try to combat this occurrence, bone stimulators have been used as a treatment option. Low-intensity, ultrasonic bone-growth stimulators are a viable and noninvasive option that provides positive outcomes for accelerating healing of Jones fractures, and they have a lower risk of complications when compared with surgery. These are easy to use and are painless. In addition, they can be the preferred option over surgery to avoid postoperative complications, and the athlete can return to play quicker if union occurs (Rhim & Hunt, 2011).

3. Identify key terms and concepts, and then research each to broaden your knowledge about the rehabilitation of foot and ankle injuries.
   - What anatomical structures might be involved in Mr. Madison's injury?

     Answer: ______
   - In which phase of healing is this injury?

     Answer: ______
   - Define *Jones fracture.*

     Answer: ______
   - Define *edema.*

     Answer: ______
   - What is the tap test? What does it test? What does a positive result indicate?

     Answer: ______
   - What is the compression test? What does it test? What does a positive result indicate?

     Answer: ______
   - What are the criteria for issuing crutches?

     Answer: ______
4. Based on the information that you currently have and what was provided by your instructor, how will you begin Mr. Madison's rehabilitation?
   - ______
   - ______
   - ______
   - ______

Why or why not?

How will Mr. Madison's rehabilitation progress? For the *why?* portion of each exercise, explain why you chose a particular exercise or activity as part of your program. Describe which rehabilitation goals the exercise or activity covers, and describe the key indicators for progression. For the *why not?* portion of each exercise, explain why other rehabilitation exercises or activities were not chosen and what to avoid during rehabilitation for this injury. Gather details from the textbook, your own research, and data from Mr. Madison's scenario to help formulate your answer.

Why?

- ______
- ______
- ______
- ______

Why not?

- ______
- ______

What do you think?

1. Based on your rehabilitation protocol, discuss the indicators for a limited or full return to play. Include a rough timeline for return to play, if applicable, which is impacted by the athlete's compliance with the rehabilitation program.
   - ______
   - ______
   - ______
   - ______
2. Are modifications or personal protective equipment needed to return to play?
   - ______
   - ______

STUDENT SCENARIO 5: BRIANNA WARD

Brianna Ward rolled her ankle at basketball practice yesterday. Her left ankle went into inversion, and she sustained a grade 1 lateral ankle sprain of the anterior talofibular ligament. She has a history of lateral ankle sprains. On evaluation, Ms. Ward's signs and symptoms include edema over the anterior talofibular ligament (Fig. 11-7), pain with her gait but no limp, full but painful active ROM, and a positive anterior drawer test result.

1. Based on this scenario, what do you know about Ms. Ward's injury?
   - ______________________________
   - ______________________________
   - ______________________________
   - ______________________________

2. To rehabilitate Ms. Ward's injury effectively, you will need to gather additional information. What questions should you ask in addition to what is presented in this scenario?
   - ______________________________
   - ______________________________
   - ______________________________
   - ______________________________

3. Identify key terms and concepts, and then research each to broaden your knowledge about rehabilitation of ankle and foot injuries.
   - What anatomical structures might be involved in Ms. Ward's injury?

     Answer: ______________________________

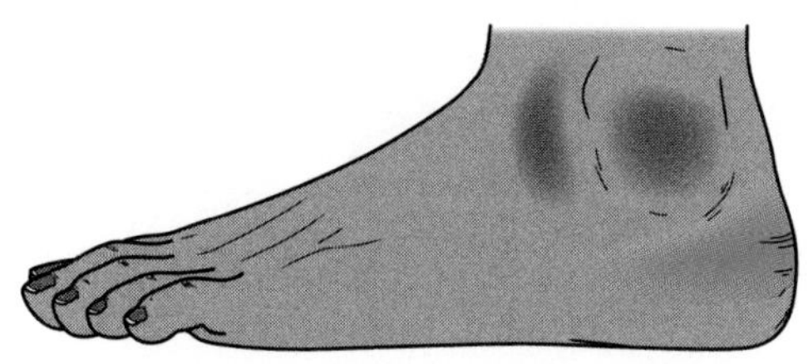

Figure 11-7: Brianna Ward's ankle.

   - In which phase of healing is this injury?

     Answer: ______________________________
   - Define *edema.*

     Answer: ______________________________
   - Define *active range of motion.*

     Answer: ______________________________
   - What is a grade 1 ankle sprain to the anterior talofibular ligament?

     Answer: ______________________________
   - Where is the anterior talofibular ligament located?

     Answer: ______________________________
   - What is the anterior drawer test? What does it test? What does a positive result indicate?

     Answer: ______________________________

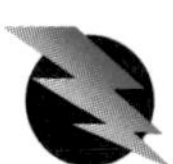

Brain Jolt

Edema can increase or lead to pain. If you can control the edema, you will increase the chances of a faster recovery for the athlete.

4. Based on the information that you currently have and what was provided by your instructor, how will you begin Ms. Ward's rehabilitation?
   - ______________________________
   - ______________________________
   - ______________________________
   - ______________________________

Why or why not?

How will Ms. Ward's rehabilitation progress? For the *why?* portion of each exercise, explain why you chose a particular exercise or activity as part of your program. Describe which rehabilitation goals the exercise or activity covers, and describe the key indicators for progression. For the *why not?* portion of each exercise, explain why other rehabilitation exercises or activities were not chosen and what to avoid during rehabilitation for this injury. Gather details from the textbook, your own research, and data from Ms. Ward's scenario to help formulate your answer.

Why?

- ______________________________
- ______________________________
- ______________________________
- ______________________________

Why not?

- ______________________________
- ______________________________

What do you think?

1. Based on your rehabilitation protocol, discuss the indicators for a limited or full return to play. Include a rough timeline for return to play, if applicable, which is affected by the athlete's compliance with the rehabilitation program.
   - ______________________________
   - ______________________________
   - ______________________________
   - ______________________________
2. Are modifications or personal protective equipment needed to return to play?
   - ______________________________
   - ______________________________

STUDENT SCENARIO 6: MILES MCCLURG

Miles McClurg is a senior on the basketball team and has recently been placed on limited participation because of Achilles tendonitis. After having completed daily rehabilitation for 2 weeks, he has been allowed to participate at a full status. As Mr. McClurg jumps to rebound a ball, he feels an excruciating pain and then a pop sensation at the back of his right calcaneus. He falls to the ground. On evaluation, the signs and symptoms include indention near the posterior calcaneus causing an observable deformity distal to the gastrocnemius, as well as a positive Thompson test result. He is unable to plantar flex his foot actively, and an Achilles tendon rupture is diagnosed (Fig. 11-8).

1. Based on this scenario, what do you know about Mr. McClurg's injury?
   - ______________________________
   - ______________________________
   - ______________________________
   - ______________________________

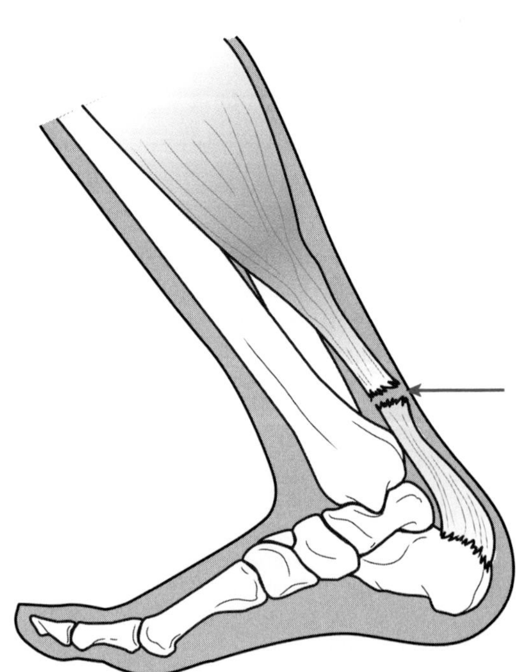

Figure 11-8: Miles McClurg's injury.

2. To rehabilitate Mr. McClurg's injury effectively, you will need to gather additional information. What questions should you ask in addition to what is presented in this scenario?
   - ______________________________
   - ______________________________
   - ______________________________
   - ______________________________

Brain Jolt
Remember what muscles insert into the Achilles tendon. Be sure to rehabilitate all the muscles involved once the patient is referred for rehabilitation.

Brain Jolt
Before rehabilitation is permitted on the lower leg, try to maintain upper-leg strength to reduce the athlete's recovery time.

Conversation Buffer
Achilles tendon ruptures can be repaired in one of two ways: immobilization using a cast or surgical repair of the rupture. Once the patient has consulted with a physician, ensure that he or she understands the treatment options. An athletic trainer is a liaison between the athlete and the physician, and it is important for patients to understand their health options and make informed decisions.

3. Identify any key terms and concepts, and research each to broaden your knowledge about the rehabilitation of ankle and foot injuries.
   - What anatomical structures might be involved in Mr. McClurg's injury?

     Answer: ______________________________
   - In which phase of healing is this injury?

     Answer: ______________________________
   - Define *Achilles tendon rupture*.

     Answer: ______________________________
   - Define *Achilles tendonitis*.

     Answer: ______________________________
   - Define *active plantar flexion*.

     Answer: ______________________________
   - Why is there an indentation at the back of Mr. McClurg's calcaneus?

     Answer: ______________________________
   - Why is there a deformity in Mr. McClurg's gastrocnemius?

     Answer: ______________________________
   - What is the Thompson test? What does it test? What does a positive result indicate?

     Answer: ______________________________

4. Based on the information that you currently have and what was provided by your instructor, how will you begin Mr. McClurg's rehabilitation?
   - ______________________________
   - ______________________________
   - ______________________________
   - ______________________________

Why or why not?

How will Mr. McClurg's rehabilitation progress? For the *why?* portion of each exercise, explain why you chose a particular exercise or activity as part of your program. Describe which rehabilitation goals the exercise or activity covers, and describe the key indicators for progression. For the *why not?* portion of each exercise, explain why other rehabilitation exercises or activities were not chosen and what to avoid during rehabilitation for this injury. Gather details from the textbook, your own research, and data from Mr. McClurg's scenario to help formulate your answer.

Why?

- ______________________________
- ______________________________
- ______________________________
- ______________________________

Why not?

- ______________________________
- ______________________________

What do you think?

1. Based on your rehabilitation protocol, discuss the indicators for a limited or full return to play. Include a rough timeline for return to play, if applicable, which is affected by the athlete's compliance with the rehabilitation program.
   - ______________________________
   - ______________________________
   - ______________________________
   - ______________________________
2. Are modifications or required protective equipment needed to return to play?
   - ______________________________
   - ______________________________

STUDENT SCENARIO 7: NICHOLAS BRYER

Nicholas Bryer is a varsity soccer player who performed a slide tackle into an opponent, which caused the opposing player to land on his right ankle. Mr. Bryer is point tender over the tip of his right lateral malleolus and has mild edema. He has a positive compression test and a positive percussion test. He is able to walk with only a slight limp. As a result of the positive special test results and Ottawa ankle rules, he is referred for a radiographic examination, which indicates a fibular fracture at the lateral malleolus (Fig. 11-9).

1. Based on this scenario, what do you know about Mr. Bryer's injury?

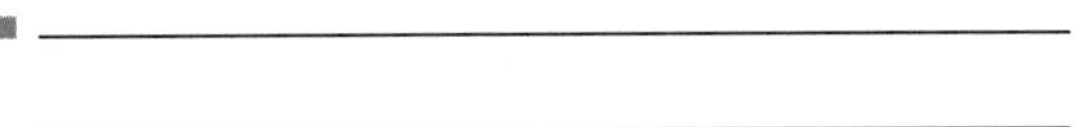

   - ______________________________
   - ______________________________
   - ______________________________

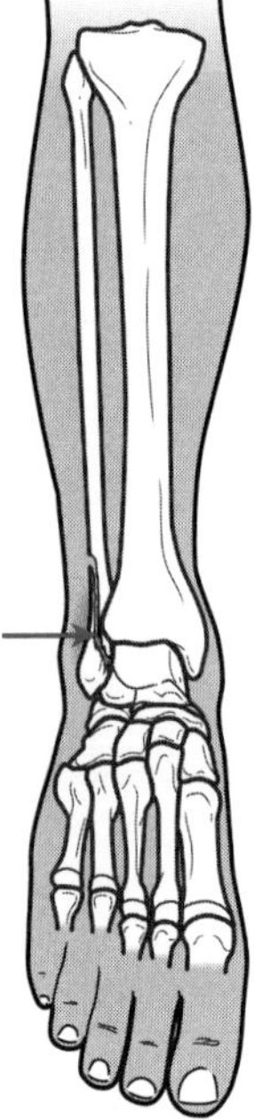

Figure 11-9: Nicholas Bryer's fibular fracture.

2. To rehabilitate Mr. Bryer's injury effectively, you will need to gather additional information. What questions should you ask in addition to what is presented in this scenario?
   - ______________________________
   - ______________________________
   - ______________________________
   - ______________________________

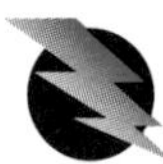

Brain Jolt

Casting causes atrophy, which requires that you begin and continue strengthening exercises in rehabilitation at a slower rate, because the patient's previous strength is diminished.

3. Identify key terms and concepts, and then research each to broaden your knowledge about the rehabilitation of ankle and foot injuries.
   - What anatomical structures might be involved in Mr. Bryer's injury?

     Answer: ______________________________

- In which phase of healing is this injury?

  Answer: ______________________________
- Define *fibular fracture.*

  Answer: ______________________________
- Define *edema.*

  Answer: ______________________________
- What are the different types of fracture patterns in the ankle and foot?

  Answer: ______________________________
- What is the compression test? What does it test? What does a positive result indicate?

  Answer: ______________________________
- What is the percussion test? What does it test? What does a positive result indicate?

  Answer: ______________________________

4. Based on the information that you currently have and what was provided by your instructor, how will you begin Mr. Bryer's rehabilitation?

- ______________________________
- ______________________________
- ______________________________
- ______________________________

Why or why not?

How will Mr. Bryer's rehabilitation progress? For the *why?* portion of each exercise, explain why you chose a particular exercise or activity as part of your program. Describe which rehabilitation goals the exercise or activity covers, and describe the key indicators for progression. For the *why not?* portion of each exercise, explain why other rehabilitation exercises or activities were not chosen and what to avoid during rehabilitation for this injury. Gather details from the textbook, your own research, and data from Mr. Bryer's scenario to help formulate your answer.

Why?

- ______________________________
- ______________________________
- ______________________________
- ______________________________

Why not?

- ______________________________
- ______________________________

What do you think?

1. Based on your rehabilitation protocol, discuss the indicators for a limited or full return to play. Include a rough timeline for return to play, if applicable, which is affected by the athlete's compliance with the rehabilitation program.

- ______________________________
- ______________________________
- ______________________________
- ______________________________

2. Are modifications or personal protective equipment needed to return to play?

- ______________________________
- ______________________________

STUDENT SCENARIO 8: MADISON CUMMINGS

Madison Cummings is a gymnast with a history of forefoot sprains and a lateral ankle sprain to her right foot. After forcefully going up on her toes, her weight comes down onto her toes and her foot goes into pronation. She feels pain at her first and second metatarsals. On examination, there is point tenderness and a positive glide test result. After this incident, a radiographic examination of her right foot is positive for a Lisfranc fracture (Fig. 11-10). She is given crutches and is referred for rehabilitation.

1. Based on this scenario, what do you know about Ms. Cummings' injury?
   - ______________________________
   - ______________________________
   - ______________________________
   - ______________________________
2. To rehabilitate Ms. Cummings' injury effectively, you will need to gather additional information. What questions should you ask in addition to what is presented in this scenario?
   - ______________________________
   - ______________________________
   - ______________________________
   - ______________________________

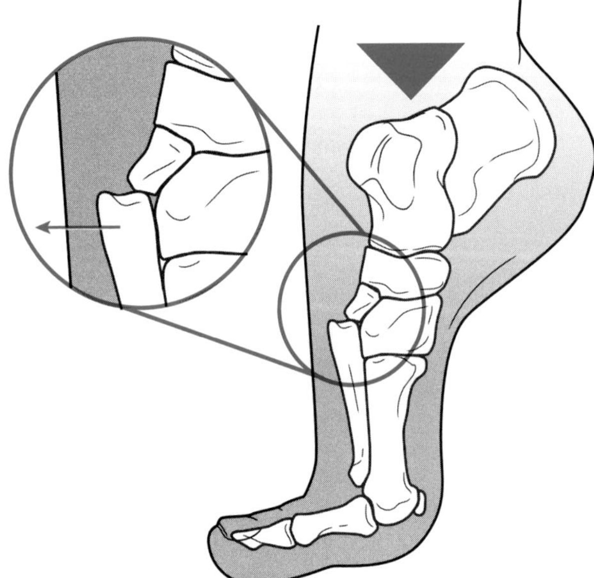

Figure 11-10: Madison Cummings' injury.

3. Identify key terms and concepts, and then research each to broaden your knowledge about rehabilitation of ankle and foot injuries.
   - What anatomical structures might be involved in Ms. Cummings' injury?

     Answer: ______________________________
   - In which phase of healing is this injury?

     Answer: ______________________________
   - Define *Lisfranc fracture.*

     Answer: ______________________________
   - Are there any other diagnostic tests needed?

     Answer: ______________________________
   - How do Ms. Cummings' previous injuries affect her current injury?

     Answer: ______________________________
   - What other body part can be injured with this type of fracture?

     Answer: ______________________________
4. Based on the information that you currently have and what was provided by your instructor, how will you begin Ms. Cummings' rehabilitation?
   - ______________________________
   - ______________________________
   - ______________________________
   - ______________________________

Why or why not?

How will Ms. Cummings' rehabilitation progress? For the *why?* portion of each exercise, explain why you chose a particular exercise or activity as part of your program. Describe which rehabilitation goals the exercise or activity covers, and describe the key indicators for progression. For the *why not?* portion of each exercise, explain why other rehabilitation exercises or activities were not chosen and what to avoid during rehabilitation for this injury. Gather details from the textbook, your own research, and data from Ms. Cummings' scenario to help formulate your answer.

Why?

- __________
- __________
- __________
- __________

Why not?

- __________
- __________

What do you think?

1. Based on your rehabilitation protocol, discuss the indicators for a limited or full return to play. Include a rough timeline for return to play, if applicable, which is affected by the athlete's compliance with the rehabilitation program.
   - __________
   - __________
   - __________
   - __________
2. Are modifications or personal protective equipment needed to return to play?
   - __________
   - __________

STUDENT SCENARIO 9: RUBEN GOLD

Ruben Gold is a cyclist. He takes 30-mile rides twice per week and then 15-mile rides three additional days per week. He normally has a day of rest between each ride, but he has had to cycle consecutive days for the last 2 weeks. He is now experiencing a burning feeling on the plantar surface of his right foot, located over the third and fourth metatarsal heads, when standing up on his bike to pedal. He finds that the pain is relieved when not bearing weight. Because of the pain, Mr. Gold visits a podiatrist who diagnoses Morton neuroma (Fig. 11-11). The podiatrist has ruled out that Mr. Gold has a metatarsal fracture.

1. Based on this scenario, what do you know about Mr. Gold's injury?
   - __________
   - __________
   - __________
   - __________
2. To rehabilitate Mr. Gold's injury effectively, you will need to gather additional information. What questions should you ask in addition to what is presented in this scenario?
   - __________

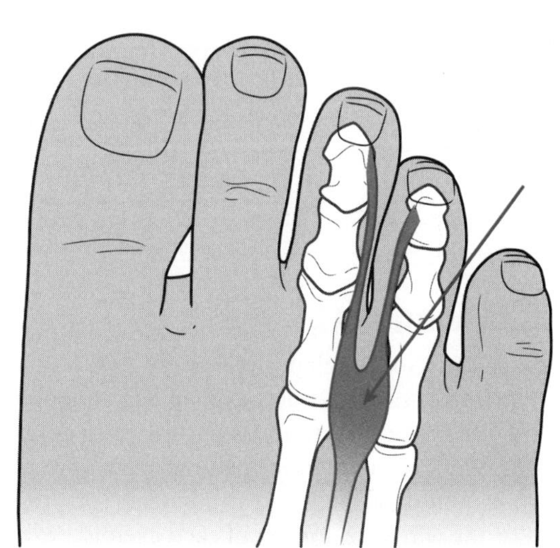

Figure 11-11: Ruben Gold's neuroma.

- ______________________
- ______________________
- ______________________

3. Identify key terms and concepts, and then research each to broaden your knowledge about the rehabilitation of ankle and foot injuries.
   - What anatomical structures might be involved in Mr. Gold's injury?

     Answer: ______________________
   - In which phase of healing is this injury?

     Answer: ______________________
   - Define *Morton neuroma.*

     Answer: ______________________
   - Define *podiatrist.*

     Answer: ______________________
   - Define *plantar surface.*

     Answer: ______________________
   - Why is Mr. Gold's pain relieved when he is not bearing weight?

     Answer: ______________________
   - Why is it necessary for the athletic trainer to be familiar with cycling mechanics?

     Answer: ______________________
4. Based on the information that you currently have and what was provided by your instructor, how will you begin Mr. Gold's rehabilitation?
   - ______________________
   - ______________________
   - ______________________
   - ______________________

Why or why not?

How will Mr. Gold's rehabilitation progress? For the *why?* portion of each exercise, explain why you chose a particular exercise or activity as part of your program. Describe which rehabilitation goals the exercise or activity covers, and describe the key indicators for progression. For the *why not?* portion of each exercise, explain why other rehabilitation exercises or activities were not chosen and what to avoid during rehabilitation for this injury. Gather details from the textbook, your own research, and data from Mr. Gold's scenario to help formulate your answer.

Why?

- ______________________
- ______________________
- ______________________
- ______________________

Why not?

- ______________________
- ______________________

What do you think?

1. Based on your rehabilitation protocol, discuss the indicators for a limited or full return to play. Include a rough timeline for return to play, if applicable, which is affected by the athlete's compliance with the rehabilitation program.
   - ______________________
   - ______________________
   - ______________________
   - ______________________
2. Are modifications or required protective equipment needed to return to play?
   - ______________________
   - ______________________

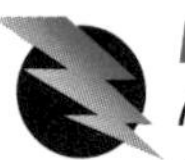

Brain Jolt

A teardrop-shaped pad works the best to decrease pressure and symptoms.

knowledge checklist

Table 11-2 offers a checklist that can be used by a peer, instructor, or preceptor to evaluate each part of the athlete's rehabilitation plan. Use this checklist as a tool to ensure that the rehabilitation plan is complete and to assess your knowledge of the competencies that apply to this chapter.

TABLE 11-2 ■ Lower Extremity: The Ankle and Foot Rehabilitation and Therapeutic Exercise Competency Checklist

	Proficient *Can demonstrate and execute the skill properly*	**Proficient With Assistance** *Can demonstrate and execute the skill with minimal guidance or tips*	**Not Proficient** *Unable to demonstrate and execute the skill properly; need to be reevaluated at another time after further study and practice*
Controlling Edema			
PRICE			
Modalities			
Controlling Pain			
Pain scales			
Medications			
Modalities			
Establishes Core Stability			
Reestablishes Neuromuscular Control			
Restores Postural Control and Balance			
Restoring Range of Motion			
Passive range of motion			
Active range of motion			
Resistive range of motion			
Goniometry			
Normal range of motion limits			
Restore Muscular Strength, Endurance, and Power			
Open kinetic chain			
Closed kinetic chain			
Isometric			
Isotonic			
Isotonic (concentric and eccentric)			
Isokinetic			
Plyometric			
Agility			
Functional or Sport-Specific Activities			
Maintains Cardiorespiratory Fitness			
Functional Testing			
Return-to-Play Criteria			
Proper Documentation			

PRICE, prevention, rest, ice, compression, and elevation.

REFERENCES

Higgins, M. (2011). *Therapeutic exercise from theory to practice.* Philadelphia, PA: F.A. Davis.

Looney, B., Srokose, T., Fernández-de-las-Peñas, C., & Cleland, J. A. (2011). Graston instrument soft tissue mobilization and home stretching for the management of plantar heel pain: A case series. *Journal of Manipulative and Physiological Therapeutics, 34*, 138–142.

Prentice, W. (2011). *Rehabilitation techniques for sports medicine and athletic training* (5th ed.). New York, NY: McGraw-Hill.

Rhim, B., & Hunt, J. C. (2011). Lisfranc injury and Jones fracture in sports. *Clinics in Podiatric Medicine and Surgery, 28*, 69–86.

Starkey, C. (2004). *Therapeutic modalities* (3rd ed.). Philadelphia, PA: F.A. Davis.

Starkey, C., Brown, S. D., & Ryan, J. (2010). *Examination of orthopedic and athletic injuries* (3rd ed.). Philadelphia, PA: F.A. Davis.

Venes, D. (Ed.) (2009). *Taber's cyclopedic medical dictionary* (21st ed.). Philadelphia, PA: F.A. Davis.

Williams, G. N., Jones, M. H., & Amendola, A. (2007). Syndesmotic ankle sprains in athletes. *The American Journal of Sports Medicine, 35*, 1197–1207.

chapter 12

Lower Extremity: The Knee

chapter outline

athletic trainer's corner

Here is what one athletic trainer experienced with an athlete's rehabilitation from injury:

I worked with an athlete who tore the anterior cruciate ligament (ACL) in his right knee, which ended his season. I was fortunate to have the experience of watching this young man progress from a college freshman who viewed the surgery and rehabilitation process like it was an insurmountable climb to a confident starter and leader of his team. I learned that the results of an athlete's rehabilitation process are determined mainly by the mentality of both the athlete and the athletic trainer. I set small goals so that he could see his progress, which gave him the motivation to continue to work hard. I also kept the rehabilitation exercises new and fresh. I noticed that he became bored with exercises after doing them for a long period of time. Therefore, it was important for me to change the exercises to keep the workout fun and to keep him interested. It was also essential for me as an athletic trainer to remain positive and verbally reward the athlete between exercises and at the end of a rehabilitation session. It was rewarding for me to see this athlete, who at one point needed my assistance to lift his leg off the table, start as a safety for his college football team.

Andrea Anderson, ATC
Adena Health System

learning outcomes

After working through this chapter, you will be able to:

1. Describe seven different goals of rehabilitation and the importance each plays in the overall rehabilitation protocol.
2. Verbalize indications for performing knee rehabilitative techniques.
3. Discuss modifications and progressions that are used during a rehabilitation program for the knee.
4. Discuss outcome measures used to identify activity levels and return-to-play guidelines for knee injuries.
5. Explain what modality is proper for rehabilitation by using indications, contraindications, and the principles and theory related to the physiological response of the intervention.

MODEL SCENARIO 1: ALVIN SAVILLE

Alvin Saville is a defensive player on his school's hockey team. During practice, there is an offensive break toward the goal that leaves Mr. Saville as the last defender. The offensive center makes a move to the outside to pass. In an effort to prevent the pass, Mr. Saville sticks out his right leg to stop the center. He absorbs a hard blow to the medial side of his right knee and immediately drops to the ice. On evaluation, Mr. Saville tests positive for laxity during a varus stress test, is point tender over the lateral epicondyle, and has moderate edema on the lateral side of the right knee. The certified athletic trainer's assessment is a grade 3 lateral collateral ligament (LCL) tear and the concurrent MRI results indicate a complete LCL tear (Fig. 12-1).

1. Based on this scenario, what do you know about Mr. Saville's injury?
   - *Male athlete*
   - *Hockey player*
   - *Mechanism of injury: direct hit to the medial knee*
   - *Positive varus stress test for laxity*
   - *Point tender over lateral epicondyle*
   - *Moderate edema*
   - *MRI positive for LCL tear*

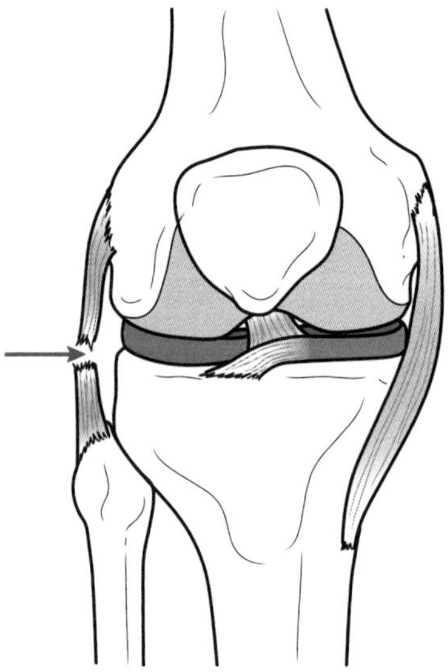

Figure 12-1: Alvin Saville's lateral collateral ligament tear.

2. To rehabilitate Mr. Saville's injury effectively, you will need to gather additional information. What questions should you ask in addition to what is presented in this scenario?
   - *Are there any preexisting injuries? If yes, what are they?*
   - *How long has the athlete experienced this pain?*
   - *What is the athlete's pain level and type of pain felt?*
   - *What is the level of strength at the knee?*
   - *What is the range of motion (ROM) at the knee?*
   - *Does the athlete have any numbness or paraesthesia?*
   - *Are there any deformities?*
   - *Is ecchymosis present?*
3. Identify key terms and concepts, and then research each to broaden your knowledge about the rehabilitation of knee injuries.
   - What anatomical structures might be involved in Mr. Saville's injury?
     Tibia
     Femur
     Fibula
     LCL
     Medial collateral ligament (MCL)
     Condyles
   - What is an LCL tear?
     A tear in the lateral collateral ligament of the knee
   - In which phase of healing is this injury?
     This injury occurs at the inflammatory response phase.
   - Define *edema*.
     Swelling; a localized or general condition that causes body tissues to contain an excessive amount of fluid
   - Define *lateral*.
     Directional term meaning to the outside
   - What does the abbreviation *MRI* stand for?
     Magnetic resonance imaging

- What is an MRI used for?
  An MRI is valuable for showing images of soft tissue for the central nervous and musculoskeletal systems. Occasionally MRIs are used for other disorders determined by a doctor.
- What is a varus stress test? What does it test? What does a positive result indicate?
  The varus stress test is performed by stressing the lateral collateral ligament of the knee by placing one hand on the medial side of the knee and the other hand on the lateral side of the ankle, and then forcing the knee laterally. It tests the integrity of the LCL by testing for laxity and pain. If laxity is present, the lateral knee joint space will open, indicating a positive test result.
- What is the healing process and timeframe for a ligament?
  Ligament healing will follow the typical phases of healing going through each phase in a timeframe dependent on the severity of injury. This typically takes anywhere from 7 days to 8 weeks; however, grade 3 LCL tears can require surgery.

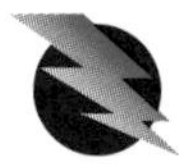

Brain Jolt
Sometimes ROM should be avoided in the early phases of rehabilitation, depending on the injury.

4. Based on the information that you currently have and what was provided by your instructor, how will you begin Mr. Saville's rehabilitation?
First assess edema, pain, and ROM. Place the athlete on crutches and non–weight-bearing restrictions, and instruct the athlete to use a compression wrap to control edema outside of the rehabilitation session. Next, begin mild ROM exercises to get some movement in the knee. Implement simple stretching exercises of the hamstrings and calves to maintain flexibility. Next, add two sets of 30 repetitions of quad sets to activate the quadriceps. If pain is present, implement electrical stimulation with ice therapy and elevation of the affected area for 20 min.

Brain Jolt
It is important to keep the muscles surrounding the knee as strong as possible after injury, especially if surgery is in the treatment plan. The stronger a patient is before surgery, the easier it is to regain strength postoperatively.

Why or why not?

How will Mr. Saville's rehabilitation progress? For the *why?* portion of each exercise, explain why you chose a particular exercise or activity as part of your program. Describe which rehabilitation goals the exercise or activity covers, and describe the key indicators for progression. For the *why not?* portion of each exercise, explain why other rehabilitation exercises or activities were not chosen and what to avoid during rehabilitation for this injury. Gather details from the textbook, your own research, and data from Mr. Saville's scenario to help formulate your answer.

Why?

- ***Towel stretching.*** *This activity helps with the rehabilitation goal of increasing flexibility and ROM in the hamstrings and calves. Once the stretching becomes easy for the athlete, progress to the traditional modes of hamstring stretches and stretching of the calves on the incline board.*
- ***Heel slides.*** *This activity helps with the rehabilitation goal of increasing ROM by gaining active ROM. If a lack of ROM continues to be a problem, perform gravity-assisted wall slides or cycle for 5 minutes on a stationary bike to gain ROM. If the athlete cannot move the full circle while pedaling, he or she can do pendulum swings until able to master the stationary bike.*
- ***Quad sets.*** *This exercise helps with the rehabilitation goal of increasing strength by activating the quadriceps muscle. Once good contraction is gained, move to short arc quad sets to work on the vastus medialis oblique. Next, move to straight-leg raises in all four directions and then implement total knee extensions over the table. This exercise improves overall strength of the thigh and buttock.*
- ***Single-leg stance.*** *Once weight-bearing is allowed, focus on proprioception of the knee. Have the athlete stand on the injured leg for 20 seconds at first, and increase the time as tolerated. Progress to having the athlete close his or her eyes while standing on an unsteady surface to improve proprioception.*
- ***Modality.*** *Use ice and electrical stimulation to reduce pain and edema.*

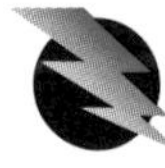

Brain Jolt
When icing the lateral aspect of the knee, be cautious of the superficial nature of the peroneal nerve, which could be damaged with prolonged icing.

Why not?

- *Avoid any closed kinetic chain exercises until the athlete is cleared by the physician and is strong enough to handle weight-bearing exercises. Avoid increasing weight or number of repetitions if they could increase any edema that is present.*

What do you think?

1. Based on your rehabilitation protocol, discuss the indicators for limited or full return to play with the athlete. Include a rough timeline for return to play, if applicable, which is affected by the athlete's compliance with the rehabilitation program.

- ***Limited return to play.*** *His status depends on whether he regains full ROM, strength, and proprioception in the injured leg. Once he achieves these goals and can perform simple functional tasks without pain or compensation, he will be able to engage in some drills and noncontact activities with the team.*
- ***Full return to play.*** *If all the exercises for limited return to play are performed without pain and compensation, and the athlete does not experience edema or any setbacks, then he can return to play without restrictions.*

2. Are modifications or required protective equipment needed to return to play?
   - *Hinge knee brace for support*

MODEL SCENARIO 2: **DON HARPER**

Don Harper is a high school baseball player who complains of pain in his right knee. He recently noticed a bump over the anterior portion of his knee and an increase in pain. On evaluation, he has a deformity on his right tibial tuberosity, is point tender over the inferior patella, and has point tenderness over the tibial tuberosity. After further discussion, he states that it is most painful when he performs squats and box jumps. He also mentions that he has had a recent growth spurt. As a result, the diagnosis is Osgood-Schlatter disease (Fig. 12-2).

1. Based on this scenario, what do you know about Mr. Harper's injury?
   - *Male athlete*
   - *High school baseball player*
   - *Knee pain*
   - *Deformity at tibial tuberosity*
   - *Point tender over tibial tuberosity and inferior patella*
   - *Pain worse with squats and box jumps*
   - *Recent growth spurt*

Figure 12-2: Don Harper's Osgood-Schlatter disease.

2. To rehabilitate Mr. Harper's injury effectively, you will need to gather more information. What questions should you ask in addition to what is presented in this scenario?
   - *Are there any preexisting injuries? If yes, what are they?*
   - *How long has the athlete experienced this pain?*
   - *What is the athlete's pain level and type of pain felt?*
   - *What is the strength at the knee?*
   - *What is the ROM at the knee?*
   - *Does the athlete have any numbness or paraesthesia?*
   - *Is edema present?*
   - *Is ecchymosis present?*
   - *How old is the athlete?*

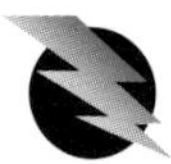

Brain Jolt

When working with athletes who have Osgood-Schlatter disease, be mindful of activities that exert stress on the tibial tuberosity via the patellar tendon.

3. Identify key terms and concepts, and then research each to broaden your knowledge about the rehabilitation of knee injuries.
   - What anatomical structures might be involved in Mr. Harper's injury?
     Quadriceps
     Patella
     Patellar tendon
     Tibial tuberosity
     Tibia
     Femur
   - What is Osgood-Schlatter disease?
     An overuse injury predominant in youth and early adolescence caused by repetitive pull of the patellar tendon at the tibial tuberosity
   - In what phase of healing is this injury?
     Acute inflammatory phase
   - Why is it painful for the athlete at the tibial tuberosity when jumping and during exercises that use the quadriceps?
     The quadriceps muscle group inserts at the tibial tuberosity via the patellar tendon; therefore, the point of pain is from the use of that muscle group.

- Why is there deformity at the tibial tuberosity?
  The traction of the patellar tendon at the tibial tuberosity sometimes involves an avulsion from the tibial tuberosity.
- Why is the athlete's age and growth spurt important?
  This disease is prevalent in the younger and early adolescent years when growth spurts occur. Enduring a growth spurt leaves the knee area more susceptible to this injury.

4. Based on the information that you currently have and from the information provided by your instructor, how will you begin Mr. Harper's rehabilitation?
Unfortunately, there are not many treatment options that help this condition. To achieve relief, begin with icing the area after activity and refraining from jumping and explosive activities. Symptoms will subside once the athlete's growth spurt has stopped.

Why or why not?

How will Mr. Harper's rehabilitation progress? For the *why?* portion of each exercise, explain why you chose a particular exercise or activity as part of your program. Describe which rehabilitation goals the exercise or activity covers, and describe the key indicators for progression. For the *why not?* portion of each exercise, explain why other rehabilitation exercises or activities were not chosen and what to avoid during rehabilitation for this injury. Gather details from the textbook, your own research, and data from Mr. Harper's scenario to help formulate your answer.

Why?

- ***Ice.*** *Ice helps with the rehabilitation goal of reducing pain and edema.*
- ***Quadriceps stretching.*** *This exercise helps with the rehabilitation goal of increasing ROM by increasing flexibility. Increasing flexibility in the quadriceps can decrease the tension on the tibial tuberosity.*
- ***Ultrasound.*** *This modality can help with flexibility of the patellar tendon. Applying ultrasound over the patellar tendon can help to reduce tension at the tibial tuberosity.*
- ***Rest or modified activity.*** *Rest and a reduction in jumping and explosive activities are needed to decrease stress on the tibial tuberosity.*

Why not?

- *Avoid any exercises that include jumping and explosive activities to decrease stress on the tibial tuberosity.*

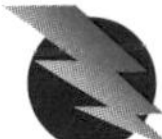

Brain Jolt
You can still strengthen the quadriceps muscles and limit pain by using exercises that limit extensive repetitive knee flexion.

What do you think?

1. Based on your rehabilitation protocol, discuss the indicators for limited return to play and full return to play. Include a rough timeline for return to play, if applicable, which is affected by the athlete's compliance with the rehabilitation program.

- ***Limited return to play.*** *His status depends on whether he regains full strength and ROM; however, activities would need to limit jumping and explosive activities until the pain subsides.*
- ***Full return to play.*** *The athlete can return to play as tolerated if full strength and ROM are achieved; however, activities would need to limit jumping and explosive activities to ensure that symptoms do not return.*

2. Are modifications or personal protective equipment needed to return to play?

- *A patellar tendon strap to help lessen pain*

STUDENT SCENARIO 1: AMANDA GOODBARR

Amanda Goodbarr is a forward on her collegiate soccer team. It has been 24 hours since she injured her left knee during a soccer game. The injury occurred as she advanced toward the goal and got into shooting position, at which point an opponent approached from her right side and kicked her tibia, forcing it posteriorly. Amanda Goodbarr fell into a lunged position with all her weight coming down onto her left knee. Her knee was forced into hyperflexion, and the ankle was plantar flexed (Fig. 12-3), creating a *pop* sensation over the posterior side of her left knee. She has moderate edema and point tenderness over the popliteal fossa. The following special test results were positive: posterior sag, posterior drawer, and recurvatum. The diagnosis is a grade 2 posterior cruciate ligament (PCL) tear.

1. Based on this scenario, what do you know about Ms. Goodbarr's injury?

- ____________________________________
  ____
- ____________________________________
  ____

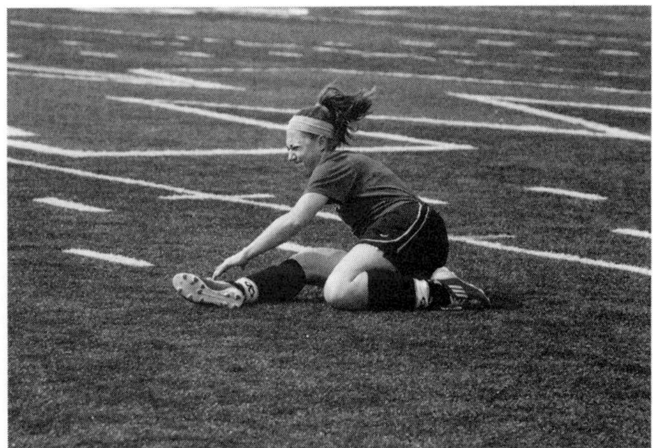

Figure 12-3: Amanda Goodbarr's mechanism of injury.

- ______________________________
- ______________________________

2. To rehabilitate Ms. Goodbarr's injury effectively, you will need to gather more information. What questions should you ask in addition to what is presented in this scenario?

- ______________________________
- ______________________________
- ______________________________
- ______________________________

Brain Jolt

A posterior cruciate ligament tear is often called the dashboard injury.

Conversation Buffer

Many people assume that the recovery time for a PCL injury is similar to that for an ACL injury. You need to communicate to the athlete, coaches, and parents that a PCL injury has a long rehabilitation time and that there are debates over the success of surgery for PCL injuries.

3. Identify key terms and concepts, and then research each to broaden your knowledge about the rehabilitation of knee injuries.

- What anatomical structures might be involved in Ms. Goodbarr's injury?

  Answer: ______________________________
- What is a grade 2 PCL tear?

  Answer: ______________________________
- In which phase of healing is this injury?

  Answer: ______________________________
- Define *hyperflexion of the knee.*

  Answer: ______________________________
- Define *plantar flexion of the ankle.*

  Answer: ______________________________
- Define *edema.*

  Answer: ______________________________
- What is a posterior sag test? What does it test? What does a positive result indicate?

  Answer: ______________________________
- What is a posterior drawer test? What does it test? What does a positive result indicate?

  Answer: ______________________________
- What is a recurvatum test? What does it test? What does a positive result indicate?

  Answer: ______________________________
- Why is it important that the ankle be in a plantar flexed position for the injury to damage the PCL?

  Answer: ______________________________

4. Based on the information that you currently have and what was provided by your instructor, how will you begin Ms. Goodbarr's rehabilitation?

- ______________________________
- ______________________________
- ______________________________
- ______________________________

Treatment Detour

Treatment methods for PCL injuries have been a point of debate because of infrequent prevalence rates and a lack of research. One group of researchers has data to suggest that conservative nonoperative treatment is successful. In addition, it has been found that open kinetic chain-resisted knee flexion generates high stress on the PCL; therefore, exercises involving these parameters should be performed only after the PCL is adequately healed, usually 4 to 6 months after injury. This treatment is important to remember when you are choosing your rehabilitation protocols for your athletes. You will still want to increase strength but avoid these types of activities until it is safe for the athlete to proceed (Fanelli, Beck, & Edson, 2010).

Why or why not?

How will Ms. Goodbarr's rehabilitation progress? For the *why?* portion of each exercise, explain why you chose a particular exercise or activity as part of your program. Describe which rehabilitation goals the exercise or activity covers, and describe the key indicators for progression. For the *why not?* portion of each exercise, explain why other rehabilitation exercises or activities were not chosen and what to avoid during rehabilitation for this injury. Gather details from the textbook, your own research, and data from Ms. Goodbarr's scenario to help formulate your answer.

Why?

- ______________________________
- ______________________________
- ______________________________
- ______________________________

Why not?

- ______________________________
- ______________________________

What do you think?

1. Based on your rehabilitation protocol, discuss the indicators for a limited or full return to play. Include a rough timeline for return to play, if applicable, which is affected by the athlete's compliance with the rehabilitation program.
   - ______________________________
   - ______________________________
   - ______________________________
   - ______________________________
2. Are modifications or personal protective equipment needed to return to play?
   - ______________________________
   - ______________________________

STUDENT SCENARIO 2: CHARLIE REED

Charlie Reed is a runner for his high school cross-country team. His main goal this season is to achieve a personal best of 18 min for 5 km. To reach this goal, he has been running an additional 2 to 3 miles each day to improve his physical endurance. However, he recently noticed a pain in his right knee, inferiorly, just distal to the patella (Fig. 12-4). Initially, the irritation was present only after practice, but it is now occurring during and after practice. He is evaluated by his high school certified athletic trainer, who diagnoses patella tendonitis. The right knee has a thickened patellar tendon and mild edema over the anterior surface of the knee. He also has tight hamstrings and quadriceps. Contracting the quadriceps produces pain at the patellar tendon.

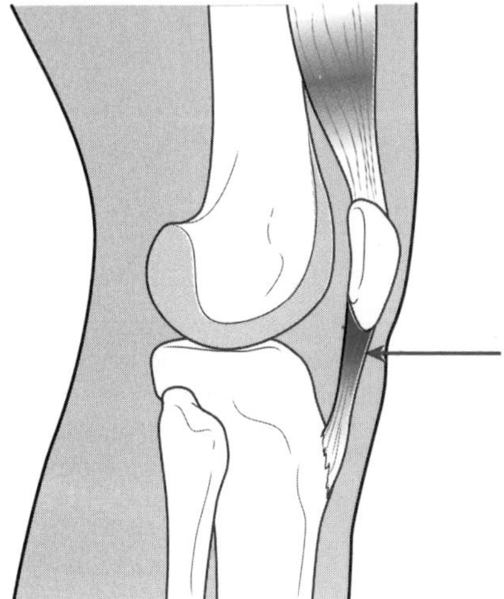

Figure 12-4: Charlie Reed's point of pain.

1. Based on this scenario, what do you know about Mr. Reed's injury?

- ____________________
- ____________________
- ____________________
- ____________________

2. To rehabilitate Mr. Reed's injury effectively, you will need to gather more information. What questions should you ask in addition to what is presented in this scenario?

- ____________________
- ____________________
- ____________________
- ____________________

3. Identify any key terms and concepts, and then research each to broaden your knowledge about knee injuries.

- What anatomical structures might be involved in Mr. Reed's injury?

  Answer: ____________________
- What is patellar tendonitis?

  Answer: ____________________
- In which phase of healing is this injury?

  Answer: ____________________
- Explain a thickened patellar tendon.

  Answer: ____________________
- Define *edema.*

  Answer: ____________________
- Describe the stages of tendonitis.

  Answer: ____________________
- Why is pain produced at the patella tendon when contracting the quadriceps muscle?

  Answer: ____________________

4. Based on the information that you currently have and what was provided by your instructor, how will you begin Mr. Reed's rehabilitation?

- ____________________
- ____________________
- ____________________
- ____________________

Brain Jolt

When rehabilitating athletes with patellar tendonitis, be sure to prevent any forceful, explosive movements, such as plyometrics, so there is not an increased risk for a patellar tendon rupture.

Why or why not?

How will Mr. Reed's rehabilitation progress? For the *why?* portion of each exercise, explain why you chose a particular exercise or activity as part of your program. Describe which rehabilitation goals the exercise or activity covers, and describe the key indicators for progression. For the *why not?* portion of each exercise, explain why other rehabilitation exercises or activities were not chosen and what to avoid during rehabilitation for this injury. Gather details from the textbook, your own research, and data from Mr. Reed's scenario to help formulate your answer.

Why?

- ____________________
- ____________________
- ____________________
- ____________________

Why not?

- ______________________________
- ______________________________
- ______________________________
- ______________________________
- ______________________________

What do you think?

1. Based on your rehabilitation protocol, discuss the indicators for a limited or full return to play. Include a rough timeline for return to play, if applicable, which is affected by the athlete's compliance with the rehabilitation program.
   - ______________________________

2. Are modifications or personal protective equipment needed to return to play?
   - ______________________________
   - ______________________________

STUDENT SCENARIO 3: HOWARD BOYCOTT

Howard Boycott is a shortstop on his school's baseball team. During the game today, Mr. Boycott pivots toward his left, placing his weight on the ball of his right foot while trying to catch a line drive between second and third base. As Mr. Boycott pivots, his right knee rotates into a valgus stress and he feels a popping sensation. Mr. Boycott tries to alleviate the pain by flexing and extending his right knee, but notices a catching sensation during this movement. He also has a history of mild medial collateral ligament sprains. On evaluation, Mr. Boycott has mild effusion along the medial joint line, a positive McMurry test result, and an occasional occurrence of the knee giving out. He states that sometimes his knee locks up, and he is unable to flex or extend the joint. The diagnosis is a medial meniscus tear (Fig. 12-5).

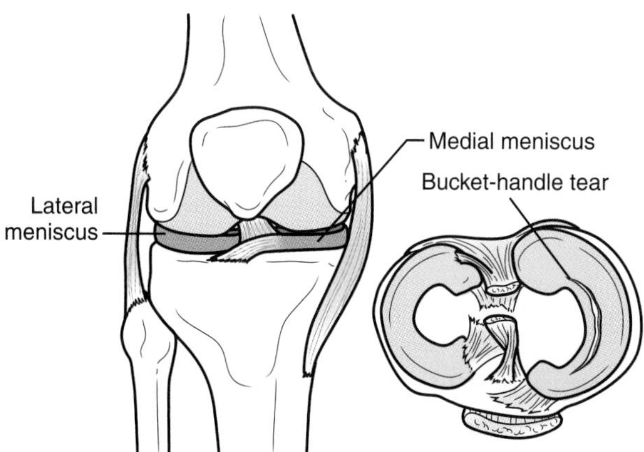

Figure 12-5: Howard Boycott's medial meniscus tear.

1. Based on this scenario, what do you know about Mr. Boycott's injury?
   - ______________________________
   - ______________________________
   - ______________________________
   - ______________________________

2. To rehabilitate Mr. Boycott's injury effectively, you will need to gather more information. What questions should you ask in addition to what is presented in this scenario?
   - ______________________________
   - ______________________________
   - ______________________________
   - ______________________________

3. Identify key terms and concepts, and then research each to broaden your knowledge about knee injuries.

- What anatomical structures are involved?

  Answer: __________
- What is a medial meniscus tear?

  Answer: __________
- In which phase of healing is this injury?

  Answer: __________
- Define *flexion*.

  Answer: __________
- Define *extension*.

  Answer: __________
- Define *effusion*.

  Answer: __________
- What is a valgus stress on the knee?

  Answer: __________
- What might a popping sensation in the knee indicate?

  Answer: __________
- Why does the knee have occasional occurrences of giving out?

  Answer: __________
- What are possible mechanisms for a medial meniscus tear?

  Answer: __________
- What is a McMurry test? What does it test? What does a positive result indicate?

  Answer: __________

Brain Jolt

A "buckle-handle tear" is one type of tear that can occur with the meniscus.

4. Based on the information that you currently have and what was provided by your instructor, how will you begin Mr. Boycott's rehabilitation?

- __________
- __________
- __________
- __________

Why or why not?

How will Mr. Boycott's rehabilitation progress? For the *why?* portion of each exercise, explain why you chose a particular exercise or activity as part of your program. Describe which rehabilitation goals the exercise or activity covers, and describe the key indicators for progression. For the *why not?* portion of each exercise, explain why other rehabilitation exercises or activities were not chosen and what to avoid during rehabilitation for this injury. Gather details from the textbook, your own research, and data from Mr. Boycott's scenario to help formulate your answer.

Why?

- __________
- __________
- __________
- __________

Why not?

- __________
- __________

What do you think?

1. Based on your rehabilitation protocol, discuss the indicators for a limited or full return to play. Include a rough timeline for return to play, if applicable, which is affected by the athlete's compliance with the rehabilitation program.

- __________
- __________
- __________
- __________

2. Are modifications or personal protective equipment needed to return to play?

- __________
- __________

STUDENT SCENARIO 4: **LAMAR NIXON**

Lamar Nixon is a receiver on his school football team. He has been on a limited playing status because of a recent left quadriceps strain. Today is his second day at full return to play. As he is completing a pass route, he quickly decelerates his forward movement, plants his left foot, and cuts to the right. He notices that his quadriceps strains, producing pain and discomfort at his patella, and he falls to the ground in agony. Mr. Nixon notices a lateral deformity at his left knee joint (Fig. 12-6). The team physician is able to relocate the dislocated patella by applying mild pressure in a medial direction to the lateral side of the patella. The leg is slowly extended while applying the medial stress to the patella. After the patella is relocated, Mr. Nixon is referred for radiographs, and the results are negative for any type of patella or femoral condyle fracture.

1. Based on this scenario, what do you know about Mr. Nixon's injury?

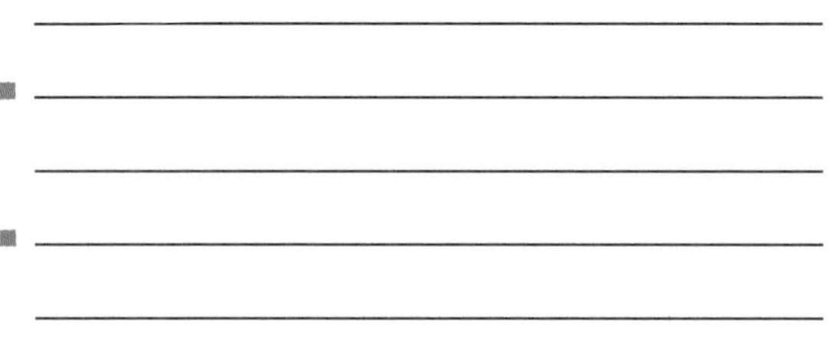

2. To rehabilitate Mr. Nixon's injury effectively, you will need to gather more information. What questions should you ask in addition to what is presented in this scenario?

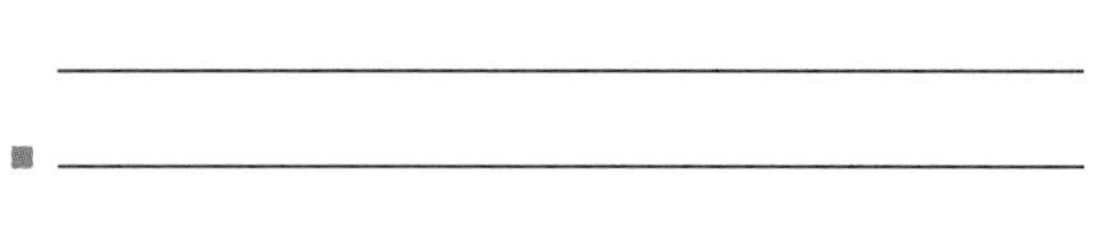

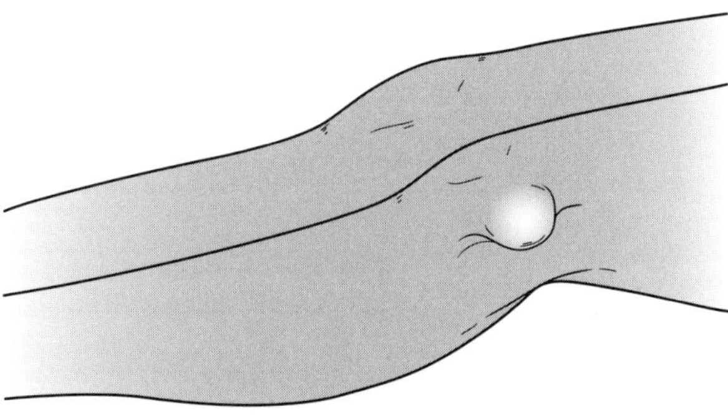

Figure 12-6: Lamar Nixon's deformity.

- ______________________________
- ______________________________

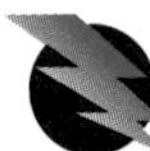

Brain Jolt

A lateral release is a procedure that can be used for an athlete with a history of chronic dislocations or subluxations from a lateral tracking patella.

Conversation Buffer

Be sure to discuss with your coaches that a patella dislocation always needs to be imaged because of the possibility of a fracture that can accompany a dislocation. Even if the athlete is experiencing minimal discomfort and pain, the coach still needs to be aware that a second injury can occur as a result of the initial trauma.

3. Identify any key terms and concepts, and research each to broaden your knowledge about the knee injuries.
   - What anatomical structures might be involved in Mr. Nixon's injury?

     Answer: ______________________________
   - What is a patellar dislocation?

     Answer: ______________________________
   - In which phase of healing is this injury?

     Answer: ______________________________
   - Define *relocation*.

     Answer: ______________________________
   - Define *decelerates*.

     Answer: ______________________________
   - What happens to a muscle during the decelerate process?

     Answer: ______________________________
   - To what does a *limited or full return-to-play status* refer?

     Answer: ______________________________
   - What does lateral deformity indicate in terms of the patella?

     Answer: ______________________________
   - What does applying a medial stress mean?

     Answer: ______________________________
   - Why is a history of a quadriceps strain important in this scenario?

     Answer: ______________________________

4. Based on the information that you currently have and what was provided by your instructor, how will you begin Mr. Nixon's rehabilitation?

- ____________________
- ____________________
- ____________________
- ____________________

Why or why not?

How will Mr. Nixon's rehabilitation progress? For the *why?* portion of each exercise, explain why you chose a particular exercise or activity as part of your program. Describe which rehabilitation goals the exercise or activity covers, and describe the key indicators for progression. For the *why not?* portion of each exercise, explain why other rehabilitation exercises or activities were not chosen and what to avoid during rehabilitation for this injury. Gather details from the textbook, your own research, and data from Mr. Nixon's scenario to help formulate your answer.

Why?

- ____________________
- ____________________
- ____________________
- ____________________

Why not?

- ____________________
- ____________________

What do you think?

1. Based on your rehabilitation protocol, discuss the indicators for a limited or full return to play. Include a rough timeline for return to play, if applicable, which is affected by the athlete's compliance with the rehabilitation program.

- ____________________
- ____________________
- ____________________
- ____________________

2. Are modifications or personal protective equipment needed to return to play?

- ____________________
- ____________________

STUDENT SCENARIO 5: CHASE WOODLEE

Chase Woodlee is the sweeper on the soccer team. He is dribbling the ball when an opponent slide tackles and hits Mr. Woodlee's left knee. The direct blow forces the knee into a valgus stress, while the lower leg is still externally rotated to strike the ball. He immediately falls to the ground while holding his left knee. The on-field evaluation reveals positive valgus, Lachman, and anterior drawer test results. He is unable to bear weight on his left knee, after which he heard and felt a popping sensation. The diagnosis is a tear of the ACL, MCL, and medial meniscus, known as an *unhappy triad* (Fig. 12-7).

1. Based on this scenario, what do you know about Mr. Woodlee's injury?

- ____________________
- ____________________
- ____________________

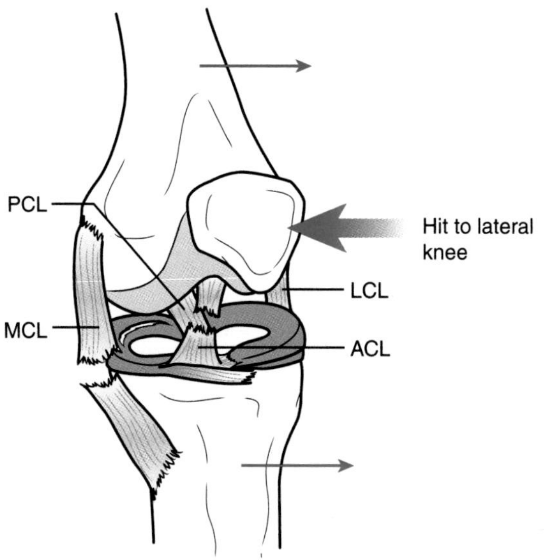

Figure 12-7: Chase Woodlee's unhappy triad.

- ______________________________

2. To rehabilitate Mr. Woodlee's injury effectively, you will need to gather more information. What questions should you ask in addition to what is presented in this scenario?
   - ______________________________
   - ______________________________
   - ______________________________
   - ______________________________

3. Identify any key terms and concepts, and research each to broaden your knowledge about the rehabilitation of knee injuries.
   - What anatomical structures might be involved in Mr. Woodlee's injury?

     Answer: ______________________________
   - What is an unhappy triad? Does it always involve the same three structures?

     Answer: ______________________________
   - In which phase of healing is this injury?

     Answer: ______________________________
   - Define *external rotation.*

     Answer: ______________________________
   - What is a valgus stress of the knee?

     Answer: ______________________________
   - Why is it important to do an on-field evaluation of an injury?

     Answer: ______________________________
   - What might a popping sensation in the knee indicate?

     Answer: ______________________________
   - What is a Lachman test? What does it test? What does a positive result indicate?

     Answer: ______________________________
   - What is an anterior drawer test? What does it test? What does a positive result indicate?

     Answer: ______________________________
   - What is a valgus stress test? What does it test? What does a positive result indicate?

     Answer: ______________________________

Brain Jolt

The extent of any injury is determined by the angle and force of the blow.

4. Based on the information that you currently have and what was provided by your instructor, how will you begin Mr. Woodlee's rehabilitation?
   - ______________________________
   - ______________________________
   - ______________________________
   - ______________________________

Why or why not?

How will Mr. Woodlee's rehabilitation progress? For the *why?* portion of each exercise, explain why you chose a particular exercise or activity as part of your program. Describe which rehabilitation goals the exercise or activity covers, and describe the key indicators for progression. For the *why not?* portion of each exercise, explain why other rehabilitation exercises or activities were not chosen and what to avoid during rehabilitation for this injury. Gather details from the textbook, your own research, and data from Mr. Woodlee's scenario to help formulate your answer.

Why?

- ______________________________

- ____________________
- ____________________
- ____________________

Why not?

- ____________________
- ____________________

Conversation Buffer

Depending on the severity of the ACL and MCL, an unhappy triad is normally an injury that ends an athlete's playing season. Be sure to be supportive, positive, and honest when discussing the severity of the injury and the treatment to the athlete, coaches, and the athlete's parents.

What do you think?

1. Based on your rehabilitation protocol, discuss the indicators for a limited or full return to play. Include a rough timeline for return to play, if applicable, which is affected by the athlete's compliance with the rehabilitation program.
   - ____________________
   - ____________________
   - ____________________
   - ____________________
2. Are modifications or personal protective equipment needed to return to play?
   - ____________________
   - ____________________
   - ____________________
   - ____________________

STUDENT SCENARIO 6: WANDA BARKLEY

Wanda Barkley plays midfield on her collegiate soccer team. She has always had trouble with her right knee, because of genu valgum, and she has corrective orthotics for her shoes to help with leg alignment problems. During a weekend soccer tournament in which the team plays two games each day on Friday, Saturday, and Sunday, Ms. Barkley plays both 45-minute halves of the games. She notices pain on her medial right knee just below the medial joint line on the tibia. Mild edema develops over the anterior medial aspect of the tibia. By Sunday, however, she experiences moderate edema on the medial aspect of the tibia and has tightness on the posterior side of her knee. On evaluation, pes anserine bursitis is diagnosed (Fig. 12-8).

1. Based on this scenario, what do you know about Ms. Barkley's injury?
   - ____________________
   - ____________________

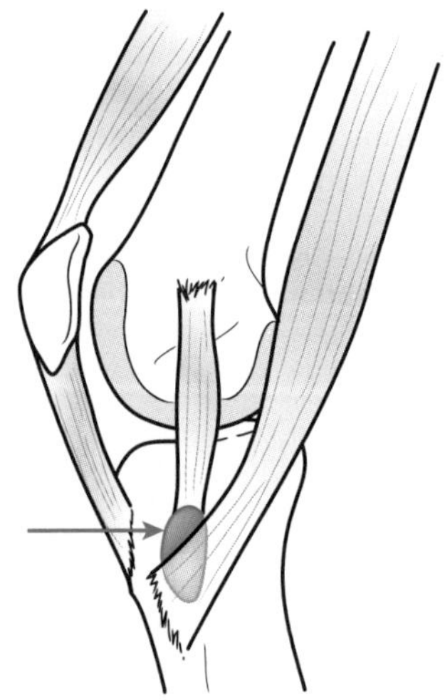

Figure 12-8: Wanda Barkley's pes anserine bursitis.

2. To rehabilitate Ms. Barkley's injury effectively, you will need to gather more information. What questions should you ask in addition to what is presented in this scenario?

- ______________________________
- ______________________________
- ______________________________
- ______________________________

Brain Jolt
If an athlete's hamstrings are tight, the pes anserine muscle group can pull at the insertion point on the tibia.

Conversation Buffer
An inflamed bursa can look worse than it actually is because of the buildup of watery fluid. Recovery is relatively quick and easy. With proper treatment, the athlete will return to the playing field with minimal time loss.

3. Identify any key terms and concepts, and research each to broaden your knowledge about knee injuries.
   - What anatomical structures might be involved in Ms. Barkley's injury?

     Answer: ______________________________
   - What is pes anserine bursitis?

     Answer: ______________________________
   - In which phase of healing is this injury?

     Answer: ______________________________
   - Define *genu valgum*.

     Answer: ______________________________
   - Define *orthotics*.

     Answer: ______________________________
   - Define *edema*.

     Answer: ______________________________
   - What is the difference between mild and moderate edema?

     Answer: ______________________________
   - Describe the appearance and feel of an inflamed bursa.

     Answer: ______________________________

4. Based on the information that you currently have and what was provided by your instructor, how will you begin Ms. Barkley's rehabilitation?

- ______________________________
- ______________________________
- ______________________________
- ______________________________

Why or why not?

How will Ms. Barkley's rehabilitation progress? For the *why?* portion of each exercise, explain why you chose a particular exercise or activity as part of your program. Describe which rehabilitation goals the exercise or activity covers, and describe the key indicators for progression. For the *why not?* portion of each exercise, explain why other rehabilitation exercises or activities were not chosen and what to avoid during rehabilitation for this injury. Gather details from the textbook, your own research, and data from Ms. Barkley's scenario to help formulate your answer.

Why?

- ______________________________
- ______________________________
- ______________________________
- ______________________________

Why not?

- ______________________________
- ______________________________

What do you think?

1. Based on your rehabilitation protocol, discuss the indicators for a limited or full return to play. Include a rough timeline for return to play, if

applicable, which is affected by the athlete's compliance with the rehabilitation program.

- ______________________
- ______________________
- ______________________
- ______________________

2. Are modifications or personal protective equipment needed to return to play?
   - ______________________
   - ______________________

STUDENT SCENARIO 7: TABATHA KNIGHT

Tabatha Knight is a point guard for her high school basketball team. She is in her senior year and has had no prior injuries. A new play is being implemented during today's practice. However, a fellow teammate executes the wrong shift and runs into Ms. Knight. Upon contact, Ms. Knight is hit from her lateral left side, forcing her knee into a valgus stress (Fig. 12-9). As her knee is forced inward, her foot is rotated externally. She feels a pulling sensation on the medial side of her knee, causing her to limp with any activity. She is removed from practice and evaluated, revealing the following symptoms: a positive valgus stress test result, mild effusion over the medial joint line, decreased ability to fully extend the knee while bearing weight, and a negative McMurry test result. The diagnosis is a grade 2 medial collateral ligament sprain.

1. Based on this scenario, what do you know about Ms. Knight's injury?
   - ______________________
   - ______________________
   - ______________________
   - ______________________

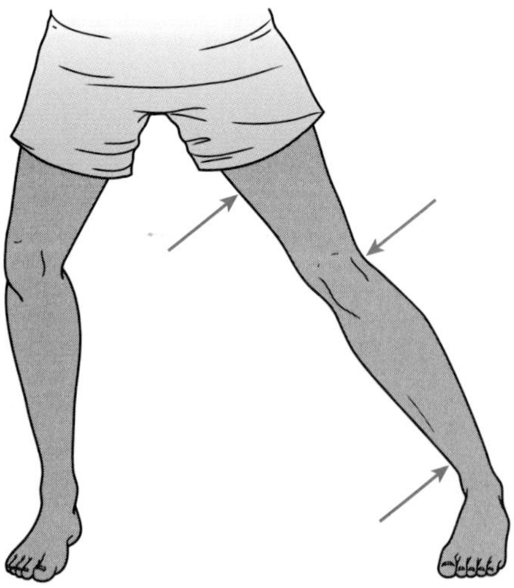

Figure 12-9: Tabatha Knight's point of force.

2. To rehabilitate Ms. Knight's injury effectively, you will need to gather more information. What questions should you ask in addition to what is presented in this scenario?
   - ______________________
   - ______________________
   - ______________________
   - ______________________

Brain Jolt
Strong muscles surrounding the knee joint help to support weak ligaments at the knee joint.

3. Identify key terms and concepts, and then research each to broaden your knowledge about knee injuries.
   - What anatomical structures might be involved in Ms. Knight's injury?

     Answer: ______________________
   - What is a grade 2 MCL sprain?

     Answer: ______________________
   - In which phase of healing is this injury?

     Answer: ______________________
   - Define *effusion*.

     Answer: ______________________

- What is a valgus stress of the knee?

Answer: ______

- With a valgus stress and a foot internally rotated, what structure is being stressed? Why is the medial meniscus not involved?

Answer: ______

- What is a valgus stress test? What does it test? What does a positive result indicate?

Answer: ______

- What is the McMurry test? What does it test? What does a positive result indicate?

Answer: ______

4. Based on the information that you currently have and what was provided by your instructor, how will you begin Ms. Knight's rehabilitation?

- ______
- ______
- ______
- ______

Conversation Buffer

Some coaches are so focused on maintaining practice for the entire designated time, repeating drills and focusing on conditioning, that they often forget about strength training. If a muscle is weak, the stress falls onto the surrounding joint structures, such as the ligaments. Remind the coaches about the importance of implementing a weight room routine within their normal practice schedule.

Why or why not?

How will Ms. Knight's rehabilitation progress? For the *why?* portion of each exercise, explain why you chose a particular exercise or activity as part of your program. Describe which rehabilitation goals the exercise or activity covers, and describe the key indicators for progression. For the *why not?* portion of each exercise, explain why other rehabilitation exercises or activities were not chosen and what to avoid during rehabilitation for this injury. Gather details from the textbook, your own research, and data from Ms. Knight's scenario to help formulate your answer.

Why?

- ______
- ______
- ______
- ______

Why not?

- ______
- ______

What do you think?

1. Based on your rehabilitation protocol, discuss the indicators for a limited or full return to play. Include a rough timeline for return to play, if applicable, which is affected by the athlete's compliance with the rehabilitation program.

- ______
- ______
- ______
- ______

2. Are modifications or personal protective equipment needed to return to play?

- ______
- ______

STUDENT SCENARIO 8: JORDAN COLLETT

Jordan Collett is a freestyle swimmer for her collegiate team with an irritation in her left knee. Most of her pain occurs over the patella when she performs a flip-turn off the pool wall. When she flips, she has slight flexion in her legs before forcefully extending her legs when pushing off the wall. On evaluation, she has pain at the inferior pole of her patella, the vastus medialis oblique muscle is weak and atrophied (Fig. 12-10), and the patella grind test result is positive. When the patella is stabilized on either side while performing a quadriceps contraction, the patella tracks properly in the femoral groove. Her pain then decreases with active extension. The diagnosis is patella femoral syndrome.

1. Based on this scenario, what do you know about Ms. Collett's injury?
   - ______________________________
   - ______________________________
   - ______________________________
   - ______________________________
2. To rehabilitate Ms. Collett's injury effectively, you will need to gather more information. What questions should you ask in addition to what is presented in this scenario?
   - ______________________________
   - ______________________________
   - ______________________________
   - ______________________________

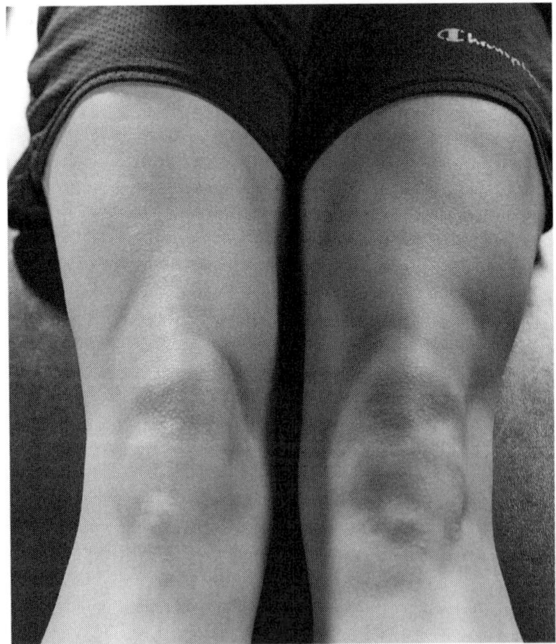

Figure 12-10: Jordan Collett's atrophied vastus medialis oblique.

Brain Jolt

Sometimes patella femoral syndrome is a catch-all phrase for unexplained knee pain. Be sure to perform a thorough examination so that you do not overlook something that might not be apparent on a quick assessment.

3. Identify key terms and concepts, and then research each to broaden your knowledge about knee injuries.
   - What anatomical structures might be involved in Ms. Collett's injury?

     Answer: ______________________________
   - What is patellar femoral syndrome?

     Answer: ______________________________
   - In which phase of healing is this injury?

     Answer: ______________________________
   - Define *inferior pole of the patella.*

     Answer: ______________________________
   - Define *atrophied.*

     Answer: ______________________________
   - What does the tracking of the patella in the femoral groove imply?

     Answer: ______________________________
   - What is the patella grind test? What does it test? What does a positive result indicate?

     Answer: ______________________________
4. Based on the information that you currently have and what was provided by your instructor, how will you begin Ms. Knight's rehabilitation?
   - ______________________________
   - ______________________________

- ______________________________
  ____
- ______________________________
  ____

Why or why not?

How will Ms. Knight's rehabilitation progress? For the *why?* portion of each exercise, explain why you chose a particular exercise or activity as part of your program. Describe which rehabilitation goals the exercise or activity covers, and describe the key indicators for progression. For the *why not?* portion of each exercise, explain why other rehabilitation exercises or activities were not chosen and what to avoid during rehabilitation for this injury. Gather details from the textbook, your own research, and data from Ms. Knight's scenario to help formulate your answer.

Why?

- ______________________________
  ____
- ______________________________
  ____
- ______________________________
  ____
- ______________________________
  ____

Why not?

- ______________________________
  ____
- ______________________________
  ____

What do you think?

1. Based on your rehabilitation protocol, discuss the indicators for a limited or full return to play. Include a rough timeline for return to play, if applicable, which is affected by the athlete's compliance with the rehabilitation program.
   - ______________________________
     ____
   - ______________________________
     ____
   - ______________________________
     ____
   - ______________________________
     ____
2. Are modifications or personal protective equipment needed to return to play?
   - ______________________________
     ____
   - ______________________________
     ____

STUDENT SCENARIO 9: GRETCHEN THOMAS

Gretchen Thomas is a forward and leading scorer on a women's collegiate soccer team. After practice each day, Ms. Thomas remains on the field to practice her outside shot on the goal, and today is no exception. Practice was hard, and Ms. Thomas feels more tired than on previous days, but she decides to persevere and take three more shots on goal. As she dribbles down to the goal on the right side of the field, she plants her left foot and kicks the ball with her right foot. She feels a pop in her left knee and drops to the ground. On evaluation, the certified athletic trainer notes that the foot is externally rotated and the knee has a valgus stress (Fig. 12-11). She has mild to moderate edema over the entire joint line and a lack of full extension. While trying to get up and proceed to the medical cart, Ms. Thomas feels like her knee will "give out" and thus is unable to bear weight on her left leg. The certified athletic trainer diagnoses an anterior cruciate ligament tear.

1. Based on this scenario, what do you know about Ms. Thomas' injury?
   - ______________________________
     ____
   - ______________________________
     ____
   - ______________________________
     ____
   - ______________________________
     ____

Treatment Detour

Researchers performed a randomized control trial involving 121 young active adults with an acute

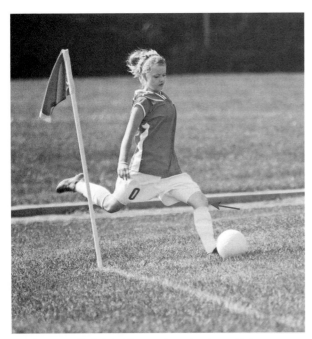

Figure 12-11: Gretchen Thomas' mechanism of injury. (© Thinkstock)

ACL injury. The results indicated that in young active adults with an acute ACL tear, a treatment option of "structured rehabilitation plus early ACL reconstruction" is not shown to be more effective than the treatment option of "rehabilitation plus optional delayed ACL reconstruction" in patient outcomes at 2 years after injury. This knowledge is important for your treatment protocol, because there could be a reason to rehabilitate the injury initially and completely before the athlete commits to surgery: reconstruction of the knee might not be necessary (Frobell, Roos, Roos, Ranstam, & Lohmander, 2010).

2. To rehabilitate Ms. Thomas' injury effectively, you will need to gather more information. What questions should you ask in addition to what is presented in this scenario?

- ____________________
- ____________________
- ____________________
- ____________________

Brain Jolt

Always consider the mechanism of injury with an ACL injury because there could be additional structures involved in the injury.

3. Identify key terms and concepts, and then research each to broaden your knowledge about knee injuries.

- What anatomical structures might be involved in Ms. Thomas' injury?

  Answer: ____________________
- What is an ACL tear?

  Answer: ____________________
- In which phase of healing is this injury?

  Answer: ____________________
- Define *edema*.

  Answer: ____________________
- Describe what *normal leg extension* means.

  Answer: ____________________
- How could Ms. Thomas possibly have torn her ACL without any type of contact with another player?

  Answer: ____________________
- Why would Ms. Thomas experience a "giving out" sensation?

  Answer: ____________________

4. Based on the information that you currently have and what was provided by your instructor, how will you begin Ms. Thomas' rehabilitation?

- ____________________
- ____________________
- ____________________
- ____________________

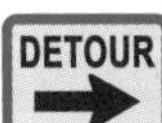

Treatment Detour

Research indicates that both concentric and eccentric open kinetic chain and closed kinetic chain exercises are safe and necessary for effective rehabilitation in post-ACL reconstruction patients. These exercises are important because they mimic actions found in sports and other daily activities. The most effective equipment to use in the rehabilitation process, in progressive succession, is the total gym, leg press, and squat rack. It is important to use these exercises in succession to avoid reinjury caused by a lack of strength and an inability to withstand the forces in each activity (Lorenz & Reiman, 2011).

Why or why not?

How will Ms. Thomas' rehabilitation progress? For the *why?* portion of each exercise, explain why you chose a particular exercise or activity as part of your program. Describe which rehabilitation goals the exercise or activity covers, and describe the key indicators for progression. For the *why not?* portion of each exercise, explain why other rehabilitation exercises or activities were not chosen and what to avoid during rehabilitation for this injury. Gather details from the textbook, your own research, and data from Ms. Thomas' scenario to help formulate your answer.

Why?

- ____________________
  ____
- ____________________
  ____
- ____________________
  ____
- ____________________
  ____

Why not?

- ____________________
  ____
- ____________________
  ____

What do you think?

1. Based on your rehabilitation protocol, discuss the indicators for a limited or full return to play. Include a rough timeline for return to play, if applicable, which is affected by the athlete's compliance with the rehabilitation program.
   - ____________________
     ____
   - ____________________
     ____
   - ____________________
     ____
   - ____________________
     ____
2. Are modifications or required protective equipment needed to return to play?
   - ____________________
     ____
   - ____________________
     ____

knowledge checklist

Table 12-1 offers a checklist that can be used by a peer, instructor, or preceptor to evaluate each part of the athlete's rehabilitation plan. Use this checklist as a tool to ensure that the rehabilitation plan is complete and to assess your knowledge of the competencies that apply to this chapter.

TABLE 12-1 ■ Lower Extremity: The Knee Rehabilitation and Therapeutic Exercise Competency Checklist

	Proficient *Can demonstrate and execute the skill properly*	**Proficient With Assistance** *Can demonstrate and execute the skill with minimal guidance or tips*	**Not Proficient** *Unable to demonstrate and execute the skill properly; need to be reevaluated at another time after further study and practice*
Controlling Edema			
PRICE			
Modalities			
Controlling Pain			
Pain scales			
Medications			
Modalities			
Establishes Core Stability			
Reestablishes Neuromuscular Control			
Restores Postural Control and Balance			
Restoring Range of Motion			
Passive range of motion			
Active range of motion			
Resistive range of motion			
Goniometry			
Normal range of motion limits			
Restore Muscular Strength, Endurance, and Power			
Open kinetic chain			
Closed kinetic chain			
Isometric			
Isotonic			
Isotonic (concentric and eccentric)			
Isokinetic			
Plyometric			
Agility			
Functional or Sport-Specific Activities			
Maintains Cardiorespiratory Fitness			
Functional Testing			
Return-to-Play Criteria			
Proper Documentation			

PRICE, prevention, rest, ice, compression, and elevation.

REFERENCES

Fanelli, G. C., Beck, J. D., & Edson C. J. (2010). Current concepts review: The posterior cruciate ligament. *The Journal of Knee Surgery, 23*, 61–72.

Frobell, R. B., Roos, E. M., Roos, H. P., Ranstam J., & Lohmander, L. S. (2010). A randomized trial of treatment for acute anterior cruciate ligament tears. *The New England Journal of Medicine, 363*, 331–342.

Higgins, M. (2011). *Therapeutic exercise from theory to practice.* Philadelphia, PA: F.A. Davis.

Lorenz, D., & Reiman, M. (2011). The role and implementation of eccentric training in athletic rehabilitation: Tendinopathy, hamstring strains, and ACL reconstruction. *International Journal of Sports Physical Therapy, 6*, 27–44.

National Athletic Training Association. (2011). *Athletic training education competencies* (5th ed.). Retrieved from http://www.nata.org/sites/default/files/5th-Edition-Competencies-2011-PDF-Version.pdf

Prentice, W. (2010). *Arnheim's principles of athletic training: A competency-based approach* (14th ed.). New York, NY: McGraw-Hill.

Prentice, W. (2011). *Rehabilitation techniques for sports medicine and athletic training* (5th ed.). New York, NY: McGraw-Hill.

Starkey, C. (2004). *Therapeutic modalities* (3rd ed.). Philadelphia PA: F.A. Davis.

Starkey, C., Brown, S. D., & Ryan, J. (2010). *Examination of orthopedic and athletic injuries* (3rd ed.). Philadelphia, PA: F.A. Davis.

Venes, D. (Ed.). (2009). *Taber's cyclopedic medical dictionary* (21st ed.). Philadelphia, PA: F.A. Davis.

chapter 13

Lower Extremity: The Hip, Thigh, and Lower Leg

chapter outline

athletic trainer's corner

Here is what one athletic trainer experienced while rehabilitating an athlete's injury:

As an athletic training student, I had the privilege of fulfilling my senior rehabilitation requirement by caring for a football receiver. He sustained a tibia-fibular fracture that resulted in further complications including compartment syndrome in the lateral chamber of his lower leg. Because this was my first experience with a rehabilitation program from start to finish, I learned a lot about the psychological aspect of rehabilitation. I realized that a rehabilitation program can be complicated. The goal is to push the athlete in his or her program, yet you cannot push him or her any faster than the body and postoperative protocol can handle. I also realized that it is important to try to expect the unexpected. I found that we cannot always control what our athletes do outside of the rehab and school setting. The athlete in my care almost jeopardized his recovery progress because of his extracurricular activities. He worked through his rehabilitation and is now able to function in sports, but he decided not to play anymore because of his injury. We always have to remember that serious injuries can affect athletes in many ways, and we have to keep that in focus when rehabilitating an athlete.

Darren Howard, AT, ATC
Graduate Assistant Athletic Trainer
Miami University
Oxford, Ohio

learning outcomes

After working through this chapter, you will be able to:

1. Describe seven different goals of rehabilitation and the importance of each in the overall rehabilitation protocol.
2. Verbalize indications for performing hip, thigh, and lower-leg rehabilitative techniques.
3. Discuss modifications and progressions that are used during a rehabilitation program for the hip, thigh, and lower leg.
4. Discuss the outcome measures used to identify activity levels and return-to-play guidelines for hip, thigh, and lower-leg injuries.
5. Explain what modality choice is proper for rehabilitation by using indications, contraindications, and the principles and theory related to the physiological response of the intervention.

MODEL SCENARIO 1: DARRYLL HUBER

Darryll Huber is an offensive lineman on his college football team who plays left tackle. During a home game, the football is hiked and Mr. Huber blocks his opponent. Unfortunately, his fellow teammate is pushed from the line of scrimmage, falls into Mr. Huber, and lands on Mr. Huber's left lower leg. Mr. Huber feels a cracking sensation and then falls to the ground. He notices an obvious deformity at the midshaft of his left lower leg. As Mr. Huber's left leg is vacuum splinted for transport, it is determined that he has a tibia-fibular fracture (Fig. 13-1). Mr. Huber is transported to the hospital for radiographs and the necessary course of action.

1. Based on this scenario, what do you know about Mr. Huber's injury?
   - *Male athlete*
   - *Football player, offensive line, left tackle*
   - *Mechanism of injury: direct blow by a fellow teammate*
   - *Cracking sensation on impact*
   - *Deformity at the midshaft of the tibia and fibula*
   - *Vacuum splinted and transported to the hospital*

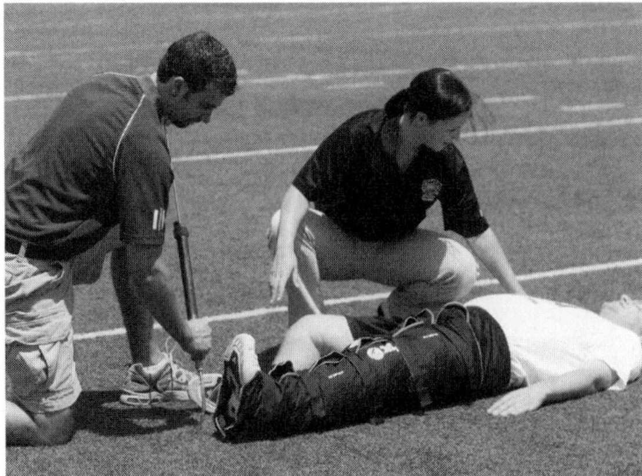

Figure 13-1: Darryll Huber's tibia-fibular fracture. (From Starkey, C., Brown, S. D., & Ryan, J. (2010). *Examination of orthopedic and athletic injuries.* Philadelphia, PA, F.A. Davis, p. 41.)

Conversation Buffer

Any type of injury is traumatic for an athlete; therefore, always be sure to assess for signs of shock. In some states, coaches must be certified to perform cardiopulmonary resuscitation (CPR); however, even if not required, it is always a good idea to study CPR and first aid, as these areas also cover information about how to treat shock. In addition, it is always a good idea to review CPR information before the season begins.

2. To rehabilitate Mr. Huber's injury effectively, you will need to gather additional information. What questions should you ask in addition to what has been presented in the previous scenario?
   - *Are there any preexisting injuries? If yes, what are they?*
   - *How long has the athlete experienced this pain?*
   - *What is this athlete's pain level and type of pain felt?*
   - *What is the strength at the ankle?*
   - *What is the range of motion (ROM) in the ankle?*
   - *Does the athlete have any numbness or paraesthesia?*
   - *Is there edema or ecchymosis?*
   - *Are there any signs of shock?*
   - *Are there any other deformities?*
   - *What treatment was given at the hospital?*
   - *Was the injury a compound fracture?*
3. Identify key terms and concepts, and then research each to broaden your knowledge about the rehabilitation of hip, thigh, and lower-leg injuries.
   - What anatomical structures might be involved in Mr. Huber's injury?
     Tibia
     Fibula
     Lower-leg muscle compartments
     Lower-leg nerves
   - What is a tibia-fibular fracture?
     A fracture that occurs at both of the lower-leg bones: the tibia and the fibula

- In which phase of healing is this injury?
  This injury occurs at the inflammatory response phase.
- Define *deformity*.
  Alteration or distortion of a body part
- What is a vacuum splint?
  A vacuum splint is a type of device that is used to help stabilize a fracture site. This cuff is placed over the injured area, securing the joint above and the joint below the fracture site. The air is removed with suction, providing full compression to any area that the cuff encompasses.
- What does midshaft of the lower leg mean?
  This is the portion of the bone that is injured: the middle or mid part of the tibia and fibula. To describe a location of an injury to a bone, the terms proximal, distal, and mid are used to describe a point of reference.
- What is a complication of a tibia-fibular fracture?
  Acute compartment syndrome

4. Based on the information that you currently have and what was provided by your instructor, how will you begin Mr. Huber's rehabilitation?
   Mr. Huber is going to be in a cast for at least 6 weeks, depending on how the fracture site heals. Check with the physician before beginning any rehabilitation program; however, the athlete can be cleared to do exercises involving the noninjured area before the injured area is cleared for rehab. Once the cast is removed, flexibility and strengthening exercises for the lower leg are the focus, along with any type of ankle-strengthening exercise.

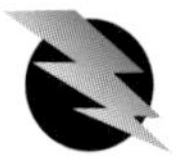

Brain Jolt
Strengthening the muscles above and below the affected joint during rehabilitation is just as important as stabilizing the areas above and below the affected joint at the time of injury.

Why or why not?

How will Darryll Huber's rehabilitation progress? For the *why?* portion of each exercise, explain why you chose a particular exercise or activity as part of your program. Describe which rehabilitation goals the exercise or activity covers, and describe the key indicators for progression. For the *why not?* portion of each exercise, explain why other rehabilitation exercises or activities were not chosen and what to avoid during rehabilitation for this injury. Gather details from the textbook, your own research, and data from Mr. Huber's scenario to help formulate your answer.

Why?

- ***Towel stretching.*** *This activity will help with the rehabilitation goal of increasing ROM. However, it is not intense enough to cause injury, thus keeping the athlete safe. This activity can progress to an inclined board once the athlete is no longer feeling the stretch with the towel and pain levels decrease.*
- ***Calf raises.*** *This activity will help with the rehabilitation goal of increasing strength. This activity strengthens the superficial compartment of the lower leg. Like leg stances, calf raises can progress by beginning with a double-leg calf raise and then moving on to single-leg calf raises. These exercises can be made more difficult by moving from a flat surface to an uneven surface or by holding weights.*
- ***Ankle exercises.*** *These exercises will help the rehabilitation goals of increasing ROM and strength. Because the athlete's ankle joint is immobilized in a cast, the ankle is an area of concern. Adding range of motion exercises like ankle pumps and by using the biomechanical ankle platform system board, including strengthening exercises that use rubber tubing where the athlete moves the area being rehabilitated in all directions, and adding flexibility exercises to the regime will help. These exercises can be progressed by increasing repetitions or exercise time and increasing the resistance of the tubing once they are performed with ease.*
- ***Double- and single-leg stance.*** *This activity will help with the rehabilitation goal of increasing proprioception and can be initiated once weight-bearing is allowed to improve proprioception of the lower leg and increase neuromuscular control. These exercises can be performed by having the athlete first stand with the legs together and eyes closed for a determined period of time. Next, instruct the athlete to stand in the double-leg stance on an uneven surface. Once the athlete is able to do this with ease and no pain, progress to single-leg stance exercises. The athlete stands on the injured leg on a flat surface with eyes closed for a determined period of time. After accomplishing this, the athlete progresses to standing on an unsteady surface to challenge his or her proprioception.*
- ***Modality.*** *Ice will help with the rehabilitation goal of reducing pain and edema. The method used to set the tibia-fibula (surgical or nonsurgical setting) will determine whether you are able to use any type of electrical modality to help achieve the rehabilitation goals. Remember that electrical stimulation cannot be used over metal, such as if the athlete has a metal implant.*

Why not?

- Avoid any closed kinetic chain exercises until they are approved by the athlete's surgeon and the athlete is strong enough to handle weight-bearing exercises.

What do you think?

1. Based on your rehabilitation protocol, discuss the indicators for a limited and full return to play with the athlete. Include a rough timeline for return to play, if applicable, which is affected by the athlete's compliance with the rehabilitation program.
   - ***Limited return to play.*** *His status depends on whether he regains full ROM, strength, and proprioception in the injured leg. Once the athlete achieves these goals and can perform simple functional tasks without pain or compensation, he will be able to engage in some drills and noncontact activities with the team.*
   - ***Full return to play.*** *If all of the previously noted exercises are performed without pain and compensation, and the athlete does not experience excessive edema or any setbacks, then he can return to play without restrictions.*
2. Are modifications or personal protective equipment needed to return to play?
   - *No*

MODEL SCENARIO 2: LISA WILLIAMS

Lisa Williams is a pitcher on her college softball team. She enters the game in the fifth inning, when she faces an opponent who has hit two home runs today. As she releases the softball, she knows that the ball is going to be hit by the batter. The batter hits a line drive straight back to Ms. Williams, and it hits her left lower leg directly over her anterior tibia. She falls and is assisted off the field because of the pain. Within 10 min of the injury, she has moderate edema and a tight feeling of pressure in her lower leg. She is unable to perform active dorsiflexion and has a decreased dorsal pedal pulse. She is transported immediately to the hospital, where it is determined that she has acute compartment syndrome of the anterior compartment (Fig. 13-2). Acute compartment syndrome is a medical emergency; therefore, Ms. Williams is scheduled for surgery.

1. Based on this scenario, what do you know about Ms. Williams' injury?
   - *Female athlete*
   - *Softball pitcher*
   - *Mechanism of injury: direct hit to the anterior tibia*
   - *Moderate edema*
   - *Decreased dorsal pedal pulse*
   - *No active dorsiflexion of the ankle*
   - *Transported to the hospital and scheduled for surgery*

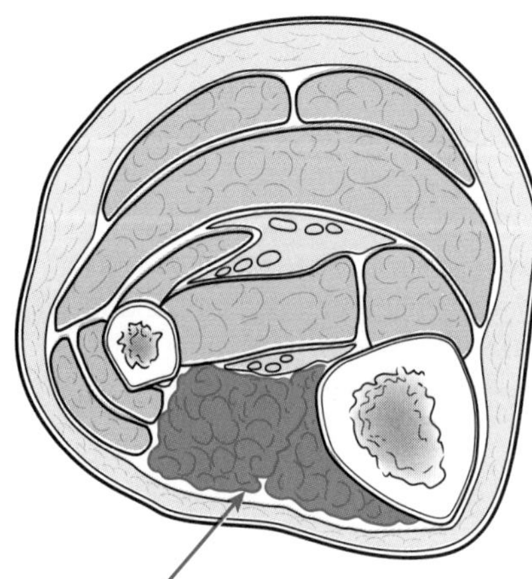

Figure 13-2: Lisa Williams' edema.

2. To rehabilitate Ms. Williams' injury effectively, you will need to gather additional information. What questions should you ask in addition to what is presented in the previous scenario?
   - *Are there any preexisting injuries? If yes, what are they?*
   - *How long has the athlete experienced this pain?*
   - *What is the athlete's pain level and type of pain felt?*
   - *What is the strength in the ankle?*
   - *What is the ROM in the ankle?*
   - *Is there any numbness or paraesthesia?*
   - *What specifically was done in surgery? Are there complications from the surgery?*

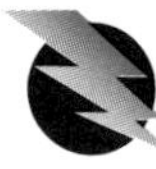

Brain Jolt

The surgery that repairs compartment syndrome is a fasciotomy. There are a few different variations of this surgical procedure; therefore, be sure to obtain the operative details and the surgeon's recommended treatment before beginning the athlete's rehabilitation.

3. Identify key terms and concepts, and research each to broaden your knowledge about the rehabilitation of hip, thigh, and lower-leg injuries.
   - What anatomical structures might be involved in Ms. Williams' injury?
     Tibialis anterior muscle
     Anterior compartment
     Tibia
     Fibula
     Anterior tibial artery
     Deep peroneal nerve
   - What is acute compartment syndrome?
     Acute means that the injury has rapid onset, and compartment syndrome is an elevation of tissue pressure within a closed fascial compartment. Acute compartment syndrome is usually caused by hemorrhage or edema within the compartment from a direct hit or other trauma to the area.

- In which phase of healing is this injury?
  This injury occurs in the inflammatory response phase.
- Define *edema.*
  Swelling; a localized or general condition that causes the body tissues to contain an excessive amount of fluid
- Define *dorsiflexion of the foot.*
  Directional term; movement of a body part toward the posterior aspect of the body; of the foot, moving backward in which the foot moves toward its top
- Define *pedal pulse.*
  The pedal pulse, the pulse of the foot, is located just on top of the foot above the talus.
- What is meant by *tightness* or *pressure* in the lower leg?
  The lower leg is divided into compartments. When these compartments are injured, edema occurs and closes off or compresses the compartment, creating a tight feeling.

4. Based on the information that you currently have and what was provided by your instructor, how will you begin Ms. Williams' rehabilitation?
   Ms. Williams will be out of activity for 2 to 4 months after surgery. The initial 4 to 6 weeks are going to be limited regarding any type of rehabilitation as a result of the surgery. To prevent any edema from developing in the anterior compartment, elevation and ice is the best treatment. Be sure to keep a barrier between the ice and the athlete's skin to prevent any burning to the surgical area, especially if a skin graft was necessary. Ensure proper wound care of the surgical site to decrease the risk of infection. Mildly stretch the ankle, calves, and hamstrings and perform ROM exercises for the lower leg.

Why or why not?

How will Ms. Williams' rehabilitation progress? For the *why?* portion of each exercise, explain why you chose a particular exercise or activity as part of your program. Describe which rehabilitation goals the exercise or activity covers, and describe the key indicators for progression. For the *why not?* portion of each exercise, explain why other rehabilitation exercises or activities were not chosen and what to avoid during rehabilitation for this injury. Gather details from the textbook, your own research, and data from Ms. Williams' scenario to help formulate your answer.

Why?

- ***Ice and elevation.*** *These two treatments will help with the rehabilitation goal of reducing edema in the compartment, which decreases pain, edema, and inflammation; this is a critical goal of the rehabilitation of postoperative compartment syndrome.*
- ***Wound care.*** *Proper care will reduce the risk of infection of the surgical incision. Aqua therapy is initiated when the surgical incision is healed and clearance is obtained from the doctor.*
- ***Towel stretching.*** *This activity will help with the rehabilitation goal of increasing ROM in plantar flexion. This activity is not intense enough to cause injury, thus keeping the athlete safe.*
- ***ROM.*** *Ankle pumps will help with the rehabilitation goal of increasing ROM at the ankle. Cotton ball pick-ups and towel scrunches will help increase the ROM and strength of the toes.*

Why not?

- *Avoid any activities that increase the compartment pressure. Remember to increase repetitions before increasing weight to gain endurance because you do not want a lot of muscle girth to increase the compartment pressure. Pool workouts are a good choice later in the rehabilitation process; however, avoid them early in treatment because of the surgical site wound and skin graft, if applicable.*

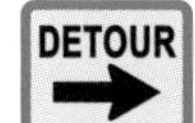

Treatment Detour

The second most common cause of acute compartment syndrome is a blunt soft tissue injury, as seen in the current scenario. Once the diagnosis is made, immediate surgical decompression is needed. Skin closure can be performed only after swelling decreases. Vacuum-assisted wound closure is a new popular method of wound management and treatment performed after a skin graft. As a result, during rehabilitation, wound care and skin graft considerations are essential to a successful recovery and to avoid setbacks from infection (Shadgen et al., 2010).

What do you think?

1. Based on your rehabilitation protocol, discuss the indicators for a limited and full return to play. Include a rough timeline for return to play, if applicable, which is affected by the athlete's compliance with the rehabilitation program.
   - ***Limited return to play.*** *Her status depends on whether she regains full ROM, strength, and proprioception in the injured leg. Once the athlete achieves these and can perform simple functional tasks without pain or compensation, she will be able to engage in some drills and noncontact activities with the team.*
   - ***Full return to play.*** *If all the previously noted exercises are performed without pain and compensation, and the athlete does not experience excessive edema or any setbacks, then she can return to play without restrictions.*
2. Are modifications or personal protective equipment needed to return to play?
   - *No*

STUDENT SCENARIO 1: ALLISON HUNTER

Allison Hunter is a cross-country runner. She is 4 weeks into preseason conditioning and has been running 4 to 7 miles daily when she notices an anterior pain on her right tibia after practice. She continues her routine of soaking in the cold whirlpool after practice and hopes that the pain will subside. Two weeks later, she experiences pain before and after running, but she is still able to run the required mileage. She is evaluated by the certified athletic trainer who diagnoses medial tibial stress syndrome (MTSS), also known as *shin splints* (Fig. 13-3). On evaluation, she displays a tight Achilles tendon, a pronated right foot with walking and running, and improperly fitted running shoes.

1. Based on this scenario, what do you know about Ms. Hunter's injury?
   - ____________________
   - ____________________
   - ____________________
   - ____________________

2. To effectively rehabilitate Ms. Hunter's injury, you will need to gather more information. What questions should you ask in addition to what is presented in this scenario?
   - ____________________
   - ____________________
   - ____________________
   - ____________________

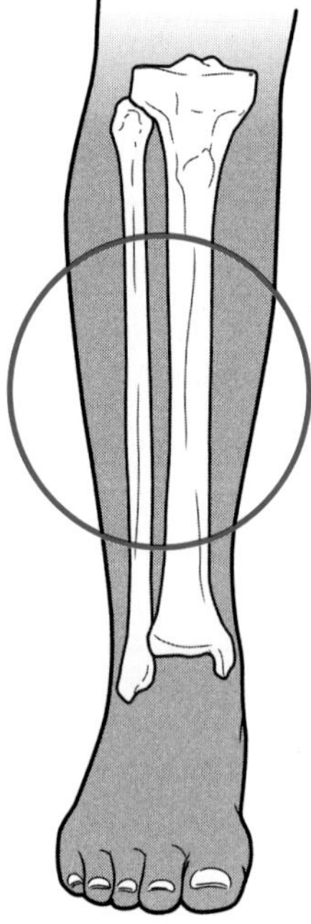

Figure 13-3: Allison Hunter's medial tibial stress syndrome.

Brain Jolt

Early detection of shin splints is the key to maintaining an athlete's performance. Determine the cause to decrease the symptoms of shin splints.

Brain Jolt

Many people do not realize the importance of wearing proper footwear when running. Be sure to suggest that athletes be fitted by a trained professional for their running shoes. This helps to ease or possibly correct any foot abnormalities that may exist, which can lead to injury.

3. Identify key terms and concepts, and then research each to broaden your knowledge about the rehabilitation of hip, thigh, and lower-leg injuries.
   - What anatomical structures might be involved in Ms. Hunter's injury?

     Answer: __________
   - What is MTSS?

     Answer: __________
   - In which phase of healing is this injury?

     Answer: __________
   - Define *pronate*.

     Answer: __________
   - What does a tight Achilles tendon indicate?

     Answer: __________
   - What are the different grades of MTSS? What are the symptoms of each grade?

     Answer: __________
   - What are the two different types of conditions that result from MTSS?

     Answer: __________

4. Based on the information that you currently have and what was provided by your instructor, how will you begin Ms. Hunter's rehabilitation?

- ______
- ______
- ______
- ______

Why or why not?

How will Ms. Hunter's rehabilitation progress? For the *why?* portion of each exercise, explain why you chose a particular exercise or activity as part of your program. Describe which rehabilitation goals the exercise or activity covers, and describe the key indicators for progression. For the *why not?* portion of each exercise, explain why other rehabilitation exercises or activities were not chosen and what to avoid during rehabilitation for this injury. Gather details from the textbook, your own research, and data from Ms. Hunter's scenario to help formulate your answer.

Why?

- ______
- ______
- ______
- ______

Why not?

- ______
- ______

What do you think?

1. Based on your rehabilitation protocol, discuss the indicators for a limited and full return to play. Include a rough timeline for return to play, if applicable, which is affected by the athlete's compliance with the rehabilitation program.

- ______
- ______
- ______
- ______

2. Are modifications or required protective equipment needed to return to play?

- ______
- ______

STUDENT SCENARIO 2: MARGARET MAYS

Margaret Mays is a midfielder on her college soccer team. While running after an opponent to get the ball, Ms. Mays lunges forward with her left leg to reach the ball. Upon doing so, she feels a pull or tearing sensation at the anterior portion of her right hip. However, she continues to play without any apparent signs of injury. After the game, she experiences pain with walking and flexion of her right hip, and she has weakness with active hip flexion and pain with hip extension. The results of an Ely test and a Kendall test are positive. The diagnosis is a grade 1 hip flexor strain, and the iliopsoas is the isolated injured muscle (Fig. 13-4).

1. Based on this scenario, what do you know about Ms. Mays' injury?

- ______
- ______
- ______

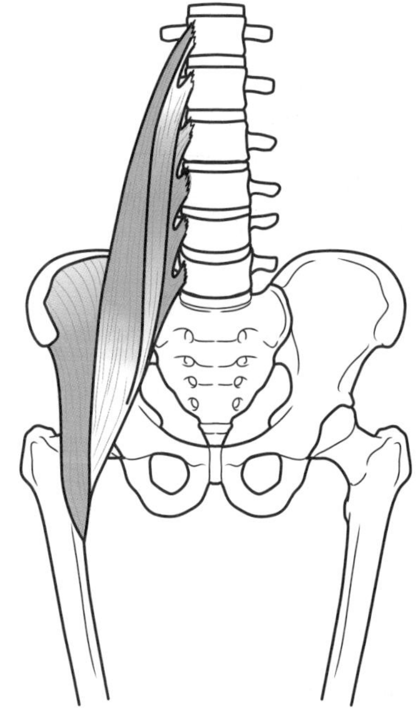

Figure 13-4: Margaret Mays' iliopsoas muscle.

- ______________________________

2. To rehabilitate Ms. Mays' injury effectively, you will need to gather additional information. What questions should you ask in addition to what is presented in this scenario?
   - ______________________________
   - ______________________________
   - ______________________________
   - ______________________________

3. Identify key terms and concepts, and then research each to broaden your knowledge about hip, thigh, and lower-leg injuries.
   - What anatomical structures might be involved in Ms. Mays' injury?

     Answer: ____________________
   - What is a hip flexor strain?

     Answer: ____________________
   - In which phase of healing is this injury?

     Answer: ____________________
   - What might a tearing sensation of a muscle indicate?

     Answer: ____________________
   - Explain a grade 1 hip flexor strain. What are the symptoms?

     Answer: ____________________
   - What types of symptoms do you see with a grade 2 and grade 3 hip flexor strain?

     Answer: ____________________
   - How do you isolate the individual hip flexor muscles in testing?

     Answer: ____________________
   - What is an Ely test? What does it test for? What does a positive test indicate?

     Answer: ____________________
   - What is a Kendall test? What does it test for? What does a positive result indicate?

     Answer: ____________________

4. Based on the information that you currently have and what was provided by your instructor, how will you begin Ms. Mays' rehabilitation?
   - ______________________________
   - ______________________________
   - ______________________________
   - ______________________________

Brain Jolt

If you can isolate the injured muscle, then rehabilitating that muscle will accelerate recovery.

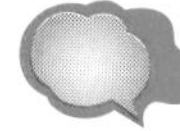

Conversation Buffer

A hip flexor strain can often be a chronic injury. Be sure to communicate with the athlete and coach that no matter how minor the injury may seem, proper treatment and compliance is extremely important to the healing process and return to play.

Why or why not?

How will Ms. Mays' rehabilitation progress? For the *why?* portion of each exercise, explain why you chose a particular exercise or activity as part of your program. Describe which rehabilitation goals the exercise or activity covers, and describe the key indicators for progression. For the *why not?* portion of each exercise, explain why other rehabilitation exercises or activities were not chosen and what to avoid during rehabilitation for this injury. Gather details from the textbook, your own research, and data from Ms. Mays' scenario to help formulate your answer.

Why?

- ______________________________
- ______________________________
- ______________________________
- ______________________________

Why not?

- ______________________________
- ______________________________

What do you think?

1. Based on your rehabilitation protocol, discuss the indicators for a limited and full return to play. Include a rough timeline for return to play, if applicable, which is affected by the athlete's compliance with the rehabilitation program.
   - ______________________________
   - ______________________________
   - ______________________________
   - ______________________________
2. Are modifications or personal protective equipment needed to return to play?
   - ______________________________
   - ______________________________

STUDENT SCENARIO 3: NEAL RIVERA

Neal Rivera is a senior who plays shortstop on the high school baseball team. The baseball team is scrimmaging and a fellow teammate is up to bat; he is known as the team's heavy hitter and has extremely powerful line drives. As the batter makes contact with the ball, Mr. Rivera glances to his left because a player is running toward third base. During that split second, Mr. Rivera loses sight of the baseball and it strikes him in the left quadriceps muscle. He is helped off the field as a result of the acute trauma, pain, and muscle weakness. The following day, Neal Rivera displays signs of edema, ecchymosis, and decreased quadriceps muscle function. For the next 2 weeks, he fails to care for the injury properly and begins to develop a hard knot at the site of the injury. Because of his negligence, the ecchymosis advances to myositis ossificans. In the months following the injury, he continues to have pain at his anterior thigh with decreased quadriceps muscle function and ROM owing to the calcification (Fig. 13-5).

1. Based on this scenario, what do you know about Mr. Rivera's injury?
   - ______________________________
   - ______________________________
   - ______________________________
   - ______________________________

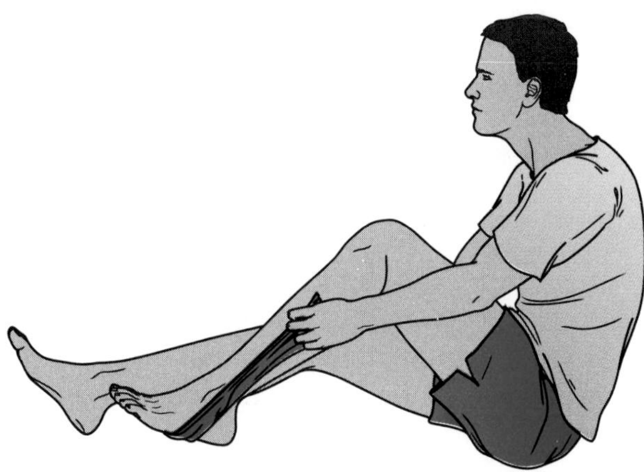

Figure 13-5: Neal Rivera's decreased ROM.

2. To rehabilitate Mr. Rivera's injury effectively, you will need to gather additional information. What questions should you ask in addition to what is presented in this scenario?

- ______________________________
- ______________________________
- ______________________________
- ______________________________

3. Identify key terms and concepts, and then research each to broaden your knowledge about hip, thigh, and lower-leg injuries.
   - What anatomical structures might be involved in Mr. Rivera's injury?

     Answer: ______________________________
   - What is myositis ossificans?

     Answer: ______________________________
   - In which phase of healing is this injury?

     Answer: ______________________________
   - Define *edema*.

     Answer: ______________________________
   - Define *ecchymosis*.

     Answer: ______________________________
   - What causes muscle weakness and decreased muscle function with this injury?

     Answer: ______________________________
   - Why is Mr. Rivera's calcification causing the decreased muscle function months after the injury?

     Answer: ______________________________

Brain Jolt
Not controlling the initial or acute edema and ecchymosis after an injury or receiving a second blow before the injury is fully healed can predispose an athlete to develop myositis ossificans.

4. Based on the information that you currently have and what was provided by your instructor, how will you begin Mr. Rivera's rehabilitation?

- ______________________________
- ______________________________
- ______________________________
- ______________________________

Why or why not?

How will Mr. Rivera's rehabilitation progress? For the *why?* portion of each exercise, explain why you chose a particular exercise or activity as part of your program. Describe which rehabilitation goals the exercise or activity covers, and describe the key indicators for progression. For the *why not?* portion of each exercise, explain why other rehabilitation exercises or activities were not chosen and what to avoid during rehabilitation for this injury. Gather details from the textbook, your own research, and data from Mr. Rivera's scenario to help formulate your answer.

Why?

- ______________________________
- ______________________________
- ______________________________
- ______________________________

Why not?

- ______________________________
- ______________________________

What do you think?

1. Based on your rehabilitation protocol, discuss the indicators for a limited or full return to play. Include a rough timeline for return to play, if applicable, which is affected by the athlete's compliance with the rehabilitation program.

- ______________________________

- ____________________
- ____________________
- ____________________

2. Are modifications or personal protective equipment needed to return to play?
   - ____________________
   - ____________________

STUDENT SCENARIO 4: ROSE KELLEY

Rose Kelley is a marathon runner who just celebrated her 40th birthday. She completed a marathon with a personal best time 1 week ago. She has been experiencing left anterior tibial pain for the past two months, and she continues to run despite the pain without improvement. She decides to have an orthopedic physician evaluate her injury. On examination, she displays localized point tenderness at the distal third of the tibia and has a positive percussion test result. A possible tibial stress fracture is diagnosed (Fig. 13-6), and Ms. Kelley is referred for imaging to confirm the stress fracture. The results are positive.

1. Based on this scenario, what do you know about Ms. Kelley's injury?
   - ____________________
   - ____________________
   - ____________________
   - ____________________

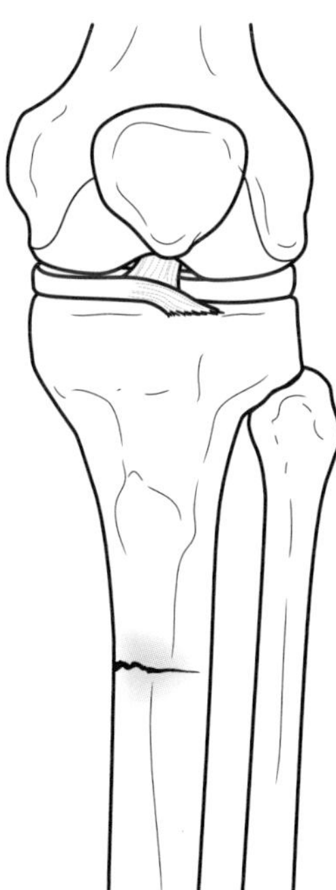

Figure 13-6: Rose Kelley's tibial stress fracture.

2. To rehabilitate Ms. Kelley's injury effectively, you will need to gather additional information. What questions should you ask in addition to what is presented in this scenario?
   - ____________________
   - ____________________
   - ____________________
   - ____________________

Brain Jolt

Stress fractures are a result of overuse and overstress of an area. Be sure to evaluate the athlete's training program, surface of the activity (e.g., dirt, grass, asphalt, concrete), and possible imbalances in the athlete's postural alignment and muscle tone.

Conversation Buffer

Advise athletes of all ages and abilities on proper training protocols and techniques, regardless of whether they compete on school teams. Those who participated in sports in high school and college frequently believe that they can continue or re-create the sport-specific activities that they did in the past, so be sure to educate them about setting realistic goals and training schedules for their fitness level today. Be sure to educate yourself about proper form, conditioning, nutrition, and preventive techniques that are age-specific, so that you can further assist this group of athletes.

3. Identify key terms and concepts, and then research each to broaden your knowledge about the rehabilitation of hip, thigh, and lower-leg injuries.
   - What anatomical structures might be involved in Ms. Kelley's injury?

     Answer: ________________
   - What is a tibial stress fracture?

     Answer: ________________
   - In which phase of healing is this injury?

     Answer: ________________
   - Define *orthopedic*.

     Answer: ________________
   - Why is a bone scan a better stress fracture indicator than a radiograph?

     Answer: ________________
   - Is the distal third of the anterior tibia a common place for a stress fracture? If so, why?

     Answer: ________________
   - Could Ms. Kelley's age have predisposed her to develop a stress fracture?

     Answer: ________________
   - What is a percussion test? What does it test? What does a positive result indicate?

     Answer: ________________
4. Based on the information that you currently have and what was provided by your instructor, how will you begin Ms. Kelley's rehabilitation?
   - ________________
   - ________________
   - ________________
   - ________________

Why or why not?

How will Ms. Kelley's rehabilitation progress? For the *why?* portion of each exercise, explain why you chose a particular exercise or activity as part of your program. Describe which rehabilitation goals the exercise or activity covers, and describe the key indicators for progression. For the *why not?* portion of each exercise, explain why other rehabilitation exercises or activities were not chosen and what to avoid during rehabilitation for this injury. Gather details from the textbook, your own research, and data from Ms. Kelley's scenario to help formulate your answer.

Why?

- ________________
- ________________
- ________________
- ________________

Why not?

- ________________
- ________________

What do you think?

1. Based on your rehabilitation protocol, discuss the indicators for a limited or full return to play. Include a rough timeline for return to play, if applicable, which is affected by the athlete's compliance with the rehabilitation program.
   - ________________
   - ________________
   - ________________
   - ________________
2. Are modifications or personal protective equipment needed to return to play?
   - ________________
   - ________________

STUDENT SCENARIO 5: ANDY SHULTZ

Andy Shultz is a college wrestler who wrestles in the 140-lb weight class; however, he is wrestling a 150-lb teammate at practice today, and he quickly notices that he is outmatched. The teammate lifts Mr. Shultz and brings him down onto his right hip. Both Mr. Shultz's and the teammate's weight are transferred to Mr. Shultz's right hip. He has immediate pain and loss of ROM at his right hip joint. On examination, Mr. Shultz is point tender over his right iliac crest, has decreased active range of motion with hip flexion and abduction, and ecchymosis is present over the right iliac crest. This diagnosis is a hip pointer (Fig. 13-7).

1. Based on this scenario, what do you know about Mr. Shultz's injury?

- ______________________________
- ______________________________
- ______________________________
- ______________________________

2. To effectively rehabilitate Mr. Shultz's injury, you will need to gather additional information. What questions should you ask in addition to what is presented in this scenario?

- ______________________________
- ______________________________
- ______________________________
- ______________________________

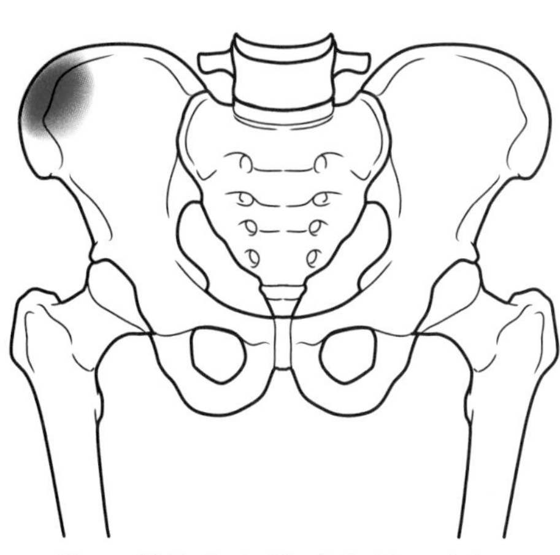

Figure 13-7: Andy Shultz's hip pointer.

3. Identify key terms and concepts, and then research each to broaden your knowledge about rehabilitation of hip, thigh, and lower-leg injuries.

- What anatomical structures might be involved in Mr. Shultz's injury?

  Answer: ______________________________
- What is a hip pointer?

  Answer: ______________________________
- In which phase of healing is this injury?

  Answer: ______________________________
- Define *hip flexion*.

  Answer: ______________________________
- Define *hip abduction*.

  Answer: ______________________________
- Define *ecchymosis*.

  Answer: ______________________________
- Why is there a loss of ROM at Mr. Shultz's right hip upon injury?

  Answer: ______________________________

Brain Jolt

Hip pointer injuries are extremely painful and can be debilitating. Protection is a major part of the treatment process and can be achieved by wearing protective equipment.

Conversation Buffer

A coach and athlete may view a hip pointer injury as merely a contusion. Because of the loss of function and the pain, edema, and ecchymosis that develop, this injury is serious. Treatment within the first 24 to 48 hours of injury is important because it affects a timely return to play.

4. Based on the information that you currently have and what was provided by your instructor, how will you begin Mr. Shultz's rehabilitation?

- ______________________________
- ______________________________

- ______________________________________
- ______________________________________

Why or why not?

How will Mr. Shultz's rehabilitation progress? For the *why?* portion of each exercise, explain why you chose a particular exercise or activity as part of your program. Describe which rehabilitation goals the exercise or activity covers, and describe the key indicators for progression. For the *why not?* portion of each exercise, explain why other rehabilitation exercises or activities were not chosen and what to avoid during rehabilitation for this injury. Gather details from the textbook, your own research, and data from Mr. Shultz's scenario to help formulate your answer.

Why?

- ______________________________________
- ______________________________________
- ______________________________________
- ______________________________________

Why not?

- ______________________________________
- ______________________________________

What do you think?

1. Based on your rehabilitation protocol, discuss the indicators for a limited or full return to play. Include a rough timeline for return to play, if applicable, which is affected by the athlete's compliance with the rehabilitation program.
   - ______________________________________
   - ______________________________________
   - ______________________________________
   - ______________________________________
2. Are modifications or personal protective equipment needed to return to play?
   - ______________________________________
   - ______________________________________

STUDENT SCENARIO 6: DAVE CRAMER

Dave Cramer is a wide receiver on his college football team. A play is called in which he sprints forward 5 yards and then cuts to his inside left to receive the football. The whistle blows and he makes the play. As he opens his arms to receive the football, with his left leg behind his right, the opposing team's defensive back puts his head down and rams Mr. Cramer in his right quadriceps. He drops to the ground in pain, and after a few minutes he limps off the field. On evaluation, he has moderate edema and ecchymosis within 15 min of the injury, along with decreased knee extension and flexion and decreased quadriceps strength and tone. The diagnosis is a right quadriceps contusion (Fig. 13-8).

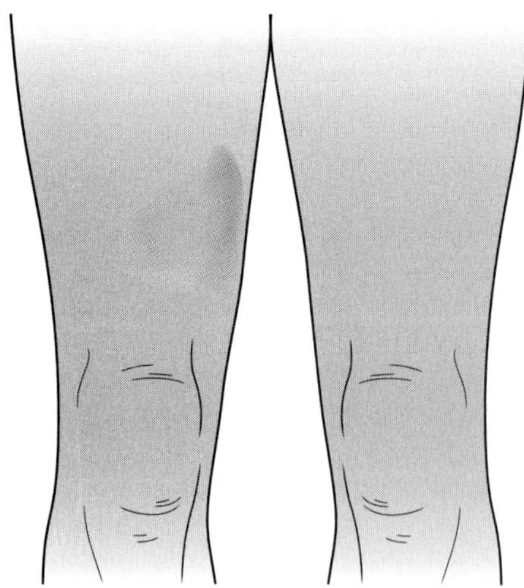

Figure 13-8: Dave Cramer's quadriceps contusion.

1. Based on this scenario, what do you know about Mr. Cramer's injury?
   -
   -
   -
   -

2. To effectively rehabilitate Mr. Cramer's injury, you will need to gather additional information. What questions should you ask in addition to what is presented in this scenario?
   -
   -
   -
   -

Brain Jolt
Throughout the treatment process, different tones of ecchymosis may be present. This is a sign of healing that should be communicated to the athlete.

3. Identify any key terms and concepts, and research each to broaden your knowledge about the rehabilitation of hip, thigh, and lower-leg injuries.
   - What anatomical structures might be involved in Mr. Cramer's injury?

     Answer:
   - What is a quadriceps contusion?

     Answer:
   - In which phase of healing is this injury?

     Answer:
   - Define *edema*.

     Answer:
   - Define *ecchymosis*.

     Answer:
   - Describe mild, moderate, and severe grades for this injury.

     Answer:
   - Why does Mr. Cramer have decreased ROM in the quadriceps muscle?

     Answer:
   - What is the importance of good quadriceps strength?

     Answer:

4. Based on the information that you currently have and what was provided by your instructor, how will you begin Mr. Cramer's rehabilitation?
   -
   -
   -
   -

Why or why not?

How will Mr. Cramer's rehabilitation progress? For the *why?* portion of each exercise, explain why you chose a particular exercise or activity as part of your program. Describe which rehabilitation goals the exercise or activity covers, and describe the key indicators for progression. For the *why not?* portion of each exercise, explain why other rehabilitation exercises or activities were not chosen and what to avoid during rehabilitation for this injury. Gather details from the textbook, your own research, and data from Mr. Cramer's scenario to help formulate your answer.

Why?

-
-
-
-

Why not?

-
-

What do you think?

1. Based on your rehabilitation protocol, discuss the indicators for a limited or full return to play. Include a rough timeline for return to play, if applicable, which is affected by the athlete's compliance with the rehabilitation program.
   - ______
   - ______
   - ______
   - ______
2. Are modifications or personal protective equipment needed to return to play?
   - ______
   - ______

STUDENT SCENARIO 7: JACKIE BRYANT

Jackie Bryant is a field hockey player at her college. The coach gives each player a summer conditioning program, and Ms. Bryant is following it as instructed. As a result, she is running more than usual. After the first 4 weeks of the conditioning schedule, she notices a pain on the lateral side of her right knee in which she has a history of a lateral meniscus tear. She thinks that this is what is causing her pain, but she continues to run despite the discomfort. Upon arriving at college for twice daily workouts, she has her right knee evaluated. She has lateral pain over the tensor fasciae latae, a negative McMurry test result, a positive Ober test result, and a tight right hamstring. The diagnosis is iliotibial band syndrome (ITBS; Fig. 13-9).

1. Based on this scenario, what do you know about Ms. Bryant's injury?
   - ______
   - ______
   - ______
   - ______

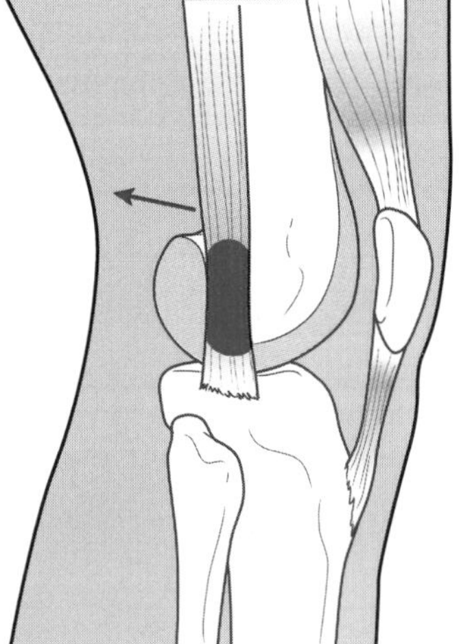

Figure 13-9: Jackie Bryant's iliotibial band syndrome.

2. To rehabilitate Ms. Bryant's injury effectively, you will need to gather additional information. What questions should you ask in addition to what is presented in this scenario?
   - ______
   - ______
   - ______
   - ______

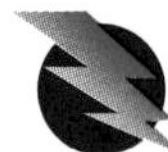

Brain Jolt

Look at the alignment of the leg and hip. By observing the natural position of the leg and surrounding structures, you may be able to determine the origin of the condition.

3. Identify key terms and concepts, and then research each to broaden your knowledge about the rehabilitation of hip, thigh, and lower-leg injuries.
   - What anatomical structures might be involved in Ms. Bryant's injury?

   Answer: ______

- What is IT band friction syndrome?

  Answer: ______
- In which phase of healing is this injury?

  Answer: ______
- Define *tensor fasciae latae.*

  Answer: ______
- What is a lateral meniscus tear?

  Answer: ______
- Does the strength of the quadriceps muscle have a role in IT band friction syndrome?

  Answer: ______
- What is an Ober test? What does it test? What does a positive result indicate?

  Answer: ______
- What is a McMurry test? What does it test? What does a positive result indicate?

  Answer: ______

4. Based on the information that you currently have and what was provided by your instructor, how will you begin Ms. Bryant's rehabilitation?

- ______
- ______
- ______
- ______

Treatment Detour

DETOUR

A recent study challenged the traditional treatments for ITBS. The cadaver-based study with an in vivo biomechanical analysis of elite rugby players with ITBS studied the players during movement to examine mechanisms and anatomical principles in which traditional treatments are based. Traditional treatments are based on decreasing inflammation of the bursa between the ITB and the lateral femoral condyle; however, this study found no bursa in any of the cadavers. Stretching exercises are traditionally performed to stretch the ITB, but the researchers found a low magnitude for stretching the ITB. Although stretching and nonsteroidal anti-inflammatory drug use for inflammation can help temporarily, treating the tensor fascia latae and the gluteus maximus with soft tissue therapy is supported as the treatment for ITBS (Falvey et al., 2010).

Why or why not?

How will Ms. Bryant's rehabilitation progress? For the *why?* portion of each exercise, explain why you chose a particular exercise or activity as part of your program. Describe which rehabilitation goals the exercise or activity covers, and describe the key indicators for progression. For the *why not?* portion of each exercise, explain why other rehabilitation exercises or activities were not chosen and what to avoid during rehabilitation for this injury. Gather details from the textbook, your own research, and data from Ms. Bryant's scenario to help formulate your answer.

Why?

- ______
- ______
- ______
- ______

Why not?

- ______
- ______

What do you think?

1. Based on your rehabilitation protocol, discuss the indicators for a limited or full return to play. Include a rough timeline for return to play, if applicable, which is affected by the athlete's compliance with the rehabilitation program.

- ______
- ______
- ______
- ______

2. Are modifications or personal protective equipment needed to return to play?
   - ____________________
   - ____________________

STUDENT SCENARIO 8: FRED GRAVES

Fred Graves is a high school sprinter with a history of hamstring strains. He warms up and is ready for the 50-yard dash during a track meet. As the gun fires, he shoots out of the blocks. Twenty-five yards into the race, he feels a pull at his right hamstring, but he is not hindered by it. As he approaches the finish line, he hears a pop, feels immediate pain, and falls to the ground. On evaluation, a deformity near his proximal right hamstring is palpated. Mild edema and ecchymosis are present. He has complete loss of function of his hamstring, and a complete hamstring rupture is diagnosed (Fig. 13-10).

1. Based on this scenario, what do you know about Mr. Graves' injury?
   - ____________________
   - ____________________
   - ____________________
   - ____________________

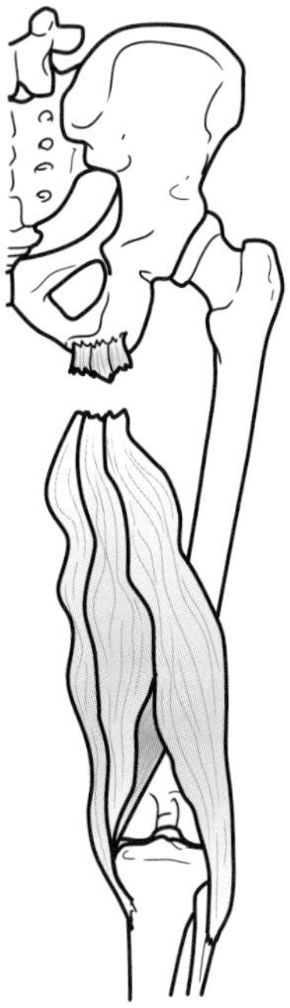

Figure 13-10: Fred Graves' hamstring rupture.

2. To rehabilitate Mr. Graves' injury effectively, you will need to gather additional information. What questions should you ask in addition to what is presented in this scenario?
   - ____________________
   - ____________________
   - ____________________
   - ____________________

Brain Jolt
Do not be alarmed by the excessive amount of ecchymosis that occurs with a hamstring rupture injury.

3. Identify key terms and concepts, and then research each to broaden your knowledge about rehabilitation of hip, thigh, and lower-leg injuries.
   - What anatomical structures might be involved in Mr. Graves' injury?

     Answer: ____________________
   - What is a hamstring rupture?

     Answer: ____________________
   - In which phase of healing is this injury?

     Answer: ____________________
   - Define *edema*.

     Answer: ____________________
   - Define *ecchymosis*.

     Answer: ____________________
   - What might a pulling sensation in the hamstring indicate?

     Answer: ____________________
   - What does a *pop* sound in the hamstring indicate?

     Answer: ____________________
   - What does the deformity with Mr. Graves' hamstring indicate?

     Answer: ____________________

- Why is there a complete loss of function of the left leg?

  Answer: ______________________________
- Could previous injuries have predisposed him to the hamstring rupture?

  Answer: ______________________________

4. Based on the information that you currently have and what was provided by your instructor, how will you begin Mr. Graves' rehabilitation?

- ______________________________
- ______________________________
- ______________________________
- ______________________________

Why or why not?

How will Mr. Graves' rehabilitation progress? For the *why?* portion of each exercise, explain why you chose a particular exercise or activity as part of your program. Describe which rehabilitation goals the exercise or activity covers, and describe the key indicators for progression. For the *why not?* portion of each exercise, explain why other rehabilitation exercises or activities were not chosen and what to avoid during rehabilitation for this injury. Gather details from the textbook, your own research, and data from Mr. Graves' scenario to help formulate your answer.

Why?

- ______________________________
- ______________________________
- ______________________________
- ______________________________

Why not?

- ______________________________
- ______________________________

What do you think?

1. Based on your rehabilitation protocol, discuss the indicators for a limited or full return to play. Include a rough timeline for return to play, if applicable, which is affected by the athlete's compliance with the rehabilitation program.

- ______________________________
- ______________________________
- ______________________________
- ______________________________

2. Are modifications or personal protective equipment needed to return to play?

- ______________________________
- ______________________________

STUDENT SCENARIO 9: PAUL SATCHWELL

Paul Satchwell is a college soccer player who is preparing for a tournament game by working on breakaway drills. As he runs beside a fellow teammate, the teammate quickly switches his running direction from the left to the right. As Mr. Satchwell quickly shifts his weight to his right leg and pushes off, he feels a pull on the inside of his leg. The irritation is mild, and he continues to play for the next 10 minutes. After returning from a water break, he notices that his adductors are now moderately sore, and he is unable to play without a limp. He is removed from practice. On evaluation, he has decreased range of motion with external and internal rotation of his hip and pain with hip flexion. He is unable to stride with a normal gait pattern, and an adductor strain is diagnosed (Fig. 13-11).

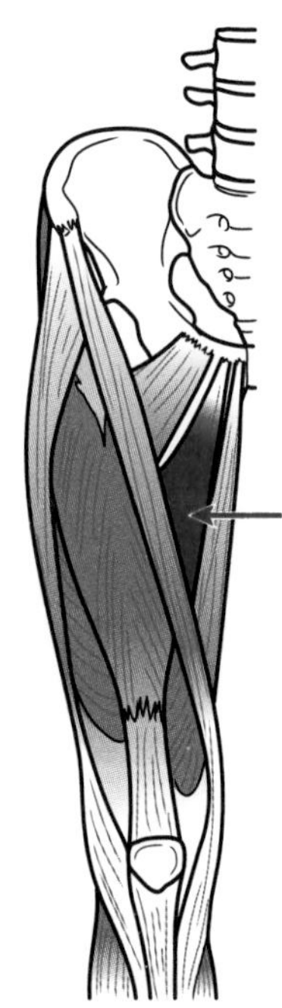

Figure 13-11: Paul Satchwell's adductor strain.

1. Based on this scenario, what do you know about Mr. Satchwell's injury?
   - ____________________
   - ____________________
   - ____________________
   - ____________________

2. To rehabilitate Mr. Satchwell's injury effectively, you will need to gather additional information. What questions should you ask in addition to what is presented in this scenario?
   - ____________________
   - ____________________
   - ____________________
   - ____________________

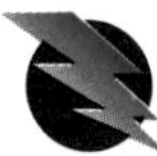

Brain Jolt

Be sure to work on an athlete's flexibility early in the season to prevent any type of muscle strains.

3. Identify key terms and concepts, and then research each to broaden your knowledge about the rehabilitation of hip, thigh, and lower-leg injuries.
   - What anatomical structures might be involved in Mr. Satchwell's injury?

     Answer: ____________________
   - What is an adductor strain?

     Answer: ____________________
   - In which phase of healing is this injury?

     Answer: ____________________
   - Define *hip adductor*.

     Answer: ____________________
   - Define *hip flexion*.

     Answer: ____________________
   - Define *external rotation of the hip*.

     Answer: ____________________
   - Define *internal rotation of the hip*.

     Answer: ____________________
   - What muscles are involved with a groin strain?

     Answer: ____________________
   - What is a normal gait pattern?

     Answer: ____________________

4. Based on the information that you currently have and what was provided by your instructor, how will you begin Mr. Satchwell's rehabilitation?
   - ____________________
   - ____________________
   - ____________________
   - ____________________

Why or why not?

How will Mr. Satchwell's rehabilitation progress? For the *why?* portion of each exercise, explain why you chose a particular exercise or activity as part of your program. Describe which rehabilitation goals the exercise or activity covers, and describe the key indicators for progression. For the *why not?* portion of each exercise, explain why other rehabilitation exercises or activities were not chosen and what to avoid during rehabilitation for this injury. Gather details from the textbook, your own research, and data from Mr. Satchwell's scenario to help formulate your answer.

Why?

- ______________________________
- ______________________________
- ______________________________
- ______________________________

Why not?

- ______________________________
- ______________________________

What do you think?

1. Based on your rehabilitation protocol, discuss the indicators for a limited or full return to play. Include a rough timeline for return to play, if applicable, which is affected by the athlete's compliance with the rehabilitation program.
   - ______________________________
   - ______________________________
   - ______________________________
   - ______________________________
2. Are modifications or personal protective equipment needed to return to play?
   - ______________________________
   - ______________________________

knowledge checklist

Table 13-1 offers a checklist that can be used by a peer, instructor, or preceptor to evaluate each part of the athlete's rehabilitation plan. Use this checklist as a tool to ensure that the rehabilitation plan is complete and to assess your knowledge of the competencies that apply to this chapter.

TABLE 13-1 ■ Lower Extremity: The Hip, Thigh, and Lower-Leg Rehabilitation and Therapeutic Exercise Competency Checklist

	Proficient *Can demonstrate and execute the skill properly*	**Proficient With Assistance** *Can demonstrate and execute the skill with minimal guidance or tips*	**Not Proficient** *Unable to demonstrate and execute the skill properly; need to be reevaluated at another time after further study and practice*
Controlling Edema			
PRICE			
Modalities			
Controlling Pain			
Pain scales			
Medications			
Modalities			
Establishes Core Stability			
Reestablishes Neuromuscular Control			
Restores Postural Control and Balance			
Restoring Range of Motion			
Passive range of motion			
Active range of motion			
Resistive range of motion			
Goniometry			
Normal range of motion limits			
Restore Muscular Strength, Endurance, and Power			
Open kinetic chain			
Closed kinetic chain			
Isometric			
Isotonic			
Isotonic (concentric and eccentric)			
Isokinetic			
Plyometric			
Agility			
Functional or Sport-Specific Activities			
Maintains Cardiorespiratory Fitness			
Functional Testing			
Return-to-Play Criteria			
Proper Documentation			

PRICE, prevention, rest, ice, compression, and elevation.

REFERENCES

Falvey, E. C., Clark, R. A., Franklyn-Miller, A., Bryant, A. L., Briggs, C., & McCrory, P. R. (2010). Iliotibial band syndrome: An examination behind a number of treatment options. *Scandinavian Journal of Medicine and Science in Sports, 20*, 580–587.

Higgins, M. (2011). *Therapeutic exercise: From theory to practice.* Philadelphia, PA: F.A. Davis.

National Athletic Training Association. (2011). *Athletic training education competencies* (5th ed.). Retrieved from http://www.nata.org/sites/default/files/5th-Edition-Competencies-2011-PDF-Version.pdf

Prentice, W. (2010). *Arnheim's principles of athletic training: A competency-based approach* (14th ed.). New York, NY: McGraw-Hill.

Prentice, W. (2011). *Rehabilitation techniques for sports medicine and athletic training* (5th ed.). New York, NY: McGraw-Hill.

Shadgen, B., Menon, M., Sanders, D., Berry, G., Martin, C. Jr., Duffy, P., . . . O'Brien, P. J. (2010). Current thinking about acute compartment syndrome of the lower extremity. *Canadian Journal of Surgery, 53*, 329–334.

Starkey, C. (2004). *Therapeutic modalities* (3rd ed.). Philadelphia, PA: F.A. Davis.

Starkey, C., Brown, S. D., & Ryan, J. (2010). *Examination of orthopedic and athletic injuries* (3rd ed.). Philadelphia, PA: F.A. Davis.

Venes, D. (Ed.). (2009). *Taber's cyclopedic medical dictionary* (21st ed.). Philadelphia, PA: F.A. Davis.

chapter 14

Upper Extremity: The Hand, Wrist, and Elbow

chapter outline

athletic trainer's corner

Here is what one athletic trainer experienced with a real world athlete's rehabilitation from injury:

One of the starting pitchers on our championship Division I baseball team underwent Tommy John surgery. Tommy John surgery is a surgical procedure to reconstruct the ulnar collateral ligament (UCL) using a tendon from the forearm. The tendon is used to recreate the damaged ligament and improve the elbow joint's stability. The player was a multisport athlete who had been competing since a young age. Because of a previous shoulder injury during high school football, his pitching mechanics were altered, thus causing more stress on his elbow. Over time and because of the repetitive motion of pitching, the amount of pitches that he threw per week decreased drastically, and he began experiencing numbness and paraesthesia radiating down his forearm and into his little finger. The player never told anyone about his pain, but it soon became evident that his performance and throwing velocity were decreasing. During a game one Friday night, one pitch practically landed at a vertical angle straight into the ground after he felt a pop in his elbow. Magnetic resonance image (MRI) confirmed a UCL tear, which led to surgery and 10 months of rehabilitation for the player. The player's typical rehabilitation day consisted of ROM exercises, followed by strengthening, and ended with ice therapy before being placed back into a functional elbow brace. I learned quickly to always place a barrier over the ulnar nerve to eliminate numbness in the little finger when using ice.

The player began a throwing program around the fourth month and then graduated to pitching off the mound around the sixth month. In this particular athlete's case, he never fully recovered from this injury. Although he felt great, and competed the next season, his pitching career was never the same. I learned that successful recovery following Tommy John surgery is dependent on ROM, time, direct observation, and outside factors. I believe that one of the most important immediate postoperative goals for these athletes is the reestablishment of ROM. Recovery can easily take up to 1 year, and the time may be shorter in some instances. Getting the athlete active as soon as possible is critical to helping him or her maintain a positive outlook during the rehabilitation process. One tool that helps the athlete is to mark a calendar with a start date (date of surgery) and a target completion date (generally 9 months later). Next, write down each day's activity so that the athlete has something to refer to when he or she has questions regarding progress. The calendar allows the athlete to see progress and to focus on the end goal that keeps motivation levels high.

J. R. Honisch, AT, ATC
OrthoIndy
Indianapolis, Indiana

learning outcomes

After working through this chapter, you will be able to:

1. Describe seven different goals of rehabilitation and the importance of each in the overall rehabilitation protocol.
2. Verbalize indications for performing hand, wrist, and elbow rehabilitative techniques.
3. Discuss modifications and progressions that are used during a rehabilitation program for the hand, wrist, and elbow.
4. Discuss outcome measures used to identify activity levels and return-to-play guidelines for hand, wrist, and elbow injuries.
5. Explain what modality choice is proper for rehabilitation by using indications, contraindications, and the principles and theory related to the physiological response of the intervention.

MODEL SCENARIO 1: TONY STEVENS

Tony Stevens is the point guard on his college basketball team and is currently in the second round of their Division tournament. The game has 1 min left to play and Mr. Stevens' team is up by one. The opposing team has the ball when Mr. Stevens commits a foul, which gives the opponent a chance to score the necessary points to win the game. Mr. Stevens feels responsible for the loss and punches the wall with his left hand upon entering the locker room. He feels a cracking sensation on the outside of his hand, but he does not pay much attention to the injury for approximately 30 minutes. Upon exiting the locker room, he notices the moderate amount of edema that has developed over his fifth metacarpal. He also finds that it is hard to flex and extend his little finger, but there is no deformity. Mr. Stevens asks the team athletic trainer to assess the injury. In addition to moderate edema and pain with active flexion and extension, he has radiating pain just below the fifth metacarpal bone with the percussion and long bone compression test. The finger is immobilized and he is referred for radiographs, with a possible diagnosis of boxer fracture. The diagnosis is confirmed as a fracture to the fifth metacarpal (Fig. 14-1) and the finger is splinted.

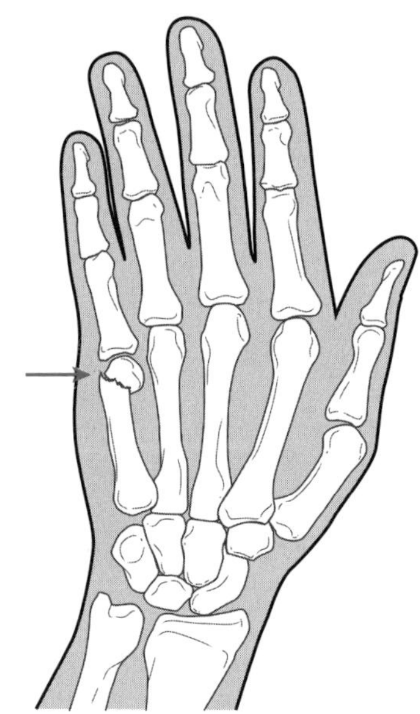

Figure 14-1: Tony Stevens' boxer fracture.

1. Based on this scenario, what do you know about Mr. Stevens' injury?
   - *Male athlete*
   - *Basketball player, point guard*
   - *Mechanism of injury: punching a wall with his fist*
   - *Feels a cracking sensation*
   - *No deformity*
   - *Moderate edema*
   - *Pain with active flexion and extension*
   - *Positive percussion and long bone compression test*
   - *Area immobilized*
   - *Radiographs positive for boxer fracture*
2. To rehabilitate Mr. Stevens' injury effectively, you will need to gather additional information. What questions should you ask in addition to what is presented in this scenario?
   - *Are there any preexisting injuries? If yes, what are they?*
   - *How long has the athlete experienced this pain?*
   - *What is the athlete's pain level and type of pain felt?*
   - *What is the level of strength at the wrist and fingers?*
   - *What is the ROM at the wrist and fingers?*

- *Does the athlete have any numbness or paraesthesia?*
- *Was there any injury to the carpal bones from the mechanism?*
- *Are there any signs of shock?*
- *What treatment was provided at the hospital?*

3. Identify key terms and concepts, and then research each to broaden your knowledge about the rehabilitation of hand, wrist, and elbow injuries.
   - What anatomical structures might be involved in Mr. Stevens' injury?
     Carpal bones
     Metacarpal bones
     Phalanges
   - What is a boxer fracture?
     A boxer fracture occurs to the fifth metacarpal bone of the hand, usually from a direct axial force or a compressive force.
   - In which phase of healing is this injury?
     This injury occurs at the inflammatory response phase.
   - Define *edema*.
     Swelling; a localized or general condition that causes body tissues to contain an excessive amount of fluid
   - Define *flexion*.
     Directional term meaning "to contract," as a muscle; to decrease the angle of a joint
   - Define *extension*.
     Directional term meaning "a movement that brings the members of a limb into or toward a straight position"
   - Define *referred pain*.
     Pain that arises in one body part or location but is perceived in another
   - What is a percussion test? What does it test? What does a positive result indicate?
     The percussion test is performed by tapping a bony prominence to test for a fracture and is positive if the person experiences radiating pain or pain at the injury site.
   - What is a long bone compression test? What does it test? What does a positive result indicate?
     The long bone compression test is performed by stressing the injured bones by pressing the bones together at a point away from the injury. It tests for a fracture and is positive if pain occurs at the injury site.
4. Based on the information that you currently have and what was provided by your instructor, how will you begin Mr. Stevens' rehabilitation?
   Mr. Stevens will be in a splint for 4 to 6 weeks. This timeframe will depend on how the fracture site heals. Besides applying ice to the injured area to help decrease the edema, ROM exercises will not be initiated until the physician orders rehabilitation. Early movement could disrupt or stress the healing process of the fracture.

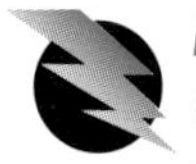

Brain Jolt

Remember that although the wrist and hand are immobilized and the athlete cannot attend practice, the athlete can still do cardio exercises to maintain fitness.

Why or why not?

How will Mr. Stevens' rehabilitation progress? For the *why?* portion of each exercise, explain why you chose a particular exercise or activity as part of your program. Describe which rehabilitation goals the exercise or activity covers, and describe the key indicators for progression. For the *why not?* portion of each exercise, explain why other rehabilitation exercises or activities were not chosen and what to avoid during rehabilitation for this injury. Gather details from the textbook, your own research, and data from Mr. Stevens' scenario to help formulate your answer.

Why?

- ***Stretching.*** *This activity will help with the rehabilitation goal of increasing ROM and is used because the passive and active ROM of the wrist, hand, and fingers have decreased since immobilizing the athlete's injured area in a splint. The goal of stretching is to achieve full, pain-free ROM. For wrist injuries, flexion, extension, and ulnar and radial deviation need to be addressed. For hand injuries, carpal and metacarpal glides need to be implemented. For the distal interphalangeal (DIP) and the proximal interphalangeal joints, flexion and extension need to be the focus. All stretching should be static.*
- ***Strengthening exercises for the wrist.*** *These exercises will help with the rehabilitation goal of increasing strength. The wrist is immobilized in the splint so that wrist weakness is present. Exercises that can be performed for strengthening the forearm musculature include weighted devices (i.e., hand weights) that can work flexion, extension, ulnar and radial deviation, pronation, and supination.*
- ***Strengthening exercises for the hand.*** *These exercises will help with the rehabilitation goal of increasing strength. Regaining normal hand strength is important for hand functions. Gripping putty, foam, and rubber balls can increase hand strength.*
- ***Strengthening exercises for the phalanges.*** *These exercises will help with the rehabilitation goal of increasing strength. Immobilization causes the fingers to decrease in strength. Using something as simple as a rubber band and focusing on finger abduction, flexion, and extension are effective exercises. The rubber web is another rehabilitation tool. Finger curls with a towel can be implemented shortly after splint removal.*

Why not?

- *Avoid any exercises that put pressure on or stress the initial fracture site. Exercises should be pain-free for the athlete to perform.*

What do you think?

1. Based on your rehabilitation protocol, discuss the indicators for limited and full return to play with the athlete. Include a rough timeline for return to play, if applicable, which is affected by the athlete's compliance with the rehabilitation program.
   - ***Limited return to play.*** *The athlete can return to play on a limited basis if the athlete regains full range of motion and strength in the wrist, hand, and phalanges. Once the athlete has achieved these functional tasks without pain, he or she can begin limited drills and contact activities with a ball.*
   - ***Full return to play.*** *If new edema or pain has not developed from limited participation, the athlete can return to play on a full status.*
2. Are modifications or required protective equipment needed to return to play?
   - *No*

MODEL SCENARIO 2: EMRY DEMOTTE

Emry Demotte is the secretary in her school's athletic office. Ms. Demotte has been doing a lot of typing for the different athletic teams and has noticed soreness at her left wrist. After several weeks, she becomes more concerned about her wrist soreness because she has numbness and paraesthesia radiating into her palm and her first and second phalanges. She decides to have her wrist evaluated, and it is noted that she has weakness in her left thumb, pain and edema at the anterior surface of her wrist joint, and a positive Phalen test result. Carpal tunnel syndrome is diagnosed (Fig. 14-2), and she is advised to begin a conservative treatment plan.

1. Based on this scenario, what do you know about Ms. Demotte's injury?
   - *Female secretary*
   - *Mechanism of injury: chronic pain from typing*
   - *Mild edema*
   - *Numbness and paraesthesia at the palm and first and second phalanges*
   - *Anterior wrist soreness*
   - *Thumb weakness*
   - *Positive Phalen test result*

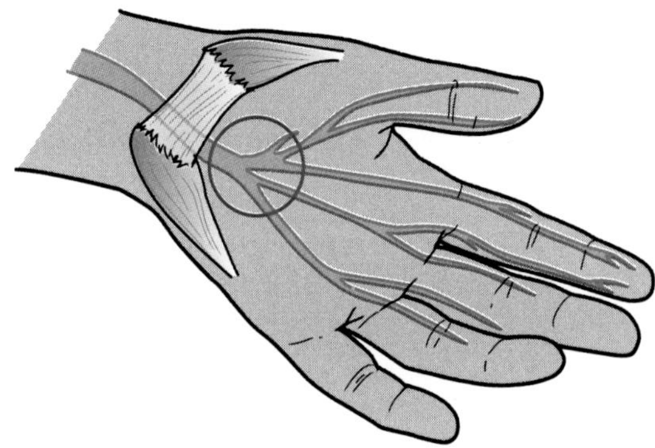

Figure 14-2: Emry Demotte's carpal tunnel.

2. To rehabilitate Ms. Demotte's injury effectively, you will need to gather additional information. What questions should you ask in addition to what is presented in this scenario?
   - *Are there any preexisting injuries? If yes, what are they?*
   - *How long has the patient experienced this pain?*
   - *What is the patient's pain level and type of pain felt?*
   - *What is the strength in the hand and wrist?*
   - *What is the ROM in the hand and wrist?*
   - *Does the patient have any numbness or paraesthesia?*

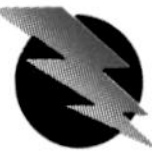

Brain Jolt
This injury is rooted in overuse and repetitive motions. Be sure to focus on more endurance exercises than on strength gains.

3. Identify key terms and concepts, and then research each to broaden your knowledge about the rehabilitation of hand, wrist, and elbow injuries.
   - What anatomical structures might be involved in Ms. Demotte's injury?
     Carpal tunnel
     Median nerve
     Flexor tendons
     Flexor tendon synovial sheaths
     Phalanges
     Thumb
   - What is carpal tunnel syndrome?
     Carpal tunnel syndrome occurs when a repetitive activity produces inflammation to the flexor tendons and the flexor tendon synovial sheaths. This inflammation fills the carpal tunnel space and exerts pressure on the median nerve. This pressure on the nerve is what brings about the sensory and motor deficits in the hand and phalanges.
   - In which phase of healing is this injury?
     This injury occurs in the subacute–chronic inflammatory response phase.

- Define *edema.*
  Swelling; a localized or general condition that causes body tissues to contain an excessive amount of fluid
- Define *anterior side of the wrist.*
  Directional term; in anatomical nomenclature, referring to the ventral or abdominal side of the body
- What is the median nerve?
  The median nerve innervates the hand through the dorsal side of the carpal tunnel space. It is the nerve root for the flexor muscles of the thumb and first and second phalanges.
- What is a Phalen test? What does it test? What does a positive result indicate?
  The Phalen test involves flexing the wrists as far as possible and then pressing them together. This position is held for 1 min. If pain is present in the carpal tunnel (anterior aspect of the wrist) region, it could indicate carpal tunnel syndrome.

4. Based on the information that you currently have and what was provided by your instructor, how will you begin Ms. Demotte's rehabilitation?
   The best course of treatment for this chronic injury is rest, ice, and immobilization. A hand-wrist splint can be worn. Nonsteroidal anti-inflammatory drugs (NSAIDs) are also recommended.

Why or why not?

How will Ms. Demotte's rehabilitation progress? For the *why?* portion of each exercise, explain why you chose a particular exercise or activity as part of your program. Describe which rehabilitation goals the exercise or activity covers, and describe the key indicators for progression. For the *why not?* portion of each exercise, explain why other rehabilitation exercises or activities were not chosen and what to avoid during rehabilitation for this injury. Gather details from the textbook, your own research, and data from Ms. Demotte's scenario to help formulate your answer.

Why?

- ***Ice and rest.*** *This will help with the rehabilitation goal of decreasing edema and pain in the inflamed area.*
- ***Stretching.*** *This will help with the rehabilitation goal of increasing ROM. If stretching is performed, it must be a gentle passive stretch. Extension movements should be the focus rather than flexion movements, because flexion movements may cause irritation.*
- ***Modality.*** *If NSAIDs are not effective, then iontophoresis is recommended to help with the rehabilitation goal of decreasing pain and inflammation. Iontophoresis is a modality that uses electrical current to drive ions from an ion solution (common ones are dexamethasone or hydrocortisone) into the inflamed tissue. The solutions are steroidal, which have the properties of decreasing inflammation.*

Why not?

- *Avoid any activity that focuses on flexion of the wrist and the phalanges. This movement specifically works the flexion muscles of the wrist and hand, which are already inflamed with this condition.*

Conversation Buffer

With carpal tunnel syndrome, the secretary's hand and wrist mechanics should be evaluated. Areas that can be examined include the heights of her desk and chair and the mobility of her keyboard. The position of her elbows, wrist, and hand has a direct effect on her recovery.

What do you think?

1. Based on your rehabilitation protocol, discuss the indicators for limited and full return to play. Include a rough timeline for return to play, if applicable, which is affected by the athlete's compliance with the rehabilitation program.
   - *Because this particular situation is not related to an athletic injury, the recommendation is movement as tolerated. Once the symptoms have decreased, the time spent using the splint can be reduced. Continue with ice therapy as a preventive measure.*
2. Are modifications or personal protective equipment needed to return to play?
   - *No*

STUDENT SCENARIO 1: TRISTEN PETERS

Tristen Peters is a sophomore in college who likes to participate in intramural sports. He is playing defensive line in a flag football game when he reaches out with his right hand to grab the running back's flag. He grabs more of the running back's belt than the flag, which causes his right fourth phalange to get caught in the belt. He feels a popping sensation at the distal end of his fourth phalange. He is immediately evaluated by the certified athletic trainer. On evaluation, Mr. Peters is unable to flex his fourth phalange at the DIP joint, the DIP joint is slightly extended, and he experiences pain and point tenderness with mild edema. He is referred to an orthopedic physician, who diagnoses a ruptured flexor digitorum profundus tendon, commonly known as *jersey finger* (Fig. 14-3).

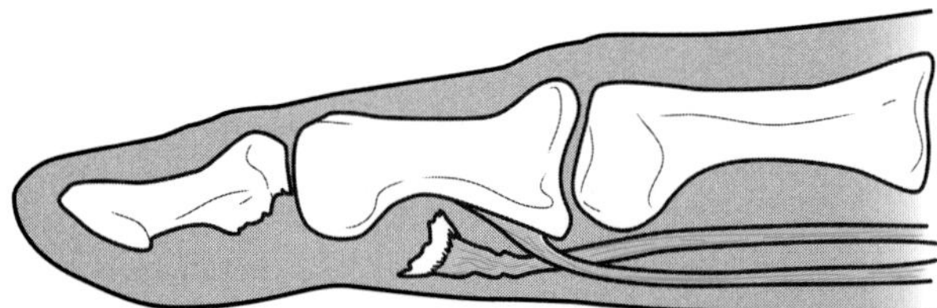

Figure 14-3: Tristen Peters' jersey finger.

1. Based on this scenario, what do you know about Mr. Peters' injury?
   - ______________________________
   - ______________________________
   - ______________________________
   - ______________________________

2. To rehabilitate Mr. Peters' injury effectively, you will need to gather additional information. What questions should you ask in addition to what is presented in this scenario?
   - ______________________________
   - ______________________________
   - ______________________________
   - ______________________________

Brain Jolt

Keeping a jersey finger injury splinted from the initial onset is extremely important in the healing process.

3. Identify key terms and concepts, and research each to broaden your knowledge about the rehabilitation of hand, wrist, and elbow injuries.
   - What anatomical structures might be involved in Mr. Peters' injury?

     Answer: ______________________________
   - What is jersey finger?

     Answer: ______________________________
   - In which phase of healing is this injury?

     Answer: ______________________________
   - Define *edema*.

     Answer: ______________________________
   - What might a popping sensation indicate?

     Answer: ______________________________
   - Why is Mr. Peters' DIP joint in slight extension?

     Answer: ______________________________
   - Can an avulsion occur with this mechanism? If so, what tendon and bone are involved?

     Answer: ______________________________
   - With this injury, is it important to test the capillary refill of the nail bed? If so, why?

     Answer: ______________________________

4. Based on the information that you currently have and what was provided by your instructor, how will you begin Mr. Peters' rehabilitation?
   - ______________________________
   - ______________________________
   - ______________________________
   - ______________________________

Why or why not?

How will Mr. Peters' rehabilitation progress? For the *why?* portion of each exercise, explain why you chose a particular exercise or activity as part of your program. Describe which rehabilitation goals the exercise or activity covers, and describe the key indicators for progression. For the *why not?* portion of each exercise, explain why other rehabilitation exercises or activities were not chosen and what to avoid during rehabilitation for this injury. Gather details from the textbook, your own research, and data from Mr. Peters' scenario to help formulate your answer.

Why?

- ______________________________
- ______________________________
- ______________________________
- ______________________________

Why not?

- ______________________________
- ______________________________
- ______________________________
- ______________________________
- ______________________________

What do you think?

1. Based on your rehabilitation protocol, discuss the indicators for limited and full return to play. Include a rough timeline for return to play, if applicable, which is affected by the athlete's compliance with the rehabilitation program.
   - ______________________________
2. Are modifications or personal protective equipment needed to return to play?
   - ______________________________
   - ______________________________

STUDENT SCENARIO 2: RYAN FISHER

Ryan Fisher is a cross-country runner who is waiting for the starting gun to begin the conference competition. Mr. Fisher is projected to place among the top three finishers if he can get in front of the pack and set a good pace. The starting gun goes off, and Mr. Fisher sprints to get in front when he tangles his feet with another runner's and falls down. He lands with all his weight on the tip of his left elbow. He experiences some pain at the tip of his elbow, attributes it to the fall, and quickly gets up to continue running. He finishes the race in second place, and upon his finish takes the time to examine his elbow. He experienced increased pain while running, and he has moderate edema over his olecranon. In addition, flexion and extension of the elbow are limited because of pain. He is referred for radiography to rule out an olecranon fracture. The results are negative, and olecranon bursitis is diagnosed (Fig. 14-4).

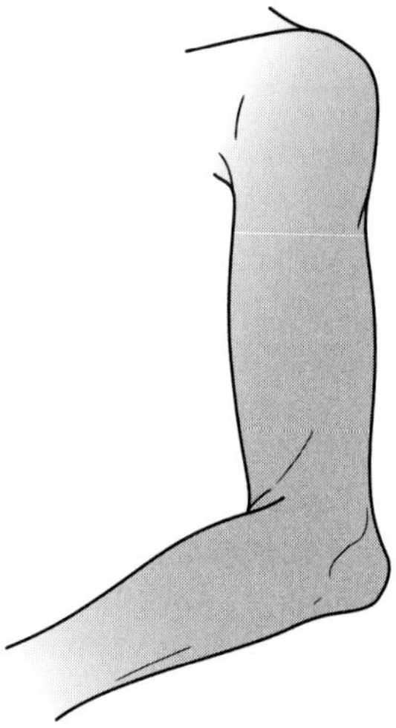

Figure 14-4: Ryan Fisher's olecranon bursitis.

1. Based on this scenario, what do you know about Mr. Fisher's injury?
   - ______________________________
   - ______________________________
   - ______________________________
   - ______________________________
2. To rehabilitate Mr. Fisher's injury effectively, you will need to gather additional information. What questions should you ask in addition to what is presented in this scenario?
   - ______________________________
   - ______________________________
   - ______________________________
   - ______________________________

3. Identify key terms and concepts, and then research each to broaden your knowledge about the rehabilitation of hand, wrist, and elbow injuries.
   - What anatomical structures might be involved in Mr. Fisher's injury?

     Answer: ______
   - What is olecranon bursitis?

     Answer: ______
   - In which phase of healing is this injury?

     Answer: ______
   - Define *edema*.

     Answer: ______
   - Why is Mr. Fisher unable to achieve full active range of motion of his elbow?

     Answer: ______
   - Because Mr. Fisher has a moderate amount of edema, should nerve impingement be of concern? If so, how is nerve involvement determined?

     Answer: ______
   - Does the edema produced by bursitis have any specific signs? If so, what might the signs be?

     Answer: ______
4. Based on the information that you currently have and what was provided by your instructor, how will you begin Mr. Fisher's rehabilitation?
   - ______
   - ______
   - ______
   - ______

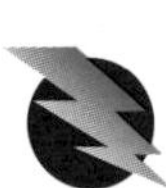

Brain Jolt

Your main rehabilitation goal with olecranon bursitis is to control edema.

Conversation Buffer

When talking with the athlete and the coach, advise them that olecranon bursitis is not a season-ending injury. The athlete should not lose much playing time because the injury can be protected properly while the athlete is still running.

Why or why not?

How will Mr. Fisher's rehabilitation progress? For the *why?* portion of each exercise, explain why you chose a particular exercise or activity as part of your program. Describe which rehabilitation goals the exercise or activity covers, and describe the key indicators for progression. For the *why not?* portion of each exercise, explain why other rehabilitation exercises or activities were not chosen and what to avoid during rehabilitation for this injury. Gather details from the textbook, your own research, and data from Mr. Fisher's scenario to help formulate your answer.

Why?

- ______
- ______
- ______
- ______

Why not?

- ______
- ______

What do you think?

1. Based on your rehabilitation protocol, discuss the indicators for limited and full return to play. Include a rough timeline for return to play, if applicable, which is affected by the athlete's compliance with the rehabilitation program.
   - ______
   - ______
   - ______
   - ______
2. Are modifications or personal protective equipment needed to return to play?
   - ______
   - ______

STUDENT SCENARIO 3: ERIN DOUGLAS

Erin Douglas is a collegiate tennis player who is playing at least four games over the next 2 days in a tournament. After two games on Friday, Ms. Douglas decides to ice the lateral side of her right elbow because of soreness in her right elbow joint. After playing three games the next day, she has pain in her elbow with wrist extension. Because of her history of elbow tendinosis, she decides to ask the certified athletic trainer to examine her elbow. On evaluation, she also has point tenderness and mild edema over the lateral epicondyle and a negative varus stress test result. The diagnosis is lateral epicondylitis (Fig. 14-5), which is commonly referred to as *tennis elbow*.

1. Based on this scenario, what do you know about Ms. Douglas' injury?
   - ______________________
   - ______________________
   - ______________________
   - ______________________

2. To rehabilitate Ms. Douglas' injury effectively, you will need to gather additional information. What questions should you ask in addition to what is presented in this scenario?
   - ______________________
   - ______________________
   - ______________________
   - ______________________

Figure 14-5: Erin Douglas' lateral epicondylitis.

3. Identify key terms and concepts, and research each to broaden your knowledge about the rehabilitation of hand, wrist, and elbow injuries.
   - What anatomical structures might be involved in Ms. Douglas' injury?

     Answer: ______________________
   - What is lateral epicondylitis?

     Answer: ______________________
   - In which phase of healing is this injury?

     Answer: ______________________
   - Define *edema*.

     Answer: ______________________
   - Define *extension*.

     Answer: ______________________
   - Define *tendinosis*.

     Answer: ______________________
   - What extensor muscles of the wrist are involved with lateral epicondylitis?

     Answer: ______________________
   - Why is this injury referred to as *tennis elbow*?

     Answer: ______________________
   - What predisposed Ms. Douglas to develop this injury in just 2 days?

     Answer: ______________________

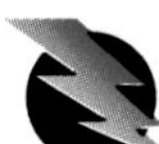

Brain Jolt

Try to limit extension and pronation movements of the wrist in lateral epicondylitis, because it causes irritation at the lateral epicondyle site.

4. Based on the information that you currently have and what was provided by your instructor, how will you begin Ms. Douglas' rehabilitation?
   - ______________________
   - ______________________
   - ______________________
   - ______________________

Treatment Detour

Lateral epicondylitis and other soft tissue injuries can be troublesome conditions to treat. When traditional treatments do not produce the desired results, implement assisted soft tissue mobilization by using the Graston technique. This technique can assist the clinician with manual therapy assessment and treatment by breaking up adhesions in the soft tissue and stimulating the healing response. There is documented research showing decreased pain and recovery time after treatment using this technique. Indications for this treatment can include medial and lateral epicondylitis, plantar fasciitis, iliotibial (IT) band friction syndrome, Achilles tendonitis, carpal tunnel syndrome, and many other soft tissue injuries (Stow, 2011).

Why or why not?

How will Ms. Douglas' rehabilitation progress? For the *why?* portion of each exercise, explain why you chose a particular exercise or activity as part of your program. Describe which rehabilitation goals the exercise or activity covers, and describe the key indicators for progression. For the *why not?* portion of each exercise, explain why other rehabilitation exercises or activities were not chosen and what to avoid during rehabilitation for this injury. Gather details from the textbook, your own research, and data from Ms. Douglas' scenario to help formulate your answer.

Why?

- ______________________________
- ______________________________
- ______________________________
- ______________________________

Why not?

- ______________________________
- ______________________________

Conversation Buffer
Be sure to talk with your team's coach about proper technique. Improper form and biomechanics can contribute to this chronic condition.

What do you think?

1. Based on your rehabilitation protocol, discuss the indicators for limited and full return to play. Include a rough timeline for return to play, if applicable, which is affected by the athlete's compliance with the rehabilitation program.
   - ______________________________
   - ______________________________
   - ______________________________
   - ______________________________
2. Are modifications or personal protective equipment needed to return to play?
   - ______________________________
   - ______________________________

STUDENT SCENARIO 4: STAN RICHARDS

Stan Richards is a pitcher for his college baseball team. He comes to the athletic training room complaining of an irritation of his right elbow. He states that he has had pain over his medial elbow for approximately 2 weeks. The pain occurred only after activity, but then increased to irritation before and after activity. Mr. Richards pitched a seven-inning game yesterday and felt a pull on the medial side of his right elbow. He now has point tenderness on the medial side of his elbow, moderate edema, a positive valgus stress test, a positive Tinel sign, and pain with active ROM. He also has a history of tight external rotators of the shoulder. After being referred to the orthopedic physician, he is scheduled for MRI. The MRI results show a grade 2 UCL tear (Fig. 14-6).

1. Based on this scenario, what do you know about Mr. Richards' injury?
   - ______________________________
   - ______________________________

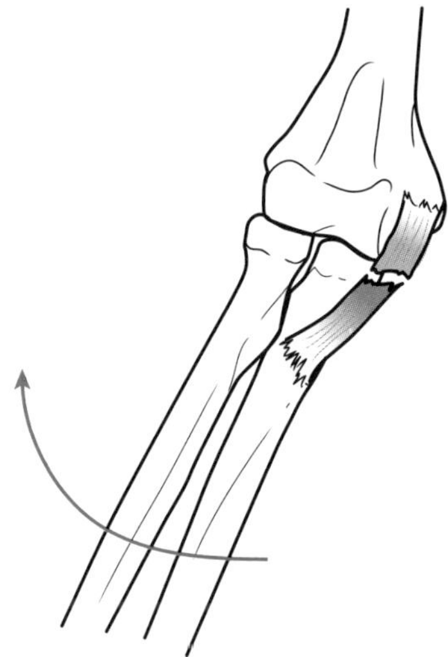

Figure 14-6: Stan Richards' ulnar collateral ligament tear.

- ______________________________

  ____
- ______________________________

  ____

2. To rehabilitate Mr. Richards' injury effectively, you will need to gather additional information. What questions should you ask in addition to what is presented in this scenario?
   - ______________________________

     ____
   - ______________________________

     ____
   - ______________________________

     ____
   - ______________________________

     ____

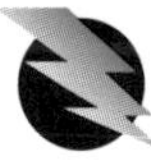

Brain Jolt

If the athlete has to undergo surgery for a UCL tear, familiarize yourself with Tommy John surgery.

Conversation Buffer

After noting that Mr. Richards already had a tight shoulder complex, implementing a stretching program for the entire baseball team is an area of interest to discuss with the head coach. Poor biomechanics can predispose an athlete to injury. You and the coach should evaluate the throwing mechanics of each athlete.

3. Identify key terms and concepts, and research each to broaden your knowledge about the rehabilitation of hand, wrist, and elbow injuries.
   - What anatomical structures might be involved in Mr. Richards' injury?

     Answer: ______________________________
   - What is a UCL tear?

     Answer: ______________________________
   - In which phase of healing is this injury?

     Answer: ______________________________
   - Define *edema*.

     Answer: ______________________________
   - Explain a UCL sprain.

     Answer: ______________________________
   - Mr. Richards had prior symptoms before the pulling sensation occurred during the game. What type of injury did he already have based on his symptoms?

     Answer: ______________________________
   - Why is it important to know about the ROM of the shoulder in this scenario?

     Answer: ______________________________
   - What symptoms are associated with a grade 2 UCL tear? What symptoms might be present with grade 1 and grade 3 tears?

     Answer: ______________________________
   - What is a valgus stress test? What does it test? What does a positive result indicate?

     Answer: ______________________________
   - What is a Tinel test? What does it test? What does a positive result indicate?

     Answer: ______________________________

Treatment Detour

Athletes who throw repeatedly subject the UCL to high repetitive loads. As a result, the UCL is often injured, frequently impairing the athletes' performance. Initially, UCL injuries are treated through conservative, nonoperative treatment; however, surgery is often the end result for competitive athletes. New operative techniques are constantly being discovered, and one study in 2011 examined long-term results of the hybrid suture anchor technique of UCL reconstruction. At a 7-year follow-up, 85% of 34 athletes had an excellent result from surgery, which meant that they returned to play at or above their preinjury level. It is important to be familiar with new operative techniques when working with injured athletes, because these techniques can potentially improve recovery time and long-term quality of life (Hechtman, Zvijac, Wells, & Botto-van Bendem, 2011).

4. Based on the information that you currently have and what was provided by your instructor, how will you begin Mr. Richards' rehabilitation?

- __________
- __________
- __________
- __________

Why or why not?

How will Mr. Richards' rehabilitation progress? For the *why?* portion of each exercise, explain why you chose a particular exercise or activity as part of your program. Describe which rehabilitation goals the exercise or activity covers, and describe the key indicators for progression. For the *why not?* portion of each exercise, explain why other rehabilitation exercises or activities were not chosen and what to avoid during rehabilitation for this injury. Gather details from the textbook, your own research, and data from Mr. Richards' scenario to help formulate your answer.

Why?

- __________
- __________
- __________
- __________

Why not?

- __________
- __________

What do you think?

1. Based on your rehabilitation protocol, discuss the indicators for limited and full return to play. Include a rough timeline for return to play, if applicable, which is affected by the athlete's compliance with the rehabilitation program.

- __________
- __________
- __________
- __________

2. Are modifications or personal protective equipment needed to return to play?

- __________
- __________

STUDENT SCENARIO 5: **KATIE FLINT**

Katie Flint is a senior on the high school volleyball team. The team is working on different blocking techniques at today's practice. Ms. Flint moves to block a shot and realizes that she is too close to the net. To ensure that she does not contact the net, she adjusts her weight backwards. This adjustment causes her to become off balance, and she falls back onto her right outstretched hand. This mechanism is known as a "foosh" injury. Ms. Flint feels a cracking sensation and has excruciating pain at her right distal forearm. She has immediate edema and deformity at her right wrist. A splint is placed above and below the deformity, and her arm is placed into a sling to be taken for radiographic imaging. The results indicate a Colles fracture (Fig. 14-7). Her arm is set in a cast with a plan to begin rehabilitation after her cast is removed.

1. Based on this scenario, what do you know about Ms. Flint's injury?

- __________
- __________

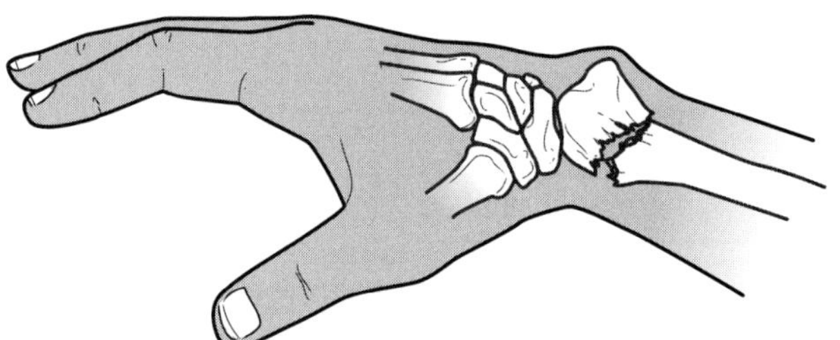

Figure 14-7: Katie Flint's Colles fracture.

- ____________________
- ____________________

2. To rehabilitate Ms. Flint's injury effectively, you will need to gather additional information. What questions should you ask in addition to what is presented in this scenario?
   - ____________________
   - ____________________
   - ____________________
   - ____________________

3. Identify key terms and concepts, and then research each to broaden your knowledge about the rehabilitation of hand, wrist, and elbow injuries.
   - What anatomical structures might be involved in Ms. Flint's injury?

     Answer: ____________________
   - What is a Colles fracture?

     Answer: ____________________
   - In which phase of healing is this injury?

     Answer: ____________________
   - Define *edema.*

     Answer: ____________________
   - Explain the term *foosh.*

     Answer: ____________________
   - What might a cracking sensation indicate?

     Answer: ____________________
   - Occasionally you will hear the phrase "dinner fork deformity" when discussing Colles fracture. What does this deformity look like and what does the term mean?

     Answer: ____________________

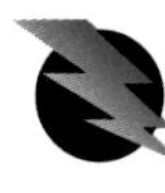

Brain Jolt

In a Colles fracture, there can be additional damage to surrounding tendons, the medial nerve, and radial or ulnar arteries because of displacement of the radius.

4. Based on the information that you currently have and what was provided by your instructor, how will you begin Ms. Flint's rehabilitation?
   - ____________________
   - ____________________
   - ____________________
   - ____________________

Why or why not?

How will Ms. Flint's rehabilitation progress? For the *why?* portion of each exercise, explain why you chose a particular exercise or activity as part of your program. Describe which rehabilitation goals the exercise or activity covers, and describe the key indicators for progression. For the *why not?* portion of each exercise, explain why other rehabilitation exercises or activities were not chosen and what to avoid during rehabilitation for this injury. Gather details from the textbook, your own research, and data from Ms. Flint's scenario to help formulate your answer.

Why?

- ____________________
- ____________________
- ____________________
- ____________________

Why not?

- ____________________
- ____________________

What do you think?

1. Based on your rehabilitation protocol, discuss the indicators for limited and full return to play. Include a rough timeline for return to play, if applicable, which is affected by the athlete's compliance with the rehabilitation program.
   - ____________________
   - ____________________
   - ____________________
   - ____________________
2. Are modifications or personal protective equipment needed to return to play?
   - ____________________
   - ____________________

STUDENT SCENARIO 6: LEAH POPE

Leah Pope is a sophomore on her college volleyball team and has a history of an ulnar collateral ligament sprain at the metacarpophalangeal joint of her left thumb. Before each practice, she tapes her left thumb using the thumb spica technique. Today at practice, she jumps up to block a ball at the net and the ball hits her thumb, abducting it forcefully. She has immediate pain resulting from the mechanism of injury and the prior soreness. The certified athletic trainer examines her left thumb, and she has a positive valgus stress test result, moderate edema over the medial side of the thumb, a positive anterior and posterior glide test result, a negative Finkelstein test result, and painful active abduction. A grade 2 UCL sprain is diagnosed, commonly known as *gamekeeper's thumb* (Fig. 14-8).

1. Based on this scenario, what do you know about Ms. Pope's injury?
   - ____________________
   - ____________________
   - ____________________
   - ____________________

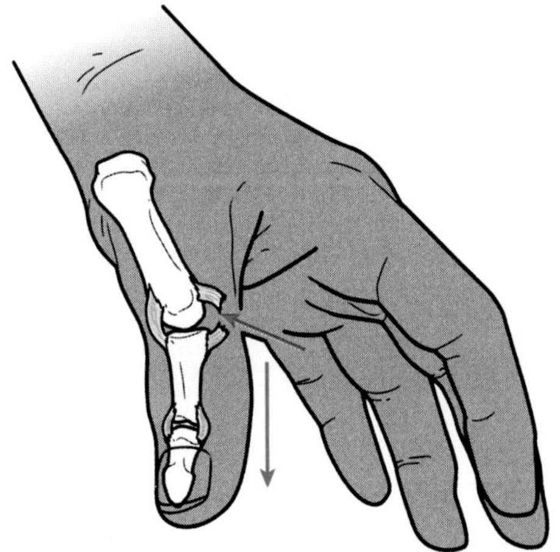

Figure 14-8: Leah Pope's gamekeeper's thumb.

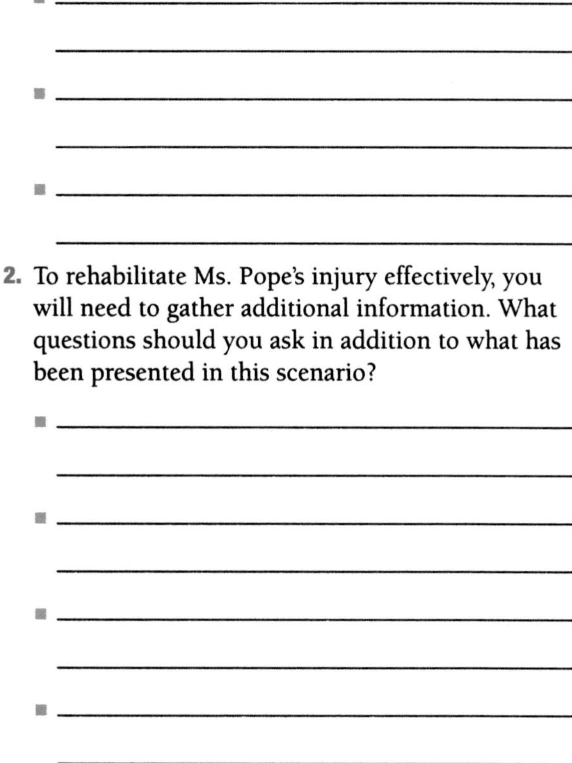

2. To rehabilitate Ms. Pope's injury effectively, you will need to gather additional information. What questions should you ask in addition to what has been presented in this scenario?
   - ____________________
   - ____________________
   - ____________________
   - ____________________

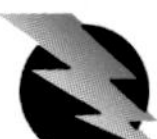

Brain Jolt

Frequently "loose" joints and hypermobility can predispose one to a UCL sprain. Remember to check the injury bilaterally, and treat the injury as a bilateral condition if required.

3. Identify any key terms and concepts, and research each to broaden your knowledge about the rehabilitation of hand, wrist, and elbow injuries.
   - What anatomical structures might be involved in Ms. Pope's injury?

   Answer: ____________________

- What is gamekeeper's thumb?

  Answer: ______________________________
- In which phase of healing is this injury?

  Answer: ______________________________
- Define *edema*.

  Answer: ______________________________
- Define *abduction*.

  Answer: ______________________________
- Describe the thumb spica tape technique.

  Answer: ______________________________
- What is a valgus stress test? What does it test? What does a positive test indicate?

  Answer: ______________________________
- What is an anterior and posterior glide test? What does it test? What does a positive test indicate?

  Answer: ______________________________
- What is a Finkelstein test? What does it test? What does a positive test indicate?

  Answer: ______________________________

4. Based on the information that you currently have and what was provided by your instructor, how will you begin Ms. Pope's rehabilitation?

- ______________________________
- ______________________________
- ______________________________
- ______________________________

Why or why not?

How will Ms. Pope's rehabilitation progress? For the *why?* portion of each exercise, explain why you chose a particular exercise or activity as part of your program. Describe which rehabilitation goals the exercise or activity covers, and describe the key indicators for progression. For the *why not?* portion of each exercise, explain why other rehabilitation exercises or activities were not chosen and what to avoid during rehabilitation for this injury. Gather details from the textbook, your own research, and data from Ms. Pope's scenario to help formulate your answer.

Why?

- ______________________________
- ______________________________
- ______________________________
- ______________________________

Why not?

- ______________________________
- ______________________________

What do you think?

1. Based on your rehabilitation protocol, discuss the indicators for limited and full return to play. Include a rough timeline for return to play, if applicable, which is affected by the athlete's compliance with the rehabilitation program.

- ______________________________
- ______________________________
- ______________________________
- ______________________________

2. Are modifications or personal protective equipment needed to return to play?

- ______________________________
- ______________________________

STUDENT SCENARIO 7: NICK VASTOLLA

Nick Vastolla is a senior on his school lacrosse team. He is running down the field, with the ball in the net of his lacrosse stick, when he passes the ball to another player and is struck by an opponent's lacrosse stick on the right forearm. Mr. Vastolla hears a pop and feels immediate pain. He is assisted off the field and is evaluated on the sidelines. He has edema, localized point tenderness, and ecchymosis where the stick struck his right forearm. The localized point tenderness is along the upper third of the ulna. Mr. Vastolla has no deformity, but percussion and compression test results are positive. He is immobilized and referred for radiography, the results of which indicate an ulnar fracture (Fig. 14-9). A cast that extends over the wrist is made for his arm.

1. Based on this scenario, what do you know about Mr. Vastolla's injury?

- ______________________________
- ______________________________
- ______________________________
- ______________________________

2. To rehabilitate Mr. Vastolla's injury effectively, you will need to gather additional information. What questions should you ask in addition to what is presented in this scenario?

- ______________________________
- ______________________________
- ______________________________
- ______________________________

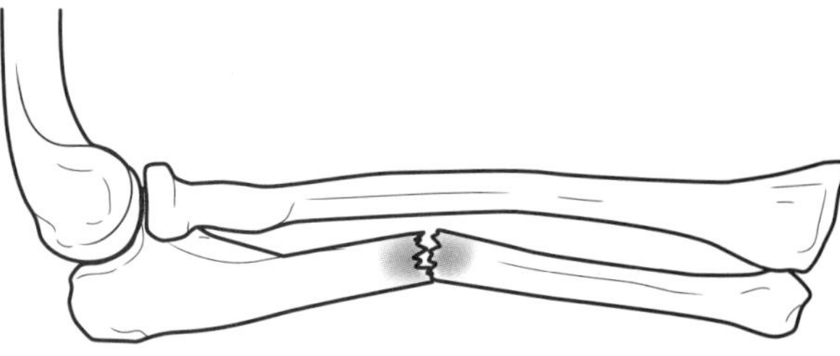

Figure 14-9: Nick Vastolla's ulnar shaft fracture.

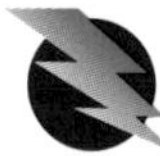

Brain Jolt

Be familiar with the type of fracture your athlete has so that you can project recovery times accurately.

3. Identify key terms and concepts, and research each to broaden your knowledge about the rehabilitation of hand, wrist, and elbow injuries.

- What anatomical structures might be involved in Mr. Vastolla's injury?

  Answer: ______________________________
- What is a forearm fracture of the ulna?

  Answer: ______________________________
- In which phase of healing is this injury?

  Answer: ______________________________
- Define *edema.*

  Answer: ______________________________
- Define *ecchymosis.*

  Answer: ______________________________
- What might a popping sensation indicate?

  Answer: ______________________________
- What is a percussion test? What does it test? What does a positive result indicate?

  Answer: ______________________________
- What is a compression test? What does it test? What does a positive result indicate?

  Answer: ______________________________
- Why would the cast extend over his wrist?

  Answer: ______________________________

4. Based on the information that you currently have and what was provided by your instructor, how will you begin Mr. Vastolla's rehabilitation?

- ______________________________
- ______________________________
- ______________________________
- ______________________________

Conversation Buffer

With physician approval, an athlete can wear a padded or soft covering over a cast and still participate in a contact sport. This topic can be discussed with the physician, coach, and athlete;

however, remember that the pad has to be approved by the officials before the game.

Why or why not?

How will Mr. Vastolla's rehabilitation progress? For the *why?* portion of each exercise, explain why you chose a particular exercise or activity as part of your program. Describe which rehabilitation goals the exercise or activity covers, and describe the key indicators for progression. For the *why not?* portion of each exercise, explain why other rehabilitation exercises or activities were not chosen and what to avoid during rehabilitation for this injury. Gather details from the textbook, your own research, and data from Mr. Vastolla's scenario to help formulate your answer.

Why?

- ______________________________
- ______________________________
- ______________________________
- ______________________________

Why not?

- ______________________________
- ______________________________

What do you think?

1. Based on your rehabilitation protocol, discuss the indicators for limited and full return to play. Include a rough timeline for return to play, if applicable, which is affected by the athlete's compliance with the rehabilitation program.
   - ______________________________
   - ______________________________
   - ______________________________
   - ______________________________
2. Are modifications or personal protective equipment needed to return to play?
   - ______________________________
   - ______________________________

STUDENT SCENARIO 8: GABE JILLIAN

Gabe Jillian is a collegiate wrestler who competes in the 175-pound weight class. He warms up for his match and goes up against the first-ranked wrestler in the conference. Mr. Jillian makes it through the first period without giving too many points to his opponent. He gets to choose his starting position for the second period and he chooses down, which puts him on the mat, sitting back on his heels with his arms positioned on the mat out in front of him. The opponent takes his position behind Mr. Jillian. The whistle blows and Mr. Jillian shoots up onto his feet, putting the majority of his weight onto his right elbow. He tries to pivot free from the opponent but feels a pop sensation at his right elbow, which causes him to fall to the mat in pain. He notices severe deformity at his elbow, and the certified athletic trainer rushes out to stabilize his dislocated elbow. Because of the twisting motion, the ulna and radius have been forced backwards, causing severe edema and ecchymosis. A splint is applied, and he is sent to the emergency department with an elbow dislocation (Fig. 14-10), where radiographic imaging is performed to rule out a possible fracture.

1. Based on this scenario, what do you know about Mr. Jillian's injury?
   - ______________________________
   - ______________________________

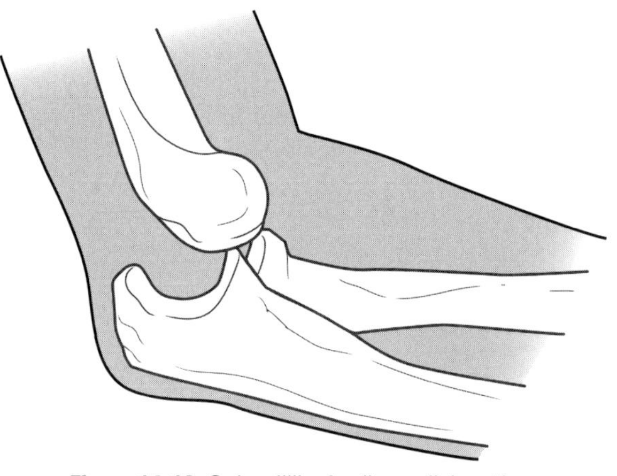

Figure 14-10: Gabe Jillian's elbow dislocation.

- ______________________________________
- ______________________________________

2. To rehabilitate Mr. Jillian's injury effectively, you will need to gather additional information. What questions should you ask in addition to what is presented in this scenario?
   - ______________________________________
   - ______________________________________
   - ______________________________________
   - ______________________________________

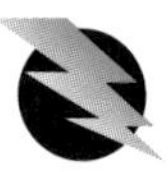

Brain Jolt

With an elbow dislocation, always be sure to check neurovascular function.

3. Identify key terms and concepts, and research each to broaden your knowledge about the rehabilitation of hand, wrist, and elbow injuries.
   - What anatomical structures might be involved in Mr. Jillian's injury?

     Answer: ____________________________
   - What is an elbow dislocation?

     Answer: ____________________________
   - In which phase of healing is this injury?

     Answer: ____________________________
   - Define *edema*.

     Answer: ____________________________
   - What might a popping sensation indicate?

     Answer: ____________________________
   - Describe the types of dislocations that can occur at the elbow joint.

     Answer: ____________________________
   - Identify structures to check when performing a neurovascular assessment distal to the injury.

     Answer: ____________________________

Conversation Buffer

A dislocated elbow can be a season-ending injury; therefore, it should be handled with the focus of still involving the athlete with the team. As long as the activity does not endanger or aggravate the prior injury, being part of the team conditioning is a great motivator for the athlete during rehabilitation. Just be sure to discuss this with the coach before you offer it to the athlete.

4. Based on the information that you currently have and what was provided by your instructor, how will you begin Mr. Jillian's rehabilitation?
   - ______________________________________
   - ______________________________________
   - ______________________________________
   - ______________________________________

Why or why not?

How will Mr. Jillian's rehabilitation progress? For the *why?* portion of each exercise, explain why you chose a particular exercise or activity as part of your program. Describe which rehabilitation goals the exercise or activity covers, and describe the key indicators for progression. For the *why not?* portion of each exercise, explain why other rehabilitation exercises or activities were not chosen and what to avoid during rehabilitation for this injury. Gather details from the textbook, your own research, and data from Mr. Jillian's scenario to help formulate your answer.

Why?

- ______________________________________
- ______________________________________

- ____________________
- ____________________

Why not?

- ____________________
- ____________________

What do you think?

1. Based on your rehabilitation protocol, discuss the indicators for limited and full return to play. Include a rough timeline for return to play, if applicable, which is affected by the athlete's compliance with the rehabilitation program.
   - ____________________
   - ____________________
   - ____________________
   - ____________________
2. Are modifications or personal protective equipment needed to return to play?
   - ____________________
   - ____________________

knowledge checklist

Table 14-1 offers a checklist that can be used by a peer, instructor, or preceptor to evaluate each part of the athlete's rehabilitation plan. Use this checklist as a tool to ensure that the rehabilitation plan is complete and to assess your knowledge of the competencies that apply to this chapter.

TABLE 14-1 ■ Upper Extremity: The Hand, Wrist, and Elbow Rehabilitation and Therapeutic Exercise Competency Checklist

	Proficient *Can demonstrate and execute the skill properly*	**Proficient With Assistance** *Can demonstrate and execute the skill with minimal guidance or tips*	**Not Proficient** *Unable to demonstrate and execute the skill properly; need to be reevaluated at another time after further study and practice*
Controlling Edema			
PRICE			
Modalities			
Controlling Pain			
Pain scales			
Medications			
Modalities			
Establishes Core Stability			
Reestablishes Neuromuscular Control			
Restores Postural Control and Balance			
Restoring Range of Motion			
Passive range of motion			
Active range of motion			
Resistive range of motion			
Goniometry			
Normal range of motion limits			
Restore Muscular Strength, Endurance, and Power			
Open kinetic chain			
Closed kinetic chain			
Isometric			
Isotonic			
Isotonic (concentric and eccentric)			
Isokinetic			
Plyometric			
Agility			
Functional or Sport-Specific Activities			
Maintains Cardiorespiratory Fitness			
Functional Testing			
Return-to-Play Criteria			
Proper Documentation			

PRICE, prevention, rest, ice, compression, and elevation.

REFERENCES

Hechtman, K. S., Zvijac, J. E., Wells, M. E., & Botto-van Bemden, A. (2011). Long-term results of ulnar collateral ligament reconstruction in throwing athletes based on a hybrid technique. *The American Journal of Sports Medicine, 39*, 342–347.

Higgins, M. (2011). *Therapeutic exercise: From theory to practice*. Philadelphia, PA: F.A. Davis.

National Athletic Training Association. (2011). *Athletic training education competencies* (5th ed.). Retrieved from http://www.nata.org/sites/default/files/5th-Edition-Competencies-2011-PDF-Version.pdf

Prentice, W. (2010). *Arnheim's principles of athletic training: A competency-based approach* (14th ed.). New York, NY: McGraw-Hill.

Prentice, W. (2011). *Rehabilitation techniques for sports medicine and athletic training* (5th ed.). New York, NY: McGraw-Hill.

Starkey, C. (2004). *Therapeutic modalities* (3rd ed.). Philadelphia, PA: F.A. Davis.

Starkey, C., Brown, S. D., & Ryan, J. (2010). *Examination of orthopedic and athletic injuries* (3rd ed.). Philadelphia, PA: F.A. Davis.

Stow, R. (2011). Instrument-assisted soft tissue mobilization. *International Journal of Athletic Therapy and Training, 16*, 5–8.

Venes, D. (Ed.). (2009). *Taber's cyclopedic medical dictionary* (21st ed.). Philadelphia, PA: F.A. Davis.

chapter 15

Upper Extremity: The Shoulder

chapter outline

athletic trainer's corner

Here is what one athletic trainer experienced with a real-world athlete's rehabilitation from injury:

At a Saturday morning boys' basketball scrimmage, two athletes collided under the basket as one intended to shoot a layup. I was informed of the injury on the following Monday. I spoke with the injured athlete's mother on the telephone the day of the injury. She stated that her son felt like his left shoulder had "gone out." The mother also mentioned that her son had a history of a left elbow dislocation. The dislocation had occurred three times in the past 3 years. When asked whether her son had ever been informed that he was double-jointed or had "loose joints," the mother replied with a chuckled "yes." He had limited range of motion (ROM) and a clicking or catching sensation in his shoulder. Generally, I would not refer an athlete to an orthopedist without having evaluated the injury myself; however, I had a unique opportunity to get this athlete to the orthopedist through a walk-in clinic that evening. Given the situation, I had concerns about the possibility of several injuries, including a tear of the labrum, a rotator cuff tear, and a fracture of the humerus or surrounding bones. The suspected dislocation and self-reduction could have easily caused any or all of these injuries. I opted to refer the athlete immediately with the hopes of starting the evaluation process. The team's first game of the season was only 4 days away. The athlete and his mother were hoping that he might be able to play. He was seen by a physician's assistant who ordered both radiographs and magnetic resonance imaging (MRI) the following day. Just 3 days after the initial evaluation (5 days post-injury), the MRI results revealed no structural damage and the radiograph was clear of any possible fracture. The orthopedic surgeon released the athlete as tolerated with the request that we work on his ROM for the next 4 days. The athlete regained full ROM and strength (compared bilaterally) and was returned to play the following week, missing only the first game of the season.

Kristen Higgins, MS, AT, ATC
Wilson Memorial Hospital
Botkins and Jackson-Center High Schools
Sidney, Ohio

learning outcomes

After working through this chapter, you will be able to:

1. Describe seven different goals of rehabilitation and the importance of each in the overall rehabilitation protocol.
2. Verbalize indications for performing shoulder rehabilitative techniques.
3. Discuss modifications and progressions that are used during a rehabilitation program for the shoulder.
4. Discuss outcome measures used to identify activity levels and return-to-play guidelines for shoulder injuries.
5. Explain what modality choice is proper for rehabilitation by using indications, contraindications, and the principles and theory related to the physiological response of the intervention.

MODEL SCENARIO 1: CASEY SPARKS

Casey Sparks is an outside hitter for the local high school volleyball team. Throughout the season, she has complained that her right shoulder is continually irritated. When examined, Ms. Sparks' strength and ROM in her shoulder are normal but painful. She ices the area after practice every day. Last night at the volleyball conference championships, she had 20 kills and her shoulder was irritated after the game. She is concerned the following day when her shoulder hurts with any type of ROM. An evaluation of her right shoulder reveals no ecchymosis or deformity. There is pain with shoulder abduction at 45 degrees, and she is unable to move her arm above 90 degrees because of the pain. Her strength is a 4/5 with external rotation, and the empty can test yields positive results. The diagnosis is with a grade 1+ supraspinatus strain of the rotator cuff (Fig. 15-1).

1. Based on this scenario, what do you know about Ms. Sparks' injury?
   - *Female athlete*
   - *Volleyball position: hitter*
   - *Mechanism of injury (MOI): overuse injury*
   - *Previous right shoulder pain*
   - *Injury occurred at end of the season*
   - *Increased number of hits this game*
   - *No deformity*
   - *No ecchymosis*
   - *Pain with range of motion*
   - *Cannot raise arm greater than 90 degrees of abduction*
   - *Decreased strength in external rotation*
   - *Positive empty can test*
   - *Grade 1+ supraspinatus strain*
2. To rehabilitate Ms. Sparks' injury effectively, you will need to gather additional information. What questions should you ask in addition to what is presented in this scenario?
   - *Are there preexisting injuries? If yes, what are they?*
   - *How long has the athlete experienced this pain?*
   - *What is the athlete's pain level and type of pain felt?*
   - *What is the strength at the shoulder?*
   - *Does the athlete have any numbness or paraesthesia?*
   - *What is the ROM at the shoulder?*
   - *Is crepitus present?*
   - *Is edema present?*
   - *Can a popping or clicking sound be heard?*

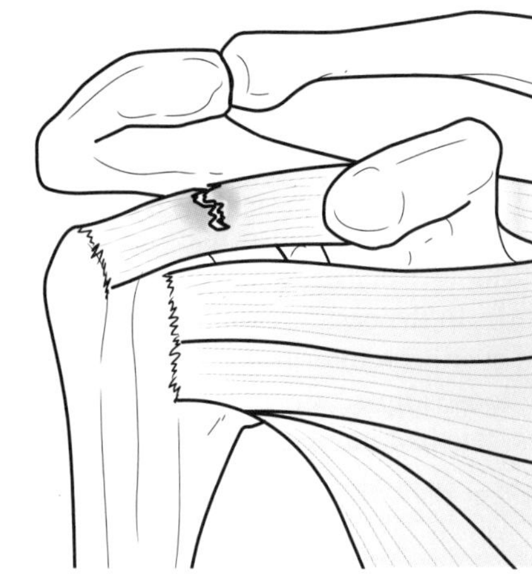

Figure 15-1: Casey Sparks' rotator cuff strain.

3. Identify key terms and concepts, and research each to broaden your knowledge about the rehabilitation of shoulder injuries.
   - What anatomical structures might be involved in Ms. Sparks' injury?
     Rotator cuff muscle group
     Scapula
     Clavicle
     Humerus
   - What is a grade 1+ supraspinatus strain?
     It is an injury to one of the rotator cuff muscles. When a muscle is strained, dependent on the degree, there are small microtears within the muscle fibers. The higher the grade of strain, the higher degree of damage. A grade 1+ strain will have mild to moderate symptoms.
   - In which phase of healing is this injury?
     Acute inflammatory phase
   - Define *ecchymosis*.
     Superficial bleeding under the skin; a bruise
   - What is the empty can test? What does it test? What does a positive test indicate?
     The empty can test is performed with the patient sitting or standing. The shoulder is fully internally rotated, abducted to 90 degrees, and placed in 30 degrees of forward flexion, as though emptying a beverage can. The patient is then instructed to resist downward pressure. Pain or the inability to maintain position against pressure, or both, indicate supraspinatus pathology.
   - Why is the pain worse with abduction?
     Abduction is the main action of the supraspinatus muscle; therefore, the pain will be worse when the muscle is actively moving the arm into abduction.
   - What muscles compose the rotator cuff?
     Supraspinatus
     Infraspinatus
     Teres minor
     Subscapularis

4. Based on the information that you currently have and what was provided by your instructor, how will you begin Ms. Sparks' rehabilitation?
   Ms. Sparks needs a rehabilitation plan that will decrease her pain and increase ROM. First, inflammation can be reduced by using ice, electrical stimulation, and nonsteroidal anti-inflammatory drugs (NSAIDs). To increase ROM, first perform passive ROM in all motions of the shoulder followed by active ROM. Initially, limit active ROM greater than 90 degrees to decrease inflammation.

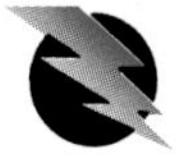

Brain Jolt

Pain with a rotator cuff strain increases with ROM activity greater than 90 degrees. Initially, rehabilitate this injury using exercises at less than 90 degrees.

Why or why not?

How will Ms. Sparks' rehabilitation progress? For the *why?* portion of each exercise, explain why you chose a particular exercise or activity as part of your program. Describe which rehabilitation goals the exercise or activity covers, and describe the key indicators for progression. For the *why not?* portion of each exercise, explain why other rehabilitation exercises or activities were not chosen and what to avoid during rehabilitation for this injury. Gather details from the textbook, your own research, and data from Ms. Sparks' scenario to help formulate your answer.

Why?

- ***Ice.*** *This will help with the rehabilitation goal of decreasing pain and inflammation. NSAIDs also help decrease pain and inflammation.*
- ***Electrical stimulation.*** *This modality will help the goal of pain management.*
- ***ROM exercises.*** *This activity will help the rehabilitation goal of increasing flexibility and ROM of the shoulder. Initially, passive ROM is performed by the athletic trainer, but the athlete can also accomplish this using cane exercises. Once the exercises are performed with ease, active ROM can be performed in all shoulder motions by implementing wall walks. Once the athlete accomplishes these exercises, resistive exercises may be implemented.*
- ***Strengthening exercises.*** *Theraband exercises will help with the rehabilitation goal of increasing strength by strengthening the rotator cuff muscles. These exercises are performed in all directions with no initial movement greater than 90 degrees. The athlete begins with the least resistive color delineated by the manufacturer and progresses to subsequent colored bands once the current band's resistance becomes too easy.*
- ***Rhythmic stabilization.*** *This activity helps with the rehabilitation goal of regaining proprioception of the shoulder. The patient begins with manual perturbations performed by the clinician and progresses to the body blade through all shoulder motions.*

Why not?

- *Avoid any exercises greater than 90 degrees. All exercises should be performed pain-free by the athlete. The athlete may have some discomfort, but pain is a contraindication to the exercise or the amount of resistance being used.*

What do you think?

1. Based on your rehabilitation protocol, discuss the indicators for limited and full return to play with

the athlete. Include a rough timeline for return to play, if applicable, which is affected by the athlete's compliance with the rehabilitation program.

- ***Limited return to play.*** *Regarding a rotator cuff strain injury, limited return to play is determined by normal pain-free ROM and strength at the shoulder. Once these are achieved, the patient can return to some functional activities with the team but nothing "live."*
- ***Full return to play.*** *Full return-to-play status is determined once the patient masters limited return to play, does not have an increase in symptoms from the initial injury, and participates in simulated "live" activities with the clinician to ensure the lowest risk of re-injury.*

2. Are modifications or personal protective equipment needed to return to play?
   - *A shoulder spica or brace could be used.*

MODEL SCENARIO 2: ELI HOFFMAN

Eli Hoffman is a baseball player on his high school team. He often complains of bilateral shoulder pain. Mr. Hoffman attributes the bilateral shoulder pain to the preseason training, but decides to visit the athletic trainer for an evaluation. On evaluation, it is determined that Mr. Hoffman has weakness bilaterally in his serratus anterior and middle and lower trapezius muscles. Considering the serratus anterior weakness, the athletic trainer instructs Mr. Hoffman to perform a wall push-up and notes bilateral winging of the scapulae (Fig. 15-2), which could be attributing to his decreased shoulder ROM.

1. Based on this scenario, what do you know about Mr. Hoffman's injury?
   - *Male athlete*
   - *Baseball player*
   - *Bilateral shoulder pain*
   - *Weakness at the shoulder*
   - *Winging scapulae, bilaterally*
   - *Weak serratus anterior and middle and lower trapezius muscles*

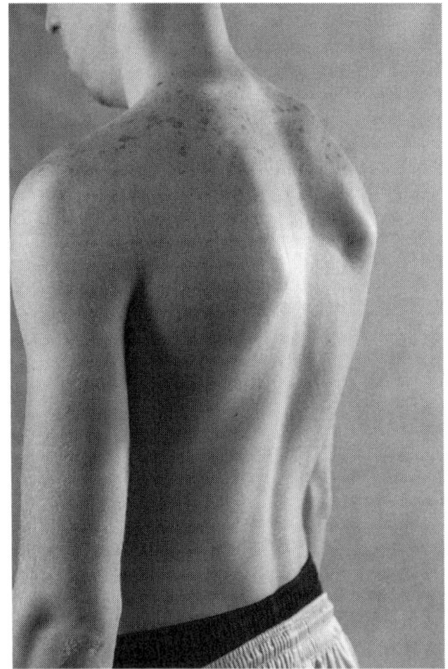

Figure 15-2: Eli Hoffman's winging of the scapula.

2. To rehabilitate Mr. Hoffman's injury effectively, you will need to gather additional information. What questions should you ask in addition to what is presented in this scenario?
   - *Are there preexisting injuries? If yes, what are they?*
   - *How long has the athlete experienced this pain?*
   - *What is the athlete's pain level and type of pain felt?*
   - *What is the strength in the shoulder?*
   - *Does the athlete have any numbness or paraesthesia?*
   - *What is the ROM in the shoulder?*

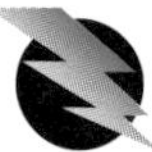

Brain Jolt

Winging of the scapula can occur secondary to injury to the long thoracic nerve. If strengthening of the scapular stabilizer muscles does not seem to improve the issue, be sure to address the nerve.

3. Identify key terms and concepts, and research each to broaden your knowledge about the rehabilitation of shoulder injuries.
   - What anatomical structures might be involved in Mr. Hoffman's injury?
     Scapula
     Humerus
     Serratus anterior
     Trapezius
     Long thoracic nerve
   - What is winging of the scapula?
     Winging of the scapula occurs when there is posterior protrusion of the vertebral or medial border of the scapula.
   - In which phase of healing is this injury?
     Chronic phase
   - Injury to what nerve can cause winging of the scapula?
     Long thoracic nerve
   - Is it more or less concerning when the issue is bilateral?
     It is less concerning because it means that there is no imbalance.
   - Define *bilateral.*
     Affecting two or both sides

4. Based on the information that you currently have and what was provided by your instructor, how will you begin Mr. Hoffman's rehabilitation?

Initially, Mr. Hoffman's strength needs to be increased at the shoulder and scapular stabilizers. His pain stems from incorrect biomechanics used to compensate for his weaknesses. He needs to begin with serratus punches, scapular retraction exercises, and exercises that work the middle and lower trapezius muscles. When doing these exercises, proper form and scapular motion are crucial to retraining and properly strengthening these muscles. Instruct Mr. Hoffman to exercise in front of a mirror when possible and provide verbal cues to ensure correct form.

Why or why not?

How will Mr. Hoffman's rehabilitation progress? For the *why?* portion of each exercise, explain why you chose a particular exercise or activity as part of your program. Describe which rehabilitation goals the exercise or activity covers, and describe the key indicators for progression. For the *why not?* portion of each exercise, explain why other rehabilitation exercises or activities were not chosen and what to avoid during rehabilitation for this injury. Gather details from the textbook, your own research, and data from Mr. Hoffman's scenario to help formulate your answer.

Why?

- ***Serratus punches.*** *This activity will help with the rehabilitation goal of increasing strength by strengthening the serratus anterior muscle, which helps to increase the strength of the scapular stabilizers. To advance this exercise, the patient can hold weights or the clinician can provide manual resistance.*
- ***Rhythmic stabilization.*** *This activity helps with the rehabilitation goal of regaining proprioception of the shoulder. The patient begins with manual perturbations by the clinician and progresses to the body blade through all shoulder motions. Ensure that the scapula is "set" for all motions.*
- ***Push-ups.*** *This activity will help with the rehabilitation goal of increasing strength by working the serratus anterior and trapezius muscles. To begin, the push-ups can be performed on a wall, then progressed to a table, and finally progressed to the floor. Once these exercises are accomplished, push-ups with a plus (a push-up with an emphasis on full extension and scapular protraction in the up phase) can be performed to further strengthen these muscles.*

Why not?

- *Avoid any activity in which the scapula is not in the proper position throughout the entire motion. By allowing improper positioning of the scapula while performing exercises, the muscles are not being retrained and strengthened in a position to promote the best shoulder biomechanics.*

What do you think?

1. Based on your rehabilitation protocol, discuss the indicators for limited and full return to play. Include a rough timeline for return to play, if applicable, which is affected by the athlete's compliance with the rehabilitation program.

- *Regarding the winging of the scapula injury, the athlete can play throughout the rehabilitation process as long as the athlete experiences nothing more than minimal pain. Pain takes time to subside, so unless the athlete experiences a tremendous lack of strength or ROM, the athlete can continue playing.*

2. Are modifications or personal protective equipment needed to return to play?

- *No*

STUDENT SCENARIO 1: DEXTER ARES

Dexter Ares is a collegiate wrestler who is currently winning his match by one point. As the third period begins, he is caught off guard by an opponent's move that quickly puts him in a pinned position. He tries to rotate his body to the right, away from the opponent, but as he does this his right shoulder is horizontally abducted and externally rotated around the opponent's body. Mr. Ares gives one last forceful twist of his body and feels a popping sensation at the center of his upper chest, on his right side. He experiences immediate pain and discomfort that prevents him from finishing the match. On evaluation, he has an upward and anterior deformity at the sternoclavicular (SC) joint (Fig. 15-3), as well as moderate edema, and he is unable to abduct his shoulder past 90 degrees without pain. A diagnosis of grade 2 SC joint sprain is made, and the area is immobilized. Mr. Ares is referred for radiographic imaging, the results of which confirm an SC joint sprain.

1. Based on this scenario, what do you know about Mr. Ares' injury?

- ______________________________

____

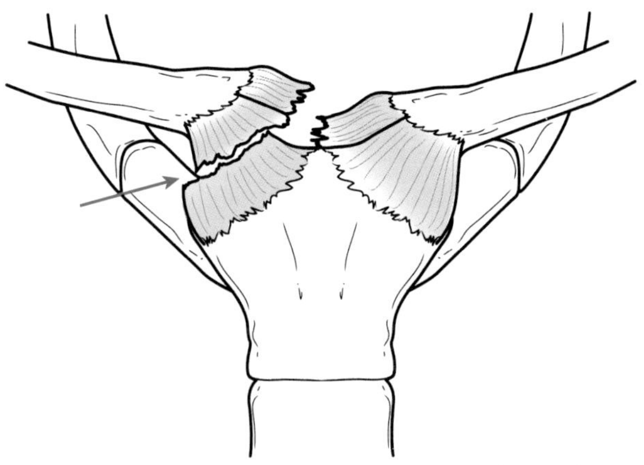

Figure 15-3: Dexter Ares' sternoclavicular joint sprain.

- ______________________
- ______________________
- ______________________

2. To rehabilitate Mr. Ares' injury effectively, you will need to gather additional information. What questions should you ask in addition to what is presented in this scenario?

- ______________________
- ______________________
- ______________________
- ______________________

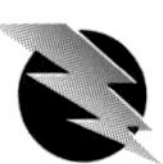

Brain Jolt
If the clavicle displaces posteriorly, it can exert pressure on the esophagus, making a SC joint sprain a life-threatening injury.

3. Identify key terms and concepts, and then research each to broaden your knowledge about the rehabilitation of shoulder injuries.
   - What anatomical structures might be involved in Mr. Ares' injury?

     Answer: ______________________
   - What is a grade 2 SC joint sprain?

     Answer: ______________________
   - In which phase of healing is this injury?

     Answer: ______________________
   - What does a popping sensation indicate?

     Answer: ______________________
   - Define *edema*.

     Answer: ______________________
   - What are the different grades of injury, with the corresponding signs and symptoms that can occur with this joint?

     Answer: ______________________
   - Describe *horizontal abduction with external rotation*.

     Answer: ______________________
   - Why is Mr. Ares unable to abduct his shoulder past 90 degrees without pain?

     Answer: ______________________

Brain Jolt
Immobilization of this joint can last 3 to 5 weeks.

4. Based on the information that you currently have and what was provided by your instructor, how will you begin Mr. Ares' rehabilitation?

- ______________________
- ______________________
- ______________________
- ______________________

Why or why not?

How will Mr. Ares' rehabilitation progress? For the *why?* portion of each exercise, explain why you chose a particular exercise or activity as part of your program. Describe which rehabilitation goals the exercise or activity covers, and describe the key indicators for progression. For the *why not?* portion of each exercise, explain why other rehabilitation exercises or activities were not chosen and what to avoid during rehabilitation for this injury. Gather details from the textbook, your own research, and data from Mr. Ares' scenario to help formulate your answer.

Why?

- ______________________
- ______________________
- ______________________

Why not?

What do you think?

1. Based on your rehabilitation protocol, discuss the indicators for limited and full return to play. Include a rough timeline for return to play, if applicable, which is affected by the athlete's compliance with the rehabilitation program.

2. Are modifications or personal protective equipment needed to return to play?

STUDENT SCENARIO 2: DICK TAYLOR

Dick Taylor is a collegiate basketball player who is currently in the conditioning phase of the preseason workout. He is in the gym doing functional drills. At the current station, the team members are doing 10 push-ups and then quickly exploding into the air to do 10 wall jumps. As Mr. Taylor is doing his push-ups, the teammate next to him stumbles while exploding up and catches himself by putting all his weight onto Mr. Taylor's back. As the weight comes down onto Mr. Taylor's back, he pushes his body up to the start position of his push-up. Mr. Taylor feels a sharp pain and popping sensation in his left pectoralis muscle that prevents him from finishing the push-ups. The certified athletic trainer determines that Mr. Taylor has a left grade 2 pectoralis major tear. He has moderate edema, complete loss of function with adduction, and deformity of the pectoralis major muscle close to the insertion point (Fig. 15-4). His shoulder is placed in a sling, and he is referred to the team physician.

1. Based on this scenario, what do you know about Mr. Taylor's injury?

2. To rehabilitate Mr. Taylor's injury effectively, you will need to gather additional information. What questions should you ask in addition to what is presented in this scenario?

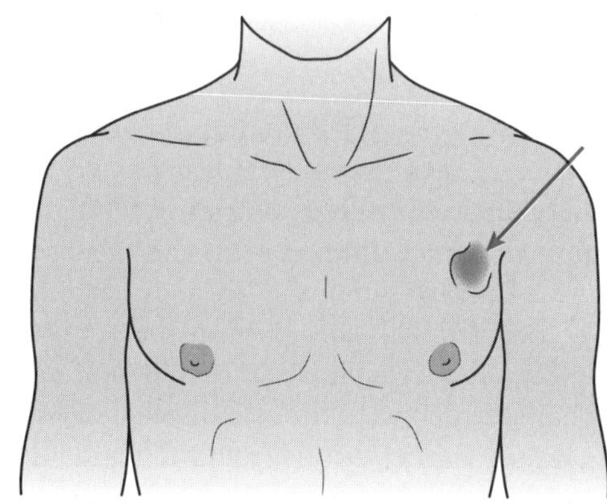

Figure 15-4: Dick Taylor's pectoralis major tear.

- ______________________________

3. Identify key terms and concepts, and then research each to broaden your knowledge about the rehabilitation of shoulder injuries.
   - What anatomical structures might be involved in Mr. Taylor's injury?

     Answer: ______________________
   - What is a grade 2 pectoralis major tear?

     Answer: ______________________
   - In which phase of healing is this injury?

     Answer: ______________________
   - Why does Mr. Taylor have decreased range of motion with adduction?

     Answer: ______________________
   - What are the origin and insertion points of the pectoralis major and minor muscles?

     Answer: ______________________
   - Define *edema*.

     Answer: ______________________
4. Based on the information that you currently have and what was provided by your instructor, how will you begin Mr. Taylor's rehabilitation?
   - ______________________________
   - ______________________________
   - ______________________________
   - ______________________________

Brain Jolt
With a pectoralis major tear, there is often a moderate amount of ecchymosis.

Why or why not?

How will Mr. Taylor's rehabilitation progress? For the *why?* portion of each exercise, explain why you chose a particular exercise or activity as part of your program. Describe which rehabilitation goals the exercise or activity covers, and describe the key indicators for progression. For the *why not?* portion of each exercise, explain why other rehabilitation exercises or activities were not chosen and what to avoid during rehabilitation for this injury. Gather details from the textbook, your own research, and data from Mr. Taylor's scenario to help formulate your answer.

Why?

- ______________________________
- ______________________________
- ______________________________
- ______________________________

Why not?

- ______________________________
- ______________________________

DETOUR

Treatment Detour

Typically, nonoperative treatment is reserved for lower-demand athletes or those with a possible partial or muscle belly rupture. Operative treatment should be considered for athletes who participate in activities that predispose them to use the pectoralis major muscle tendon unit. In nonoperative treatment, only 27% of patients have excellent results. Often, near full strength can be restored, but a cosmetic deformity often remains. If you are treating a nonoperative injury, the patient will need additional, ongoing, in-depth evaluations to prevent injury, because the specific location and extent of injury are not as concise as they would be after surgical repair (Provencher et al., 2010).

What do you think?

1. Based on your rehabilitation protocol, discuss the indicators for limited and full return to play. Include a rough timeline for return to play, if applicable, which is affected by the athlete's compliance with the rehabilitation program.
   - ______________________________
   - ______________________________
   - ______________________________
   - ______________________________

2. Are modifications or personal protective equipment needed to return to play?

■ ______________________________

■ ______________________________

STUDENT SCENARIO 3: TRAVIS MANN

Travis Mann is a receiver on his high school football team. Today at practice, the team is working on a route that has them catching the football while in an extended position. During practice, Mr. Mann performs the route, cuts to his left, and extends his body out to reach for the ball. As he does this, another teammate comes from behind him, grabs the ball, and also grabs Mr. Mann's right hand. As Mr. Mann's body makes contact with the ground, his right arm is abducted and externally rotated away from his body. This movement is due to the teammate's hold of Mr. Mann's right hand, which is clutching the ball. Mr. Mann feels a popping sensation and intense pain. An on-field examination reveals palpable anterior deformity of the humeral head and a flattened deltoid. The athletic trainer is reminded of Mr. Mann's history of right shoulder subluxation in which he completed a rehabilitation program, but which continues to cause soreness after practice. A diagnosis of an anterior shoulder dislocation is made (Fig. 15-5), the shoulder is immobilized, and he is referred for radiographic imaging.

1. Based on this scenario, what do you know about Mr. Mann's injury?

■ ______________________________

■ ______________________________

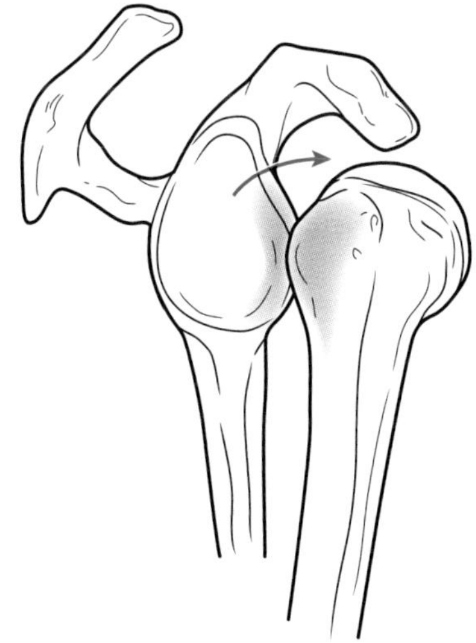

Figure 15-5: Travis Mann's anterior shoulder dislocation.

■ ______________________________

■ ______________________________

2. To rehabilitate Mr. Mann's injury effectively, you will need to gather additional information. What questions should you ask in addition to what is presented in this scenario?

■ ______________________________

■ ______________________________

■ ______________________________

■ ______________________________

3. Identify key terms and concepts, and research each to broaden your knowledge about the rehabilitation of shoulder injuries.
   - What anatomical structures might be involved in Mr. Mann's injury?

     Answer: ______________________________
   - What is an anterior shoulder dislocation?

     Answer: ______________________________
   - In which phase of healing is this injury?

     Answer: ______________________________
   - Why is there a flattened deltoid?

     Answer: ______________________________
   - In what other directions can shoulder dislocations occur?

     Answer: ______________________________
   - Did Mr. Mann's history predispose him for a dislocation? If yes, why?

     Answer: ______________________________
   - What type of rehabilitation program might Mr. Mann have completed prior for his subluxations?

     Answer: ______________________________

Conversation Buffer

Because of Mr. Mann's history, he is most likely a candidate for shoulder surgery to improve his shoulder stability. Anterior shoulder dislocation is a season-ending injury that requires at least 3 months of rehabilitation. While working with athletes such as Mr. Mann, remain positive and be encouraging during the rehabilitation program. Discuss short-term and long-term goals with the athlete, and always comment on the athlete's daily progress as a motivational tool.

4. Based on the information that you currently have and what was provided by your instructor, how will you begin Mr. Mann's rehabilitation?

- ____________________
- ____________________
- ____________________
- ____________________

Treatment Detour

Shoulder dislocations can occur in a number of sports and accidents. This related case study explored the conservative rehabilitation in a 20-year-old female wrestler who had an anterior shoulder dislocation. This program consisted of a four-phase protocol that progressively addressed specific rehabilitation goals, treatment parameters, and the minimal outcomes needed for progression to a new phase. In each phase, traditional exercises were performed, but modifications were made and new exercises were integrated to functionally reproduce the unique forces experienced during wrestling. This is important to remember. An athlete can be strong, but if his or her rehabilitation program is not sport-specific, it can delay return to play and increase the risk of further injury. After finishing the program, the female wrestler regained full ROM and strength, enabling her return to wrestling competition at the national championship level (Brumitt, Sproul, Lentz, McIntosh, & Rutt, 2009).

Why or why not?

How will Mr. Mann's rehabilitation progress? For the *why?* portion of each exercise, explain why you chose a particular exercise or activity as part of your program. Describe which rehabilitation goals the exercise or activity covers, and describe the key indicators for progression. For the *why not?* portion of each exercise, explain why other rehabilitation exercises or activities were not chosen and what to avoid during rehabilitation for this injury. Gather details from the textbook, your own research, and data from Mr. Mann's scenario to help formulate your answer.

Why?

- ____________________
- ____________________
- ____________________
- ____________________

Why not?

- ____________________
- ____________________

Brain Jolt

During the repair phase, "T-bar" exercises can be initiated as tolerated.

What do you think?

1. Based on your rehabilitation protocol, discuss indicators for limited or full return to play. Include a rough timeline for return to play, if applicable, which is affected by the athlete's compliance with the rehabilitation program.

- ____________________
- ____________________
- ____________________
- ____________________

2. Are modifications or personal protective equipment needed to return to play?

- ____________________
- ____________________

STUDENT SCENARIO 4: JERRY HOLCOMB

Jerry Holcomb is a javelin thrower on his college team. For the past 2 weeks, he has experienced some numbness with his left throwing arm. The numbness travels down into his fingers. When he throws the javelin, his left arm comes across his body, which causes pain around his trapezius. He states that his performance is not affected by this discomfort although he experiences atrophy in his trapezius, deltoid, and pectoralis muscles. He is evaluated by the certified athletic trainer, and thoracic outlet syndrome is diagnosed (Fig. 15-6). He exhibits muscle atrophy, positive Allen and Roos test results, numbness in his fingers, and pain.

1. Based on this scenario, what do you know about Mr. Holcomb's injury?
   - ______________________________
   - ______________________________
   - ______________________________
   - ______________________________

2. To rehabilitate Mr. Holcomb's injury effectively, you will need to gather additional information. What questions should you ask in addition to what is presented in this scenario?
   - ______________________________
   - ______________________________
   - ______________________________
   - ______________________________

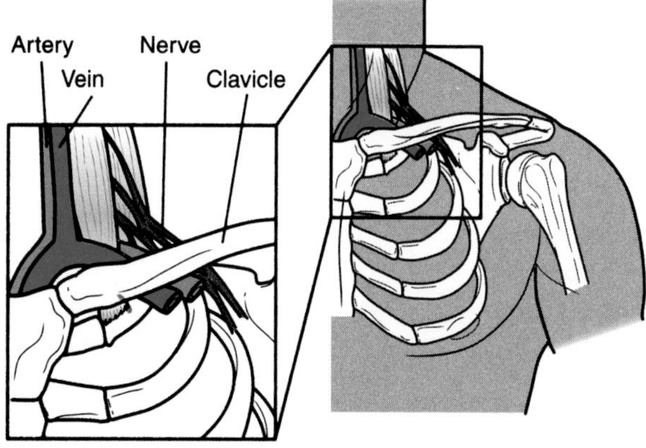

Figure 15-6: Jerry Holcomb's thoracic outlet syndrome.

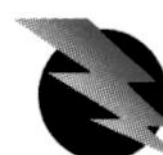

Brain Jolt

An anatomical defect could be causing this condition. Be sure to correct the anatomical condition through anterior stretching and posterior strengthening.

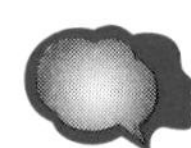

Conversation Buffer

Explain to the athlete that if a thoracic outlet syndrome injury is left untreated, it could cause permanent nerve damage. It is important to start a rehabilitation program to address the atrophy and compressive issues.

3. Identify key terms and concepts, and research each to broaden your knowledge about the rehabilitation of shoulder injuries.
   - What anatomical structures might be involved in Mr. Holcomb's injury?

     Answer: ______________________________
   - What is thoracic outlet syndrome?

     Answer: ______________________________
   - In which phase of healing is this injury?

     Answer: ______________________________
   - Define *atrophy*.

     Answer: ______________________________
   - What is the Allen test? What does it test? What does a positive sign indicate?

     Answer: ______________________________
   - What is the Roos test? What does it test? What does a positive sign indicate?

     Answer: ______________________________
   - What might numbness into the fingers indicate?

     Answer: ______________________________

4. Based on the information that you currently have and what was provided by your instructor, how will you begin Mr. Holcomb's rehabilitation?
   - ______________________________
   - ______________________________
   - ______________________________
   - ______________________________

Why or why not?

How will Mr. Holcomb's rehabilitation progress? For the *why?* portion of each exercise, explain why you chose a particular exercise or activity as part of your program. Describe which rehabilitation goals the exercise or activity covers, and describe the key indicators for progression. For the *why not?* portion of each exercise, explain why other rehabilitation exercises or activities were not chosen and what to avoid during rehabilitation for this injury. Gather details from the textbook, your own research, and data from Mr. Holcomb's scenario to help formulate your answer.

Why?

- ______________________________
- ______________________________
- ______________________________
- ______________________________

Why not?

- ______________________________
- ______________________________

What do you think?

1. Based on your rehabilitation protocol, discuss the indicators for a limited and full return to play. Include a rough timeline for return to play, if applicable, which is affected by the athlete's compliance with the rehabilitation program.
   - ______________________________
   - ______________________________
   - ______________________________
   - ______________________________
2. Are modifications or personal protective equipment needed to return to play?
   - ______________________________
   - ______________________________

STUDENT SCENARIO 5: WENDY MURPHY

Wendy Murphy is a collegiate swimmer who swims freestyle. She has experienced shoulder soreness because of decreased ROM of her right shoulder. During winter break, the swim team travels to Florida to train for 1 week. During this time, the team swims almost 10,000 m/day. Ms. Murphy is not able to do her normal activity warm-up at the different facility, which consists of stretching, heat, and massage. Upon returning to school, the certified athletic trainer learns that Ms. Murphy was held from activity for the last 2 days of winter training because of pain and soreness in her right shoulder. On examination, Ms. Murphy is point tender over the subacromial space; has atrophy of the deltoid muscle, anterior edema at the coracoacromial arch, and 3/5 decreased supraspinatus strength; and receives a positive empty can and Hawkins-Kennedy test result. A grade 2 shoulder impingement is diagnosed (Fig. 15-7).

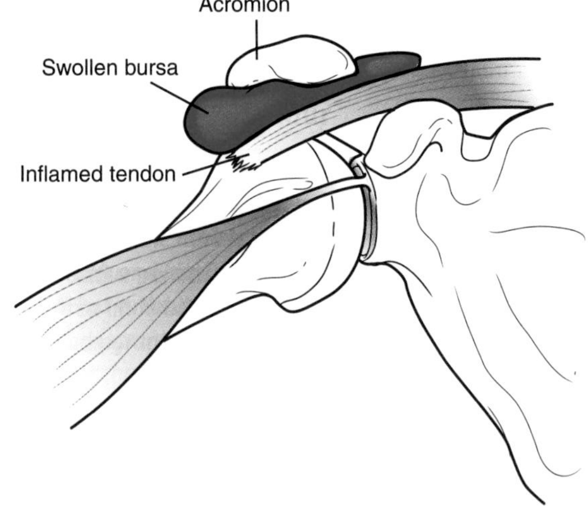

Figure 15-7: Wendy Murphy's impingement syndrome.

1. Based on this scenario, what do you know about Ms. Murphy's injury?
   - ______________________
   - ______________________
   - ______________________
   - ______________________

2. To rehabilitate Ms. Murphy's injury effectively, you will need to gather additional information. What questions should you ask in addition to what is presented in this scenario?
   - ______________________
   - ______________________
   - ______________________
   - ______________________

3. Identify key terms and concepts, and then research each to broaden your knowledge about rehabilitation of shoulder injuries.
   - What anatomical structures might be involved in Ms. Murphy's injury?

     Answer: ______________________
   - What is a grade 2 impingement syndrome?

     Answer: ______________________
   - In which phase of healing is this injury?

     Answer: ______________________
   - Define *atrophy*.

     Answer: ______________________
   - Define *edema*.

     Answer: ______________________
   - Describe the coracoacromial space.

     Answer: ______________________
   - What is the empty can test? What does it test? What does a positive test indicate?

     Answer: ______________________
   - What is a Hawkins-Kennedy test? What does it test? What does a positive test indicate?

     Answer: ______________________

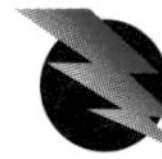

Brain Jolt

Be sure to strengthen the muscles that compress and depress the humeral head, along with the musculature that activates the scapula and external rotators.

4. Based on the information that you currently have and what was provided by your instructor, how will you begin Ms. Murphy's rehabilitation?
   - ______________________
   - ______________________
   - ______________________
   - ______________________

Treatment Detour

One group of researchers performed a study to examine the amount of muscle activation using electromyography in four scapular muscles: the serratus anterior, upper trapezius, middle trapezius, and lower trapezius in overhead athletes (athletes who carry sports items overhead or who throw sports items from an overhead position) with and without a history of impingement during three upper-extremity closed-chain exercises. These exercises included a standard push-up, a push-up on a BOSU (both sides utilized) sport-balance trainer, and the cuff link exercise using a shoulder rehabilitation device. It was concluded that the activation of the middle trapezius differs in overhead athletes with and without a history of secondary shoulder impingement during closed-chain exercises. The other muscles were similar between groups. The results suggested that closed-chain exercises are good to use in rehabilitation of this condition in overhead athletes and that clinicians should carefully select exercises that address individual muscles of interest to ensure the most effective and timely rehabilitation (Tucker, Armstrong, Gribble, Timmons, & Yeasting, 2010).

Why or why not?

How will Ms. Murphy's rehabilitation progress? For the *why?* portion of each exercise, explain why you chose a particular exercise or activity as part of your program. Describe which rehabilitation goals the exercise or activity covers, and describe the key indicators for progression. For the *why not?* portion of each exercise, explain why other rehabilitation exercises or activities were not chosen and what to avoid during rehabilitation for this injury. Gather details from the textbook, your own research, and data from Ms. Murphy's scenario to help formulate your answer.

Why?

- ______________________________
- ______________________________
- ______________________________
- ______________________________

Why not?

- ______________________________
- ______________________________

What do you think?

1. Based on your rehabilitation protocol, discuss the indicators for a limited and full return to play. Include a rough timeline for return to play, if applicable, which is affected by the athlete's compliance with the rehabilitation program.
   - ______________________________
   - ______________________________
   - ______________________________
   - ______________________________
2. Are modifications or personal protective equipment needed to return to play?
   - ______________________________
   - ______________________________

STUDENT SCENARIO 6: RICK EWING

Rick Ewing is an offensive lineman on the school football team. He has a history of right anterior shoulder dislocations and has completed a rehabilitation program, but he continues to have shoulder instability. At yesterday's practice, he experienced subluxation to his right shoulder. He is accustomed to the pain and soreness that can occur for a few days after activity, based on his history. However, this time, the pain is different and does not subside. He has limited active ROM past 90 degrees, moderate edema, and a positive clunk test. The team orthopedist orders an MRI, which shows a Bankart lesion (Fig. 15-8). Because of Mr. Ewing's history, surgery is required to mend the labrum tear.

1. Based on this scenario, what do you know about Mr. Ewing's injury?
   - ______________________________
   - ______________________________
   - ______________________________
   - ______________________________
2. To rehabilitate Mr. Ewing's injury effectively, you will need to gather additional information. What

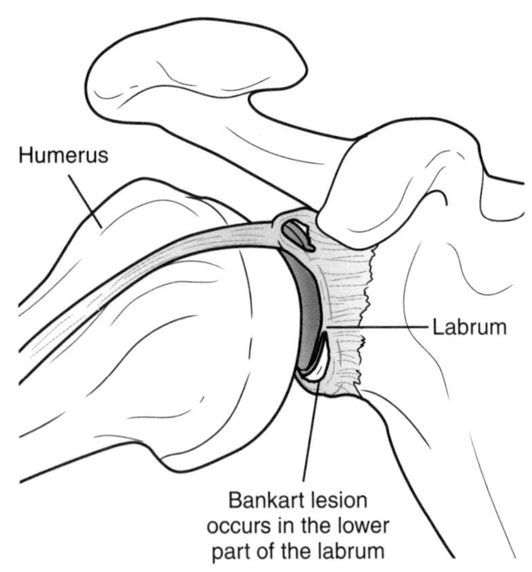

Figure 15-8: Rick Ewing's labrum tear.

questions should you ask in addition to what is presented in this scenario?

- ______________________________
- ______________________________
- ______________________________
- ______________________________

Brain Jolt
Remember that labrum tears can occur because of previous injuries; therefore, the athlete may be asymptomatic until that tear is inflamed or the labrum tear is caught with glenohumeral joint motion. Do not allow the most recent mechanism of injury to blur your current evaluation.

3. Identify any key terms and concepts, and research each to broaden your knowledge about the rehabilitation of shoulder injuries.
   - What anatomical structures might be involved in Mr. Ewing's injury?

     Answer: ______________________________
   - What is a labrum tear?

     Answer: ______________________________
   - In which phase of healing is this injury?

     Answer: ______________________________
   - Define *dislocation*.

     Answer: ______________________________
   - Define *subluxation*.

     Answer: ______________________________
   - What is a clunk test? What does it test? What does a positive test indicate?

     Answer: ______________________________
   - What is a Bankart lesion?

     Answer: ______________________________
   - What other types of lesions to the labrum can occur?

     Answer: ______________________________
   - Did Mr. Ewing's shoulder instability predispose him to injury of the labrum?

     Answer: ______________________________
   - What movements should be limited for Mr. Ewing?

     Answer: ______________________________

4. Based on the information that you currently have and what was provided by your instructor, how will you begin Mr. Ewing's rehabilitation?
   - ______________________________
   - ______________________________
   - ______________________________
   - ______________________________

Why or why not?

How will Mr. Ewing's rehabilitation progress? For the *why?* portion of each exercise, explain why you chose a particular exercise or activity as part of your program. Describe which rehabilitation goals the exercise or activity covers, and describe the key indicators for progression. For the *why not?* portion of each exercise, explain why other rehabilitation exercises or activities were not chosen and what to avoid during rehabilitation for this injury. Gather details from the textbook, your own research, and data from Mr. Ewing's scenario to help formulate your answer.

Why?

- ______________________________
- ______________________________
- ______________________________
- ______________________________

Why not?

- ______________________________
- ______________________________

What do you think?

1. Based on your rehabilitation protocol, discuss the indicators for limited and full return to play. Include a rough timeline for return to play, if

applicable, which is affected by the athlete's compliance with the rehabilitation program.

- ____________________
- ____________________
- ____________________
- ____________________

2. Are modifications or personal protective equipment needed to return to play?
   - ____________________
   - ____________________

STUDENT SCENARIO 7: PEGGY VANZANT

Peggy VanZant is a tennis player who plays singles. For the last 2 weeks, she has noticed pain at her right biceps tendon when she is performing arm flexion. The pain previously occurred just after activity, but is now occurring during activity. She ices the area after practice, which brings some relief, but the pain is still present when she is performing the forehand movement. She decides to ask the certified athletic trainer to examine her right bicep brachii. On examination, she has edema over the biceps tendon, crepitus with forward movement, a positive Yergason test result, and 4/5 decreased strength with active resistive elbow flexion. A diagnosis of grade 1 bicipital tendonitis is made (Fig. 15-9).

1. Based on this scenario, what do you know about Ms. VanZant's injury?
   - ____________________

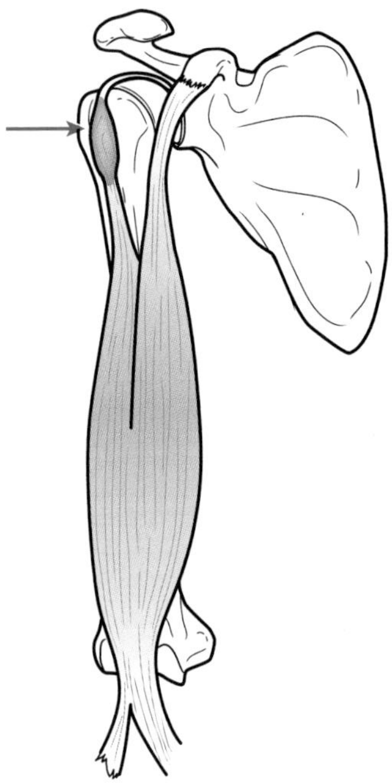

Figure 15-9: Peggy VanZant's bicipital tendonitis.

- ____________________
- ____________________
- ____________________

2. To rehabilitate Ms. VanZant's injury effectively, you will need to gather additional information. What questions should you ask in addition to what is presented in this scenario?
   - ____________________
   - ____________________
   - ____________________
   - ____________________

Brain Jolt
Your initial rehabilitation goal is to reduce the inflammation to the biceps tendon.

3. Identify key terms and concepts, and then research each to broaden your knowledge about the rehabilitation of shoulder injuries.
   - What anatomical structures might be involved in Ms. VanZant's injury?

     Answer: ____________________
   - What is grade 1 bicipital tendonitis?

     Answer: ____________________
   - In which phase of healing is this injury?

     Answer: ____________________

- Define *edema*.

  Answer: ______

- What is the Yergason test? What does it test? What does a positive test indicate?

  Answer: ______

- Define *crepitus*.

  Answer: ______

4. Based on the information that you currently have and what was provided by your instructor, how will you begin Ms. VanZant's rehabilitation?

- ______
- ______
- ______
- ______

Why or why not?

How will Ms. VanZant's rehabilitation progress? For the *why?* portion of each exercise, explain why you chose a particular exercise or activity as part of your program. Describe which rehabilitation goals the exercise or activity covers, and describe the key indicators for progression. For the *why not?* portion of each exercise, explain why other rehabilitation exercises or activities were not chosen and what to avoid during rehabilitation for this injury. Gather details from the textbook, your own research, and data from Ms. VanZant's scenario to help formulate your answer.

Why?

- ______
- ______
- ______
- ______

Why not?

- ______
- ______

What do you think?

1. Based on your rehabilitation protocol, discuss the indicators for limited and full return to play. Include a rough timeline for return to play, if applicable, which is affected by the athlete's compliance with the rehabilitation program.

- ______
- ______
- ______
- ______

2. Are modifications or personal protective equipment needed to return to play?

- ______
- ______

STUDENT SCENARIO 8: BRYCE MCDANIEL

Bryce McDaniel is a collegiate baseball player with a history of subluxations of his right shoulder. He states that he feels a forward or anterior slippage movement in his shoulder when he pitches. On examination, Mr. McDaniel has a moderate amount of effusion, a positive anterior apprehension test result, a positive clunk test result, and point tenderness over the anterior aspect of the shoulder. He is referred to the team physician who orders an MRI to confirm multidirectional instability. The MRI results show an anterior-inferior slippage of the humeral head and a SLAP (superior labrum, anterior to posterior) lesion. Because there is more than one anatomical plane that demonstrates laxity, it is determined that Mr. McDaniel has multidirectional instability (Fig. 15-10). He will need surgery to correct this injury.

1. Based on this scenario, what do you know about Mr. McDaniel's injury?

- ______________________________
- ______________________________
- ______________________________
- ______________________________

2. To rehabilitate Mr. McDaniel's injury effectively, you will need to gather additional information. What questions should you ask in addition to what is presented in this scenario?

- ______________________________
- ______________________________
- ______________________________
- ______________________________

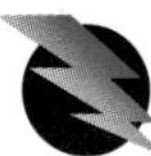

Brain Jolt

A repetitive activity or movement of the shoulder joint can produce soft tissue laxity without any traumatic event as the cause. Anterior and posterior instability are specific to the structures needing to be strengthened.

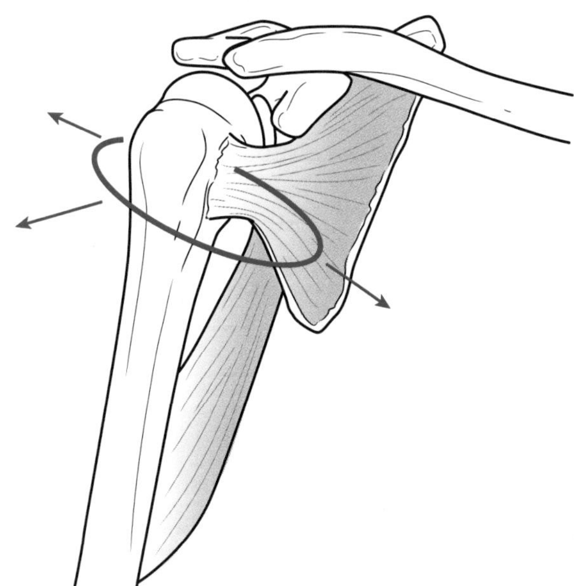

Figure 15-10: Bryce McDaniel's multidirectional instability.

3. Identify key terms and concepts, and then research each to broaden your knowledge about rehabilitation of shoulder injuries.

- What anatomical structures might be involved in Mr. McDaniel's injury?

  Answer: ______________________________
- What is multidirectional instability?

  Answer: ______________________________
- In which phase of healing is this injury?

  Answer: ______________________________
- Define *effusion*.

  Answer: ______________________________
- Explain an anterior-inferior slippage of the humeral head.

  Answer: ______________________________
- What is an anterior apprehension test? What does it test? What would a positive test indicate?

  Answer: ______________________________
- What is a clunk test? What does it test? What would a positive test indicate?

  Answer: ______________________________
- What is a SLAP lesion?

  Answer: ______________________________

4. Based on the information that you currently have and what was provided by your instructor, how will you begin Mr. McDaniel's rehabilitation?

- ______________________________
- ______________________________
- ______________________________
- ______________________________

Why or why not?

How will Mr. McDaniel's rehabilitation progress? For the *why?* portion of each exercise, explain why you chose a particular exercise or activity as part of your program. Describe which rehabilitation goals the exercise or activity covers, and describe the key indicators for progression. For the *why not?* portion of each exercise, explain why other rehabilitation exercises or activities were not chosen and what to avoid during rehabilitation for this injury. Gather details from the textbook, your own research, and data from Mr. McDaniel's scenario to help formulate your answer.

Why?

- ______________________________
- ______________________________
- ______________________________
- ______________________________

Why not?

- ______________________________
- ______________________________

What do you think?

1. Based on your rehabilitation protocol, discuss the indicators for limited and full return to play. Include a rough timeline for return to play, if applicable, which is affected by the athlete's compliance with the rehabilitation program.
   - ______________________________
   - ______________________________
   - ______________________________
   - ______________________________
2. Are modifications or personal protective equipment needed to return to play?
   - ______________________________
   - ______________________________

STUDENT SCENARIO 9: JIMMY HAMILTON

Jimmy Hamilton is a point guard on his college basketball team. He is dribbling the ball when an opposing player tries to steal it. The opposing player runs into Mr. Hamilton, catching him off guard and causing him to fall to the ground and land on his outstretched right hand. Mr. Hamilton feels a sharp pain and is unable to abduct his shoulder to 90 degrees without discomfort. He is removed from the game and is evaluated by the certified athletic trainer. On evaluation, he has pain at the acromioclavicular (AC) joint, moderate edema, inability to abduct his arm past 90 degrees without pain, and a positive AC distraction test. A diagnosis of a grade 2 AC separation is made (Fig. 15-11), and his arm is placed in a sling.

1. Based on this scenario, what do you know about Mr. Hamilton's injury?
   - ______________________________
   - ______________________________

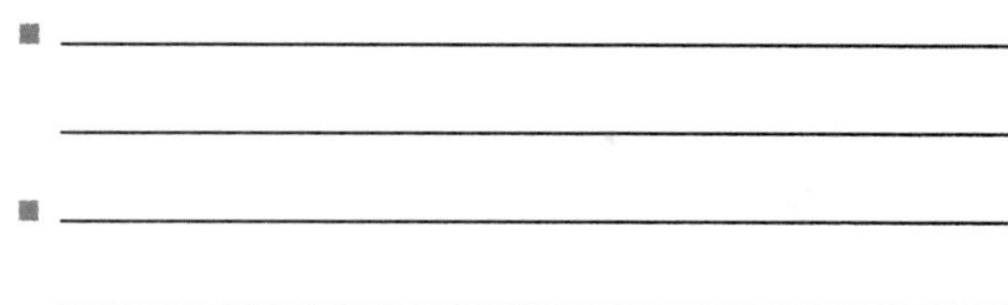

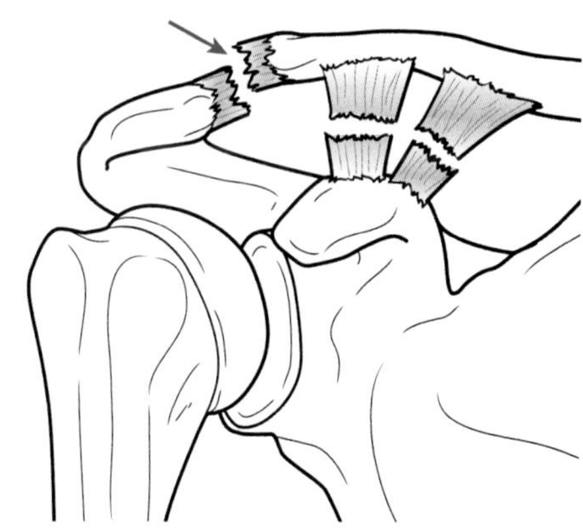

Figure 15-11: Jimmy Hamilton's acromioclavicular joint separation.

2. To rehabilitate Mr. Hamilton's injury effectively, you will need to gather additional information. What questions should you ask in addition to what is presented in this scenario?

- ______________________________
- ______________________________
- ______________________________
- ______________________________

Brain Jolt
A foosh (falling on an outstretched hand) injury can also be a mechanism of injury for an AC sprain or separation.

3. Identify key terms and concepts, and then research each to broaden your knowledge about rehabilitation of shoulder injuries.

- What anatomical structures might be involved in Mr. Hamilton's injury?

  Answer: ______________________________
- What is a grade 2 AC sprain?

  Answer: ______________________________
- In which phase of healing is this injury?

  Answer: ______________________________
- Define *edema*.

  Answer: ______________________________
- What is an AC distraction test? What does it test? What does a positive test indicate?

  Answer: ______________________________
- Why are movements past 90 degrees painful for Mr. Hamilton?

  Answer: ______________________________
- What are the different grades of AC sprains and separations? Explain each grade.

  Answer: ______________________________

4. Based on the information that you currently have and what was provided by your instructor, how will you begin Mr. Hamilton's rehabilitation?

- ______________________________
- ______________________________
- ______________________________
- ______________________________

Brain Jolt
Appropriate protection (e.g., sling or padding) should be worn until there is no pain and full ROM returns.

Why or why not?

How will Mr. Hamilton's rehabilitation progress? For the *why?* portion of each exercise, explain why you chose a particular exercise or activity as part of your program. Describe which rehabilitation goals the exercise or activity covers, and describe the key indicators for progression. For the *why not?* portion of each exercise, explain why other rehabilitation exercises or activities were not chosen and what to avoid during rehabilitation for this injury. Gather details from the textbook, your own research, and data from Mr. Hamilton's scenario to help formulate your answer.

Why?

- ______________________________
- ______________________________
- ______________________________
- ______________________________

Why not?

- ______________________________
- ______________________________

What do you think?

1. Based on your rehabilitation protocol, discuss the indicators for limited and full return to play. Include a rough timeline for return to play, if applicable, which is affected by the athlete's compliance with the rehabilitation program.
   - ______________________________
   - ______________________________
   - ______________________________
   - ______________________________

2. Are modifications or personal protective equipment needed to return to play?
   - ______________________________
   - ______________________________

knowledge checklist

Table 15-1 offers a checklist that can be used by a peer, instructor, or preceptor to evaluate each part of the athlete's rehabilitation plan. Use this checklist as a tool to ensure that the rehabilitation plan is complete and to assess your knowledge of the competencies that apply to this chapter.

TABLE 15-1 ■ Upper Extremity: The Shoulder Rehabilitation and Therapeutic Exercise Competency Checklist

	Proficient *Can demonstrate and execute the skill properly*	**Proficient With Assistance** *Can demonstrate and execute the skill with minimal guidance or tips*	**Not Proficient** *Unable to demonstrate and execute the skill properly; need to be reevaluated at another time after further study and practice*
Controlling Edema			
PRICE			
Modalities			
Controlling Pain			
Pain scales			
Medications			
Modalities			
Establishes Core Stability			
Reestablishes Neuromuscular Control			
Restores Postural Control and Balance			
Restoring Range of Motion			
Passive range of motion			
Active range of motion			
Resistive range of motion			
Goniometry			
Normal range of motion limits			
Restore Muscular Strength, Endurance, and Power			
Open kinetic chain			
Closed kinetic chain			
Isometric			
Isotonic			
Isotonic (concentric and eccentric)			
Isokinetic			
Plyometric			
Agility			
Functional or Sport-Specific Activities			
Maintains Cardiorespiratory Fitness			
Functional Testing			
Return-to-Play Criteria			
Proper Documentation			

PRICE, prevention, rest, ice, compression, and elevation.

REFERENCES

Brumitt, J., Sproul, A., Lentz, P., McIntosh, L., & Rutt, R. (2009). In season rehabilitation of a Division III female wrestler after a glenohumeral dislocation. *Physical Therapy in Sport, 10*, 112–117.

Higgins, M. (2011). *Therapeutic exercise from theory to practice.* Philadelphia, PA: F.A. Davis.

National Athletic Training Association. (2011). *Athletic training education competencies* (5th ed.). Retrieved from http://www.nata.org/sites/default/files/5th-Edition-Competencies-2011-PDF-Version.pdf

Prentice, W. (2010). *Arnheim's principles of athletic training: A competency-based approach* (14th ed.). New York, NY: McGraw-Hill.

Prentice, W. E. (2011). *Rehabilitation techniques for sports medicine and athletic training* (5th ed.). New York, NY: McGraw-Hill.

Provencher, M. T., Handfield, K., Boniquit, N. T., Reiff, S. N., Sekiya, J. K., & Romeo, A. A. (2010). Injuries to the pectoralis major muscle: Diagnosis and management. *The American Journal of Sports Medicine, 38*, 1693–1705.

Starkey, C. (2004). *Therapeutic modalities* (3rd ed.). Philadelphia, PA: F.A. Davis.

Starkey, C., Brown, S. D., & Ryan, J. (2010). *Examination of orthopedic and athletic injuries* (3rd ed.). Philadelphia, PA: F.A. Davis.

Tucker, W. S., Armstrong, C. W., Gribble, P. A., Timmons, M. K., & Yeasting, R. A. (2010). Scapular muscle activity in overhead athletes with symptoms of secondary shoulder impingement during closed chain exercises. *Archives of Physical Medicine and Rehabilitation, 91*, 550–556.

Venes, D. (Ed.). (2009). *Taber's cyclopedic medical dictionary* (21st ed.). Philadelphia, PA: F.A. Davis.

chapter 16

The Head, Neck, and Trunk

chapter outline

athletic trainer's corner

Here is what one athletic trainer experienced while rehabilitating an athlete's injury:

In the third period of Tommy Davis' wrestling match, with 30 seconds remaining, he was brought down on the back of his head and neck by the opponent. The official instantly blew his whistle to stop the match as Mr. Davis laid motionless. At first I thought he was unconscious. Was he breathing? Had he broken his neck? As I approached Mr. Davis, I saw that he was breathing, his eyes were open, and he was responsive. After evaluating him on the mat, I determined that he had no cervical spine tenderness, no numbness or paraesthesia into his extremities, and no symptoms of a concussion. However, he had point tenderness over the left upper trapezius muscle. Two days after the injury, he saw an orthopedist to rule out anything other than an upper trapezius strain. For the next 2 weeks, Mr. Davis was taught a noncontact practice regiment. He continued to have upper trapezius pain when he rotated his head from side to side. His rehabilitation program included lateral neck side bending stretches, head rotation stretches, and a gentle massage over the upper trapezius. He was also taught strengthening exercises such as shoulder shrugs, isometric neck rotation, and side bending sets. It was important for him to maintain his cardiovascular level; therefore, he was taught a stationary bike interval program. The stationary bike was brought into wrestling practice so that Mr. Davis could do his interval program while watching the team practice. As a result, Mr. Davis still felt like a part of the team. I can still see Mr. Davis lying there on the mat, but I am thankful that an upper trapezius strain was our only concern.

Lori Ulrich, AT, ATC
Head Athletic Trainer, Eaton High School
Dayton Sports Medicine Institute
Dayton, Ohio

learning outcomes

After working through this chapter, you will be able to:

1. Describe seven different goals of rehabilitation and the importance of each in the overall rehabilitation protocol.
2. Verbalize indications for performing head, neck, and trunk rehabilitative techniques.
3. Discuss modifications and progressions that are used during a rehabilitation program for the head, neck, and trunk.
4. Discuss outcome measures used to identify activity levels and return-to-play guidelines for head, neck, and trunk injuries.
5. Explain what modality choice is proper for rehabilitation by using indications and contraindications and the principles and theory related to the physiological response of the intervention.

MODEL SCENARIO 1: MIGUEL LOPEZ

Miguel Lopez is a collegiate tennis player who is currently in preseason training. While practicing his serve, he feels a sharp pain in his abdomen. He moves around a bit and then decides that he is fine, so he serves again. The pain is now worse, and he goes to see the athletic trainer. He has no history of injury. On evaluation, he is point tender over his upper abdomen, which is painful with trunk extension, and the sharp pain is reproduced with trunk flexion. There is no abdominal rigidity present and no other signs and symptoms of any general medical condition. A diagnosis of rectus abdominis strain is made (Fig. 16-1).

1. Based on this scenario, what do you know about Mr. Lopez's injury?
   - *Male athlete*
   - *Tennis player*
   - *Mechanism of injury: trunk extension during a tennis serve*
   - *No previous injury*
   - *Pain with trunk extension*

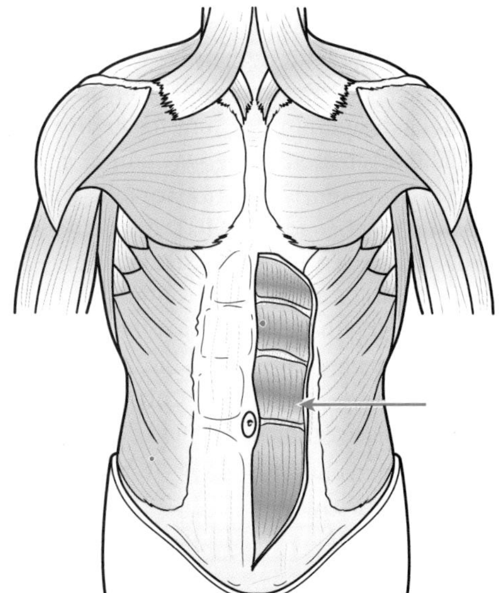

Figure 16-1: Miguel Lopez's rectus abdominis strain.

   - *Sharp pain reproduced with trunk flexion*
   - *No abdominal rigidity*
   - *No signs and symptoms of general medical condition*
2. To rehabilitate Mr. Lopez's injury effectively, you will need to gather additional information. What questions should you ask in addition to what is presented in this scenario?
   - *Are there any preexisting injuries? If yes, what are they?*
   - *How long has the athlete experienced this pain?*
   - *What is the athlete's pain level and type of pain felt?*
   - *What is the level of strength in the abdominals?*
   - *Does the athlete have any numbness or paraesthesia?*
   - *What is the range of motion (ROM) of the trunk?*
3. Identify key terms and concepts, and research each to broaden your knowledge about the rehabilitation of head, neck and trunk injuries.
   - What anatomical structures might be involved in Mr. Lopez's injury?
     Rectus abdominis
     Transverse abdominis
     Internal and external oblique
     Internal organs of abdominal cavity
   - What is a rectus abdominis strain?
     Trauma to the rectus abdominis muscle from a violent contraction or excessive force
   - In which phase of healing is this injury?
     Acute inflammatory phase
   - What part of a muscle is most often injured?
     Near the insertion point of the muscle
   - Where does the power of a tennis serve originate?
     The core
   - What other medical conditions should you rule out when abdominal pain is present?
     Appendicitis
     Acute spleen
     "Hot" gallbladder
     Gastrointestinal issues
   - Define *rigidity*.
     Tenseness, immovability, stiffness

4. Based on the information that you currently have and what was provided by your instructor, how will you begin Mr. Lopez's rehabilitation?
   The core needs to be strengthened without motion initially because pain is present. Begin with the quadruped cat-camel exercise to gain some ROM and gentle contraction while drawing the abdomen toward the spine. Once the pain has decreased, try modified planks on the knees to again increase strength without ROM.

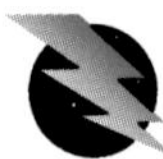

Brain Jolt

Sometimes, abdominal strains can be challenging to rehabilitate. Remember that the core is the back's main stabilizer. When strengthening the back, be sure to instruct the athlete to draw the abdominal muscles to the spine to gain the most strength while protecting the spine.

Why or why not?

How will Mr. Lopez's rehabilitation progress? For the *why?* portion of each exercise, explain why you chose a particular exercise or activity as part of your program. Describe which rehabilitation goals the exercise or activity covers, and describe the key indicators for progression. For the *why not?* portion of each exercise, explain why other rehabilitation exercises or activities were not chosen and what to avoid during rehabilitation for this injury. Gather details from the textbook, your own research, and data from Mr. Lopez's scenario to help formulate your answer.

Why?

- ***Quadruped cat-camel.*** *This activity will help with the rehabilitation goal of gaining some gentle ROM and strength without stressing the rectus abdominis too much. This activity also teaches the athlete to draw the core toward the spine to gain the best position for strengthening while protecting the spine. This exercise can be advanced by extending one arm at a time and then extending one leg at a time. Once this is no longer challenging to the athlete, it can be performed simultaneously with ipsilateral extremities.*
- ***Planks.*** *This exercise will help with the rehabilitation goal of increasing strength without a lot of ROM. It is first performed in the modified position on the knees and then progressed to the push-up position. Again, the drawing in of the abdomen toward the spine needs to be emphasized to protect the spine and maintain the neutral position.*
- ***Eccentric crunches.*** *This activity can help with the rehabilitation goal of increasing strength once the athlete has decreased pain and has pain-free ROM. This exercise is performed to increase strength, but in a slow eccentric motion that helps to restore the muscle in the motion that it was injured. Once this is performed by the athlete with ease, the concentric phase can be added to achieve the full crunch motion.*

Why not?

- *Initially, avoid any exercises that involve too much motion or that are not comfortable for the athlete to perform.*

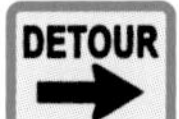

Treatment Detour

In order to return to play after an abdominal or back injury, it is crucial to have a structured core stabilization program that allows constant reevaluation and guided exercises. The authors of one study have a five-level program that gradually increases strength, endurance, and proprioception, which are the main goals of any core rehabilitation. The abdomen and back go hand-in-hand during a rehabilitation program. Initially, it is emphasized that the patient must find his or her neutral position and perform exercises holding this position isometrically. This activity trains the core muscles to protect the spine and is the cornerstone to the program, because the patient can develop proprioceptive feedback of the core muscles. The program then progresses through different levels of difficulty and then to sport-specific exercises (Schlink & Watkins, 2011).

What do you think?

1. Based on your rehabilitation protocol, discuss the indicators for limited and full return to play with the athlete. Include a rough timeline for return to play, if applicable, which is affected by the athlete's compliance with the rehabilitation program.
   - ***Limited return to play.*** *The athlete can return to play with limited participation that involves limited ROM and no large motions once the rehabilitation exercises can be performed without pain. The athlete can participate in conditioning once he or she does not experience any pain.*
   - ***Full return to play.*** *The athlete can attain full return-to-play status once he or she is pain free and exhibits ROM and good strength. Focus on strengthening the core, because this can return the athlete to functional activities.*
2. Are modifications or personal protective equipment needed to return to play?
   - *No*

MODEL SCENARIO 2: TYREESE JAMES

Tyreese James is a freshman who plays second-string defensive linebacker on his college football team. Because an upper classman has been injured, Mr. James is put on the field during today's game. He reads the offense and drops back while the wide receiver sprints and is seconds from catching the ball. Mr. James charges forward to tackle the wide receiver. As the opponent jumps up to catch the ball, Mr. James lowers his head and shoulder for the tackle. He is so focused on completing the tackle that he does not remember the basic tackling techniques that he has been taught. He lowers his head as he tackles the opponent, causing his spine to become straight as he makes contact with the opponent's thigh. (This event is known as *axial loading*.) Mr. James drops to the ground. The certified athletic trainer finds Mr. James lying face down on the field but conscious and immediately stabilizes the cervical spine. The athletic training staff members log roll Mr. James to a supine position while maintaining cervical spine stabilization. An assessment reveals that he has cervical pain, bilateral numbness in his arms, and bilateral paraesthesia in his toes. He has loss of sensation to his upper trunk, but has mild movement at his feet. The emergency action plan is activated and paramedics are called. The certified athletic trainer continues to stabilize Mr. James' cervical spine as his face mask and shoulder pads are cut away, but not removed, before he is placed on a spine board for transport. Upon arrival at the emergency department, Mr. James is assessed and prepared for imaging. The radiographs show a C5 cervical fracture (Fig. 16-2). There is no cervical dislocation. Further testing with a computed tomography scan and magnetic resonance imaging (MRI) are performed to determine the spinal cord integrity.

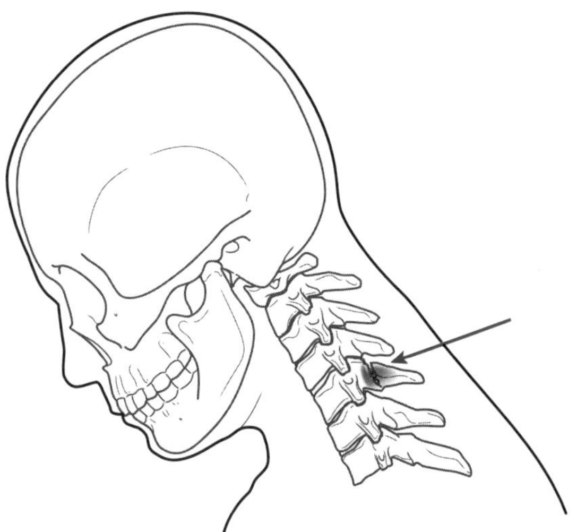

Figure 16-2: Tyreese James' cervical vertebrae fracture.

1. Based on this scenario, what do you know about Mr. James' injury?
   - *Male athlete*
   - *Football player, defensive linebacker*
   - *Mechanism of injury: head down while tackling*
   - *Cervical pain*
   - *Numbness and paraesthesia into the extremities*
   - *No loss of consciousness*
   - *Emergency action plan activated*
   - *Spine boarded and transported*
2. To rehabilitate Mr. James' injury effectively, you will need to gather additional information. What questions should you ask in addition to what is presented in this scenario?
   - *Are there any preexisting injuries? If yes, what are they?*
   - *How long has the athlete experienced this pain?*
   - *What is the athlete's pain level and type of pain felt?*
   - *What is the strength in the extremities?*
   - *Does the athlete have any numbness or paraesthesia?*
   - *Is there voluntary movement in the extremities?*
   - *Are there any signs of shock?*

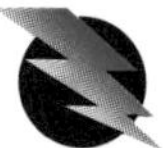

Brain Jolt

Many cervical fractures occur between C4 and C6.

3. Identify key terms and concepts, and then research each to broaden your knowledge about the rehabilitation of head, neck, and trunk injuries.
   - What anatomical structures might be involved in Mr. James' injury?
     Skull, brain
     Spinal cord
     Cervical vertebrae
     Nerve roots
   - What is a cervical fracture?
     It is a fracture that occurs to cervical vertebrae because of axial loading, twisting, or a direct blow to the cervical spine.
   - In which phase of healing is this injury?
     This injury occurs at the inflammatory response phase.
   - Explain the log roll technique.
     The log roll technique is performed with a minimum of three people, but preferably five to six people. The head is stabilized by one individual who controls the technique of the roll. Position one of the patient's arms up and by the ear, and prepare to roll the patient to that side. The shoulder, hip, lower leg, and feet are controlled by another person while turning the patient over. On the command of the individual stabilizing the patient's neck, everyone at the same time performs a smooth inline body roll. The athlete is now on his or her back and can be assessed and treated more effectively.

- Why are Mr. James' face mask and shoulder pads cut away, but not removed, while he is still on the field?
  The athletic training staff has to be prepared for any type of emergency resuscitation that might be needed because of this injury. With the face mask removed, the jaw thrust maneuver can be performed if cardiopulmonary resuscitation is necessary. The shoulder pads are cut away by cutting the strings that tighten them in the front. As a result, the chest can be exposed for any necessary application of an automated external defibrillator.
- Why are the helmet and shoulder pads not completely removed?
  Taking off the helmet and leaving the shoulder pads puts the cervical spine into extension. The opposite happens to the cervical spine if the shoulder pads are removed and the helmet is kept on. The cervical spine goes into slight flexion. With the possibility of any type of cervical injury, always maintain the cervical spine in a straight or neutral position to avoid any further injury.
- Why is it important to know that a cervical dislocation occurs?
  If a cervical dislocation occurs, then head rotation was involved at the cervical spine when contact was made. This increases the severity of the injury to the spinal column.

4. Based on the information that you currently have and what was provided by your instructor, how will you begin Mr. James' rehabilitation?
Mr. James will either be placed in a neck brace or will have surgery to help stabilize the cervical fracture. You will begin a rehabilitation program only after Mr. James is cleared by the physician. Mr. James must be asymptomatic and have no numbness or paraesthesia in the extremities, no cervical spine abnormalities on a radiograph and MRI, and no vertebral instability. Mild stretching and strengthening of the neck musculature is the area of focus for his rehabilitation program.

Why or why not?

How will Mr. James' rehabilitation progress? For the *why?* portion of each exercise, explain why you chose a particular exercise or activity as part of your program. Describe which rehabilitation goals the exercise or activity covers, and describe the key indicators for progression. For the *why not?* portion of each exercise, explain why other rehabilitation exercises or activities were not chosen and what to avoid during rehabilitation for this injury. Gather details from the textbook, your own research, and data from Mr. James' scenario to help formulate your answer.

Why?

- ***Cervical neck stretching.*** *This exercise will help with the rehabilitation goal of restoring the athlete's range of motion. The exercises should be performed gently and passively. The motions that should be addressed include cervical flexion, extension, and right- and left-sided bending (lateral flexion).*
- ***Cervical neck strengthening.*** *These exercises will help with the rehabilitation goal of increasing strength. These should be added to the program once neck range of motion is achieved. The cervical neck strength exercises should begin as basic resistance type exercises. Manual resistance can be applied by the individual's hand, a table, or an athletic trainer. The same motions for cervical neck stretching are the motions that are used with cervical neck strengthening.*
- ***Trapezius stretching and strengthening.*** *These activities will help with the rehabilitation goals of increasing ROM and strength. Stretching and strengthening can also be applied to the trapezius muscle group. The upper fibers of this muscle group originate at the cervical vertebra and help with the functioning of the scapula. If any damage occurred to the upper fibers of the trapezius during injury, these exercises should also be part of the rehabilitation program.*
- ***Levator scapulae stretching and strengthening.*** *These activities will help with the rehabilitation goals of increasing ROM and strength. The levator scapulae is another neck muscle group that originates at the cervical vertebra. As mentioned with the trapezius, if the levator scapulae suffered any type of damage during the initial injury, this muscle group should be addressed during the rehabilitation program. The levator scapulae is responsible for elevating the upper medial point of the scapula.*

Why not?

- *Any type of exercise that puts an axial load or body weight stress on the neck should not be performed after an athlete has suffered a cervical fracture. Excessive cervical extension should also be avoided because of compression of an already weak area.*

Conversation Buffer

Extreme caution should always be used when moving a patient. Further injury can occur if improper technique is used when transporting the athlete. This is why it is necessary to practice spine boarding and the proper positioning and transporting procedures with your health-care team. You want to be sure that every individual who might help with this type of situation—certified athletic trainers, coaches, physicians, and emergency medical technicians—all have the same emergency positioning and transporting procedure information.

What do you think?

1. Based on your rehabilitation protocol, discuss the indicators for limited and full return to play with the athlete. Include a rough timeline for return to play, if applicable, which is affected by the athlete's compliance with the rehabilitation program.
   - ***Limited return to play.*** *The athlete will return to limited play once a rehabilitation program has been completed and there are no symptoms that are reproduced from performing the exercises associated with the stretching and strengthening program. Performing exertional type exercises such as running, biking, and functional sport-specific exercises is a great way to allow the athlete to return to the field without being forced into full play.*
   - ***Full return to play.*** *Based on the physician's orders, an athlete may or may not be able to return to a full contact sport after suffering a cervical fracture. Return to play is based on how well the fracture site heals. If the participant is cleared to play in full contact sports, proper techniques for tackling safely should be revisited.*
2. Are modifications or personal protective equipment needed to return to play?
   - *A cowboy collar can be worn for defensive players whose neck might be forced into hyperextension.*

STUDENT SCENARIO 1: EMILIO RODRIGUEZ

Emilio Rodriguez is a wide receiver on his college football team. He reaches up for a pass and is hit by an opposing player on the right side of his chest during a home game. After catching the ball, Mr. Rodriguez notices discomfort every time he inhales and exhales. He is removed from the game when his respiratory effort increases. On evaluation, Mr. Rodriguez is point tender over his fifth and sixth ribs. A sharp pain is produced with inspiration. On palpation, he has crepitus over the fifth and sixth ribs along with localized deformity. The deformity steps inward, causing concern for a possible hemothorax. He is immediately referred for radiographic imaging, which reveals fractures of the fifth and sixth ribs (Fig. 16-3). A hemothorax is ruled out. Mr. Rodriguez is given instructions for his treatment plan.

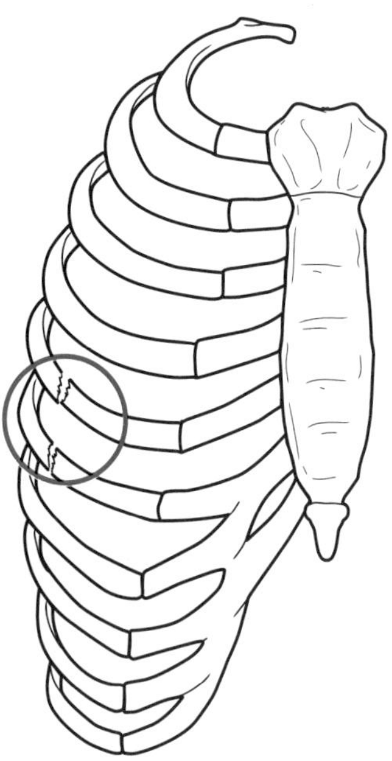

Figure 16-3: Emilio Rodriguez's rib fracture.

1. Based on this scenario, what do you know about Mr. Rodriguez's injury?
   - ______________________________
   - ______________________________
   - ______________________________
   - ______________________________
2. To rehabilitate Mr. Rodriguez's injury effectively, you will need to gather additional information. What questions should you ask in addition to what is presented in this scenario?
   - ______________________________
   - ______________________________
   - ______________________________
   - ______________________________

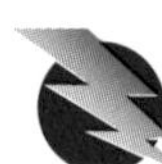

Brain Jolt

A hemothorax, which is a perforation to the pleurae tissue of the lung from a puncture, is a life-threatening emergency and requires immediate medical attention. Watch for signs of shock.

3. Identify key terms and concepts, and research each to broaden your knowledge about the rehabilitation of head, neck, and trunk injuries.
   - What anatomical structures might be involved in Mr. Rodriguez's injury?

     Answer: ______
   - What is a rib fracture?

     Answer: ______
   - In what phase of healing is this injury?

     Answer: ______
   - Explain a hemothorax. List other types of injuries that can occur with a direct blow to the chest cavity and their signs and symptoms.

     Answer: ______
   - Define *crepitus*.

     Answer: ______
   - Define *inspiration* as it relates to this subject.

     Answer: ______
   - Why was an anterior-posterior rib compression test not performed in the evaluation?

     Answer: ______
   - Explain how to perform an anterior-posterior rib compression test.

     Answer: ______
4. Based on the information that you currently have and what was provided by your instructor, how will you begin Mr. Rodriguez's rehabilitation?
   - ______
   - ______
   - ______
   - ______

Why or why not?

How will Mr. Rodriguez's rehabilitation progress? For the *why?* portion of each exercise, explain why you chose a particular exercise or activity as part of your program. Describe which rehabilitation goals the exercise or activity covers, and describe the key indicators for progression. For the *why not?* portion of each exercise, explain why other rehabilitation exercises or activities were not chosen and what to avoid during rehabilitation for this injury. Gather details from the textbook, your own research, and data from Mr. Rodriguez's scenario to help formulate your answer.

Why?

- ______
- ______
- ______
- ______

Why not?

- ______
- ______

What do you think?

1. Based on your rehabilitation protocol, discuss the indicators for limited and full return to play. Include a rough timeline for return to play, if applicable, which is affected by the athlete's compliance with the rehabilitation program.
   - ______
   - ______
   - ______
   - ______
2. Are modifications or personal protective equipment needed to return to play?
   - ______
   - ______

STUDENT SCENARIO 2: JERMAINE LEWIS

Jermaine Lewis is a running back on his college football team. He has a history of right shoulder injuries, ranging from a rotator cuff strain to a glenoid labrum tear. Mr. Lewis previously completed two different rehabilitation programs, but he continues to have weakness in his right deltoid muscle with visible atrophy. This weakness is attributed to his history of repeated injuries in high school. At practice, Mr. Lewis is handed the ball, and he runs straight up the middle of the field. As he gets through the line of scrimmage, a teammate grabs hold of his right arm and Mr. Lewis struggles to free himself. He continues to advance forward, and feels a tingling sensation radiate down his right arm while his arm is still being pulled by the teammate. Mr. Lewis is brought down to the field by multiple players, and his body and neck are forced laterally while his right shoulder remains depressed. He comes off the field with his right arm hanging limp. He has numbness and paraesthesia down his right arm and into his fingers, point tenderness over the right trapezius, a 3/5 strength test with horizontal abduction, and a positive brachial plexus stretch test result. A brachial plexus neurapraxia is diagnosed (Fig. 16-4).

1. Based on this scenario, what do you know about Mr. Lewis' injury?
   - ____________________
   - ____________________
   - ____________________
   - ____________________

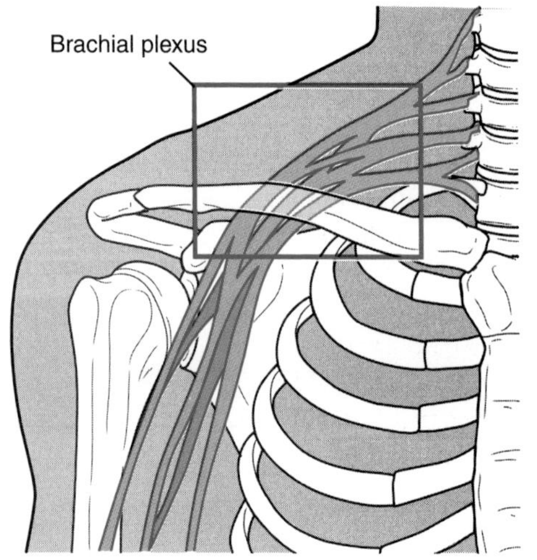

Figure 16-4: Jermaine Lewis' brachial plexus neuropraxia.

2. To rehabilitate Mr. Lewis' injury effectively, you will need to gather additional information. What questions should you ask in addition to what is presented in this scenario?
   - ____________________
   - ____________________
   - ____________________
   - ____________________

3. Identify key terms and concepts, and research each to broaden your knowledge about the rehabilitation of head, neck, and trunk injuries.
   - What anatomical structures might be involved in Mr. Lewis' injury?

     Answer: ____________________
   - What is a brachial plexus neurapraxia?

     Answer: ____________________
   - In which phase of healing is this injury?

     Answer: ____________________
   - Why does Mr. Lewis have atrophy of his right deltoid?

     Answer: ____________________
   - Where does the brachial plexus originate?

     Answer: ____________________
   - What can numbness and paraesthesia indicate?

     Answer: ____________________
   - Explain the different strength grades when assessing the strength of a muscle group.

     Answer: ____________________
   - What is the brachial plexus stretch test? What does it test? What does a positive test indicate?

     Answer: ____________________

4. Based on the information that you currently have and what was provided by your instructor, how will you begin Mr. Lewis' rehabilitation?
   - ____________________
   - ____________________

- ____________________
- ____________________

Brain Jolt

A "stinger" or "burner" pertains to a brachial plexus neurapraxia.

Conversation Buffer

A plexus neurapraxia injury can scare an athlete because sensation in the extremity does not return immediately. Explain to the athlete the rationale for experiencing the numbness and the typical course of injury progression. Knowledge and understanding will calm the athlete's nerves.

Why or why not?

How will Mr. Lewis' rehabilitation progress? For the *why?* portion of each exercise, explain why you chose a particular exercise or activity as part of your program. Describe which rehabilitation goals the exercise or activity covers, and describe the key indicators for progression. For the *why not?* portion of each exercise, explain why other rehabilitation exercises or activities were not chosen and what to avoid during rehabilitation for this injury. Gather details from the textbook, your own research, and data from Mr. Lewis' scenario to help formulate your answer.

Why?

- ____________________
- ____________________
- ____________________
- ____________________

Why not?

- ____________________
- ____________________

What do you think?

1. Based on your rehabilitation protocol, discuss the indicators for limited and full return to play. Include a rough timeline for return to play, if applicable, which is affected by the athlete's compliance with the rehabilitation program.
   - ____________________
   - ____________________
   - ____________________
   - ____________________
2. Are modifications or personal protective equipment needed to return to play?
   - ____________________
   - ____________________

STUDENT SCENARIO 3: IVANKA WRIGHT

Ivanka Wright is a midfielder on the women's soccer team. As she is dribbling the ball up the field, she is met head-on by an approaching player. Ms. Wright tries to dribble around the player, but they collide and Ms. Wright falls backwards, hitting her head. An on-field assessment shows that Ms. Wright has no changes in level of consciousness (LOC), but she does have a headache, blurred vision, and mild ringing in the ears. She has no cervical pain, and she is assisted off the field. Once off the field, her symptoms are reevaluated. She states that she no longer has blurred vision but still has a headache and ringing in her ears. She is then put through an off-field standardized assessment of concussion (SAC) test, resulting in a score of 27 out of 30 as an overall score, although she shows weakness with her concentration score. Her immediate and delayed memory recall are unaffected. After 20 minutes from the initial injury, she has only a headache, but is kept from the game because she is still symptomatic. She is reevaluated the following day with the computerized Immediate Post Concussion

Assessment and Cognitive Testing (ImPACT), resulting in a diagnosis of concussion (Fig. 16-5).

1. Based on this scenario, what do you know about Ms. Wright's injury?

- ______________________________
- ______________________________
- ______________________________
- ______________________________

2. To rehabilitate Ms. Wright's injury effectively, you will need to gather additional information. What questions should you ask in addition to what is presented in this scenario?

- ______________________________
- ______________________________
- ______________________________
- ______________________________

3. Identify key terms and concepts, and then research each to broaden your knowledge about the rehabilitation of head, neck, and trunk injuries.

- What anatomical structures might be involved in Ms. Wright's injury?

  Answer: ______________________________
- What is a concussion?

  Answer: ______________________________

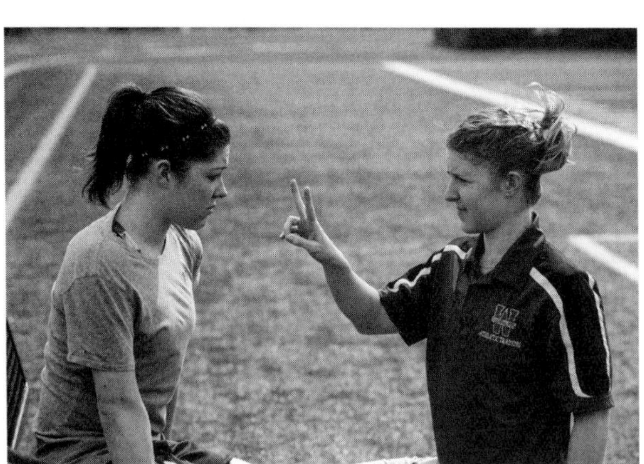

Figure 16-5: Ivanka Wright's concussion.

- In which phase of healing is this injury?

  Answer: ______________________________
- Define *LOC*.

  Answer: ______________________________
- What are the symptoms of concussion?

  Answer: ______________________________
- What is the SAC test? What does it include?

  Answer: ______________________________
- What is the ImPACT test?

  Answer: ______________________________
- What criteria are used to diagnose a concussion?

  Answer: ______________________________

Brain Jolt

Concussions should always be treated as a major injury and return-to-play guidelines should be strictly followed.

4. Based on the information that you currently have and what was provided by your instructor, how will you begin Ms. Wright's rehabilitation?

- ______________________________
- ______________________________
- ______________________________
- ______________________________

Why or why not?

How will Ms. Wright's rehabilitation progress? For the *why?* portion of each exercise, explain why you chose a particular exercise or activity as part of your program. Describe which rehabilitation goals the exercise or activity covers, and describe the key indicators for progression. For the *why not?* portion of each exercise, explain why other rehabilitation exercises or activities were not chosen and what to avoid during rehabilitation for this injury. Gather details from the textbook, your own research, and data from Ms. Wright's scenario to help formulate your answer.

Why?

- ______________________________
- ______________________________

- ____________________
- ____________________

Why not?

- ____________________
- ____________________

Conversation Buffer

Not all of Ms. Wright's symptoms persisted, making it seem that her injury was not severe. However, if an athlete is sent back into participation before being completely asymptomatic, he or she runs the risk of experiencing another concussion in addition to the existing one, which is known as *second-impact syndrome*. Second-impact syndrome is a life-threatening emergency that can result in death. Talk with your coaches and athletes about concussions, and ensure that they know the importance of being honest about their symptoms and playing symptom free.

Treatment Detour

Public awareness of concussions and the associated symptoms has increased the number of concussions being treated in today's world. However, not every concussion resolves without complications. Postconcussion syndrome (PCS) has been reported to occur in 10% of concussion cases. It is diagnosed when "three or more symptoms of concussion have persisted for at least three months after head trauma." One study found that this condition is often missed, being recognized by only 60% of general practitioners. It can affect an athletes' academic and athletic development; therefore, it is important to regularly reevaluate the athlete to avoid misdiagnosis. After a diagnosis of PCS, it is important to get proper treatment to reduce recovery time (Logan, 2010).

What do you think?

1. Based on your rehabilitation protocol, discuss the indicators for limited and full return to play. Include a rough timeline for return to play, if applicable, which is affected by the athlete's compliance with the rehabilitation program.
   - ____________________
   - ____________________
   - ____________________
   - ____________________
2. Are modifications or personal protective equipment needed to return to play?
   - ____________________
   - ____________________

STUDENT SCENARIO 4: EDWARD DEAN

Edward Dean is a senior guard on his high school basketball team and is excited about tonight's first game. Two minutes into the second quarter, he is guarding an opponent who has already received two fouls for elbowing. Mr. Dean is going for a rebound as the opponent also tries to rebound the ball. The opponent gets the ball and claims possession while throwing his elbows at chest height, hitting Mr. Dean's nose and forcing his head and neck into quick hyperextension and then immediate flexion. Mr. Dean leaves the game with an epistaxis and neck pain. Once the nasal bleeding is controlled, his neck is evaluated. He has no point tenderness over the cervical spinous processes, pain with head rotation, no cervical deformity, no numbness or paraesthesia into his arms, and a negative cervical compression and distraction test result. He is referred for radiography to rule out disc injury, such as a fracture or dislocation. The results are negative and the injury is diagnosed as whiplash (Fig. 16-6).

1. Based on this scenario, what do you know about Mr. Dean's injury?
   - ____________________
   - ____________________

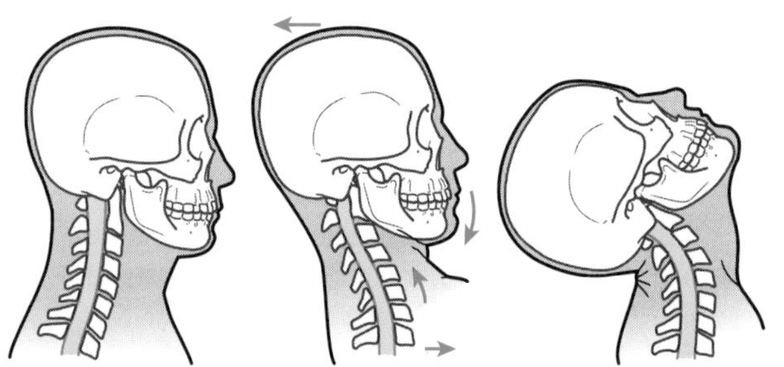

Figure 16-6: Edward Dean's whiplash.

- ______________________________
- ______________________________

2. To rehabilitate Mr. Dean's injury effectively, you will need to gather additional information. What questions should you ask in addition to what is presented in this scenario?
   - ______________________________
   - ______________________________
   - ______________________________
   - ______________________________

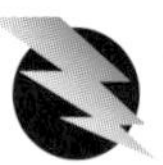

Brain Jolt

With whiplash, always be sure to rule out any spinal cord and nerve root injury before you begin a rehabilitation program.

3. Identify key terms and concepts, and research each to broaden your knowledge about the rehabilitation of head, neck, and trunk injuries.
   - What anatomical structures might be involved in Mr. Dean's injury?

     Answer: ______________________________
   - What is whiplash?

     Answer: ______________________________
   - In which phase of healing is this injury?

     Answer: ______________________________
   - Define *epistaxis*.

     Answer: ______________________________
   - What could numbness and paraesthesia indicate, if present?

     Answer: ______________________________
   - What is a cervical compression test? What does it test? What does a positive sign indicate?

     Answer: ______________________________
   - What is a cervical distraction test? What does it test? What does a positive sign indicate?

     Answer: ______________________________

4. Based on the information that you currently have and what was provided by your instructor, how will you begin Mr. Dean's rehabilitation?
   - ______________________________
   - ______________________________
   - ______________________________
   - ______________________________

Why or why not?

How will Mr. Dean's rehabilitation progress? For the *why?* portion of each exercise, explain why you chose a particular exercise or activity as part of your program. Describe which rehabilitation goals the exercise or activity covers, and describe the key indicators for progression. For the *why not?* portion of each exercise, explain why other rehabilitation exercises or activities were not chosen and what to avoid during rehabilitation for this injury. Gather details from the textbook, your own research, and data from Mr. Dean's scenario to help formulate your answer.

Why?

- ______________________________
- ______________________________
- ______________________________
- ______________________________

Why not?

- ______________________________
- ______________________________

What do you think?

1. Based on your rehabilitation protocol, discuss the indicators for limited and full return to play. Include a rough timeline for return to play, if applicable, which is affected by the athlete's compliance with the rehabilitation program.

2. Are modifications or personal protective equipment needed to return to play?

STUDENT SCENARIO 5: HOPE SANCHEZ

Hope Sanchez plays shortstop on her softball team. The coach is working on in-field drills at practice today. The current drill is to have the shortstop field the ball on the run and quickly throw to first base. Ms. Sanchez moves forward, expecting a slow roller; however, the ball takes a bad hop and hits her in the right eye. The soft tissue around her right eye immediately begins to show signs of edema. She then complains of diplopia and difficulty looking downward. Ms. Sanchez is sent for radiographic imaging to rule out a possible orbital fracture or "blowout" fracture (Fig. 16-7). The radiograph reveals a fracture, and Ms. Sanchez is prescribed antibiotics and referred to an ophthalmologist.

1. Based on this scenario, what do you know about Ms. Sanchez's injury?

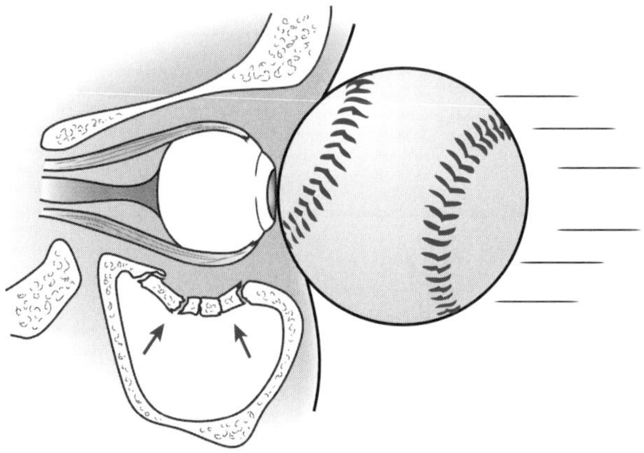

Figure 16-7: Hope Sanchez's orbital fracture.

2. To rehabilitate Ms. Sanchez's injury effectively, you will need to gather additional information. What questions should you ask in addition to what is presented in this scenario?

3. Identify key terms and concepts, and then research each to broaden your knowledge about the rehabilitation of head, neck, and trunk injuries.
   - What anatomical structures might be involved in Ms. Sanchez's injury?

     Answer:
   - What is an orbital fracture?

     Answer:
   - In which phase of healing is this injury?

     Answer:
   - Define *edema.*

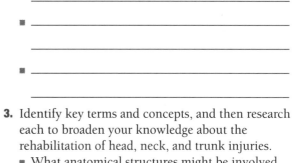

     Answer:

- Define *diplopia*.

  Answer: ______________________________
- Why does Ms. Sanchez experience restricted eye movement?

  Answer: ______________________________
- Why is Ms. Sanchez given antibiotics?

  Answer: ______________________________

Brain Jolt

Most orbital fractures are treated with surgery.

4. Based on the information that you currently have and what was provided by your instructor, how will you begin Ms. Sanchez's rehabilitation?

- ______________________________
- ______________________________
- ______________________________
- ______________________________

Why or why not?

How will Ms. Sanchez's rehabilitation progress? For the *why?* portion of each exercise, explain why you chose a particular exercise or activity as part of your program. Describe which rehabilitation goals the exercise or activity covers, and describe the key indicators for progression. For the *why not?* portion of each exercise, explain why other rehabilitation exercises or activities were not chosen and what to avoid during rehabilitation for this injury. Gather details from the textbook, your own research, and data from Ms. Sanchez's scenario to help formulate your answer.

Why?

- ______________________________
- ______________________________
- ______________________________
- ______________________________

Why not?

- ______________________________
- ______________________________

What do you think?

1. Based on your rehabilitation protocol, discuss the indicators for limited and full return to play. Include a rough timeline for return to play, if applicable, which is affected by the athlete's compliance with the rehabilitation program.

- ______________________________
- ______________________________
- ______________________________
- ______________________________

2. Are modifications or personal protective equipment needed to return to play?

- ______________________________
- ______________________________

STUDENT SCENARIO 6: MADELYN BLANFORD

Madelyn Blanford is a volleyball player with a history of head and shoulder injuries. She suffered a concussion the previous year and was treated for rotator cuff weakness. Ms. Blanford is the team's outside hitter and blocker, and she is in a rotation where she is primarily at the net. As she goes up for a block, the opposing hitter gets the ball past her hands and spikes it onto her head. She immediately drops to the ground, unconscious. As the certified athletic trainer approaches, she notices that Ms. Blanford is regaining consciousness. Her cervical spine is stabilized immediately, and she is assessed. She has no cervical neck pain and no lower extremity signs and symptoms, but she is disorientated. The emergency action plan is initiated and paramedics are called.

Ms. Blanford is transported to the emergency department for further examination. Fifteen minutes after arriving at the hospital, her condition begins to worsen. She develops a headache, begins vomiting, has dilation of one pupil, and is dizzy. She is sent for a computed tomography scan, which reveals an epidural hematoma (Fig. 16-8). Ms. Blanford is rushed into surgery.

1. Based on this scenario, what do you know about Ms. Blanford's injury?
   - ______________________________
   - ______________________________
   - ______________________________
   - ______________________________

2. To rehabilitate Ms. Blanford's injury effectively, you will need to gather additional information. What questions should you ask in addition to what is presented in this scenario?
   - ______________________________
   - ______________________________
   - ______________________________
   - ______________________________

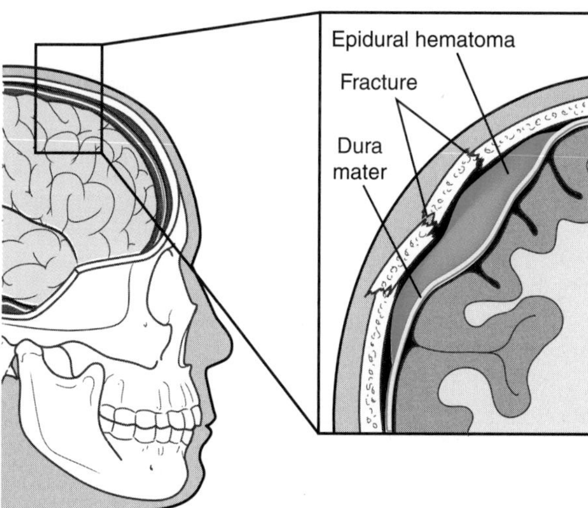

Figure 16-8: Madelyn Blanford's epidural hematoma.

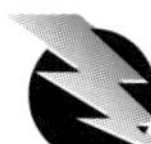

Brain Jolt

An epidural hematoma often has few head injury symptoms. As a result, constant reevaluation is crucial. This reevaluation will also help to identify a subdural hematoma.

3. Identify any key terms and concepts, and then research each to broaden your knowledge about the rehabilitation of head, neck, and trunk injuries.
   - What anatomical structures might be involved in Ms. Blanford's injury?

     Answer: ______________________________
   - What is an epidural hematoma?

     Answer: ______________________________
   - In which phase of healing is this injury?

     Answer: ______________________________
   - Describe another hematoma that can occur to the brain with a head injury.

     Answer: ______________________________
   - Did Ms. Blanford's history of concussion predispose her to an epidural hematoma? If so, explain.

     Answer: ______________________________
   - Why is an epidural hematoma a life-threatening emergency?

     Answer: ______________________________
   - What is the focus of Ms. Blanford's emergency surgery?

     Answer: ______________________________

4. Based on the information that you currently have and what was provided by your instructor, how will you begin Ms. Blanford's rehabilitation?
   - ______________________________
   - ______________________________
   - ______________________________
   - ______________________________

Why or why not?

How will Ms. Blanford's rehabilitation progress? For the *why?* portion of each exercise, explain why you chose a particular exercise or activity as part of your program. Describe which rehabilitation goals the exercise or activity covers, and describe the key indicators for progression. For the *why not?* portion of each exercise, explain why other rehabilitation exercises or activities were not chosen and what to avoid during rehabilitation for this injury. Gather details from the textbook, your own research, and data from Ms. Blanford's scenario to help formulate your answer.

Why?

- ______________________________
- ______________________________
- ______________________________
- ______________________________

Why not?

- ______________________________
- ______________________________

What do you think?

1. Based on your rehabilitation protocol, discuss the indicators for limited and full return to play. Include a rough timeline for return to play, if applicable, which is affected by the athlete's compliance with the rehabilitation program.
   - ______________________________
   - ______________________________
   - ______________________________
   - ______________________________
2. Are modifications or personal protective equipment needed to return to play?
   - ______________________________
   - ______________________________

STUDENT SCENARIO 7: BRITTANY VONDONHUGAL

Brittany Vondonhugal comes to the certified athletic trainer complaining of a chronic headache and ear pain on the left side. She has moderate edema around her left temporomandibular ligament. The athletic trainer refers her to the campus physician, who diagnoses a sinus and ear infection and prescribes antibiotics. She is told to return in 7 days if she has not improved. She returns to the athletic trainer's office on the fifth day with increased ear pain and clicking when she opens and closes her jaw. She states that she had a custom-designed removable mouthpiece that she had to wear at night, but she lost the mouthpiece 2 months ago. Her current symptoms began 1 month ago. She also states that she has a history of lockjaw. Ultimately, temporomandibular joint (TMJ) dysfunction is diagnosed (Fig. 16-9).

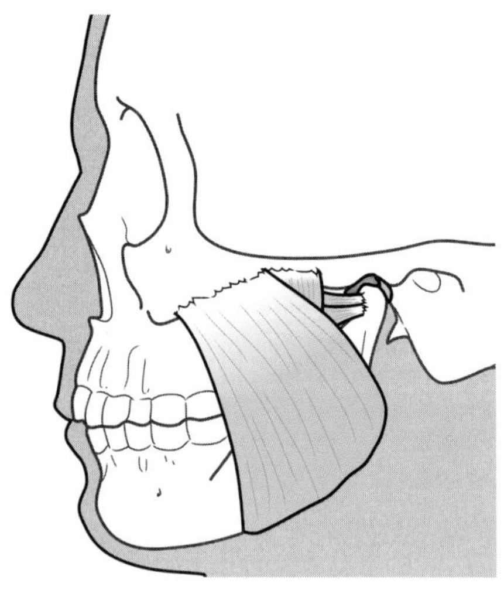

Figure 16-9: Brittany Vondonhugal's temporomandibular joint dysfunction.

1. Based on this scenario, what do you know about Ms. Vondonhugal's injury?
   - ______________________________
   - ______________________________
   - ______________________________
   - ______________________________

2. To rehabilitate Ms. Vondonhugal's injury effectively, you will need to gather additional information. What questions should you ask in addition to what is presented in this scenario?

- ______________________________
- ______________________________
- ______________________________
- ______________________________

Brain Jolt
A patient with TMJ dysfunction should be referred to a dentist for further evaluation and treatment.

3. Identify key terms and concepts, and research each to broaden your knowledge about the rehabilitation of head, neck, and trunk injuries.
   - What anatomical structures might be involved in Ms. Vondonhugal's injury?

     Answer: ______________________________
   - What is a TMJ dysfunction?

     Answer: ______________________________
   - In which phase of healing is this injury?

     Answer: ______________________________
   - Why does Ms. Vondonhugal have ear pain with this injury?

     Answer: ______________________________
   - What other types of symptoms can accompany TMJ dysfunction?

     Answer: ______________________________
   - Can TMJ dysfunction be corrected with strengthening exercises?

     Answer: ______________________________

4. Based on the information that you currently have and what was provided by your instructor, how will you begin Ms. Vondonhugal's rehabilitation?

- ______________________________
- ______________________________
- ______________________________
- ______________________________

Why or why not?

How will Ms. Vondonhugal's rehabilitation progress? For the *why?* portion of each exercise, explain why you chose a particular exercise or activity as part of your program. Describe which rehabilitation goals the exercise or activity covers, and describe the key indicators for progression. For the *why not?* portion of each exercise, explain why other rehabilitation exercises or activities were not chosen and what to avoid during rehabilitation for this injury. Gather details from the textbook, your own research, and data from Ms. Vondonhugal's scenario to help formulate your answer.

Why?

- ______________________________
- ______________________________
- ______________________________
- ______________________________

Why not?

- ______________________________
- ______________________________

What do you think?

1. Based on your rehabilitation protocol, discuss the indicators for limited and full return to play. Include a rough timeline for return to play, if applicable, which is affected by the athlete's compliance with the rehabilitation program.

- ______________________________

- ______________________________
  ____
- ______________________________
  ____
- ______________________________
  ____

2. Are modifications or personal protective equipment needed to return to play?
   - ______________________________
     ____
   - ______________________________
     ____

knowledge checklist

Table 16-1 offers a checklist that can be used by a peer, instructor, or preceptor to evaluate each part of the athlete's rehabilitation plan. Use this checklist as a tool to ensure that the rehabilitation plan is complete and to assess your knowledge of the competencies that apply to this chapter.

TABLE 16-1 ■ Head, Neck, and Trunk Rehabilitation and Therapeutic Exercise Competency Checklist

	Proficient *Can demonstrate and execute the skill properly*	**Proficient With Assistance** *Can demonstrate and execute the skill with minimal guidance or tips*	**Not Proficient** *Unable to demonstrate and execute the skill properly; need to be reevaluated at another time after further study and practice*
Controlling Edema			
PRICE			
Modalities			
Controlling Pain			
Pain scales			
Medications			
Modalities			
Establishes Core Stability			
Reestablishes Neuromuscular Control			
Restores Postural Control and Balance			
Restoring Range of Motion			
Passive range of motion			
Active range of motion			
Resistive range of motion			
Goniometry			
Normal range of motion limits			
Restore Muscular Strength, Endurance, and Power			
Open kinetic chain			
Closed kinetic chain			
Isometric			
Isotonic			
Isotonic (concentric and eccentric)			
Isokinetic			
Plyometric			
Agility			
Functional or Sport-Specific Activities			
Maintains Cardiorespiratory Fitness			
Functional Testing			
Return-to-Play Criteria			
Proper Documentation			

PRICE, prevention, rest, ice, compression, and elevation.

REFERENCES

Higgins, M. (2011). *Therapeutic exercise: From theory to practice.* Philadelphia, PA: F.A. Davis.

Logan, K. (2010). Recognition and management of post-concussion syndrome. *Athletic Therapy Today, 15*, 4–7.

National Athletic Training Association. (2011). *Athletic training education competencies* (5th ed.). Retrieved from http://www.nata.org/sites/default/files/5th-Edition-Competencies-2011-PDF-Version.pdf

Prentice, W. (2010). *Arnheim's principles of athletic training: A competency-based approach* (14th ed.). New York, NY: McGraw-Hill.

Prentice, W. (2011). *Rehabilitation techniques for sports medicine and athletic training* (5th ed.). New York, NY: McGraw-Hill.

Schlink, M., & Watkins, R. (2011). Get back in the game with core stabilization. *Rehab Management: Interdisciplinary Journal of Rehabilitation.* Aug/Sept, 20–23.

Starkey, C. (2004). *Therapeutic modalities* (3rd ed.). Philadelphia, PA: F.A. Davis.

Starkey, C., Brown, S. D., & Ryan, J. (2010). *Examination of orthopedic and athletic injuries* (3rd ed.). Philadelphia, PA: F.A. Davis.

Venes, D. (Ed.). (2009). *Taber's cyclopedic medical dictionary* (21st ed.). Philadelphia, PA: F.A. Davis.

chapter 17

Lower Back, Sacroiliac Joint, and Pelvis

chapter outline

athletic trainer's corner

Out there in the real world, one athletic trainer experienced the following:

During my junior year of college I began experiencing pain in my lower back along my posterior superior iliac spine (PSIS). My senior athletic training student (ATS) said it was from knots in my muscle from hitting and that they would resolve after the season. Later in the season, I suffered two disc herniations at L4–L5 and at L5–S1. This issue improved after many months of rehabilitation, but I still had the sacroiliac (SI) pain. Putting pressure on my lower back was the only thing that relieved this pain. Over the summer months, the pain got increasingly worse and the pain moved into my hips as well. I brought this to my ATS's attention and she diagnosed it as SI joint dysfunction. We began using muscle energy and I starting wearing an SI belt. The pain subsided after a couple of weeks. I learned that many things can contribute to low back pain; however, a proper diagnosis and a good rehabilitation plan bring success and reduce pain.

Chelcey Lyons, AT, ATC
Graduate Assistant Athletic Trainer
Valdosta State University
Valdosta, Georgia

learning outcomes

After working through this chapter, you will be able to:

1. Describe seven different goals of rehabilitation and the importance of each in the overall rehabilitation protocol.
2. Verbalize indications for performing low back, sacroiliac joint, and pelvis rehabilitative techniques.
3. Discuss modifications and progressions that are used during a rehabilitation program for the low back, sacroiliac joint, and pelvis.
4. Discuss outcome measures used to identify activity levels and return-to-play guidelines for low back, sacroiliac joint, and pelvis injuries.
5. Explain what modality choice is proper for rehabilitation by using indications, contraindications, and the principles and theory related to the physiological response of the intervention.

MODEL SCENARIO 1: CLAIRE HUTCHINS

Claire Hutchins is a collegiate distance runner who participates in both cross-country and track. She has a prior history of low back, left gluteal, and lateral thigh pain that radiates to the left knee. The pain intensifies over her summer break while she participates in a summer running program. She visits her family physician, who orders a radiograph of her low back. The results show a spondylolysis at the L4–L5 vertebrae. The physician diagnoses spondylolysis and a weak core, and he refers Claire Hutchins for physical therapy. The physical therapy sessions focus on lumbar stabilization and strengthening; however, the physical therapy sessions bring no pain relief. Her physician then orders magnetic resonance imaging (MRI), which has no significant findings. The physician recommends an epidural steroid injection to help relieve any effusion that might be present between the vertebrae, which brings about only temporary relief. She is still having a moderate amount of low back and left gluteal pain when she reports back to college for preseason cross-country practices. The team's orthopedic physician reevaluates Ms. Hutchins and notes low back pain, left gluteal pain (Fig. 17-1), a positive Trendelenburg test result, and point tenderness over the left greater trochanter and gluteal muscles. Her range of motion (ROM) is normal, but painful. Certain manual muscle testing movements reproduce the pain and symptoms. There are no neurological symptoms. The orthopedic physician reexamines the MRI results to rule out any stress fracture of the SI joint or femoral head. He finds a grade 2 gluteus medius strain and a tear at the origin of the gluteus medius. Ms. Hutchins is advised to stop her running program until symptoms disappear, and she begins a strict and conservative rehabilitation program.

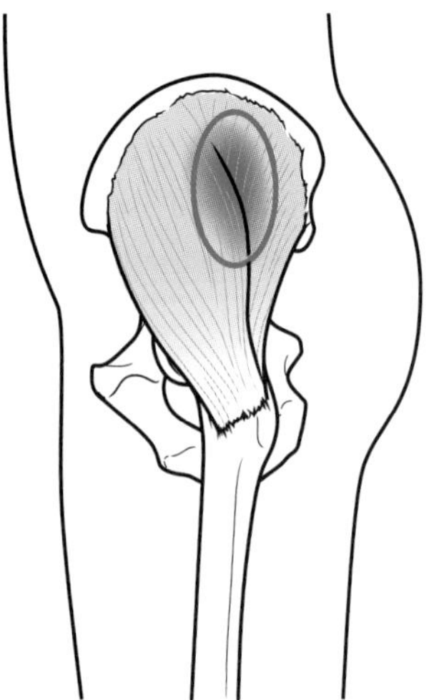

Figure 17-1: Claire Hutchins' gluteus medius tear.

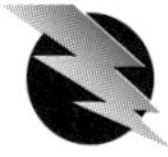

Brain Jolt

This injury is often diagnosed as a low back injury or trochanteric bursitis. It is often overlooked as a possible injury site because of the muscle's location.

1. Based on this scenario, what do you know about Ms. Hutchins' injury?
   - *Female athlete*
   - *Runner*
   - *No specific or traumatic event mechanism of injury*
   - *Low back pain, left gluteal pain, and lateral thigh pain that radiates to the knee*
   - *Spondylolysis at L4–L5*
   - *Prior history of physical therapy*
   - *Had epidural steroid injection*
   - *Positive Trendelenburg test result*
   - *Point tender over left greater trochanter*
   - *Normal ROM but painful*
   - *No neurological symptoms*
   - *Diagnosed with a grade 2 gluteus medius tear*
2. To rehabilitate Ms. Hutchins' injury effectively, you will need to gather additional information. What questions should you ask in addition to what is presented in this scenario?
   - *Are there any preexisting injuries? If yes, what are they?*
   - *How long has the athlete experienced this pain?*
   - *What is the athlete's pain level and type of pain felt?*

- *What is the level of strength in the athlete's hip?*
- *Does the athlete have any numbness or paraesthesia?*
- *What was the athlete's previous rehabilitation program?*
- *Is there any pelvic obliquity?*

3. Identify key terms and concepts, and research each to broaden your knowledge about the rehabilitation of low back, SI, and pelvis injuries.
   - What anatomical structures might be involved in Ms. Hutchins' injury?
     Pelvis
     Lumbar vertebrae
     SI joint
     Femur
   - What is a grade 2 gluteus medius tear?
     A partial tear of the gluteus medius muscle
   - In which phase of healing is this injury?
     Acute inflammatory phase
   - Explain the actions of the gluteus medius. Is this injury common?
     The action of the gluteus medius is abduction at the hip joint. It also assists with pelvic stabilization during single-leg follow-through or stance with walking and running. Injury to the gluteus medius is becoming more common because of recognition that the injured area is not always the low back or trochanter bursitis.
   - What is the Trendelenburg test? What does it test? What does a positive test indicate?
     The Trendelenburg test is used to indicate whether there is a weakness of the gluteus medius muscle on the affected side. The athlete is instructed to stand on the affected side and then flex the unaffected hip. If the pelvis or PSIS on the unaffected side is higher than on the affected side, the test result is negative. If the pelvis or PSIS on the unaffected side is lower than the affected side, the test result is positive for a weak hip abductor, known as the gluteus medius muscle.
   - What is an epidural steroid injection?
     An epidural steroid injection is an invasive procedure that is used to help relieve low back pain. A combination corticosteroid and a pain relief medication are injected into the space around the spinal cord and nerve roots. The hope is to reduce any pain and inflammation surrounding the vertebrae.
   - Define *effusion*.
     Increased fluid within a joint cavity
   - Explain manual muscle testing.
     Manual muscle testing is the bilateral comparison of the strength of the muscle or muscles in question and assignment of a numeric number grade from 0 to 5.

4. Based on the information that you currently have and what was provided by your instructor, how will you begin Ms. Hutchins' rehabilitation?
   Ms. Hutchins will be taught to use a three-point gait, assisted by a crutch. The added assistance with ambulation will help to alleviate the stress on her left gluteus medius muscle. This will also help with her pelvic stabilization. Ice is one modality that will be initiated. A mild to moderate exercise program will be started to strengthen the gluteus medius muscle, which helps with hip abduction and pelvic stabilization during single-leg stances with walking and running.

Why or why not?

How will Ms. Hutchins' rehabilitation progress? For the *why?* portion of each exercise, explain why you chose a particular exercise or activity as part of your program. Describe which rehabilitation goals the exercise or activity covers, and describe the key indicators for progression. For the *why not?* portion of each exercise, explain why other rehabilitation exercises or activities were not chosen and what to avoid during rehabilitation for this injury. Gather details from the textbook, your own research, and data from Ms. Hutchins' scenario to help formulate your answer.

Why?

- ***Leg abduction exercises.*** *This activity will help with the rehabilitation goal of increasing strength. It was chosen because this is the main action of the gluteus medius muscle. This exercise can initially be performed while side-lying and progresses to a standing single-leg stance. Ankle cuff weights or a resistive band can be added to increase the difficulty. Begin with one set of 15, and progress as tolerated.*
- ***Stretching exercises.*** *This type of activity will help with the rehabilitation goal of increasing ROM. It was chosen to focus on the flexibility of the piriformis, hamstrings, and hip flexors. This exercise will help to increase the range of motion of the anterior and posterior hip muscles and pelvic region.*
- ***Ice or cryotherapy.*** *This modality was chosen to help with the rehabilitation goal of decreasing pain and edema that may be present from the injury or any that may be produced from the rehabilitation program.*
- ***Pelvic-lumbar stabilization exercises.*** *These types of exercises were chosen to help with the rehabilitation goal of increasing strength, because the gluteus medius muscle helps with pelvic stabilization during walking and running. An example of a pelvic-lumbar stabilization exercise is the pelvic tilt. This exercise helps to strengthen the lower abdominal muscles, which assist with pelvic rotation. The stabilization exercises can be held for 2 to 5 seconds, and it is recommended to begin with a small number of repetitions.*
- ***Forward leg raises.*** *This exercise was chosen to help with the rehabilitation goal of increasing strength because of the importance of offsetting the weak or injured gluteus medius muscle. The concept is similar to how a strong core helps to take the stress off the low back. If the anterior pelvic muscles are strong, they will help to prevent a cocontraction from occurring at*

the stronger posterior muscles. The exercises can progress from a forward supine straight-leg raise to a standing hip hike. Begin with one set of 15, and progress as tolerated.

Why not?

- ***Explosive functional exercises.*** *This type of activity cannot be used until the physician is ready to allow the athlete to return to activity. Because the athlete already has a muscle tear, adding any extra quick, explosive movement on the muscle creates a risk for further damage of the already weakened muscle fibers.*
- ***Heat.*** *This type of modality should not be performed because of the possibility of increasing any edema to the injured area.*
- ***Running exercises.*** *This activity should not be performed initially because of the severity of the injury. The potential to further increase the tear to the gluteus medius is great. The strength needs to be comparable bilaterally before beginning any type of functional activity.*

What do you think?

1. Based on your rehabilitation protocol, discuss the indicators for limited and full return to play with the athlete. Include a rough timeline for return to play, if applicable, which is affected by the athlete's compliance with the rehabilitation program.
   - ***Limited return to play.*** *Limited return to play will depend on regaining full active ROM and strength to the injured hip, compared bilaterally. Once the athlete has completed the initial rehabilitation program and is asymptomatic, he or she can begin to participate in noncontact activities with the team.*
   - ***Full return to play.*** *This status is an extension of the limited return to play. If all exercises for limited return to play are performed without pain—without any type of compensation, no setbacks, and no new signs of edema—the athlete should be able to return to activity completely.*
2. Are modifications or personal protective equipment needed to return to play?
   - *No*

MODEL SCENARIO 2: MEI YANG

Mei Yang is a high school cheerleader and is the main tumbler on the squad, performing frequent back handsprings and flips. She has just returned from cheer camp to prepare for the upcoming football season. She has been complaining of back pain to her parents for approximately 4 weeks, and the pain has increased over the summer. She states that she is typically able to get through her routines, but her low back hurts the most after practice. She also says that her low back hurts after sitting through her 2-hour night class. On evaluation, her trunk ROM is good but she has pain with extension. The athletic trainer (AT) palpates her lower back and notices some point tenderness near L4 and L5 and some mild hypermobility. As a result of Ms. Yang's symptoms and repetitive hyperextension of the trunk, the AT refers her for a radiographic imaging, which shows a unilateral pars interarticularis fracture on L4, or spondylolysis (Fig. 17-2).

1. Based on this scenario, what do you know about Ms. Yang's injury?
   - *Female athlete*
   - *Cheerleader with frequent tumbling*
   - *Mechanism of injury: chronic overuse from excessive back extension*
   - *Had pain for a while that is now worse after cheer camp*
   - *Achy pain when sitting in class that is worse after practice*
   - *Good trunk ROM, pain with extension*
   - *Point tenderness and hypermobility at L4 and L5*
2. To rehabilitate Ms. Yang's injury effectively, you will need to gather additional information. What questions should you ask in addition to what is presented in this scenario?
   - *Are there any preexisting injuries? If yes, what are they?*
   - *How long has the patient experienced this pain?*
   - *What is the patient's pain level and type of pain felt?*
   - *What is the strength in the trunk (back and core)?*
   - *Does the athlete have any numbness or paraesthesia?*

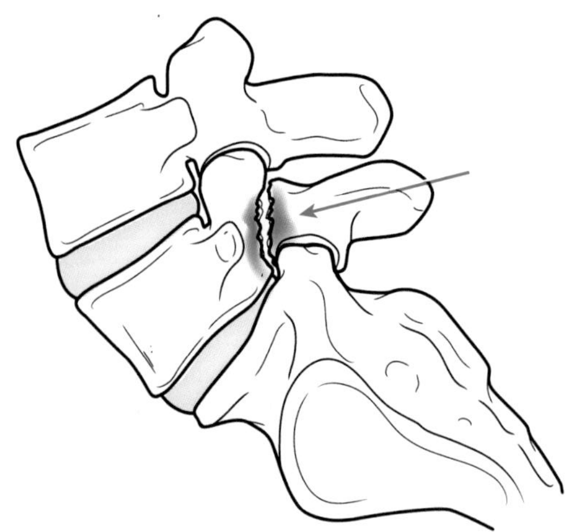

Figure 17-2: Mei Yang's spondylolysis.

- *Is any radiating pain present?*
- *Is there a positive Valsalva maneuver?*

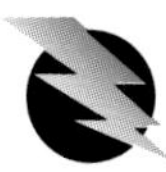

Brain Jolt
A "collared scotty dog" will be seen on a radiograph.

3. Identify key terms and concepts, and then research each to broaden your knowledge about the rehabilitation of low back, SI, and pelvis injuries.
   - What anatomical structures are involved?
     Lumbar vertebrae
     Paraspinal muscles
     Pelvis
     Sacrum
   - What is spondylolysis?
     A degeneration of the vertebrae or a fracture in the pars interarticularis of the articular process of the vertebrae
   - In what phase of healing is this injury?
     The inflammatory chronic phase
   - Define *unilateral*.
     Affecting one side
   - Define *hypermobility*.
     Increased range of motion at a joint or joint laxity
   - Define *hyperextension*.
     Extension of a limb or part beyond its normal limit
   - Why does Ms. Yang's tumbling predispose her to this condition?
     A spondylolysis can be asymptomatic until there is a disc herniation or there is a sudden trauma such as hyperextension, which occurs in back handsprings.
   - What condition can occur if Ms. Yang's fracture becomes bilateral?
     Spondylolisthesis
4. Based on the information that you currently have and what was provided by your instructor, how will you begin Ms. Yang's rehabilitation?
   Ms. Yang should be placed in a brace for her daily activities and withheld from tumbling. Next, she should begin progressive trunk strengthening exercises and core stability exercises to help stabilize the hypermobile vertebral segment. Heat would be used before her rehabilitation routine to increase flexibility in her paraspinal muscles that may be in spasm, and ice would be used afterward and whenever she has increased pain.

Why or why not?

How will Ms. Yang's rehabilitation progress? For the *why?* portion of each exercise, explain why you chose a particular exercise or activity as part of your program. Describe which rehabilitation goals the exercise or activity covers, and describe the key indicators for progression. For the *why not?* portion of each exercise, explain why other rehabilitation exercises or activities were not chosen and what to avoid during rehabilitation for this injury. Gather details from the textbook, your own research, and data from Ms. Yang's scenario to help formulate your answer.

Why?

- ***Trunk strengthening exercises.*** *These exercises are chosen to help with the rehabilitation goal of increasing strength to stabilize the hypermobile vertebral segment and to protect the injured area. Begin with low repetitions and ROM that avoids end ROMs. These exercises can be increased in repetitions and in difficulty as rehabilitation progresses.*
- ***Core stability exercises.*** *These exercises are chosen to help with the rehabilitation goal of increasing strength to stabilize the hypermobile vertebral segment and to protect the injured area. These begin with stationary isometric core exercises limiting excessive flexion and extension of the trunk. Once the patient has increased strength, these exercises can be increased in repetitions and in difficulty.*
- ***Stretching.*** *This exercise can be done to help with the rehabilitation goal of increasing ROM. Mild stretching is done for the paraspinal muscles to reduce any discomfort from muscle spasm around the area.*
- ***Heat.*** *Heat can be used to help with the rehabilitation goal of increasing ROM and is used before rehabilitation to increase the flexibility of the paraspinal muscles if there is tightness or spasm present.*
- ***Ice.*** *Ice can be used to help with the rehabilitation goal of decreasing pain and edema. It is used after rehabilitation to decrease any inflammation, edema, or pain from the exercises. It can also be used whenever there is increased pain in the injured area.*

Why not?

- *Vigorous activity is limited to reduce the risk of lumbar muscle strains and ligamentous strains as a result of the segmental hypermobility.*
- *ROM exercises and activities that reach the end range of the ROM are limited to reduce the risk of further injury.*

What do you think?

1. Based on your rehabilitation protocol, discuss the indicators for limited and full return to play with the athlete. Include a rough timeline for return to play, if applicable, which is affected by the athlete's compliance with the rehabilitation program.
   - ***Limited return to play.*** *Limited return to play is contingent on the physician's orders and requires full painless ROM and good strength in the trunk and core to protect the area. Once this is achieved, modified activity is allowed.*

- ***Full return to play.*** *A full return to play is contingent on the physician's orders and the progression of the condition. It is possible that certain movements and activities will be off limits with this condition.*

2. Are modifications or personal protective equipment needed to return to play?
   - *Ms. Yang could possibly cheer while wearing a brace to protect the area.*

STUDENT SCENARIO 1: JONATHAN GORDON

Jonathan Gordon is a lineman on his football team, and he has a history of chronic low back pain. He attributes the pain to many years of football. Mr. Gordon has had a prior rehabilitation program for his back. He believes that the program helped to relieve some weakness issues that he was having with his low back, but he was never 100% free of pain. It is the fourth quarter of the football game, and Mr. Gordon is blocking an opponent when his upper body is suddenly twisted. Afterward, he notices a sharp pain in his low back that prevents him from playing. On examination, he has low back pain, localized point tenderness at one particular vertebra, pain with lumbar extension, a positive standing stork test result, and no neurological symptoms. Mr. Gordon is referred to the team's orthopedic physician the following day. Radiographic imaging and an MRI result in a diagnosis of spondylolisthesis (Fig. 17-3).

1. Based on this scenario, what do you know about Mr. Gordon's injury?
   - ______________________________
     ____
   - ______________________________
     ____
   - ______________________________
     ____
   - ______________________________
     ____

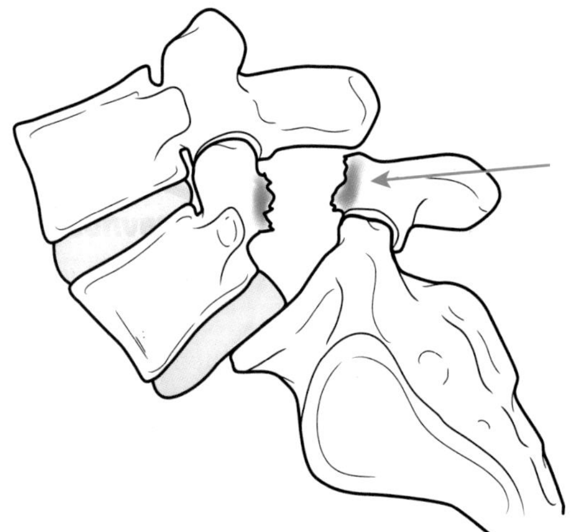

Figure 17-3: Jonathan Gordon's spondylolisthesis.

2. To rehabilitate Mr. Gordon's injury effectively, you will need to gather additional information. What questions should you ask in addition to what is presented in this scenario?
   - ______________________________
     ____
   - ______________________________
     ____
   - ______________________________
     ____
   - ______________________________
     ____

Brain Jolt
Normally, a spondylolisthesis occurs secondary to spondylolysis, creating a "decapitated scotty dog" appearance.

3. Identify key terms and concepts, and then research each to broaden your knowledge about the rehabilitation of low back, SI, and pelvis injuries.
   - What anatomical structures might be involved in Mr. Gordon's injury?

     Answer: ______________________________
   - What is spondylolisthesis?

     Answer: ______________________________
   - In which phase of healing is this injury?

     Answer: ______________________________
   - What vertebra is most commonly affected?

     Answer: ______________________________
   - Could a positive finding of the spondylolysis predispose Mr. Gordon to a spondylolisthesis?

     Answer: ______________________________
   - What is a standing stork test? What does it test? What does a positive test indicate?

     Answer: ______________________________

4. Based on the information that you currently have and what was provided by your instructor, how will you begin Mr. Gordon's rehabilitation?

- ______________________________
- ______________________________
- ______________________________
- ______________________________

Why or why not?

How will Mr. Gordon's rehabilitation progress? For the *why?* portion of each exercise, explain why you chose a particular exercise or activity as part of your program. Describe which rehabilitation goals the exercise or activity covers, and describe the key indicators for progression. For the *why not?* portion of each exercise, explain why other rehabilitation exercises or activities were not chosen and what to avoid during rehabilitation for this injury. Gather details from the textbook, your own research, and data from Mr. Gordon's scenario to help formulate your answer.

Why?

- ______________________________
- ______________________________
- ______________________________
- ______________________________

Why not?

- ______________________________
- ______________________________

What do you think?

1. Based on your rehabilitation protocol, discuss the indicators for limited and full return to play. Include a rough timeline for return to play, if applicable, which is affected by the athlete's compliance with the rehabilitation program.

- ______________________________
- ______________________________
- ______________________________
- ______________________________

2. Are modifications or personal protective equipment needed to return to play?

- ______________________________
- ______________________________

STUDENT SCENARIO 2: TITUS RAY

Titus Ray is a point guard on his college basketball team. Since the beginning of the season, Mr. Ray has been coming into the athletic training room each day with low back pain that is localized to the right side. He was started on a low back rehabilitation program, but he has not noticed any relief. The athletic trainer refers Mr. Ray to the team's orthopedic surgeon to determine the cause of his low back pain. Mr. Ray states that he has had low back pain for the last 4 to 5 years, and it started when he was a freshman in high school. His history of injury involves only a growth plate fracture of his right tibia in seventh grade. After hearing that important piece of information, the orthopedist looks for an anatomical leg-length issue. He is supine and instructed to flex his knees to 90 degrees with his feet flat on the table. The left knee appears to be higher than the right, suggesting a shortened tibia on the right side. Anatomical leg-length discrepancy is measured; in addition, any muscular imbalances are assessed. Test results for SI dysfunction are negative. The final diagnosis is anatomical leg-length discrepancy with the right leg (Fig. 17-4).

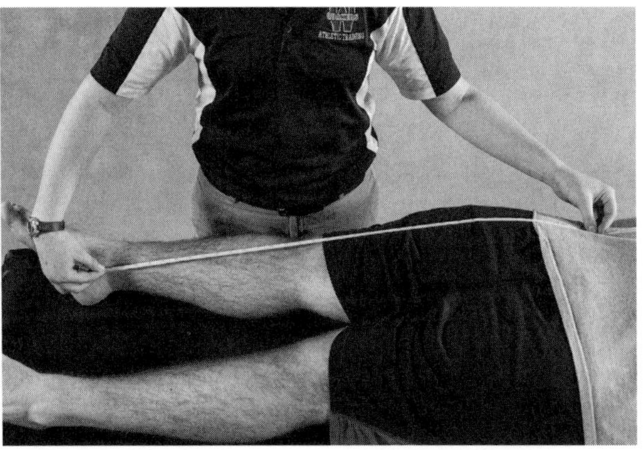

Figure 17-4: Titus Ray's anatomical leg-length discrepancy.

1. Based on this scenario, what do you know about Mr. Ray's injury?
   - ______________________________
   - ______________________________
   - ______________________________
   - ______________________________

Brain Jolt
Obtaining an athlete's complete history is vital to your success in evaluating and rehabilitating any injury.

2. To rehabilitate Mr. Ray's injury effectively, you will need to gather additional information. What questions should you ask in addition to what is presented in this scenario?
   - ______________________________
   - ______________________________
   - ______________________________
   - ______________________________

3. Identify key terms and concepts, and research each to broaden your knowledge about the rehabilitation of low back, SI, and pelvis injuries.
   - What anatomical structures might be involved in Mr. Ray's injury?

     Answer: ______________________________
   - What is an anatomical leg-length discrepancy?

     Answer: ______________________________
   - In which phase of healing is this injury?

     Answer: ______________________________
   - What type of musculature imbalances would be present with anatomical leg-length discrepancy?

     Answer: ______________________________
   - Explain a functional leg-length discrepancy.

     Answer: ______________________________
   - Explain how you measure for an anatomical and functional leg-length discrepancy.

     Answer: ______________________________
   - Why was the low back program designed for Mr. Ray not working?

     Answer: ______________________________
   - Define *supine*.

     Answer: ______________________________

4. Based on the information that you currently have and what was provided by your instructor, how will you begin Mr. Ray's rehabilitation?
   - ______________________________
   - ______________________________
   - ______________________________
   - ______________________________

Why or why not?

How will Mr. Ray's rehabilitation progress? For the *why?* portion of each exercise, explain why you chose a particular exercise or activity as part of your program. Describe which rehabilitation goals the exercise or activity covers, and describe the key indicators for progression. For the *why not?* portion of each exercise, explain why other rehabilitation exercises or activities were not chosen and what to avoid during rehabilitation for this injury. Gather details from the textbook, your own research, and data from Mr. Ray's scenario to help formulate your answer.

Why?

- ______________________________
- ______________________________

-
-

Why not?

-
-

1. Based on your rehabilitation protocol, discuss the indicators for limited and full return to play. Include a rough timeline for return to play, if applicable, which is affected by the athlete's compliance with the rehabilitation program.

-
-
-
-

2. Are modifications or personal protective equipment needed to return to play?

-
-

STUDENT SCENARIO 3: RAYMOND CLETTRIE

Raymond Clettrie, a cross-country runner, is one of the top three runners on his college team. He has a prior history of SI problems. Last season, running down hills or on any type of uneven surface irritated his low back. He was not compliant with his back rehabilitation program last season. Only 4 weeks into the current cross-country season, Mr. Clettrie is experiencing moderate low back pain, pain with walking and standing, an asymmetrical PSIS, a positive straight-leg raise at 70 to 90 degrees, and a positive FABER test result. He also has a tight iliotibial (IT) band on the left side. When examining the asymmetrical PSIS, the left PSIS is higher than the right PSIS (Fig. 17-5). The diagnosis is SI joint dysfunction, more specifically a hypermobile SI joint.

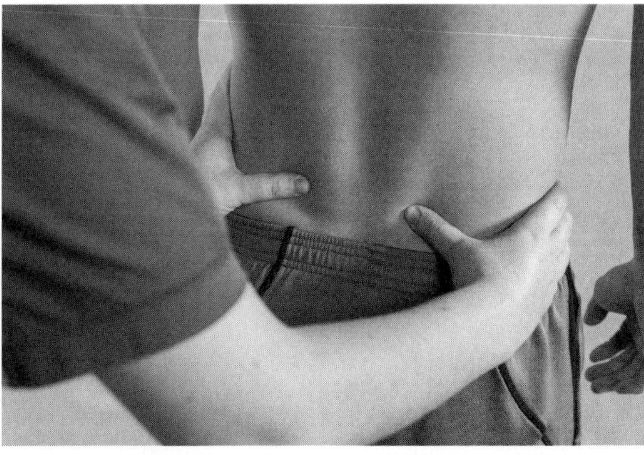

Figure 17-5: Raymond Clettrie's sacroiliac joint dysfunction.

1. Based on this scenario, what do you know about Mr. Clettrie's injury?

-
-
-
-

2. To rehabilitate Mr. Clettrie's injury effectively, you will need to gather additional information. What questions should you ask in addition to what is presented in this scenario?

-
-
-
-

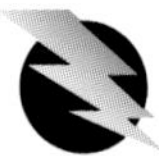

Brain Jolt

Special tests that address hypermobility and hypomobility are essential with low back injuries.

3. Identify key terms and concepts, and then research each to broaden your knowledge about the rehabilitation of low back, SI, and pelvis injuries.
   - What anatomical structures might be involved in Mr. Clettrie's injury?

     Answer: ______________________
   - What is a sacroiliac joint dysfunction?

     Answer: ______________________
   - In which phase of healing is this injury?

     Answer: ______________________
   - If Mr. Clettrie would have been more compliant with his low back rehabilitation program, would he still be having issues?

     Answer: ______________________
   - What is a straight-leg raise test above 70 to 90 degrees? What does it test? What does a positive test indicate?

     Answer: ______________________
   - What is a *FABER test*? What does it test? What does a positive test indicate?

     Answer: ______________________
   - Why is it important to know about the tight iliotibial band?

     Answer: ______________________
4. Based on the information that you currently have and what was provided by your instructor, how will you begin Mr. Clettrie's rehabilitation?
   - ______________________
   - ______________________
   - ______________________
   - ______________________

Treatment Detour

Sacroiliac joint dysfunction is an injury that can be frustrating for the clinician because of the various contributing factors to the condition. One study investigates the idea that tight hamstring muscles are a mechanism for providing sacroiliac joint stability in patients who have gluteal weakness and sacroiliac joint dysfunction. This study included 159 subjects with and without low back pain. It was found that 66% of the participants had gluteal weakness with sacroiliac joint dysfunction, whereas only 34% of the participants with low back pain without sacroiliac joint dysfunction had weakness. There was no difference in hamstring muscle length between those with and without sacroiliac joint dysfunction; however, those with sacroiliac dysfunction that had gluteal weakness did have shorter hamstring muscle length. Therefore, hamstring tightness in sacroiliac joint dysfunction could be related to gluteal muscle weakness. Clinically, it is important to remember this relationship for the patients with sacroiliac dysfunction in order to get the best results from rehabilitation and to reduce their pain (Arab, Nourbakhsh, & Mohammadifar, 2011).

Why or why not?

How will Mr. Clettrie's rehabilitation progress? For the *why?* portion of each exercise, explain why you chose a particular exercise or activity as part of your program. Describe which rehabilitation goals the exercise or activity covers, and describe the key indicators for progression. For the *why not?* portion of each exercise, explain why other rehabilitation exercises or activities were not chosen and what to avoid during rehabilitation for this injury. Gather details from the textbook, your own research, and data from Mr. Clettrie's scenario to help formulate your answer.

Why?

- ______________________
- ______________________
- ______________________
- ______________________

Why not?

- ______________________
- ______________________

What do you think?

1. Based on your rehabilitation protocol, discuss the indicators for limited and full return to play.

Include a rough timeline for return to play, if applicable, which is affected by the athlete's compliance with the rehabilitation program.

- ______________________________
- ______________________________
- ______________________________
- ______________________________

2. Are modifications or personal protective equipment needed to return to play?
   - ______________________________
   - ______________________________

STUDENT SCENARIO 4: CHEYENNE DETTRICK

Cheyenne Dettrick is a right-handed softball player who has been experiencing some posterior hip pain on her right side. She notices that her pain increases when she is batting. The pain occurs as she swings and rotates her hips, while pushing off with her right foot to run. It is produced posteriorly and radiates down her right gluteus maximus and hamstring. She also has pain when she actively rotates her hip externally, in addition to pain, numbness, and paraesthesia in her right posterior gluteus maximus when she sits for an extended period of time. She has a positive piriformis muscle test result, a negative bowstring test result, and a negative straight-leg raise test result, resulting in a diagnosis of piriformis syndrome (Fig. 17-6).

1. Based on this scenario, what do you know about Ms. Dettrick's injury?
   - ______________________________
   - ______________________________
   - ______________________________
   - ______________________________

Figure 17-6: Cheyenne Dettrick's piriformis syndrome.

2. To rehabilitate Ms. Dettrick's injury effectively, you will need to gather additional information. What questions should you ask in addition to what is presented in this scenario?
   - ______________________________
   - ______________________________
   - ______________________________
   - ______________________________

Brain Jolt

Knowing your anatomy can help you to determine the correct injury and avoid misdiagnosis.

3. Identify key terms and concepts, and research each to broaden your knowledge about the rehabilitation of low back, SI, and pelvis injuries.
   - What anatomical structures might be involved in Ms. Dettrick's injury?

     Answer: ______________________________
   - What is piriformis syndrome?

     Answer: ______________________________
   - In which phase of healing is this injury?

     Answer: ______________________________
   - Why does this condition occur more in females than males?

     Answer: ______________________________

- What is a piriformis muscle test? What does it test? What does a positive test indicate?

  Answer: ______________________________
- What is the bowstring test? What does it test? What does a positive test indicate?

  Answer: ______________________________
- What is the straight-leg raise test? What does it test? What does a positive test indicate?

  Answer: ______________________________
- Why might this injury often be diagnosed as sciatica?

  Answer: ______________________________

4. Based on the information that you currently have and what was provided by your instructor, how will you begin Ms. Dettrick's rehabilitation?

- ______________________________
- ______________________________
- ______________________________
- ______________________________

Why or why not?

How will Ms. Dettrick's rehabilitation progress? For the *why?* portion of each exercise, explain why you chose a particular exercise or activity as part of your program. Describe which rehabilitation goals the exercise or activity covers, and describe the key indicators for progression. For the *why not?* portion of each exercise, explain why other rehabilitation exercises or activities were not chosen and what to avoid during rehabilitation for this injury. Gather details from the textbook, your own research, and data from Ms. Dettrick's scenario to help formulate your answer.

Why?

- ______________________________
- ______________________________
- ______________________________
- ______________________________

Why not?

- ______________________________
- ______________________________

DETOUR **Treatment Detour**

The sciatic nerve penetrates 7% to 21% of the population's piriformis muscle, which can predispose individuals to piriformis syndrome by exerting pressure on the sciatic nerve with an injured or inflamed piriformis muscle. One case study reported a 30-year-old man with right buttock and posterior thigh pain for 2 years. Traditional treatment involves stretching or soft tissue massage of the piriformis muscle, or both. However, a biomechanical analysis revealed excessive hip adduction and internal rotation. The treatment protocol revolved around strengthening his weak right hip abductors and external rotators and movement re-education to correct his biomechanics. The patient reported a 0/10 pain scale for all activities. Therefore, when a patient has piriformis pain, it is beneficial to do movement analysis to depict the origin of the issue (Tonley et al., 2010).

What do you think?

1. Based on your rehabilitation protocol, discuss the indicators for limited and full return to play. Include a rough timeline for return to play, if applicable, which is affected by the athlete's compliance with the rehabilitation program.

- ______________________________
- ______________________________
- ______________________________
- ______________________________

2. Are modifications or personal protective equipment needed to return to play?

- ______________________________
- ______________________________

STUDENT SCENARIO 5: KATHRYN COSGROVE

Kathryn Cosgrove is the point guard on her basketball team. During the game, Ms. Cosgrove stops in the paint and takes a jump shot. The opponent forcefully boxes her out while trying to rebound, causing Ms. Cosgrove to come down hard onto her right gluteus maximus. She has some immediate discomfort, but continues to play. The next day, she has point tenderness over the gluteus maximus and numbness and paraesthesia that radiate down the posterior side of her right hamstring. She has a positive bowstring, straight-leg raise, and piriformis muscle test results. A muscle spasm is palpated at the piriformis, and a diagnosis of sciatica is made (Fig. 17-7).

1. Based on this scenario, what do you know about Ms. Cosgrove's injury?
   - ______________________________
   - ______________________________
   - ______________________________
   - ______________________________

2. To rehabilitate Ms. Cosgrove's injury effectively, you will need to gather additional information.

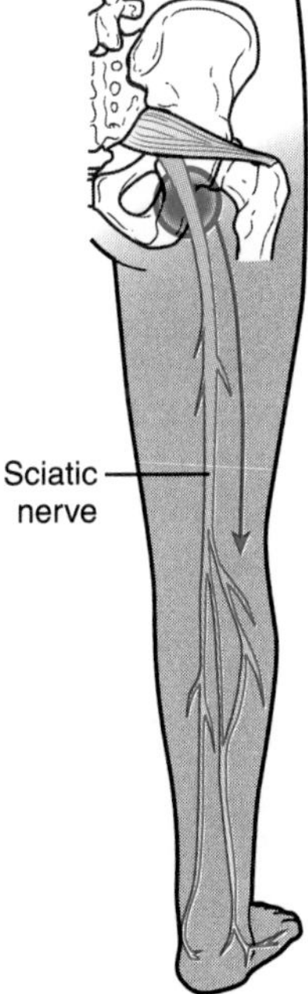

Figure 17-7: Kathryn Cosgrove's sciatica.

What questions should you ask in addition to what is presented in this scenario?
   - ______________________________
   - ______________________________
   - ______________________________
   - ______________________________

3. Identify key terms and concepts, and then research each to broaden your knowledge about the rehabilitation of low back, SI, and pelvis injuries.
   - What anatomical structures might be involved in Ms. Cosgrove's injury?

     Answer: ______________________________
   - What is sciatica?

     Answer: ______________________________
   - In which phase of healing is this injury?

     Answer: ______________________________
   - Would a spasm of the piriformis be related to sciatica?

     Answer: ______________________________
   - Between what two bony structures does the sciatic nerve travel?

     Answer: ______________________________
   - In what position (supine, prone, or side lying) is the sciatic nerve most effectively palpated?

     Answer: ______________________________
   - What is the bowstring test? What does it test? What does a positive test indicate?

     Answer: ______________________________
   - What is the straight-leg raise test? What does it test? What does a positive test indicate?

     Answer: ______________________________
   - What is the piriformis muscle test? Explain.

     Answer: ______________________________

Brain Jolt

Sciatica can occur secondary to piriformis syndrome.

4. Based on the information that you currently have and what was provided by your instructor, how will you begin Ms. Cosgrove's rehabilitation?

- ______________________________
- ______________________________
- ______________________________
- ______________________________

Why or why not?

How will Ms. Cosgrove's rehabilitation progress? For the *why?* portion of each exercise, explain why you chose a particular exercise or activity as part of your program. Describe which rehabilitation goals the exercise or activity covers, and describe the key indicators for progression. For the *why not?* portion of each exercise, explain why other rehabilitation exercises or activities were not chosen and what to avoid during rehabilitation for this injury. Gather details from the textbook, your own research, and data from Ms. Cosgrove's scenario to help formulate your answer.

Why?

- ______________________________
- ______________________________
- ______________________________
- ______________________________

Why not?

- ______________________________
- ______________________________

Conversation Buffer

Recovery from sciatica can last 2 to 3 weeks, and it can sideline an athlete for an extended period. Because of the inflammation of the nerve from the injury and the tight piriformis, the athlete must be diligent in adhering to a rehabilitation program. Remember to explain the importance of rehabilitation and to detail the consequences of noncompliance with your athlete.

What do you think?

1. Based on your rehabilitation protocol, discuss the indicators for limited and full return to play. Include a rough timeline for return to play, if applicable, which is affected by the athlete's compliance with the rehabilitation program.

- ______________________________
- ______________________________
- ______________________________
- ______________________________

2. Are modifications or personal protective equipment needed to return to play?

- ______________________________
- ______________________________
- ______________________________

STUDENT SCENARIO 6: STAN MOOREFIELD

Stan Moorefield is a quarterback on his college football team. He has a history of lumbosacral sprains attributed to the continual twisting motion that he endures when throwing the football or from receiving blind hits to the hip region. He is 2 weeks into the regular season and is already noticing some low back discomfort. The pain seems to spread across his low back around vertebras L4–L5. The movements that bother him the most are forward bending and sitting for long periods. His posture is in slight forward flexion with slight lateral flexion to his left. This posture helps to relieve some of his pain, because most of his pain is located on his right side. He has a positive straight-leg raise test and Valsalva test result. Mr. Moorefield is referred for further evaluation, and the orthopedic physician orders radiographic imaging and MRI, which reveals an L4 disc herniation (Fig. 17-8).

1. Based on this scenario, what do you know about Mr. Moorefield's injury?
   - ______________________
   - ______________________
   - ______________________
   - ______________________
2. To rehabilitate Mr. Moorefield's injury effectively, you will need to gather additional information. What questions should you ask in addition to what is presented in this scenario?
   - ______________________
   - ______________________
   - ______________________
   - ______________________

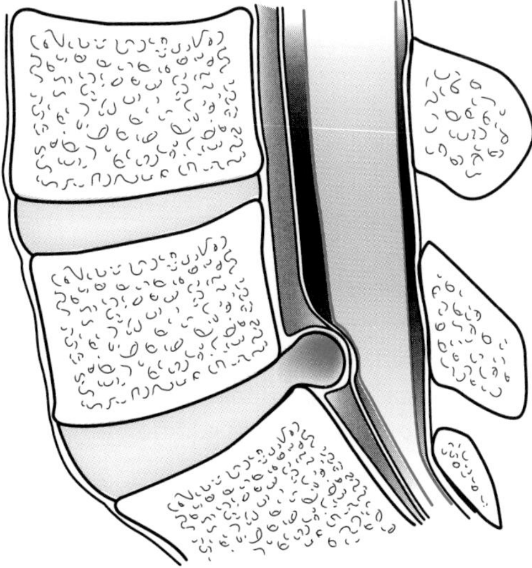
Figure 17-8: Stan Moorefield's L4 disc herniation.

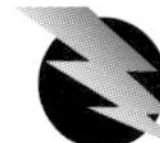

Brain Jolt

A herniated disc can produce numbness and paraesthesia down the posterior side of the affected leg. This can often be confused with sciatica, but a Valsalva maneuver can help to differentiate the conditions.

3. Identify any key terms and concepts, and then research each to broaden your knowledge about the rehabilitation of low back, SI, and pelvis injuries.
   - What anatomical structures might be involved in Mr. Moorefield's injury?

     Answer: ______________________
   - What is an L4 disc herniation?

     Answer: ______________________
   - In which phase of healing is this injury?

     Answer: ______________________
   - What are the different types of herniations?

     Answer: ______________________
   - What is the straight-leg raise test? What does it test? What does a positive test indicate?

     Answer: ______________________
   - What is a Valsalva test? What does it test? What does a positive test indicate?

     Answer: ______________________
4. Based on the information that you currently have and what was provided by your instructor, how will you begin Mr. Moorefield's rehabilitation?
   - ______________________
   - ______________________
   - ______________________
   - ______________________

Why or why not?

How will Mr. Moorefield's rehabilitation progress? For the *why?* portion of each exercise, explain why you chose a particular exercise or activity as part of your program. Describe which rehabilitation goals the exercise or activity covers, and describe the key indicators for progression. For the *why not?* portion of each exercise, explain why other rehabilitation exercises or activities were not chosen and what to avoid during rehabilitation for this injury. Gather details from the textbook, your own research, and data from Mr. Moorefield's scenario to help formulate your answer.

Why?

Why not?

What do you think?

1. Based on your rehabilitation protocol, discuss the indicators for limited and full return to play. Include a rough timeline for return to play, if applicable, which is affected by the athlete's compliance with the rehabilitation program.

2. Are modifications or personal protective equipment needed to return to play?

STUDENT SCENARIO 7: LANA YOUNG

Lana Young is a softball player who plays center field. As a ball is hit hard and high to center field, Ms. Young takes off running toward the fence, and the ball drops just short of the fence line. She quickly bends forward to pick up the ball and then quickly twists her torso to throw the ball to the cutoff person near second base (Fig. 17-9). During this motion, she feels a sharp, deep pain at her low back. She leaves the field holding the left side of her low back. On evaluation, she has point tenderness just lateral to her lumbar vertebra, pain with lateral flexion and any lumbar rotation, no numbness and paraesthesia, and a positive FADIR test result. The injury is diagnosed as a lumbar strain.

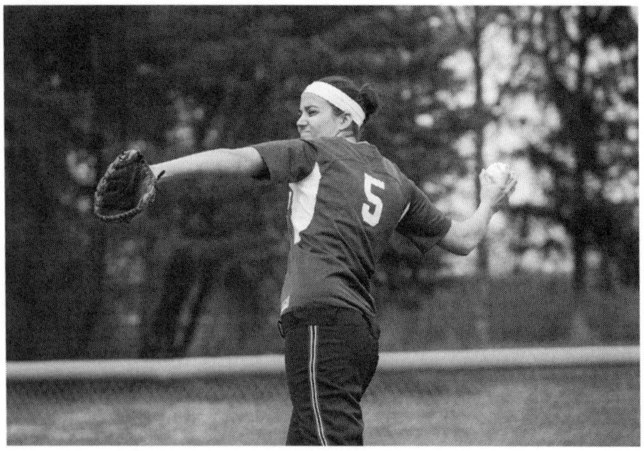

Figure 17-9: Lana Young's lumbar strain.

1. Based on this scenario, what do you know about Ms. Young's injury?

2. To rehabilitate Ms. Young's injury effectively, you will need to gather additional information. What questions should you ask in addition to what is presented in this scenario?

- ____________________
- ____________________
- ____________________

Brain Jolt
The FADIR test is in the same family as the FABER test.

3. Identify key terms and concepts, and then research each to broaden your knowledge about the rehabilitation of low back, SI, and pelvis injuries.
   - What anatomical structures might be involved in Ms. Young's injury?

     Answer: ____________________
   - What is a lumbar strain?

     Answer: ____________________
   - In which phase of healing is this injury?

     Answer: ____________________
   - What is a FADIR test? What does it test? What does a positive test indicate?

     Answer: ____________________
   - Why does Ms. Young have pain with lateral flexion and lumbar rotation?

     Answer: ____________________
4. Based on the information that you currently have and what was provided by your instructor, how will you begin Ms. Young's rehabilitation?
   - ____________________
   - ____________________
   - ____________________
   - ____________________

Why or why not?

How will Ms. Young's rehabilitation progress? For the *why?* portion of each exercise, explain why you chose a particular exercise or activity as part of your program. Describe which rehabilitation goals the exercise or activity covers, and describe the key indicators for progression. For the *why not?* portion of each exercise, explain why other rehabilitation exercises or activities were not chosen and what to avoid during rehabilitation for this injury. Gather details from the textbook, your own research, and data from Ms. Young's scenario to help formulate your answer.

Why?

- ____________________
- ____________________
- ____________________
- ____________________

Why not?

- ____________________
- ____________________

What do you think?

1. Based on your rehabilitation protocol, discuss the indicators for limited and full return to play. Include a rough timeline for return to play, if applicable, which is affected by the athlete's compliance with the rehabilitation program.
   - ____________________
   - ____________________
   - ____________________
   - ____________________
2. Are modifications or personal protective equipment needed to return to play?
   - ____________________
   - ____________________

STUDENT SCENARIO 8: YOLANDA BORNHORST

Yolanda Bornhorst is a soccer player with a history of L4 disc herniation. When treated for this injury 1 year ago, MRI was used to determine the extent of the herniation. The results indicated that her disc was bulging, and it was diagnosed as a disc protrusion. At that time, there was no numbness or paraesthesia radiating into her lower extremities, and she was experiencing only low back pain. She completed a low back rehabilitation program and remained pain free until the game 2 days ago. During the game she was side tackled, and her feet were taken out from underneath her, causing her to come down hard onto her low back. Since that time, she has experienced localized point tenderness, a sharp deep pain, and numbness and paraesthesia radiating into her left gluteus maximus and hamstring. She has positive Valsalva test and Milgram test results and is referred for further evaluation. Radiographs and MRI show a positive herniated disc at L4, but the disc has progressed to a disc extrusion, exerting pressure on the nerve. The disc extrusion is causing spinal stenosis, which is causing a nerve root impingement (Fig. 17-10).

1. Based on this scenario, what do you know about Ms. Bornhurst's injury?
   - ______________________________
   - ______________________________
   - ______________________________
   - ______________________________

2. To rehabilitate Ms. Bornhurst's injury effectively, you will need to gather additional information.

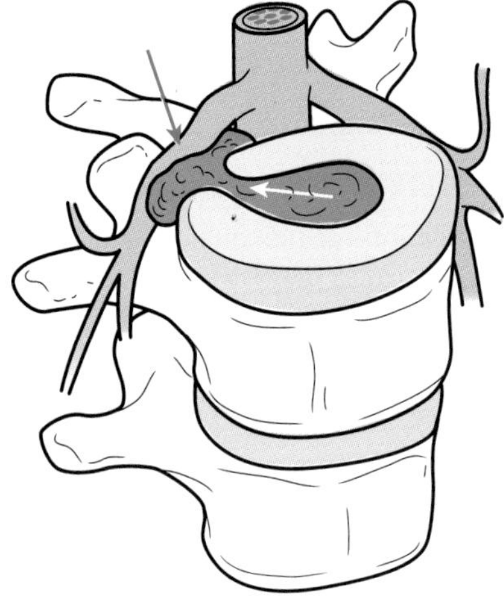

Figure 17-10: Yolanda Bornhorst's lumbar strain.

What questions should you ask in addition to what is presented in this scenario?

- ______________________________
- ______________________________
- ______________________________
- ______________________________

Brain Jolt
Nerve root impingement is most common in the cervical and lumbar vertebrae.

3. Identify key terms and concepts, and then research each to broaden your knowledge about the rehabilitation of low back, SI, and pelvis injuries.
   - What anatomical structures might be involved in Ms. Bornhurst's injury?

     Answer: ______________________________
   - What is nerve root impingement?

     Answer: ______________________________
   - In which phase of healing is this injury?

     Answer: ______________________________
   - Why did she not have numbness and paraesthesia with her initial low back pain or injury?

     Answer: ______________________________
   - Define *herniated disc.*

     Answer: ______________________________
   - Describe the different types of herniation.

     Answer: ______________________________
   - Define *spinal stenosis.*

     Answer: ______________________________
   - What is the Valsalva test? What does it test? What does a positive result indicate?

     Answer: ______________________________
   - What is the Milgram test? What does it test? What does a positive result indicate?

     Answer: ______________________________

4. Based on the information that you currently have and what was provided by your instructor, how will you begin Ms. Bornhurst's rehabilitation?
   - ______________________________

-
-
-

Conversation Buffer
Initially with nerve root impingement, you should focus on reducing inflammation to the injured area. Once that is addressed, progress with a stretching and strengthening program that will help to restore flexion to the joints and musculature involved, while improving stability to the spine. The rehabilitation process can range from 4 to 12 weeks, depending on severity. Therefore, it is essential to set goals with your athletes to keep them engaged during what could be a prolonged rehabilitation. Be sure to discuss these goals and to give them objective progress points to help them see progress in their symptoms.

Why or why not?

How will Ms. Bornhurst's rehabilitation progress? For the *why?* portion of each exercise, explain why you chose a particular exercise or activity as part of your program. Describe which rehabilitation goals the exercise or activity covers, and describe the key indicators for progression. For the *why not?* portion of each exercise, explain why other rehabilitation exercises or activities were not chosen and what to avoid during rehabilitation for this injury. Gather details from the textbook, your own research, and data from Ms. Bornhurst's scenario to help formulate your answer.

Why?

-
-
-
-

Why not?

-
-

What do you think?

1. Based on your rehabilitation protocol, discuss the indicators for limited and full return to play. Include a rough timeline for return to play, if applicable, which is affected by the athlete's compliance with the rehabilitation program.
   -
   -
   -
   -
2. Are modifications or personal protective equipment needed to return to play?
   -
   -

knowledge checklist

Table 17-1 offers a checklist that can be used by a peer, instructor, or preceptor to evaluate each part of the athlete's rehabilitation plan. Use this checklist as a tool to ensure that the rehabilitation plan is complete and to assess your knowledge of the competencies that apply to this chapter.

TABLE 17-1 ■ Low Back, Sacroiliac, and Pelvis Rehabilitation and Therapeutic Exercise Competency Checklist

	Proficient *Can demonstrate and execute the skill properly*	**Proficient With Assistance** *Can demonstrate and execute the skill with minimal guidance or tips*	**Not Proficient** *Unable to demonstrate and execute the skill properly; need to be reevaluated at another time after further study and practice*
Controlling Edema			
PRICE			
Modalities			
Controlling Pain			
Pain scales			
Medications			
Modalities			
Establishes Core Stability			
Reestablishes Neuromuscular Control			
Restores Postural Control and Balance			
Restoring Range of Motion			
Passive range of motion			
Active range of motion			
Resistive range of motion			
Goniometry			
Normal range of motion limits			
Restore Muscular Strength, Endurance, and Power			
Open kinetic chain			
Closed kinetic chain			
Isometric			
Isotonic			
Isotonic (concentric and eccentric)			
Isokinetic			
Plyometric			
Agility			
Functional or Sport-Specific Activities			
Maintains Cardiorespiratory Fitness			
Functional Testing			
Return-to-Play Criteria			
Proper Documentation			

PRICE, prevention, rest, ice, compression, and elevation.

REFERENCES

Arab, A. M., Nourbakhsh, M. R., & Mohammadifar, A. (2011). The relationship between hamstring length and gluteal muscle strength individuals with sacroiliac joint dysfunction. *Journal of Manual and Manipulative Therapy*, *19*, 5–6.

Higgins, M. (2011). *Therapeutic exercise: From theory to practice*. Philadelphia, PA: F.A. Davis.

National Athletic Training Association. (2011). *Athletic training education competencies* (5th ed.). Retrieved from http://www.nata.org/sites/default/files/5th-Edition-Competencies-2011-PDF-Version.pdf

Prentice, W. (2010). *Arnheim's principles of athletic training: A competency-based approach* (14th ed.). New York, NY: McGraw-Hill.

Prentice, W. (2011). *Rehabilitation techniques for sports medicine and athletic training* (5th ed.). New York, NY: McGraw-Hill.

Starkey, C., Brown, S. D., & Ryan, J. (2010). *Examination of orthopedic and athletic injuries* (3rd ed.). Philadelphia, PA: F.A. Davis.

Starkey, C. (2004). *Therapeutic modalities* (3rd ed.). Philadelphia, PA: F.A. Davis.

Tonley, J. C., et al. (2010). Treatment of an individual with piriformis syndrome focusing on hip muscle strengthening and movement reeducation: A case report. *Journal of Orthopaedic and Sports Physical Therapy*, *40*, 103–111.

Venes, D. (Ed.). (2009). *Taber's cyclopedic medical dictionary* (21st ed.). Philadelphia, PA: F.A. Davis.

part four

Medical Interventions

[illegible]

Figure 10-6

MODEL SCENARIO — ELI HOFFMAN

[illegible]

Why or why not?

[illegible]

Brain Jolt

[illegible]

Why?

[illegible]

Why not?

[illegible]

chapter 18

General Medical Conditions

chapter outline

athletic trainer's corner

Out there in the real world, one nurse witnessed the following:

During halftime of the high school championship basketball game, Cara Beckwith began to exhibit shaking in her hands and arms. She was sweating profusely, which she thought was related to the intensity of the game and her unusual level of aggression on the court. She was unable to focus on the coach's instructions and became agitated when addressed. When she complained about a headache and paraesthesia in her hands, the coach summoned the athletic trainer (AT), who realized that Ms. Beckwith might be showing signs of hypoglycemia related to her recently diagnosed diabetes. Ms. Beckwith was instructed to test her blood glucose level, which was found to be 60 mg/dL. She needed to eat something with at least 15 g of carbohydrates and retest her blood glucose in 15 min. She was given 4 oz of orange juice, a handful of jellybeans, and half of a protein bar. In 15 min, her glucose level was 90 mg/dL and her symptoms improved. If her symptoms had not improved, she would have required emergent evaluation by a physician, because severe hypoglycemia is a medical emergency that could lead to loss of consciousness and coma if left untreated. It is important to be able to recognize signs and symptoms early to treat conditions properly.

Jodi Nili, RN, BSN
Patient Safety Manager
Community Regional Medical Center
Fresno, California

learning outcomes

After working through this chapter, you will be able to:

1. Obtain a thorough medical history that includes identifying pertinent past medical conditions and injuries related to the present condition.
2. Communicate the reasoning for differential diagnosis of general medical conditions.
3. Explain the medical terminology associated with general medical condition assessments.

introduction

As an athletic trainer (AT), you will see numerous issues other than orthopedic injuries. Throughout this section, you are presented with many signs and symptoms of general medical conditions to help you fine-tune your assessment skills. You will also be presented with various situations that require medication, referral, or both. Beyond observing visual characteristics of the condition, you will need to determine whether the injury is severe enough to prevent the athlete from returning to play or to affect the athlete's activities. By implementing all the information you have learned in the classroom and then applying it by looking at the big picture in terms of what is going on with the athlete, you can determine the effective treatment for the injury to create the best possible outcome for the athlete.

MODEL SCENARIO 1: RAYMOND OLIVER

Raymond Oliver has a history of eczema. He often notices patches of dry skin and has irritation during the winter months that subsides when he begins using moisturizing cream. However, Mr. Oliver has noticed a spot on his left gastrocnemius that is not responding to his normal eczema treatment. He decides to show the AT the irritated patch of skin. After taking a brief history of Mr. Oliver, the AT notes that he participates on the college wrestling team. The circular spot on his gastrocnemius is red and inflamed around the edges, but with a normal skin appearance in the center of the irritated area. The irritated spot is itchy and slightly raised (Fig. 18-1). He is unable to participate in any contact sports until the skin condition can be identified and treated. Mr. Oliver is referred to the team physician for further examination.

1. Based on this scenario, what do you know about Mr. Oliver's injury or condition?
   - *Male athlete*
   - *Wrestler*

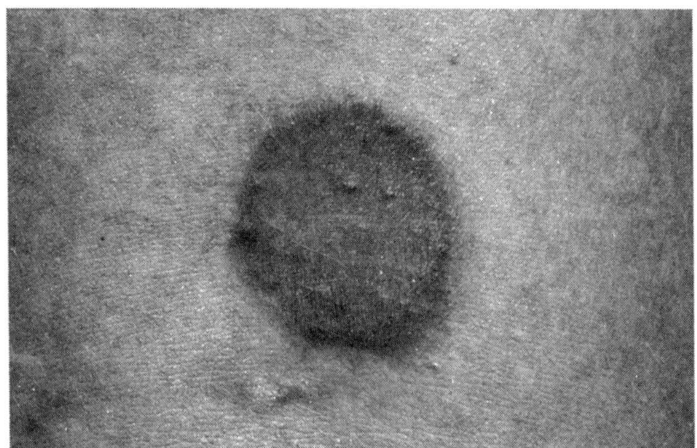

Figure 18-1: Raymond Oliver's skin condition. (© Thinkstock)

   - *History of chronic eczema*
   - *Circular spot on left gastrocnemius*
   - *Irritated spot: red, inflamed, itchy, and slightly raised*
   - *Center of affected area is normal in appearance*
   - *Unable to participate in wrestling until diagnosis is confirmed*

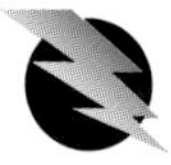

Brain Jolt
This condition is highly contagious and can spread quickly.

2. To evaluate Mr. Oliver's injury or condition effectively, you will need to gather additional information. What questions should you ask yourself in addition to what is presented in this scenario?
   - *Is this injury a medical emergency?*
   - *Are there any preexisting injuries? If yes, what are they?*
   - *Has Mr. Oliver ever been diagnosed with a viral or bacterial skin condition?*
   - *Was there any hypersensitivity or new sensation at the irritated skin spot a few days before the outbreak?*
   - *Has Mr. Oliver been exposed to any contagious skin conditions recently?*
   - *Are there any other irritated circular spots on Mr. Oliver?*
   - *What type of ointment has Mr. Oliver been applying? Is it antifungal or antibacterial ointment?*
   - *Has Mr. Oliver been ill, fatigued, or stressed recently?*
3. Identify key terms and concepts, and then research each to broaden your knowledge of general medical conditions.
   - What anatomical structures might be involved in Mr. Oliver's injury or condition?
     Gastrocnemius
     Dermis layer of the skin

- Define *eczema*.

  Eczema is a chronic skin condition where the skin becomes itchy, red, cracked, and dry.
- What causes eczema, and is it contagious?

  The exact cause is unknown, but eczema is a reaction to an internal or external allergen and is not contagious.
- Why is Mr. Oliver held from participation in a contact sport? Will he need any paperwork to return to wrestling?

  Mr. Oliver is unable to participate in a contact sport with an unknown skin condition because of the possibility of that skin condition being highly contagious through skin-to-skin contact. Mr. Oliver could put the health of an opposing player, or possibly a whole team, at risk. Mr. Oliver will need a form completed by the physician, marking the placement of the spot, along with the treatment plan. The type of skin condition the athlete has will determine the length of time that the athlete will not be able to participate.

4. Based on the information that you currently have and what was provided by your instructor, what are the possible assessments for Mr. Oliver's injury or condition?

   Impetigo

   Ringworm

   Methicillin-resistant Staphylococcus aureus (MRSA)

   Herpes simplex infection

Why or why not?

For each assessment or diagnosis, write *why?* or *why not?* statements identifying why the information is correct or incorrect. Take details from your textbook, your own research, and data from Mr. Oliver's scenario to help you formulate an answer.

1. *Mr. Oliver does not have impetigo because of the absence of the small vesicles or pustules that normally form with impetigo. The pustules will rupture and leave a yellow crust over the spots. Impetigo is not an infection that forms in a perfect circular pattern. It is a highly contagious bacterial infection that needs to be treated with an antibacterial ointment.*
2. *Mr. Oliver has ringworm because of the perfect circular spot formation. Ringworm is itchy and red with raised red edges on the periphery of the circle. The center is a normal or pale skin color. This skin condition is highly contagious and needs to be treated with an antifungal cream.*
3. *Mr. Oliver does not have MRSA infection. Frequently, MRSA infection first appears as a small pustule with a white head to it almost resembling a pimple or boil. The area around the pustule is red, inflamed, and tender to the touch. When the pustule pops, a pus-colored liquid drains from it. MRSA is highly contagious and needs to be treated immediately by a physician with oral or intravenous antibiotics. MRSA can become a life-threatening condition if not treated properly.*
4. *Mr. Oliver does not have herpes simplex infection. Herpes simplex is normally brought on by fatigue, illness, or stress. It could be attributed to a low immune system. Normally the infection manifests as a blister around the mouth, genitals, or rectum. It leaves painful sores after the blister breaks. The virus remains inactive in the body until a certain stressor makes it active again. A topical viral cream is often prescribed by a physician.*

What do you think?

1. What is your assessment of Mr. Oliver's injury or condition?

   Answer: *Ringworm*
2. Was your assessment of Mr. Oliver's injury or condition correct?

   Answer: *Yes*
3. If not, explain what you did incorrectly and how you could have performed a better assessment.

   Answer: ______________________________

MODEL SCENARIO 2: LELAND BENNETT

Leland Bennett plays third base on his college baseball team. Today's game is nearing completion and the score is tied. During the bottom of the ninth inning, with runners on first and second base, an opposing batter hits a ground ball to the third base side. As Mr. Bennett attempts to field the ball, it takes a bad hop and hits him in the face. The AT rushes onto the field after the play is stopped to help control the resulting bleeding. Mr. Bennett also complains of a headache and blurred vision, but no neck pain. After being helped off the field, Mr. Bennett is evaluated further. He is point tender over the inferior orbit of the eye socket and has redness within the anterior chamber of the right eye (Fig. 18-2). He has normal eye movement, reactive pupils to light, and an eyelid that is swollen shut. Mr. Bennett's headache is subsiding, but his vision in the right eye has diminished. He is referred to the team physician for further treatment. A computed tomography (CT) scan is performed, and the results are negative for any type of orbital fracture.

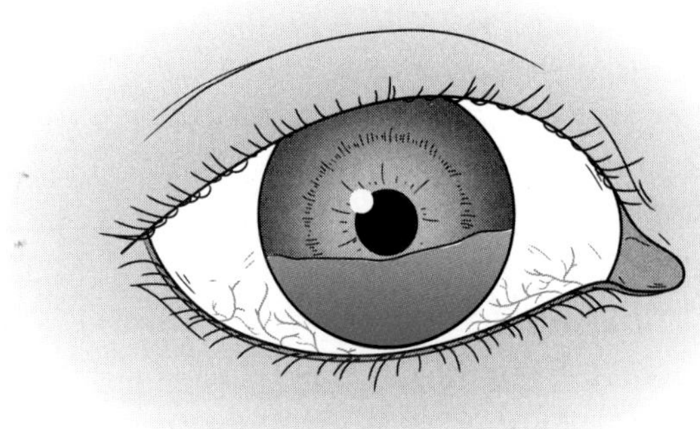

Figure 18-2: Leland Bennett's eye.

1. Based on this scenario, what do you know about Mr. Bennett's injury or condition?
   - *Male athlete*
   - *Baseball player*
   - *Mechanism of injury: direct hit with a baseball to the right eye*
   - *Point tenderness over the right inferior eye orbit*
   - *Redness within the anterior chamber of the right eye*
   - *Edema over the right eyelid*
   - *Bleeding*
   - *No neck pain*
   - *Initially headache that is subsiding*
   - *Normal eye movement*
   - *Initial blurry vision that is diminishing*
   - *Reactive pupils to light*
   - *Negative CT scan for orbital fracture*

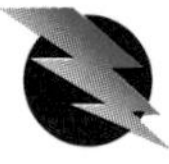

Brain Jolt
This injury is an eye emergency that can result in irreversible vision damage if not handled properly.

Conversation Buffer
You will need to express to the athlete that body position is crucial for proper treatment of this injury. If this injury is not treated quickly and correctly, significant vision damage could result. Therefore, it is vital that the athlete adhere to your guidelines en route to the hospital and follow the physician's orders.

2. To evaluate Mr. Bennett's injury or condition effectively, you will need to gather additional information. What questions should you ask yourself in addition to what has been presented in this scenario?
   - *Is this injury a medical emergency?*
   - *Are there any preexisting injuries? If yes, what are they?*
   - *Does Mr. Bennett have a dilated pupil?*
   - *Is there the possibility of a concussion?*
   - *Is there complete or partial loss of vision?*
   - *Has the redness pooled inferiorly in the anterior chamber of the eye?*
   - *What is the origin of the bleeding?*
3. Identify key terms and concepts, and then research each to broaden your knowledge of general medical conditions.
   - What anatomical structures might be involved in Mr. Bennett's injury or condition?
     Nasal bone
     Right eye and orbit
     Eyelid
   - What does the redness in the eye indicate?
     It indicates that there is some type of bleeding occurring in the eye from the trauma.
   - Why does Mr. Bennett have impaired vision?
     The blood pooling inferiorly in the anterior chamber of the eye is blocking his field of vision.
   - What are the signs and symptoms of a concussion?
     Headache, dizziness, blurred vision, nausea, tinnitus, impaired coordination, impaired balance, impaired memory, nystagmus, photophobia, and tinnitus
   - What is the PERLA or PEARL standard for eye health?
     PERLA = pupils equal and reactive to light and accommodation; PEARL = pupils are equal and reactive to light when examined.
4. Based on the information that you currently have and what was provided by your instructor, what are the possible assessments of Mr. Bennett's injury or condition?
   Orbital fracture
   Hyphema
   Concussion
   Rupture of the eye globe

Why or why not?

For each assessment or diagnosis, write *why?* or *why not?* statements identifying why the information is correct or incorrect. Take details from your textbook, your own research, and data from Mr. Bennett's scenario to help you formulate an answer.

1. *Mr. Bennett does not have an orbital fracture because the CT results were negative and there was no compromised eye movement. Inferior eye movement is often restricted with an orbital fracture.*
2. *Mr. Bennett has a hyphema. The redness that developed as a result of the initial contact with the ball suggests that there is bleeding in the eye from the trauma. One to two hours after the injury, the anterior chamber will have prominent pooling of blood that will settle inferiorly.*
3. *Mr. Bennett also has a concussion. The initial symptoms of concussion subsided approximately 15 min after the initial injury. However, any symptoms of a concussion indicate that a concussion is present and proper treatment should follow.*
4. *Mr. Bennett does not have a ruptured eye globe. A ruptured eye globe occurs when an object smaller than*

the eye orbit, such as a golf ball, strikes the eye. An athlete with a ruptured eye globe will have diplopia, orbital discharge, and a dilated pupil.

What do you think?

1. What is your assessment of Mr. Bennett's injury?
Answer: *Hyphema with an accompanying concussion*

2. Was your assessment of Mr. Bennett's injury correct?
Answer: *Yes*

3. If not, explain what you did incorrectly and how you could have performed a better assessment.

Answer: ______________________________

STUDENT SCENARIO 1: CLAIRE O'SULLIVAN

Claire O'Sullivan is a senior on her high school soccer team. During a home game, an opposing player has the ball. As Ms. O'Sullivan approaches the opponent to steal the ball, the opponent forcefully kicks the ball toward the opposite side of the field. Ms. O'Sullivan jumps up in hopes of heading the ball, but instead the ball hits her directly over her left eye. She falls to one knee, holding her face. When approached by the AT, she states that she is not disoriented and has no headache or neck pain. She is concerned about seeing floaters in her field of vision in her left eye (Fig. 18-3). She has no prior injuries to the left eye. Ms. O'Sullivan does not wear contact lenses, but she does wear reading glasses for an extreme case of myopia. She is assisted off the field and examined with an ophthalmoscope.

Brain Jolt
Floaters, a dark curtain, or flashes of light are common with this injury.

1. Based on this scenario, what do you know about Ms. O'Sullivan's injury or condition?
   - ______________________________
   - ______________________________
   - ______________________________
   - ______________________________

Figure 18-3: Claire O'Sullivan's vision.

2. To evaluate Ms. O'Sullivan's injury or condition effectively, you will need to gather additional information. What questions should you ask yourself in addition to what has been presented in this scenario?
   - ______________________________
   - ______________________________
   - ______________________________
   - ______________________________

3. Identify key terms and concepts, and then research each to broaden your knowledge of general medical conditions.
   - What anatomical structures might be involved in Ms. O'Sullivan's injury?

     Answer: ______________________________
   - Define *myopia.*

     Answer: ______________________________
   - What could the presence of floaters in her field of vision imply?

     Answer: ______________________________
   - What are the signs and symptoms of a concussion?

     Answer: ______________________________
   - Define *ophthalmoscope* and explain its purpose.

     Answer: ______________________________

4. Based on the information that you currently have and what was provided by your instructor, what are the possible assessments for Ms. O'Sullivan's injury?

- ______________________________
- ______________________________
- ______________________________
- ______________________________

Conversation Buffer

An athlete with this eye injury needs to be referred immediately to a physician or the emergency department with follow-up within 24 to 72 hours by an ophthalmologist. Surgery may be indicated to prevent further damage or possible vision loss. Ensure that the athlete, parents, and coaches are informed of all treatment possibilities.

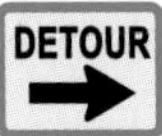

Treatment Detour

Tears or perforations in this anatomical structure can be nontraumatic and asymptomatic. However, these breaks can become symptomatic and lead to detachment, which is the most significant complication. A small percentage of breaks are traumatic and are more prone to detachment and vision complications. In one case study, a 20-year-old male college basketball player sustained a blunt trauma to his right eye from an opponent's finger. He experienced immediate, intense pain and blurred vision. He was sent to the emergency department, where he experienced decreased visual acuity, decreased pupil reactivity, and photophobia. On follow-up with an ophthalmologist, the patient still experienced no floaters or flashes of light. A specialist was consulted about the symptoms, and a mild tear of this anatomical structure was found. After treatment, the athlete returned to play. It is important to follow up with all eye injuries. Although there are common signs for injuries and conditions, these signs will not always be present. Therefore, any vision or eye issue needs to be evaluated by a physician and followed up with an ophthalmologist within 24 to 72 hours to prevent complications (Robinson, Wadsworth, & Feman, 2011).

Why or why not?

For each assessment or diagnosis, write *why?* or *why not?* statements identifying why the information is correct or incorrect. Take details from your textbook, your own research, and data from Ms. O'Sullivan's scenario to help you formulate an answer.

1. ______________________________
2. ______________________________
3. ______________________________
4. ______________________________

What do you think?

1. What is your assessment of Ms. O'Sullivan's injury or condition?

   Answer: ______________________________

2. Was your assessment of Ms. O'Sullivan's injury or condition correct?

   Answer: ______________________________

3. If not, explain what you did incorrectly and how you could have performed a better assessment.

   Answer: ______________________________

STUDENT SCENARIO 2: LUIGI RUSSO

Luigi Russo is a semiprofessional soccer player who recently traveled to Chile to participate in a weekend soccer tournament. During the first day of competition, Mr. Russo strained his right iliopsoas muscle. As a result, he experienced constant pain and soreness near his anterior superior iliac spine. After the injury, Mr. Russo noticed that he did not feel well and had a low-grade fever during the last day of competition. He was unable to play because of the injury to his iliopsoas and the fever. Upon arriving home, he began vomiting. He disregarded the symptoms and surmised he had caught a "stomach bug." Thirty-six hours later, Mr. Russo consulted a physician when his lower right abdominal pain intensified. On palpation, the physician noted abdominal rigidity in the lower right quadrant of the abdomen and rebound tenderness (Fig. 18-4).

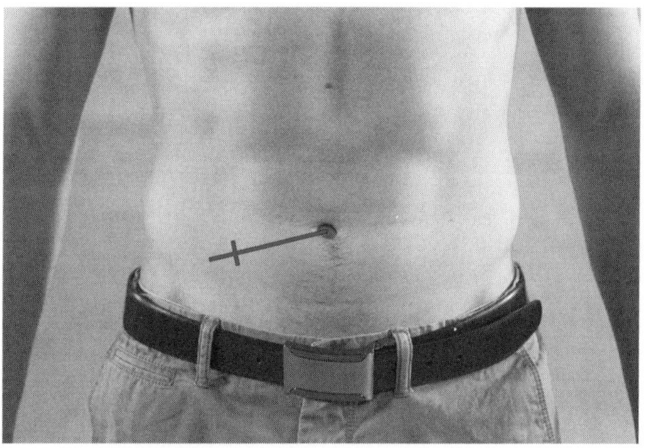

Figure 18-4: Luigi Russo's area of pain.

Brain Jolt

Palpate McBurney's point to help you determine the issue.

1. Based on this scenario, what do you know about Mr. Russo's injury or condition?
   - ______________________________
   - ______________________________
   - ______________________________
   - ______________________________

2. To evaluate Mr. Russo's injury or condition effectively, you will need to gather additional information. What questions should you ask yourself in addition to what has been presented in this scenario?
   - ______________________________
   - ______________________________
   - ______________________________
   - ______________________________

3. Identify key terms and concepts, and research each to broaden your knowledge of general medical conditions.
   - What anatomical structures might be involved in Mr. Russo's injury or condition?

     Answer: ______________________________
   - What two muscles compose the iliopsoas muscle, and what are their origin and insertion points?

     Answer: ______________________________
   - Define *abdominal rigidity*.

     Answer: ______________________________
   - Define *rebound tenderness*.

     Answer: ______________________________
   - Name the four quadrants of the abdomen and the corresponding organs in each quadrant.

     Answer: ______________________________
   - What anatomical landmark is located between the anterior superior iliac spine and the umbilicus?

     Answer: ______________________________

4. Based on the information that you currently have and what was provided by your instructor, what are the possible assessments for Mr. Russo's injury or condition?
   - ______________________________
   - ______________________________
   - ______________________________
   - ______________________________

Why or why not?

For each assessment or diagnosis, write *why?* or *why not?* statements identifying why the information is correct or incorrect. Take details from your textbook, your own research, and data from Mr. Russo's scenario to help you formulate an answer.

1. ______________________________
2. ______________________________
3. ______________________________
4. ______________________________

Treatment Detour

This condition is the most common emergency requiring surgical intervention in children aged 3 to 18 years. It is estimated that in the United States, more than 341,000 operations resolving this condition are performed each year. One concern involving this condition is that children tend to have higher rates of rupture than adults. In one study of 197 patients undergoing this operation, it was found that the risk of rupture increases in a linear fashion during the time between the onset of symptoms and surgery. The risk of rupture within 24 hours of onset is 7.7%, a substantial risk that continues to increase with time. Therefore, this study shows that it is critical to recognize the symptoms of this condition quickly and to refer the athlete for medical treatment quickly to reduce the risk of rupture (Narsule, Kahle, Kim, Anderson, & Luks, 2011).

What do you think?

1. What is your assessment of Mr. Russo's injury or condition?

   Answer: ______________________________

2. Was your assessment of Mr. Russo's injury or condition correct?

   Answer: ______________________________

3. If not, explain what you did incorrectly and how you could have performed a better assessment.

   Answer: ______________________________

STUDENT SCENARIO 3: CARINA ZIMMERMAN

Carina Zimmerman is a catcher on her college softball team. The AT has observed that Ms. Zimmerman is experiencing some left eye irritation during warm-ups. She continues to take her mask off to rub her eye throughout the game, which has caused her to miss two throws to third base. She is removed from the game to have her left eye evaluated by the AT. She wears daily disposable contact lenses and has been wearing the same pair for the past week. On examination, the eyelid appears swollen, and the conjunctiva lining is red. The athlete states that the eye is itchy, but there is no purulent discharge from the eye or complaint of photophobia. However, there seems to be an excessive amount of a clear, watery liquid draining from the eye. Ms. Zimmerman puts a clean contact lens in her left eye and returns to the game. The next day, Ms. Zimmerman arrives in the training room with a yellow discharge oozing from her left eye that now itches (Fig. 18-5). The athlete states that her eye was "matted" shut that morning when she woke up. The conjunctiva shows signs of hyperemia, and Ms. Zimmerman is referred to the optometrist.

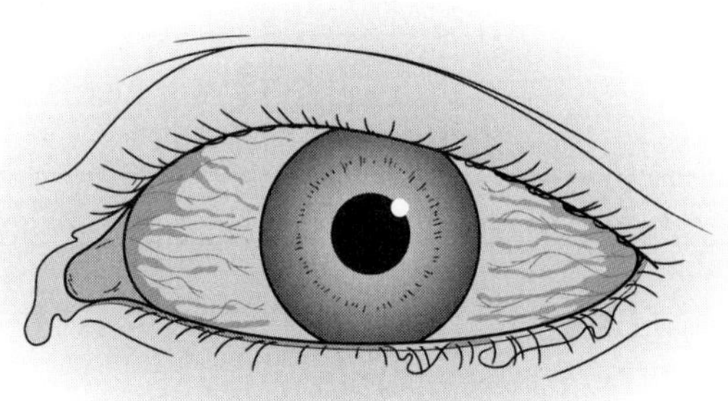

Figure 18-5: Carina Zimmerman's eye.

1. Based on this scenario, what do you know about Ms. Zimmerman's injury or condition?

   - ______________________________
   - ______________________________
   - ______________________________
   - ______________________________

2. To evaluate Ms. Zimmerman's injury or condition effectively, you will need to gather additional information. What questions should you ask in addition to what has been presented in this scenario?

   - ______________________________
   - ______________________________
   - ______________________________
   - ______________________________

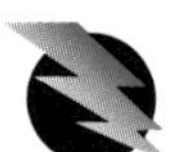

Brain Jolt

A pink sclera is a sign of this highly contagious condition.

3. Identify key terms and concepts, and research each to broaden your knowledge of general medical conditions.
   - What anatomical structures might be involved in Ms. Zimmerman's injury or condition?

     Answer: ____________________
   - Define *conjunctiva.*

     Answer: ____________________
   - Define *photophobia.*

     Answer: ____________________
   - Define *purulent.*

     Answer: ____________________
   - What does a yellow discharge from the eye indicate?

     Answer: ____________________
   - Is this condition contagious?

     Answer: ____________________
   - Define *hyperemia.*

     Answer: ____________________
   - Do Ms. Zimmerman's contact lenses play a role in this condition?

     Answer: ____________________
4. Based on the information you currently have and what was provided by your instructor, what are the possible assessments for Ms. Zimmerman's injury or condition?
   - ____________________
   - ____________________
   - ____________________
   - ____________________

Why or why not?

For each assessment or diagnosis, write *why?* or *why not?* statements identifying why the information is correct or incorrect. Gather details from the textbook, your own research, and data from Ms. Zimmerman's scenario to help formulate your answer.

1. ____________________
2. ____________________
3. ____________________
4. ____________________

What do you think?

1. What is your assessment of Ms. Zimmerman's injury or condition?

   Answer: ____________________
2. Was your assessment of Ms. Zimmerman's injury or condition correct?

   Answer: ____________________
3. If not, explain what you did incorrectly and how you could have performed a better assessment.

   Answer: ____________________

STUDENT SCENARIO 4: JULIANA BERGER

Juliana Berger is a senior in high school who has noticed that for the past 2 months she has been overly tired and has unintentionally lost 8 lb. Ms. Berger is also a basketball player on the girls' team and a cheerleader for the boys' basketball team. She attributes her symptoms to being active and not receiving adequate rest. She decides to approach her high school AT when she experiences blurred vision (Fig. 18-6) and her teammates comment that she looks pale during basketball practice. She has no history of injuries or conditions, but she does have a family history of metabolic disease. She has always tried to be a healthy athlete in regard to diet and hydration. When the AT examines Ms. Berger, it is noted that she has a 20-oz water bottle and has to excuse herself to go to the bathroom twice within the hour. She states that she drinks six to eight of the 20-oz bottles of water a day and seems to be thirsty a fair amount of the time. The AT decides to refer Ms. Berger to her family physician for further blood work.

1. Based on this scenario, what do you know about Ms. Berger's injury or condition?
   - ____________________

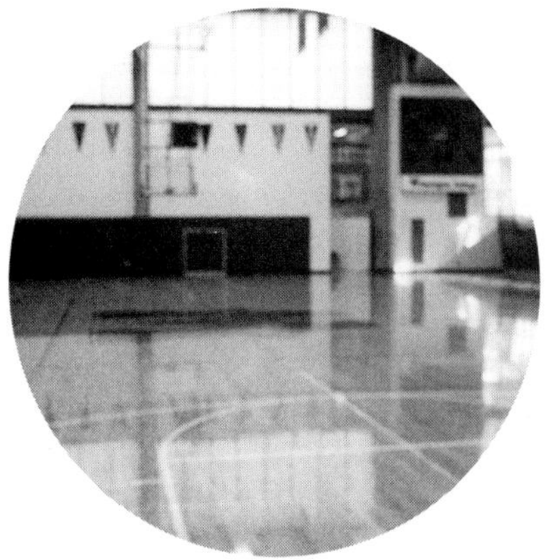

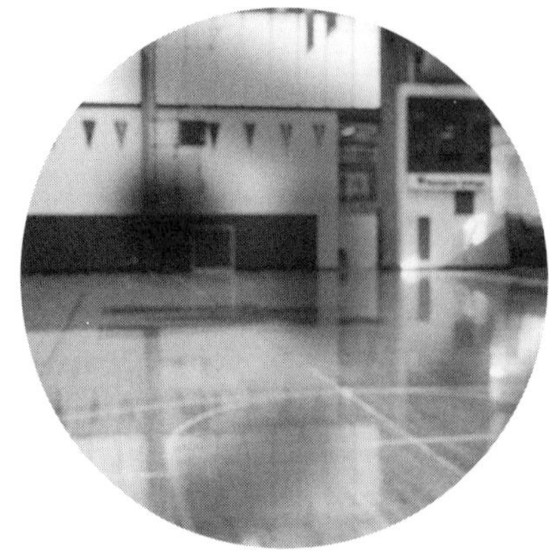

Figure 18-6: Juliana Berger's blurred vision.

- ______________________________
- ______________________________
- ______________________________

2. To evaluate Ms. Berger's injury or condition effectively, you will need to gather additional information. What questions should you ask yourself in addition to what has been presented in this scenario?
   - ______________________________
   - ______________________________
   - ______________________________
   - ______________________________

Brain Jolt
This condition has two subtypes with one requiring medication and another requiring only lifestyle and nutritional changes.

3. Identify key terms and concepts, and research each to broaden your knowledge of general medical conditions.
   - What anatomical structures might be involved in Ms. Berger's injury or condition?

     Answer: ______________________________
   - Why is Ms. Berger's family history important?

     Answer: ______________________________
   - Define *metabolic disease.*

     Answer: ______________________________
   - Why is it important to observe Ms. Berger's diet and hydration pattern?

     Answer: ______________________________
   - What could blurred vision and pale skin during sports practice indicate?

     Answer: ______________________________
   - What type of blood work is needed to determine Ms. Berger's condition?

     Answer: ______________________________
   - What other tests could be performed to diagnose this condition?

     Answer: ______________________________
4. Based on the information you currently have and what was provided by your instructor, what are the possible assessments for Ms. Berger's injury or condition?
   - ______________________________
   - ______________________________
   - ______________________________
   - ______________________________

Why or why not?

For each assessment or diagnosis, write *why?* or *why not?* statements identifying why the information is correct or incorrect. Take details from your textbook, your own research, and data from Ms. Berger's scenario to help you formulate an answer.

1. ______________________________

2. ______________________________

____

3. ______________________________

____

4. ______________________________

____

DETOUR

Treatment Detour

It is important that the athlete and the AT properly monitor and manage this disease. Frequent monitoring of the athlete's blood glucose levels is required. Continuous, moderately intense aerobic exercise frequently causes hypoglycemia, or a decline in blood glucose concentration, in people with type 1 of this particular condition. Authors of one study found that continuous exercise, either with or without intermittent high-intensity exercise in athletes with type 1 of this condition, does in fact cause similar decreases in glucose levels during the activity itself. However, it was also found that with the addition of the intermittent high-intensity exercise, there is a decrease in the risk of having late-onset decreases in blood glucose after exercising. This is important because athletes with this condition often have trouble regulating their blood glucose when they are not supervised by their AT. These findings indicate that if the exercise regimen is modified by adding intermittent, high-intensity exercise versus continuous exercise, the athlete has a better chance of accurately monitoring his or her condition (Iscoe & Riddell, 2011).

What do you think?

1. What is your assessment of Ms. Berger's injury or condition?

Answer: ______________________________

2. Was your assessment of Ms. Berger's injury or condition correct?

Answer: ______________________________

3. If not, explain what you did incorrectly and how you could have performed a better assessment.

Answer: ______________________________

STUDENT SCENARIO 5: SETH FLAHERTY

Seth Flaherty is a running back on his college football team. The opposing team that Mr. Flaherty is playing has won the Division III playoffs the last three years. This team is big, physical, and hard-hitting. It is only the first quarter of the game and Mr. Flaherty already feels lethargic after having the flu earlier in the week. As Mr. Flaherty hands off the ball, he runs toward an opening and a linebacker hits him from the left side. He is hit in the upper left quadrant of the abdomen, which results in immediate pain. He tries to continue playing despite the discomfort, but after 10 min he is nauseated and has to leave the game. He is point tender over the upper left abdominal quadrant and has palpable abdominal rigidity (Fig. 18-7), normal bowel sounds, and a positive Kehr's sign. An ambulance is called, and Mr. Flaherty is transported to the hospital for further evaluation.

1. Based on this scenario, what do you know about Mr. Flaherty's injury or condition?

- ______________________________

  ____

- ______________________________

  ____

- ______________________________

  ____

- ______________________________

  ____

2. To evaluate Mr. Flaherty's injury or condition effectively, you will need to gather additional information. What questions should you ask yourself in addition to what has been presented in this scenario?

- ______________________________

  ____

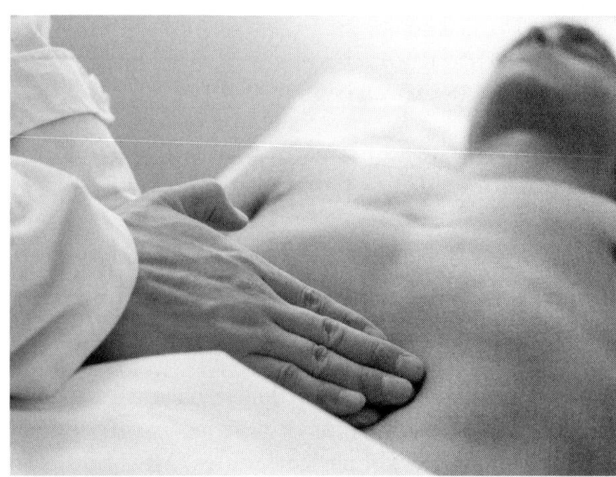

Figure 18-7: Seth Flaherty's area of rigidity. (From Ryan McVay, © Ryan McVay)

- ______________________________
  ____
- ______________________________
  ____
- ______________________________
  ____

3. Identify key terms and concepts, and research each to broaden your knowledge of general medical conditions.
   - What anatomical structures might be involved in Mr. Flaherty's injury or condition?

     Answer: ______________________________
   - What organ is located in the upper left quadrant of the abdomen?

     Answer: ______________________________
   - What might rigidity indicate?

     Answer: ______________________________
   - Why are bowel sounds important?

     Answer: ______________________________
   - How do you evaluate bowel sounds?

     Answer: ______________________________
   - Explain a positive Kehr's sign. What does it indicate?

     Answer: ______________________________
4. Based on the information that you currently have and what was provided by your instructor, what are the possible assessments for Mr. Flaherty's injury or condition?
   - ______________________________
     ____
   - ______________________________
     ____
   - ______________________________
     ____
   - ______________________________
     ____

Brain Jolt

The injured internal organ in this scenario can be affected by the illness mononucleosis.

Conversation Buffer

One of the dangers with this injury is the organ's ability to splint itself and therefore delay hemorrhage, which can mask the original injury. If the athlete returns to competition too soon, the healing process could be disrupted. The athlete and coaches need to be informed that the initial return-to-play timeframe is 3 to 4 weeks, which is a lengthy recovery.

Why or why not?

For each assessment or diagnosis, write *why?* or *why not?* statements identifying why the information is correct or incorrect. Take details from your textbook, your own research, and data from Mr. Flaherty's scenario to help you formulate an answer.

1. ______________________________
   ____
2. ______________________________
   ____
3. ______________________________
   ____
4. ______________________________
   ____

What do you think?

1. What is your assessment of Mr. Flaherty's injury or condition?

   Answer: ______________________________
2. Was your assessment of Mr. Flaherty's injury or condition correct?

   Answer: ______________________________
3. If not, explain what you did incorrectly and how you could have performed a better assessment.

   Answer: ______________________________

STUDENT SCENARIO 6: GAVIN MIDDLETON

Gavin Middleton is a senior quarterback on his high school football team. Today's practice is full contact as the team works on passing routes. Mr. Middleton drops back to pass the ball when a linebacker hits him with the helmet below the shoulder pads lateral to the vertebral column (Fig. 18-8). Mr. Middleton falls down onto the field after the hit and is unable to move. He shows signs of shock and has palpable rigid back muscles. An ambulance is called, and Mr. Middleton is prepared for transport to the hospital. While waiting on

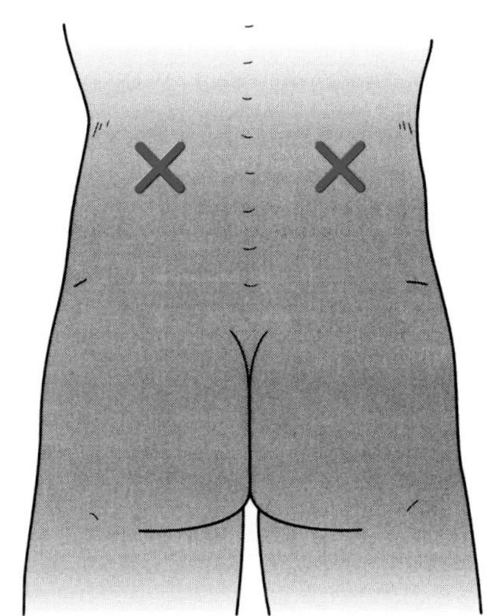

Figure 18-8: Gavin Middleton's point of impact.

the ambulance to arrive, he is log rolled onto his side into a recovery position because he begins vomiting.

1. Based on this scenario, what do you know about Mr. Middleton's injury or condition?
   - ______
   - ______
   - ______
   - ______
2. To evaluate Mr. Middleton's injury or condition effectively, you will need to gather additional information. What questions should you ask in addition to what has been presented in this scenario?
   - ______
   - ______
   - ______
   - ______

Brain Jolt
Injury to this organ can produce hematuria.

3. Identify key terms and concepts, and then research each to broaden your knowledge of general medical conditions.
   - What anatomical structures might be involved in Mr. Middleton's injury or condition?

     Answer: ______
   - Explain the signs of shock.

     Answer: ______
   - What are vital signs?

     Answer: ______
   - How do you take vital signs?

     Answer: ______
   - What are normal ranges for vital signs?

     Answer: ______
   - Explain what rigid back muscles could indicate.

     Answer: ______
   - Explain the log roll procedure.

     Answer: ______
   - Explain the recovery position.

     Answer: ______
   - Define *hematuria.*

     Answer: ______
4. Based on the information that you currently have and what was provided by your instructor, what are the possible assessments for Mr. Middleton's injury or condition?
   - ______
   - ______
   - ______
   - ______

Why or why not?

For each assessment or diagnosis, write *why?* or *why not?* statements identifying why the information is correct or incorrect. Take details from your textbook, your own research, and data from Mr. Middleton's scenario to help you formulate an answer.

1. ______
2. ______

3. ____

____

4. ____

____

What do you think?

1. What is your assessment of Mr. Middleton's injury or condition?

   Answer: ______________________________

2. Was your assessment of Mr. Middleton's injury or condition correct?

   Answer: ______________________________

3. If not, explain what you did incorrectly and how you could have performed a better assessment.

   Answer: ______________________________

STUDENT SCENARIO 7: MARCUS GRAY

Marcus Gray throws shot put for his college outdoor track and field team. The official start to the season began 3 weeks ago. Since the beginning of the season, Mr. Gray has noticed a deep pain around his groin region during the twisting motion of his throw. The pain intensifies during practice when he increases the shot put weight while warming up. Because the pain has not been consistent and has not affected his throwing, he has not mentioned this discomfort to the AT. In addition, he is preparing for this week's first competition and does not want anything to deter his ability to compete. The size shot put that he typically uses is 7.26 kg (16 lb). The coach believes that interval-type training using a rubber-weighted ball weighing 18 lb is beneficial. Mr. Gray believes that the additional 2 lb will make a noticeable difference, but he does agree that his normal shot put weight will seem lighter if he can successfully throw the 18-lb ball. During the warm-up, he notices a mild amount of deep groin pain. The discomfort subsides until he takes his first throw with the 18-lb ball. As Mr. Gray begins the initial twisting motion (Fig. 18-9) of his throw, he immediately feels a sharp pain that is located on his lower left side that radiates into the groin region. He states that it feels like a tearing sensation. On evaluation, he has point tenderness just proximal to a normal groin strain. He has a small palpable deformity that is tender to palpate and that elicits pain during a sit-up. He also experiences referred pain to the testicular region. Mr. Gray is referred to the team physician for further evaluation.

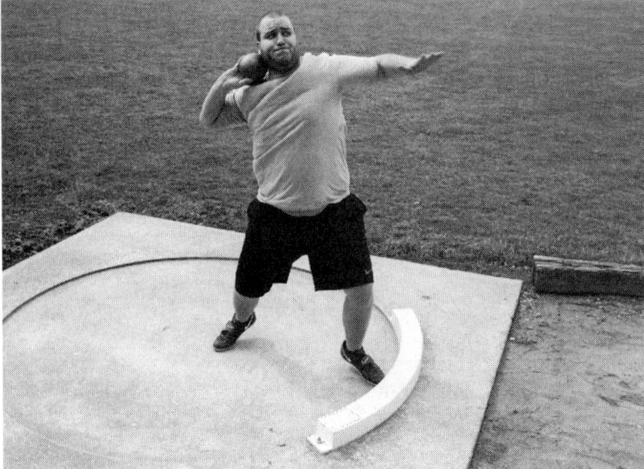

Figure 18-9: Marcus Gray's mechanism of injury.

1. Based on this scenario, what do you know about Mr. Gray's injury or condition?
   - ____
   - ____
   - ____
   - ____

2. To evaluate Mr. Gray's injury or condition effectively, you will need to gather additional information. What questions should you ask in addition to what has been presented in this scenario?
   - ____
   - ____
   - ____
   - ____

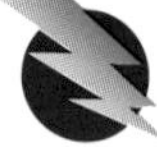

Brain Jolt

This condition is often confused with a groin strain or abdominal strain.

3. Identify key terms and concepts, and research each to broaden your knowledge of general medical conditions.
   - What anatomical structures might be involved in Mr. Gray's injury or condition?

     Answer: ______
   - Explain *interval training.*

     Answer: ______
   - What does a tearing sensation imply?

     Answer: ______
   - Why is pain experienced with a sit-up or cough?

     Answer: ______
   - Why is there referred pain to the testicular region?

     Answer: ______
   - What could a palpable lump indicate?

     Answer: ______
4. Based on the information that you currently have and what was provided by your instructor, what are the possible assessments for Mr. Gray's injury or condition?
   - ______
   - ______
   - ______
   - ______

Why or why not?

For each assessment or diagnosis, write *why?* or *why not?* statements identifying why the information is correct or incorrect. Take details from your textbook, your own research, and data from Mr. Gray's scenario to help you formulate an answer.

1. ______
2. ______
3. ______
4. ______

What do you think?

1. What is your assessment of Mr. Gray's injury or condition?

   Answer: ______
2. Was your assessment of Mr. Gray's injury or condition correct?

   Answer: ______
3. If not, explain what you did incorrectly and how you could have performed a better assessment.

   Answer: ______

STUDENT SCENARIO 8: SAMPSON JUSTUS

Sampson Justus is a forward on his rugby team where he is frequently involved in scrums. He comes to the athletic training room with a noticeable skin lesion on his left cheek near his zygomatic bone that reaches up toward his temple. On examination, this skin lesion is filled with pus and has a yellow tinted outline that is crusted. The AT refers Mr. Justus to the team physician for treatment (Fig. 18-10).

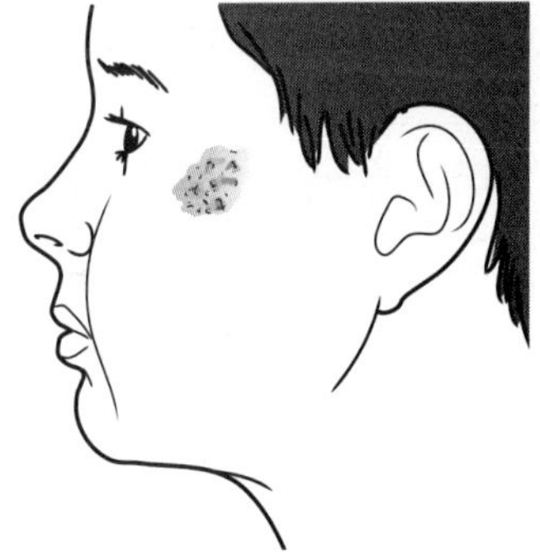

Figure 18-10: Sampson Justus' skin lesion.

1. Based on this scenario, what do you know about Mr. Justus' injury or condition?
   - ______

- ______________________________
- ______________________________
- ______________________________

2. To evaluate Mr. Justus' injury or condition effectively, you will need to gather additional information. What questions should you ask yourself in addition to what has been presented in this scenario?
   - ______________________________
   - ______________________________
   - ______________________________
   - ______________________________

Brain Jolt

This skin lesion is a highly contagious bacterial infection.

3. Identify key terms and concepts, and research each to broaden your knowledge of general medical conditions.
   - What anatomical structures might be involved in Mr. Justus' injury or condition?

     Answer: ______________________________
   - What is a bacterial infection?

     Answer: ______________________________
   - How is this skin lesion contracted? Does Mr. Justus' sport increase the risk of transference?

     Answer: ______________________________
   - Can Mr. Justus return to play?

     Answer: ______________________________
4. Based on the information that you currently have and what was provided by your instructor, what are the possible assessments for Mr. Justus' injury or condition?
   - ______________________________
   - ______________________________
   - ______________________________
   - ______________________________

Why or why not?

For each assessment or diagnosis, write *why?* or *why not?* statements identifying why the information is correct or incorrect. Take details from your textbook, your own research, and data from Mr. Justus' scenario to help you formulate an answer.

1. ______________________________
2. ______________________________
3. ______________________________
4. ______________________________

What do you think?

1. What is your assessment of Mr. Justus' injury or condition?

   Answer: ______________________________
2. Was your assessment of Mr. Justus' injury or condition correct?

   Answer: ______________________________
3. If not, explain what you did incorrectly and how you could have performed a better assessment.

   Answer: ______________________________

knowledge checklist

Table 18-1 offers a checklist that can be used by a peer, instructor, or preceptor to evaluate your skills related to general medical conditions. Use this checklist as a tool to ensure that the proper evaluation plan is complete and to assess your knowledge of the competencies that apply to this chapter.

TABLE 18-1 ■ General Medical Conditions Skills Assessment Competency Checklist

	Proficient *Can demonstrate and execute the skill properly*	**Proficient With Assistance** *Can demonstrate and execute the skill with minimal guidance or tips*	**Not Proficient** *Unable to demonstrate and execute the skill properly; need to be reevaluated at another time after further study and practice*
Athlete's Health History			
Medical history			
History of injury or conditions			
Type of sport and position played			
When did the injury or condition occur?			
Mechanisms of Injury			
How did the injury or condition occur?			
When does the pain occur?			
What makes the pain better or worse?			
Visual Observations			
Bleeding			
Edema			
Ecchymosis			
Deformity, misalignment			
Asymmetrical eye issues			
General Medical Skills: Clinical Examination			
Abdominal assessment: rigidity, percussion, bowel sounds, auscultation, organ positions			
Respiratory assessment: auscultation, respirations, breath sounds, peak-flow meter			
Circulatory assessment: pulse, blood pressure, auscultation			
Ocular assessment: eye tracking, PERLA, PEARL, vision, ophthalmoscope			
Dermatological assessment			
Ear, nose, and throat assessment: otoscope			
Other: urinalysis, glucometer, temperature			
Final Assessment			
Referral?			

PERLA = pupils equal and reactive to light andaccommodation; PEARL = pupils are equal andreactive to light when examined.

REFERENCES

Iscoe, K. E., & Riddell, M. C. (2011). Continuous moderate-intensity exercise with or without intermittent high-intensity work: Effects on acute and late glycaemia in athletes with type 1 diabetes mellitus. *Diabetic Medicine*, *28*, 824–832.

Narsule, C. K., Kahle, E. J., Kim, D. S., Anderson, A. C., & Luks, F. I. (2011). Effect of delay in presentation on rate of perforation in children with appendicitis. *American Journal of Emergency Medicine*, *29*, 890–893.

National Athletic Training Association. (2011). *Athletic training education competencies* (5th ed.). Retrieved from http://www.nata.org/sites/default/files/5th-Edition-Competencies-2011-PDF-Version.pdf

Prentice, W. (2010). *Arnheim's principles of athletic training: A competency-based approach* (14th ed.). New York, NY: McGraw-Hill.

Robinson, R. T., Wadsworth, L. T., & Feman, S. S. (2011). Traumatic retinal tear in a basketball player. *Current Sport Medicine Reports, 10*, 129–130.

Starkey, C., Brown, S. D., & Ryan, J. (2010). *Examination of orthopedic and athletic injuries* (3rd ed.). Philadelphia, PA: F.A. Davis.

Toy, B. J., & Healy, P. F. (2009). *Primary care for sports and fitness: A lifespan approach*. Philadelphia, PA: F.A. Davis.

Venes, D. (Ed.). (2009). *Taber's cyclopedic medical dictionary* (21st ed.). Philadelphia, PA: F.A. Davis.

chapter 19

Pharmacology

chapter outline

athletic trainer's corner

Out there in the real world, one athletic trainer experienced the following:

When working with high school athletes, you never know what you may encounter. I usually sit between the soccer benches to be more accessible to both teams during the game. During one of these games, I watched one of my female players ask to come off the field. I didn't notice any symptoms or injury that would require her to leave the game, so I attributed it to a need for a water break. A minute into her break, I looked over at our team bench to find her using a fellow teammate's inhaler. I quickly approached her and informed her that she should never use a prescription that is not meant for her. The athlete proceeded to tell me that she was slightly short of breath, and that her fellow teammate recommended trying her inhaler to help improve her own breathing. I informed the athlete of the dangers associated with using someone else's prescription. A prescription is intended for the patient only, based on his or her individual symptoms. I asked the athlete to take notice of the current weather conditions, which included 70% humidity. I explained that the dense air could contribute to her shortness of breath symptoms. After the game, I spoke with the entire team about the proper use of individual prescriptions.

Melissa Noble, AT, ATC
Wilson Memorial Hospital
Sidney, Ohio

learning outcomes

After working through this chapter, you will be able to:

1. Explain the federal, state, and local laws, regulations, and procedures for dispensing, administering (when appropriate), and documenting commonly used prescription and nonprescription medications.
2. Describe the common routes used to administer medications and the advantages and disadvantages for each.
3. Properly instruct patients in the use of medications, including interactions and side effects, and the proper use of metered-dose medications.
4. Describe how pharmacological agents influence pain and healing.

MODEL SCENARIO 1: CASSIDY WARD

Cassidy Ward is a freshman in college who does not participate in sports; however, she has recently joined the campus health club. She has a 2-hour block between classes and is able to exercise and shower before going back to class. Two weeks into her workout regimen, Ms. Ward notices that the plantar sides of her feet are dry and scaly. She attributes it to her eczema and puts extra lotion on the affected area. After another week, the symptoms do not go away, and now the plantar sides of her feet are red, dry, itchy, and scaly. The symptoms have also migrated between her toes (Fig. 19-1). Cassidy Ward is diagnosed with tinea pedis, also called *athlete's foot*.

1. Based on this scenario, what do you know about tinea pedis?
   - *Signs and symptoms: red, dry, itchy, and scaly patches on feet, often between the toes*
   - *Recently has been in campus health club locker room to shower*
   - *Can mimic eczema*
2. Identify key terms and concepts, and then research each to broaden your knowledge of pharmacology.
   - What is tinea pedis?
     Tinea pedis is a fungal infection on the foot.
   - Is tinea pedis a fungal, bacterial, or viral skin condition?
     It is a fungal condition.
   - What is an OTC medication?
     Over the counter: drugs and devices that are available without a prescription
   - Define *eczema.*
     Eczema is a chronic skin condition in which the skin becomes itchy, red, cracked, and dry.
   - How is tinea pedis contracted, and is it contagious?
     Tinea pedis is contagious and is contracted through direct contact with an infected source.
   - What are the possible complications of not treating the condition?
     The condition can spread to other parts of the body and progress from itching to cracked skin and bleeding with pain in the area.
   - What are the differences between a fungal, bacterial, and viral skin condition?
     A fungal infection is produced from a fungus and is treated with an antifungal medication. A bacterial condition is produced by bacteria and is treated with an antibiotic. A viral condition is produced by a virus and is treated with an antiviral drug to lessen the symptom intensity but not cure the virus.
3. Based on the information that you currently have and what was provided by your instructor, what are the possible treatments for Ms. Ward's condition?
   Ms. Ward needs to treat the affected area with an antifungal cream or spray following the treatment dosage of the chosen medication. In addition to the medication, she needs to keep her feet dry as much as possible and avoid walking barefoot in public areas. This is important not only to avoid spreading the fungus, but also to avoid contracting the fungus again.

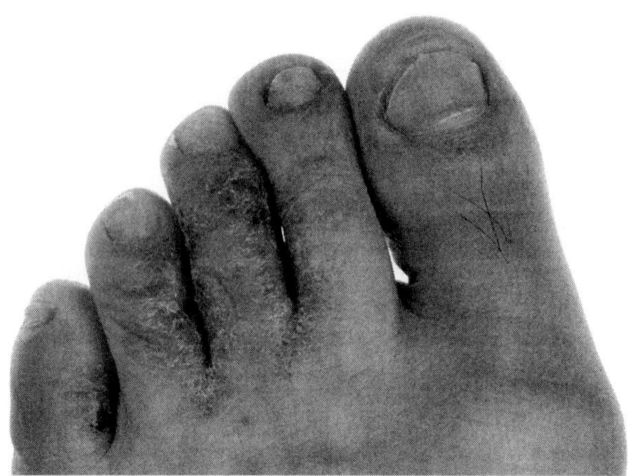

Figure 19-1: Cassidy Ward's skin condition. (© Thinkstock)

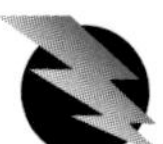

Brain Jolt

This condition can be contracted on numerous body parts, but this type is often contracted from not having a barrier between the feet and the floor in a community shower.

MODEL SCENARIO 2: AMBER LYKINS

Amber Lykins is a newly certified athletic trainer (AT) and has just taken a job at a small community college in her hometown. After meeting with the athletic director, she is given a budget for the year. After researching and making a list of supplies that she will need to stock the athletic training room, she realizes that her budget is small and money is tight. She wants to be able to have some OTC medications on hand for simple things like injury pain relief, common cold symptoms, allergies, and upset stomach, but the individual packs of brand name drugs are a bit pricey for her college's athletic training budget. To save money, Ms. Lykins decides to buy generic medications instead of name brands (Fig. 19-2), and she buys the medications in bulk containers instead of single-dose packages.

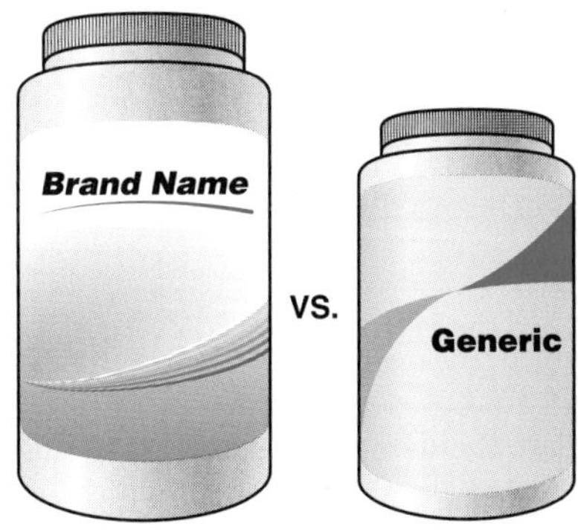

Figure 19-2: Amber Lykin's generic medications.

1. Based on this scenario, what do you know about Ms. Lykins' situation?
   - *In charge of ordering supplies for the athletic training room*
   - *Laboring under a small budget*
   - *Desires OTC medications for common ailments*
   - *Buys generic drugs in bulk to decrease costs*

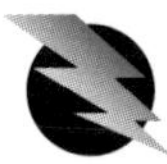

Brain Jolt

The right consultation and proper packaging of OTC drugs can decrease the risk of liability.

2. Identify key terms and concepts, and research each to broaden your knowledge of pharmacology.
   - Define *generic drug*.
     Drugs not protected by a commercial trademark that are typically less expensive
   - Is it safe to take generic drugs for illness symptoms?
     Yes, these are drugs manufactured and sold without the brand name.
   - Can an AT distribute drugs?
     Yes, an AT can distribute OTC drugs within certain guidelines.
   - What are drug distribution guidelines?
     Each state has its own guidelines for the dispensing, acquiring, and storing of drugs. Every AT should check all state and federal laws to ensure that they are within their scope of practice. In general, ATs administer OTC medications for general pain relief and cold symptoms. These drugs need to be in a secured area and administered in single-dose packages with the proper directions for use, expiration date, and side effects related to the drug. Each drug administered needs to be documented in a log book, and no drug can be administered to a minor (younger than 18 years).
   - Is there any violation in storing medications in bulk in the athletic training room?
     If medications are stored in bulk, then they are to be administered in single-dose, sealed envelopes with the athlete's name and appropriate directions for use.
   - What steps should an AT take before administering medication to an athlete?
     When an OTC medication is administered, the AT should review the patient's medical history to ensure there are no potential drug interactions or allergies related to the drug in question. Proper directions for use and the potential side effects related to the drug should also be discussed.
3. Based on the information that you currently have and what was provided by your instructor, what are the possible solutions for Ms. Lykins' situation?
   Ms. Lykins has a few options. For example, she can choose not to have OTC medications stocked in the athletic training room. However, if bulk is the only type she can afford in her budget and she wants to have OTC drugs available, Ms. Lykins can buy generic medications to save money and prepare the medications into single-dose, sealed envelopes with the proper directions for use on the envelope. Then when she is administering the medications, she can write the athlete's name on the envelope, review all the information about the drug with the athlete, and then document the drug in her log book. This will keep her in compliance with drug policy and allow her to have OTC drugs available to administer to the athletes.

Treatment Detour

Within the athletic training world, the topic of medications is frequently debated. ATs have to obtain drugs, administer them, and consult patients regarding prescription and OTC medications. A 5-year review was conducted examining the practices of ATs in collegiate athletic training rooms. In general, it was found that most collegiate athletic training rooms had poor compliance with federal law regulating the administration of medications. The research found that only 55.5% of ATs stored medications in a locked cabinet and that 44% of ATs administered OTC drugs in any amount that they believed was needed to relieve symptoms. Approximately 3.6% of ATs allowed athletes to have access to OTCs without any consultation about allergies, drug indications, or directions of use. This finding shows that education about the guidelines regarding OTC drug administration is still needed within the collegiate athletic training room. If the proper guidelines are not followed, the ATs are at risk for legal issues (Kahanov, Roberts, & Wughalter, 2010).

STUDENT SCENARIO 1: JASIME QUSAEM

Jasime Qusaem is a high school AT. One of her 16-year-old athletes has been struggling with seasonal allergies. The athlete experiences a mild headache, rhinorrhea, and frequent sneezing, but has no history of being sick or any medical conditions. The athlete has a softball double header this afternoon and is asking for some medication for her symptoms. The athlete states that she forgot to take her Allegra today and asks Ms. Qusaem for some medication (Table 19-1).

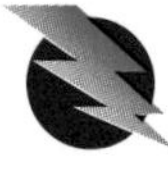

Brain Jolt

Although ATs can administer OTC medications, there are specific guidelines about administering medications to children and young adults.

1. Based on this scenario, what do you know about Ms. Qusaem's situation?

- ______________________________
- ______________________________
- ______________________________
- ______________________________

2. Identify key terms and concepts, and then research each to broaden your knowledge of pharmacology.

- What health conditions could have symptoms similar to allergy symptoms?

  Answer: ______________________________
- What is Allegra?

  Answer: ______________________________
- Where can you find information regarding the side effects and dosage for Allegra?

  Answer: ______________________________
- What are the side effects and dosage of Allegra?

  Answer: ______________________________
- What are the determining factors to distribute medications?

  Answer: ______________________________
- What are the different categories of antihistamines?

  Answer: ______________________________
- What are common side effects of antihistamines?

  Answer: ______________________________
- Can Ms. Qusaem give her athlete the medication?

  Answer: ______________________________

3. Based on the information that you currently have and what was provided by your instructor, what are the possible solutions for Ms. Qusaem's situation?

- ______________________________
- ______________________________
- ______________________________
- ______________________________

TABLE 19-1 ■ Allergy Symptoms
• Sneezing • Itchy, watery eyes • Runny nose • Itchy nose • Nasal congestion

Conversation Buffer

When dealing with any medications in the high school setting, unless the athlete is 18 years old, you will need to consult with the athlete's parent or legal guardian. Be sure to discuss the athlete's medical history, directions for use of the drug, and any side effects of the drug to allow the parent or legal guardian to decide whether or not to administer the medication.

STUDENT SCENARIO 2: LEIM DUNNIGAN

Leim Dunnigan is a basketball player who is currently enjoying the offseason. He is playing a pick-up game with his friends on the college recreational court when he inverts his ankle. He is still able to play but experiences minor pain when sprinting. He ices his ankle to ease the mild edema and takes some Tylenol. A few days later, Mr. Dunnigan is still experiencing minor pain and edema. He has been doing some simple range-of-motion and strengthening exercises while still taking Tylenol; however, Mr. Dunnigan wonders what else he can do to improve his condition (Table 19-2).

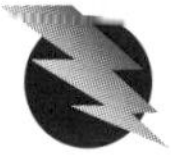

Brain Jolt

NSAIDs can be more helpful in managing pain and inflammation than an analgesic only.

1. Based on this scenario, what do you know about Mr. Dunnigan's injury?
   - ______
   - ______
   - ______
   - ______

2. Identify key terms and concepts, and research each to broaden your knowledge of pharmacology.
   - What is an analgesic?

     Answer: ______

   - What is an NSAID?

     Answer: ______

   - What is Tylenol?

     Answer: ______

   - What medications are NSAIDs?

     Answer: ______

   - What clinical situation calls for the use of an analgesic versus an NSAID?

     Answer: ______

   - Can an analgesic and NSAID be taken together?

     Answer: ______

   - What are the possible consequences of long-term use of both analgesics and NSAIDs?

     Answer: ______

   - What medical history would influence the use of an analgesic versus an NSAID?

     Answer: ______

3. Based on the information that you currently have and what was provided by your instructor, what are the possible solutions for Mr. Dunnigan's injury?
   - ______
   - ______
   - ______
   - ______

TABLE 19-2 ■ Common Analgesics
• Acetaminophen • Ibuprofen • Aspirin • Naproxen sodium

STUDENT SCENARIO 3: ALEJANDRO SANTOS

Alejandro Santos is a freshman collegiate soccer player. Although he has good skills, his coach has told him he needs to get stronger and faster in order to be a starting player next year. Over the summer, Mr. Santos has been going to the gym to work on his speed and strength, but he has been frustrated with his results. He is thinking about taking supplements to enhance his muscle mass and give him more energy to get through longer, harder training sessions. He comes to the AT's office for advice on what supplements to take to avoid National Collegiate Athletic Association (NCAA) violations (Fig. 19-3).

1. Based on this scenario, what do you know about Mr. Santos' situation?
   - ______

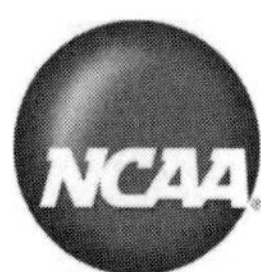

2013-14 NCAA Banned Drugs

It is your responsibility to check with the appropriate or designated athletics staff before using any substance

The NCAA bans the following classes of drugs:

a. Stimulants
b. Anabolic Agents
c. Alcohol and Beta Blockers (banned for rifle only)
d. Diuretics and Other Masking Agents
e. Street Drugs
f. Peptide Hormones and Analogues
g. Anti-estrogens
h. Beta-2 Agonists

Note: Any substance chemically related to these classes is also banned.
The institution and the student-athlete shall be held accountable for all drugs within the banned drug class regardless of whether they have been specifically identified.

Drugs and Procedures Subject to Restrictions:

a. Blood Doping.
b. Local Anesthetics (under some conditions).
c. Manipulation of Urine Samples.
d. Beta-2 Agonists permitted only by prescription and inhalation.
e. Caffeine if concentrations in urine exceed 15 micrograms/ml.

NCAA Nutritional/Dietary Supplements Warning:

Before consuming any nutritional/dietary supplement product, review the product with the appropriate or designated athletics department staff!

Dietary supplements are not well regulated and may cause a positive drug test result.
Student-athletes have tested positive and lost their eligibility using dietary supplements.
Many dietary supplements are contaminated with banned drugs not listed on the label.
Any product containing a dietary supplement ingredient is taken at your own risk.

Note to Student-Athletes: There is no complete list of banned substances.
Do not rely on this list to rule out any supplement ingredient.

Check with your athletics department staff prior to using a supplement.

Some Examples of NCAA Banned Substances in Each Drug Class

Stimulants:
amphetamine (Adderall); caffeine (guarana); cocaine; ephedrine; fenfluramine (Fen); methamphetamine; methylphenidate (Ritalin); phentermine (Phen); synephrine (bitter orange); methylhexaneamine, "bath salts" (mephedrone), etc. exceptions: phenylephrine and pseudoephedrine are not banned.

Anabolic Agents (sometimes listed as a chemical formula, such as 3,6,17-androstenetrione): boldenone; clenbuterol; DHEA (7-Keto); nandrolone; stanozolol; testosterone; methasterone; androstenedione; norandrostenedione; methandienone; etiocholanolone; trenbolone; etc.

Alcohol and Beta Blockers (banned for rifle only): alcohol; atenolol; metoprolol; nadolol; pindolol; propranolol; timolol; etc.

Diuretics (water pills) and Other Masking Agents: bumetanide; chlorothiazide; furosemide; hydrochlorothiazide; probenecid; spironolactone (canrenone); triameterene; trichlormethiazide; etc.

Street Drugs:
heroin; marijuana; tetrahydrocannabinol (THC); synthetic cannabinoids (e.g., spice, K2, JWH-018, JWH-073)

Peptide Hormones and Analogues:
growth hormone (hGH); human chorionic gonadotropin (hCG); erythropoietin (EPO); etc.

Anti-Estrogens:
anastrozole; tamoxifen; formestane; 3,17-dioxo-etiochol-1,4,6-triene (ATD),etc.

Beta-2 Agonists:
bambuterol; formoterol; salbutamol; salmeterol; etc.

Any substance that is chemically related to the class, even if it is not listed as an example, is also banned!

Information about ingredients in medications and nutritional/dietary supplements can be obtained by **contacting the Resource Exchange Center, REC, 877-202-0769 or** www.drugfreesport.com/rec **password ncaa1, ncaa2, or ncaa3.**

It is your responsibility to check with the appropriate or designated athletics staff before using any substance.

The National Collegiate Athletic Association
June 2012 MEW

Figure 19-3: NCAA banned substance list. (With permission from The National Collegiate Athletic Association, June 2012)

- ___
- ___
- ___
- ___
- ___
- ___

2. Identify key terms and concepts, and then research each to broaden your knowledge of pharmacology.
   - What are ergogenic aids?

     Answer: ___
   - What is the FDA?

     Answer: ___
   - Are supplements regulated by the FDA?

     Answer: ___
   - What is the attraction of athletes to supplements?

     Answer: ___
   - Are there any concerns with taking supplements? If so, what?

     Answer: ___
   - Are supplements safe to take?

     Answer: ___
   - Are there other options for Mr. Santos to get his desired results?

     Answer: ___
   - What specific risks do supplements pose for athletes?

     Answer: ___
3. Based on the information that you currently have and what was provided by your instructor, what are the possible solutions for Mr. Santos' situation?
   - ___

Treatment Detour

Athletes are always trying to improve their performance. One way some athletes do this is by taking nutritional supplements. One study that followed track and field athletes found that two-thirds of all the track and field athletes reported using one or more supplements, and nearly half used at least one medication. These supplements were reportedly used to help with recovery from training and to optimize performance. This finding increases concerns about athletes taking supplements because of the risk for a positive drug test for a banned substance. The supplements can be cross-contaminated because they are not regulated by the FDA. In addition, inappropriate use of these supplements can lead to health issues; therefore, proper research and consultation regarding supplements is needed to maintain safety for athletes (Tscholl et al., 2010).

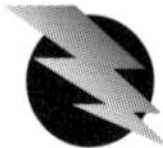

Brain Jolt

Supplements are not regulated by the FDA; therefore, an athlete may be susceptible to taking a supplement that can lead to a positive drug test for a banned substance.

STUDENT SCENARIO 4: NICOLE COTTRELL

Nicole Cottrell is a senior basketball player. Since the beginning of the season, which has been underway for 1 month, Ms. Cottrell has been having difficulty making it through daily practices owing to shortness of breath, extreme fatigue, and painful chest tightness. After Ms. Cottrell rests for 30 to 60 minutes, his symptoms subside. Ms. Cottrell had bronchitis before the start of the season, and he was prescribed an antibiotic. The AT suggests that Ms. Cottrell see his family physician. On examination, the family physician concludes that Ms. Cottrell has a complication resulting from bronchoconstriction, and exertion from exercise seems to trigger an increase in this type of condition (Fig. 19-4). Ms. Cottrell is given a prescription for a fast acting medication that is to be taken when he experiences symptoms.

1. Based on this scenario, what do you know about Ms. Cottrell's condition?
   - ___
   - ___

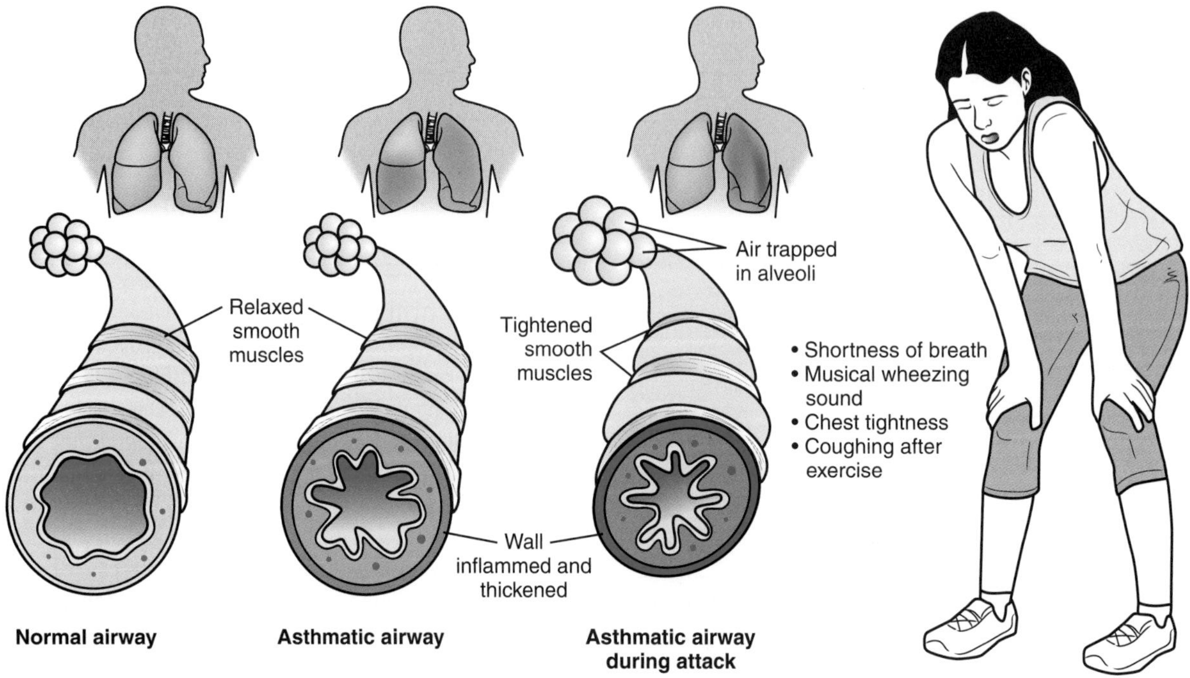

Figure 19-4: Nicole Cottrell's symptoms of exercise-induced asthma.

- ______________________________
- ______________________________

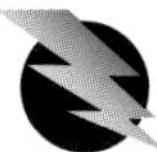

Brain Jolt

Often two puffs of this "rescue" medication will help an athlete breathe better.

Treatment Detour

Exercise-induced asthma is a common condition among athletes. Typically, these athletes will be prescribed a metered-dose inhaler (MDI) to treat and prevent short-term bronchoconstriction. However, the fact that these inhalers are self-administered and used for self-perceived symptoms creates the risk for misuse and abuse of the MDI. The most often prescribed MDI bronchodilator is albuterol. MDIs are often stored in an AT's medical kit, which can increase the risk of misuse. This situation can be dangerous because the medication specificity for the prescribed patient might not be appropriate for the person who is using the medication without a prescription. The other issue with MDIs is that the athlete might not administer the medication properly, which compromises the effectiveness of the medication delivery. It is important for the AT to monitor the MDI's use and administration and properly instruct the athlete in the medication's correct use. If abuse or misuse is suspected, a referral to the prescribing physician is warranted (Wennerberg & Adams, 2010).

2. Identify key terms and concepts, and then research each to broaden your knowledge of pharmacology.

- Explain exercise-induced asthma.

  Answer: ______________________________
- What medication would Ms. Cottrell have been given by the family physician?

  Answer: ______________________________
- Why does exercise cause Ms. Cottrell's symptoms to develop?

  Answer: ______________________________
- Define *bronchitis*.

  Answer: ______________________________
- Define *bronchoconstriction*.

  Answer: ______________________________
- What are the side effects of this medication?

  Answer: ______________________________
- How is this medication administered?

  Answer: ______________________________

3. Based on the information that you currently have and what was provided by your instructor, what are the possible solutions for Ms. Cottrell's condition?

- ______________________________

- ____________________
- ____________________
- ____________________

STUDENT SCENARIO 5: CHAVEZ LOPEZ

Chavez Lopez is a college swimmer. At the end of this season, he qualifies to go to nationals in the butterfly stroke. For the next 2 weeks, Mr. Lopez continues to work on his speed, while still tapering for optimal performance. The athletic training staff members who work with Mr. Lopez are expected to have all of the necessary personal information on Mr. Lopez properly documented by the team physician before he leaves for nationals. Mr. Lopez uses an inhaler that contains a beta-2 agonist, which is banned by the NCAA. As a result, he is sure to obtain a written document by the team physician to take with him. On the morning preceding the start of the competition, the NCAA administers a random drug test. Mr. Lopez is one of the random names selected. His paperwork, including the inhaler documentation, is given to the appropriate people. Later that afternoon, Mr. Lopez is informed that he is unable to participate because of a banned substance that was found in his urine sample. Mr. Lopez states that he has the necessary documents for his inhaler, but he is informed that this is not the substance in question. The substance in question is a stimulant that he takes each day to help him focus. Mr. Lopez then realizes that he forgot to add a list of daily medications to the paperwork. He has been taking this medication since he was in junior high. Unfortunately, Mr. Lopez is not allowed to add this medication to the list at this point, and he is disqualified from competition (Fig. 19-5).

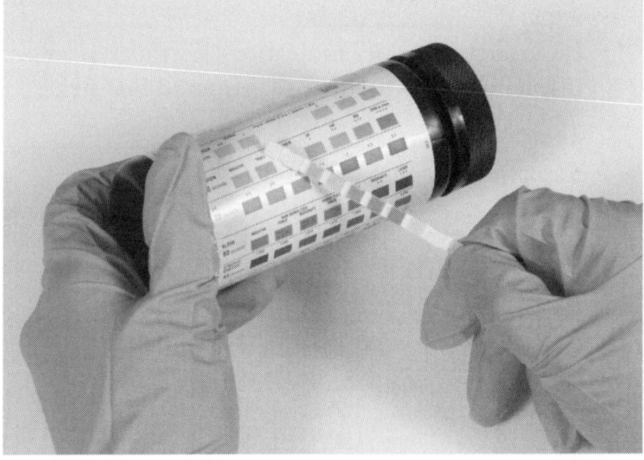

Figure 19-5: Chavez Lopez's drug testing. (© Thinkstock)

1. Based on this scenario, what do you know about Mr. Lopez's situation?

- ____________________
- ____________________
- ____________________
- ____________________

Brain Jolt

Always be sure to take a thorough health history during each athlete's physical examination.

Conversation Buffer

Many athletes and coaches are unaware of what substances are included on the banned substance list by the NCAA. At the start of each season, this list should be addressed with the team. Frequently a substance that an athlete or coach does not think would be on the list, such as caffeine, is overlooked. Be sure to educate your team.

2. Identify key terms and concepts, and research each to broaden your knowledge of pharmacology.

- Explain what *tapering* means in reference to an athlete's performance.

  Answer: ____________________
- What type of information is required on Mr. Lopez's inhaler documentation to be accepted by the NCAA?

  Answer: ____________________
- Discuss your institution's drug policy. Does it mirror the NCAA drug testing procedures?

  Answer: ____________________
- What type of stimulant, taken daily by Mr. Lopez to help him focus, is most likely in question?

  Answer: ____________________

- What are the side effects of this stimulant medication?

Answer: ______________________

3. Based on the information that you currently have and what was provided by your instructor, what are the possible solutions for Mr. Lopez's situation?
   - ______________________
   - ______________________
   - ______________________
   - ______________________

STUDENT SCENARIO 6: TRACY NUSS

Tracy Nuss is a collegiate freshman cross-country runner. She has a history of exercise-induced asthma, and she has been instructed to use her albuterol inhaler 30 minutes before activity. She has performed this routine for the past 2 years. Since the start of this cross-country season, Ms. Nuss has used her inhaler as instructed, but she is now noticing some other daily symptoms. She develops a throat irritation while running, and later in the evenings she begins coughing, experiences shortness of breath, and has a headache. She is now using an albuterol inhaler twice a day. This routine continues for 3 weeks, and Ms. Nuss is instructed by the AT to see the team physician. Ms. Nuss informs the team physician that she takes an antihistamine medication occasionally during the fall season for her allergy symptoms. It is noted that, during her high school career, Ms. Nuss ran through the neighborhood, but now her college team runs through an arboretum. The team physician prescribes a corticosteroid oral medication to be used once per day and a long-acting inhaler medication. She is instructed to use her albuterol inhaler only when necessary (Table 19-3).

1. Based on this scenario, what do you know about Ms. Nuss' condition?
   - ______________________
   - ______________________
   - ______________________
   - ______________________

TABLE 19-3 ■ Common Asthma Medications

Anti-inflammatory Agents	Steroidal
	• Metered-dose inhaler: Flovent, Azmacort • Oral: prednisone
	Nonsteroidal • Metered-dose inhaler: Intal, Tilade • Oral: Singulair, Accolate
Bronchodilators	Beta agonists
	• Short acting: Albuterol • Long acting: Serevent

*Refer to competency list link in front of the book.

Brain Jolt

The surrounding environment can affect an athlete's airway.

2. Identify key terms and concepts, and then research each to broaden your knowledge of pharmacology.
   - What anatomical structures might be involved in Ms. Nuss' condition?

     Answer: ______________________
   - Define *exercise-induced asthma*. What are the symptoms?

     Answer: ______________________
   - What is the function of albuterol?

     Answer: ______________________
   - What are the side effects of albuterol?

     Answer: ______________________
   - Describe the proper indications for this type of inhaler and how frequently it should be used.

     Answer: ______________________
   - Explain the technique for using an inhaler.

     Answer: ______________________
   - What is an antihistamine?

     Answer: ______________________
   - Why is it important to note the change of running environment in which Ms. Nuss exercises?

     Answer: ______________________

- What is a nonsteroidal oral medication? What is its purpose? What are some common names of nonsteroidal medications?

  Answer: ______
- What long-acting inhaler can be prescribed for Ms. Nuss?

  Answer: ______

3. Based on the information that you currently have and what was provided by your instructor, what are the possible solutions for Ms. Nuss' condition?
   - ______
   - ______
   - ______
   - ______

STUDENT SCENARIO 7: SHAWN FITZGERALD

Shawn Fitzgerald is a college football player who is second string on his team. He has decent skills, but he is always being told that he is too small, needs to gain muscle mass, and needs to get tougher. He has been exercising in the weight room all summer and has seen a noticeable improvement in muscle bulk. Mr. Fitzgerald returns to school and reports for football pre-season camp. He has bulked up and is significantly larger than he was when he left school, causing the athletic training staff to question his workout regimen and any use of supplements or muscle enhancers. He does well with camp training and is able to perform the skills needed to gain a first string spot. However, the coaches and AT have noticed that he has severe mood swings and is short-tempered on the field when he is being critiqued by his coaches. There are rumors that Mr. Fitzgerald is using anabolic steroids.

Signs and Symptoms

- Conflicts with the legal system for violence
- Depression
- Hypotension
- Impotence
- Masculinization
- Mood swings (rage)
- Retarded growth in children

1. Based on this scenario, what do you know about Mr. Fitzgerald's condition?
   - ______
   - ______
   - ______
   - ______

Brain Jolt
"Roid rage" is often a sign of steroid abuse.

2. Identify key terms and concepts, and then research each to broaden your knowledge of pharmacology.
   - What are anabolic steroids?

     Answer: ______
   - What are the effects of anabolic steroids?

     Answer: ______
   - Are steroids a banned substance?

     Answer: ______
   - What is the AT's role when he or she suspects steroid use in athletes?

     Answer: ______
3. Based on the information that you currently have and what was provided by your instructor, what are the possible solutions for Mr. Fitzgerald's situation?
   - ______
   - ______
   - ______
   - ______

knowledge checklist

Table 19-4 offers a checklist that can be used by a peer, instructor, or preceptor to evaluate an athlete's treatment plan. Use this checklist as a tool to ensure that the treatment plan is complete and to assess your knowledge of the competencies that apply to this chapter.

TABLE 19-4 ■ Pharmacology Competency Checklist

	Proficient *Can demonstrate and execute the skill properly*	**Proficient With Assistance** *Can demonstrate and execute the skill with minimal guidance or tips*	**Not Proficient** *Unable to demonstrate and execute the skill properly; need to be reevaluated at another time after further study and practice*
Athlete's Health History			
Medical history			
Current medications			
Medical allergies			
Pharmacology Knowledge			
Demonstrates understanding of pharmacologic agents			
Demonstrates understanding of drug distribution guidelines			
Demonstrates use of drug resources, electronic and print, to find drug information			
Demonstrates understanding of pharmacological concepts			
Describes common routes used to administer medications			
Properly demonstrates use of: Inhaler Blood glucose test Nebulizers Insulin pumps Peak flow meter			

REFERENCES

Kahanov, L., Roberts, J., & Wughalter, E. (2010). Adherence to drug-dispensation and drug-administration laws and guidelines in collegiate athletic training rooms: A 5-year review. *Journal of Athletic Training, 45*, 299–305.

Mangus, B. C., & Miller, M. G. (2005). *Pharmacology application in athletic training*. Philadelphia, PA: F.A. Davis.

National Athletic Training Association. (2011). *Athletic training education competencies* (5th ed.). Retrieved from http://www.nata.org/sites/default/files/5th-Edition-Competencies-2011-PDF-Version.pdf

Prentice, W. (2010). *Arnheim's principles of athletic training: A competency-based approach* (14th ed.). New York, NY: McGraw-Hill.

Tscholl, P., et al. (2010). The use of drugs and nutritional supplements in top-level track and field athletes. *American Journal of Sports Medicine, 38*, 133–140.

Venes, D. (Ed.). (2009). *Taber's cyclopedic medical dictionary* (21st ed.). Philadelphia, PA: F.A. Davis.

Wennerberg, D. K., & Adams, A. B. (2010). Metered dose inhaler use and misuse by athletes. *Athletic Therapy Today, 15*, 30–33.

chapter 20

Psychosocial Intervention

chapter outline

athletic trainer's corner

Out there in the real world, one athletic trainer experienced the following:

While working in the athletic training room one day, I made a referral to the college counselor for an athlete who suffered from severe depression. This athlete had just suffered an unhappy triad in his knee and was struggling with a season-ending injury. He also had personal issues at home that he was dealing with prior to the injury, which seemed to compound after the surgery on his knee. The athlete missed several rehabilitation appointments, and when he did show up his mood was low and he made comments that I found alarming. I remember thinking that he couldn't mean these disparaging statements about his life, but I knew that I had to err on the side of caution and report his psychological condition to the college counselor, the college doctor, and the coach. After receiving counseling and further medical care for his knee, he made a full recovery from his knee surgery and was able to achieve emotional stability. This situation taught me that sometimes athletes endure emotional stress caused by situations in their life that are not always apparent to others. Therefore, always be empathetic toward your athletes and refer anyone who might be struggling emotionally or might be in danger of harming himself or herself or others.

Kim Isaac, MS, AT, ATC
Wilmington College
Wilmington, Ohio

learning outcomes

After working through this chapter, you will be able to:

1. Identify and explain the warning signs of patients exhibiting abnormal social, emotional, and mental behaviors.
2. Describe the psychology of an injury and techniques that can be used to help a patient during injury rehabilitation and return to activity.
3. Identify and properly refer patients to various mental health-care providers when patients are in need of mental health care.
4. Identify the signs and symptoms of patients with eating disorders, the psychological factors associated with each disorder, and the appropriate management and referral.

MODEL SCENARIO 1: **BRENDA KROHN**

Brenda Krohn is a collegiate women's basketball coach. Her team's record this year is 15–2 with only 3 weeks left in the regular season. The team members have done everything that she has asked of them and more. Ms. Krohn should be a coach that is basking in her team's success, but instead she has noticed a lack of concentration, fatigue, and episodes of drowsiness in the afternoon. She also has a history of clinical depression. Being concerned about her symptoms, she talks with the team's athletic trainer. They discuss her medical history and the possibility of her having seasonal affective disorder (SAD; Fig. 20-1).

1. Based on this scenario, what do you know about Ms. Krohn's condition?
- *History of clinical depression*
- *Lack of concentration*
- *Fatigue*
- *Drowsiness in the afternoon*
- *Seasonal affective disorder*
- *Reason to be happy owing to team's success*

2. Identify key terms and concepts, and then research each to broaden your knowledge of psychosocial interventions.
- Define *seasonal affective disorder (SAD).*
  A mood disorder characterized by depression in the winter and fall months
- What are the symptoms of SAD? Is it more common in men or women?
  The symptoms are more common in women and include fatigue, diminished concentration, and daytime drowsiness.
- Is this disorder more common in those with a history of depression?
  Yes, if a diagnosis of clinical depression has already been made, then the onset of SAD symptoms may be more intense and can more easily affect the patient.

3. Based on the information that you currently have and what was provided by your instructor, what are the possible treatment plans for Ms. Krohn's condition?
Ms. Krohn should look into stress management techniques to manage any outside stress she may be feeling. A regular exercise program might help to elevate her mood. If Ms. Krohn's symptoms do not improve, she can try an antidepressant medication prescribed by her physician, as well as light therapy.

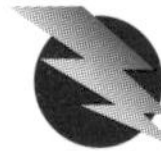

Brain Jolt
The symptoms of this disorder are most prevalent in the winter months.

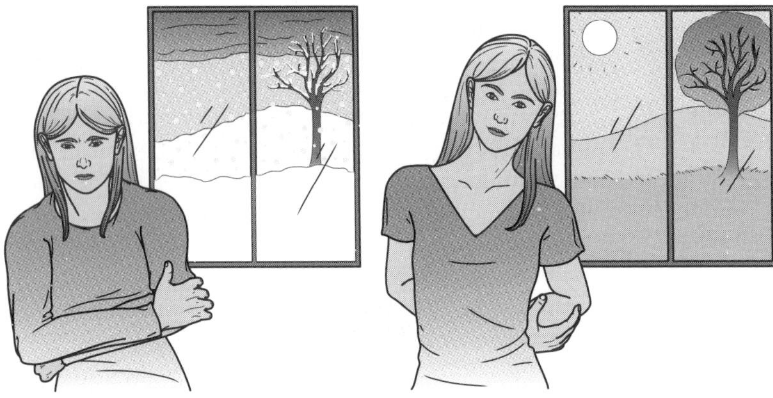

Figure 20-1: Seasonal affective disorder.

MODEL SCENARIO 2: **ZEB SHARP**

Zeb Sharp is a sophomore running back on his college football team. With 2 min left in the game, Mr. Sharp inverts his left ankle. He is evaluated on the sideline and is told that he has a grade 2 lateral ankle sprain. Based on Mr. Sharp's current symptoms, he should be able to return to play within 4 weeks. Mr. Sharp is unable to accept that he will be out of participation for that long. He had to miss three games last season because of a shoulder injury, and denies that this is happening to him again. He takes out his frustration by punching a locker. One week after the injury, Mr. Sharp's edema, range of motion, and strength in his left ankle improve each day. However, he is still unable to walk without a limp 2 weeks after his injury, and it takes all of Mr. Sharp's energy and focus to come to practice. He tries to bargain with the athletic trainer to let him do some jogging with the team, but is not cleared to do so. He even tells the athletic training staff that he might quit the team because he cannot bear to just watch practice and not participate. The athletic trainer meets with the coaching staff, all of whom have expressed their concerns regarding Mr. Sharp's emotional state. Mr. Sharp is approached by the head coach and is asked if he would like to help him call in the plays. This helps him begin to feel like a part of the team again, and he returns to practice the next day with a better outlook. Mr. Sharp finds that the remaining 2 weeks pass quickly (Fig. 20-2).

1. Based on this scenario, what do you know about Mr. Sharp's situation?
   - *Running back on his college football team*
   - *Sustained a grade 2 lateral left ankle sprain*
   - *Out of competition for 4 weeks*
   - *Previously missed games because of a shoulder injury*
   - *Experiences many emotions as a result of his current situation*
   - *Mood tends to improve after he is asked to help coach with team*

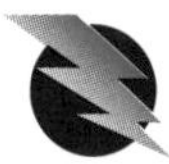

Brain Jolt

The Kübler-Ross stages can occur in any order in response to a stressful or traumatic event.

Conversation Buffer

An athlete's mental well-being is an area of concern after a traumatic event or injury. It is important for the athletic training staff and the coaching staff to include the injured athlete in team activities. Many athletes associate their identity with their particular sport or team. When that is interrupted, athletes can experience a series of emotional stages. Therefore, talk with your coaches and others who are closely involved in the situation and advise them to monitor the injured athlete's state of mind and to notify you if they observe any behavior that is unusual for that individual. In addition, talk with athletes about how they feel and about their importance to the team by discussing how they can stay involved with the team.

2. Identify key terms and concepts, and then research each to broaden your knowledge of psychosocial interventions.
   - What are the Kübler-Ross stages of reaction?
     Denial, anger, bargaining, depression, and acceptance
   - What is the time frame for each stage?
     A person can go through these stages in any order and in any time frame. Some will go through these stages in days to years depending on the level of trauma experienced and perceived by the patient.
   - What other factors can influence these stages and psychological reactions to injury?
     The athlete's coping skills, history of injury, amount of emotional support received from others, and individual personality traits
   - How can the AT help with these issues?
     The AT can be a support system if the athlete does not have one. The AT can also be a good listener and try to create a safe place for the athlete to share feelings about the situation, keep the athlete educated about the injury and the rehabilitation process, and help the athlete return to play. In addition, the AT should refer the patient to a mental health-care professional once the issues extend beyond the AT's scope of practice.

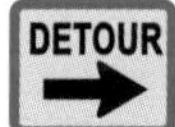

Treatment Detour

Participating in athletics demands a high level of determination, hard work, and physical skill. However, athletics also demand a high level of psychological skill to overcome injury and the stress of competition. One study examined professional soccer players from Sweden because it is estimated that 65% to 91% of elite soccer players in Sweden have at least one injury per year. The results of this study indicate

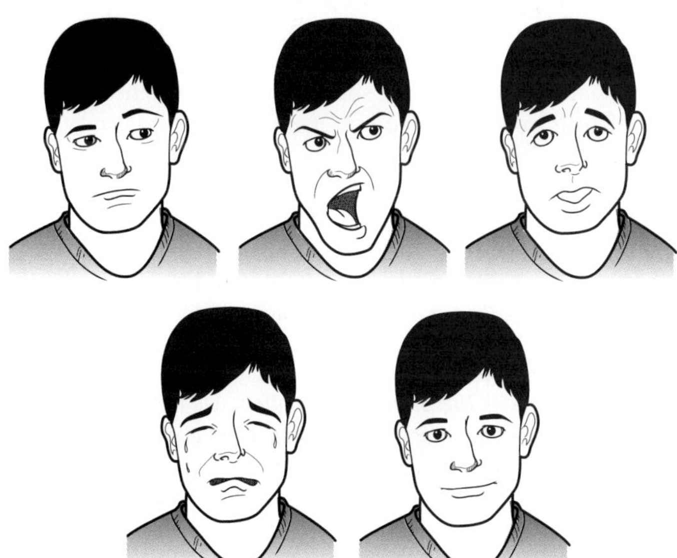

Figure 20-2: Kübler-Ross reactions.

that personality traits are good predictors of injury risk. It showed that somatic trait anxiety, psychic trait anxiety, stress susceptibility, and trait irritability are high predictors of an increased injury risk. This risk is important to ATs because, when an athlete is observed to have one of these traits, the AT might need to alter the athlete's rehabilitation goals and monitor them closely throughout the season for proper injury prevention, stress management, or relaxation techniques (Ivarsson & Johnson, 2010).

3. Based on the information that you currently have and what was provided by your instructor, what are the possible treatment plans for Mr. Sharp's situation?

To help Mr. Sharp, talk with him about his injury. It is helpful to put the injury in the perspective of the entire season and the season to come. Keep Mr. Sharp informed about his injury and his progress in rehabilitation. This will hopefully increase his motivation during rehabilitation because he will see that he is getting closer to returning to play. In addition, find things that he can do with the team during his recovery, such as calling plays with the coach and helping teammates with skill observation and critique during practice. This allows the athlete to feel like a part of the team and see that the team needs him to return to play, which serves as an additional motivation to comply with rehabilitation.

STUDENT SCENARIO 1: ELOISA DOMINGO

Eloisa Domingo has received a scholarship to play soccer this year at a Division III college. She receives the summer conditioning program in the mail from her new coach. Ms. Domingo has always strived to be the best at anything she tries. Last year, she participated in 2-hour practices followed by an additional 1-hour workout. She believed that this helped to keep her physically fit and aided with her weight problem. At the time, she weighed 135 lb; currently she is 5 feet, 4 inches tall and weighs 115 lb. She is excited by her weight loss and believes that the only time that she is in control of herself is when she is working out. She still envisions herself as having a thick, athletic build. After looking over the summer conditioning program sent by her coach, Ms. Domingo personally sets her own goals, in addition to the ones set by the coach. She hopes that losing an additional 8 lb will help to increase her energy level. She has already reduced her food portions, and she will cut an additional 500 calories from her diet. Ms. Domingo reports to summer camp weighing 103 lb, and it is noted in her preparticipation physical that she has primary amenorrhea, fainting episodes, and low energy levels. It is also observed in the dining hall that she eats very little and pushes her food around on the plate before returning her tray. The AT believes that Ms. Domingo might have anorexia nervosa (Fig. 20-3) and schedules a meeting to discuss the health concerns indicated on her physical examination form.

Brain Jolt

Often with this disorder, the patient will avoid eating with others. When eating alone is not an option, the patient will try to make it look as though food has been eaten by moving food around on the plate.

1. Based on this scenario, what do you know about Ms. Domingo's situation?

- ______________________________
- ______________________________
- ______________________________
- ______________________________
- ______________________________

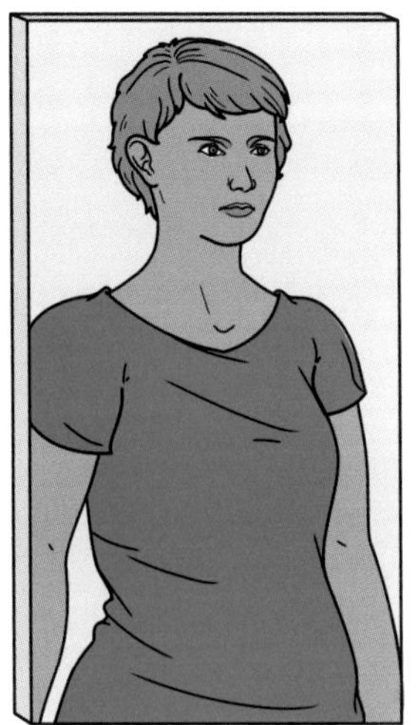
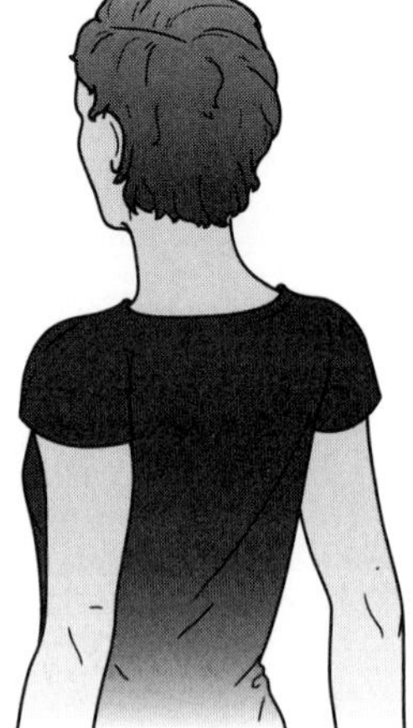

Figure 20-3: Body image of anorexia nervosa.

- ______________________________

  ____

2. Identify key terms and concepts, and research each to broaden your knowledge of psychosocial interventions.
   - What is anorexia nervosa?

     Answer: ______________________________
   - What are the signs and symptoms of anorexia nervosa?

     Answer: ______________________________
   - What steps need to be taken to address this issue?

     Answer: ______________________________
   - Who is privy to patient information about this condition without violating privacy laws?

     Answer: ______________________________

DETOUR **Treatment Detour**
Eating disorders can be present in collegiate athletes and are seen more frequently in participants of sports with a strong emphasis on body image. However, the prevalence rates vary throughout the literature. One study interviewed 17 female collegiate athletes who experienced eating disorders and the factors that they believed contributed to their eating disorders. The reported internal factors included negative mood states, low self-esteem, perfectionism, drive for achievement, and a high desire for control. In addition, external factors included negative influences on their self-esteem, hurtful relationships, hurtful role models, and athletic performance. As a result, ATs can use this knowledge to assist athletes with these traits as a means to detect and prevent eating disorders early (Arthur-Cameselle & Quatromoni, 2010).

3. Based on the information that you currently have and what was provided by your instructor, what are the possible treatment plans for Ms. Domingo's situation?
   - ______________________________

     ____
   - ______________________________

     ____
   - ______________________________

     ____
   - ______________________________

     ____

STUDENT SCENARIO 2: WENDY VOSLER

Wendy Vosler is a junior setter on her collegiate volleyball team. The coach has recruited a freshman setter to learn the team's plays and slowly blend in with the team to take Ms. Vosler's spot when she graduates. Ms. Vosler has always been a player who needs to be reassured of her athletic ability because she continually doubts herself in most facets of her life. She is 5 feet, 8 inches tall and weighs 135 lb, and she is an above average student; however, she perceives herself weighing 170 lb. The freshman setter is 6 feet tall and weighs 140 lb. Ms. Vosler sees her teammate as someone who could easily take her position on the team, because she is quicker and more agile. The freshman's presence psychologically takes a toll on Ms. Vosler. Midway through the season, Ms. Vosler's roommate (who is also a teammate) confidentially approaches the athletic trainer and says she is concerned about Ms. Vosler because she has been observed going to the bathroom shortly after lunch and dinner each day. In addition, Ms. Vosler has been seen taking pills throughout the day and stating that she is not hungry. However, Ms. Volser has also been seen eating two bags of chips and a cheeseburger in her dorm room. The AT is concerned that Ms. Vosler is having binging (Fig. 20-4) and purging episodes and could have bulimia nervosa.

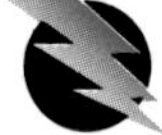

Brain Jolt
The frequent purging associated with bulimia nervosa can cause tooth decay and a chronically inflamed lining of the mouth and throat.

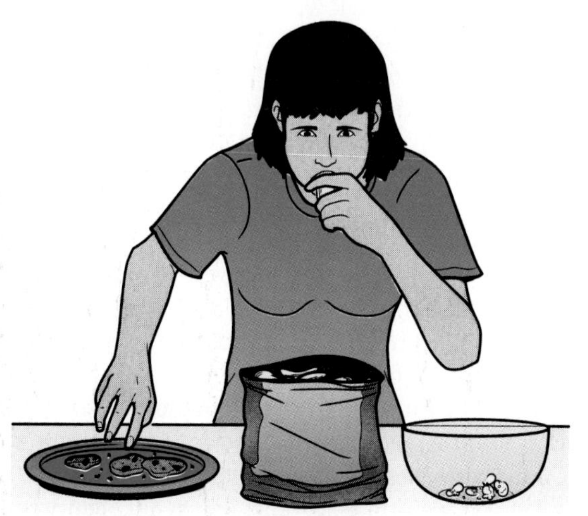

Figure 20-4: Binge eating associated with bulimia nervosa.

Conversation Buffer

When an eating disorder is suspected, the AT should intervene early. This matter should be confronted in a kind, empathic, and nonjudgmental manner to ensure that the athlete does not feel threatened. It is important to avoid overwhelming the athlete and thus inadvertently isolating him or her. The AT could be the only one who can get through to the athlete and thus be the catalyst for change.

1. Based on this scenario, what do you know about Ms. Vosler's situation?
   - ______________________________
   - ______________________________
   - ______________________________
   - ______________________________

2. Identify key terms and concepts, and research each to broaden your knowledge of psychosocial interventions.
   - What is bulimia nervosa?

     Answer: ______________________________
   - Define *binging.*

     Answer: ______________________________
   - Define *purging.*

     Answer: ______________________________
   - What are the signs and symptoms of bulimia nervosa?

     Answer: ______________________________
   - What pills might Ms. Vosler be taking that contribute to her disordered eating?

     Answer: ______________________________
   - What steps should be taken to maintain Ms. Vosler's privacy?

     Answer: ______________________________

3. Based on the information that you currently have and what was provided by your instructor, what are the possible treatment plans for Ms. Vosler's situation?
   - ______________________________
   - ______________________________
   - ______________________________
   - ______________________________

STUDENT SCENARIO 3: JILL BOGUSKI

Jill Boguski is a 35-year-old woman whose passion is running. She has set a goal of running a marathon every other year and is presently training for her fifth marathon. Her love of running began when she ran cross-country and track while in high school and college. When she is not training for a marathon, she runs an average of 42 miles per week. She would like to incorporate strength training into her workout routine, but she currently lacks the time. Between working full time, raising two teenagers who are active in sports, and having a husband who travels a fair amount, she usually has time to run only 6 to 7 miles per day. The marathon is 8 weeks away when Ms. Boguski notices a "hot spot" on her right shin. She attributes it to a shin splint. She treats it with ice, stretches of the gastrocnemius and soleus muscles, and a gel foot insert in her shoe. She previously had a stress fracture on her right tibia 6 months ago. After 3 weeks of her symptoms not improving, she inquires with her friend who is an AT. The AT recommends that with her symptoms, training regimen, and history of injury she should see an orthopedist. The doctor recommends radiographic and magnetic resonance imaging. The results of the tests are positive for a stress fracture of the right tibia and a diminished percentage of bone density. It is also revealed that Ms. Boguski has a history of secondary amenorrhea (Fig. 20-5).

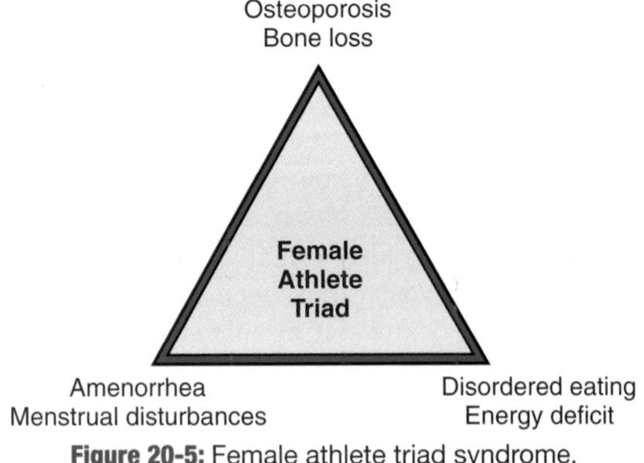

Figure 20-5: Female athlete triad syndrome.

1. Based on this scenario, what do you know about Ms. Boguski's situation?
   - ______________________________
   - ______________________________
   - ______________________________
   - ______________________________

2. Identify key terms and concepts, and research each to broaden your knowledge of psychosocial intervention.
   - What is the female athlete triad?

     Answer: ______________________________
   - What are the symptoms of the female athlete triad?

     Answer: ______________________________
   - What is the term for decreased bone density?

     Answer: ______________________________
   - Would adding a strength-training program help this condition?

     Answer: ______________________________
   - Define *secondary amenorrhea.*

     Answer: ______________________________
   - What other aspect of Ms. Boguski's life should be examined?

     Answer: ______________________________

DETOUR

Treatment Detour

According to Thein-Nissenbaum et al. (2012), the female athlete triad is the interrelatedness of decreased energy availability owing to an eating disorder; menstrual irregularity including primary amenorrhea, secondary amenorrhea, or oligomenorrhea; and decreased bone density. This study examined the relationship between menstrual irregularity and musculoskeletal injury in female high school athletes. The authors found that there is a high incidence rate of menstrual issues at the high school level in addition to a high prevalence in musculoskeletal injuries. It was concluded that female athletes who reported having menstrual irregularities sustained more severe injuries than athletes who had a regular menstrual cycle. Proper education about menses is important and should be provided to young women so that irregularities can be identified and thus managed properly (Thein-Nissenbaum et al., 2012).

3. Based on the information that you currently have and what was provided by your instructor, what are the possible treatment plans for Ms. Boguski's situation?
   - ______________________________
   - ______________________________
   - ______________________________
   - ______________________________

Brain Jolt

This disorder can be potentially fatal if it is not recognized and treated.

STUDENT SCENARIO 4: BRUCE HECKLER

Bruce Heckler is a freshman on his college baseball team. He has played baseball since he was 5 years old, and is the first in his family to ever attend college, let alone play a collegiate sport. Mr. Heckler cannot understand why he has sweaty palms, shortness of breath, and indigestion on the first day of fall baseball practice. He attributes the symptoms to the new team, coach, and environment. Through the first week of practice Mr. Heckler experiences occasional headaches and has difficulty sleeping. In addition, he is finding his class load to be challenging. When he goes home for winter break, his family notices that he has lost weight, seems fatigued, and has lost his normal appetite. When he returns to school, he discusses his symptoms with the AT, who suspects that Mr. Heckler is suffering from anxiety and refers him to the campus physician (Fig. 20-6).

1. Based on this scenario, what do you know about Mr. Heckler's condition?
   - ______________________________
   - ______________________________
   - ______________________________

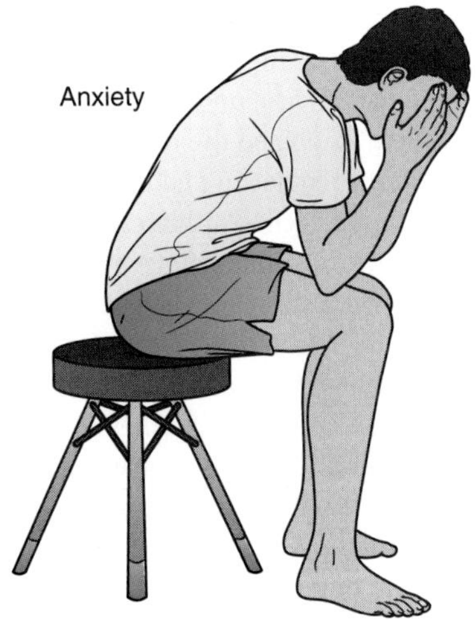

Figure 20-6: Anxiety.

- ______________________________
  ____

Brain Jolt
General anxiety can last 6 months or longer and can progress to more severe anxiety disorders.

2. Identify key terms and concepts, and research each to broaden your knowledge of psychosocial interventions.
   - What is anxiety?

     Answer: ______________________________
   - What are the signs and symptoms of anxiety?

     Answer: ______________________________
   - What are the different anxiety disorders?

     Answer: ______________________________
   - What are the various treatments for anxiety?

     Answer: ______________________________
3. Based on the information that you currently have and what was provided by your instructor, what are the possible treatment plans for Mr. Heckler's condition?
   - ______________________________
     ____
   - ______________________________
     ____
   - ______________________________
     ____
   - ______________________________
     ____

Conversation Buffer
In today's society, there is a high expectation for athletes to succeed. When individuals are put in challenging situations or environments, the pressure can often become overwhelming. This emotional uncertainty can present itself through physical symptoms. Anxiety is a real condition that can be debilitating for some individuals. Be sure to educate those close to the individual that this condition needs to be addressed and handled in a professional manner. Seek a physician or counseling assistance if the patient's needs extend beyond your scope of practice.

STUDENT SCENARIO 5: BAYLA CLUTTER

Bayla Clutter is a freshman college baseball player who is typically quiet but recently has had some trouble in classes with intermittent episodes of rowdiness and class disruptions. The baseball team is going on a weeklong training trip to Florida. Two days into the trip, a few of Mr. Clutter's teammates notice some behavioral changes in him. He seems overly excited and unable to sleep at night in the hotel. He starts breaking team rules and is preoccupied with being the life of the party in the hotel. He begins to portray the personality traits that have gotten him in trouble in classes. However, within 24 hours of his unruly behavior, he then displays a lack of interest in the team and training, is irritable, and exhibits aggression. In addition, he complains of a headache. His teammates express their concerns to the AT, and Mr. Clutter is pulled aside after practice to talk (Fig. 20-7). Bipolar depression disorder is suspected.

1. Based on this scenario, what do you know about Mr. Clutter's situation?
   - ______________________________
     ____

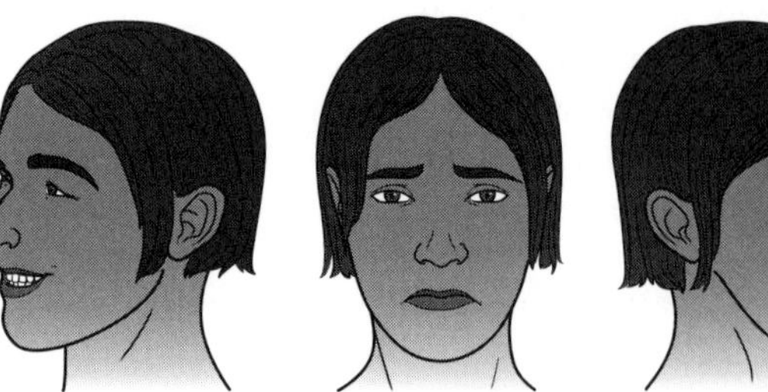

Figure 20-7: Bipolar depression disorder.

- ______________________________________

  ____
- ______________________________________

  ____
- ______________________________________

  ____

Brain Jolt
This disease is associated with extreme emotional highs and lows.

2. Identify key terms and concepts, and research each to broaden your knowledge of psychosocial interventions.
   - What is bipolar depression disorder?

     Answer: ______________________________
   - What are the signs and symptoms of this disorder?

     Answer: ______________________________
   - How does it differ from clinical depression?

     Answer: ______________________________
   - Can prescription medication help?

     Answer: ______________________________
   - What other treatments can help?

     Answer: ______________________________
3. Based on the information that you currently have and what was provided by your instructor, what are the possible treatment plans for Mr. Clutter's situation?
   - ______________________________________

     ____
   - ______________________________________

     ____
   - ______________________________________

     ____
   - ______________________________________

     ____

STUDENT SCENARIO 6: SEBASTIAN CRUZE

Sebastian Cruze is a senior in college who has just completed his final season of swimming. Mr. Cruze is proud of his swimming career, during which he has set three school records. He is equally proud of being able to keep his grade point average at a 3.2 in the athletic training major, while still meeting the demands of a hectic swimming schedule. Swimming has always been Mr. Cruze's stress reliever. Now that swimming is over, he can focus on continuing the application process for graduate school and preparing for the athletic training Board of Certification examination. It is the first of March, and Mr. Cruze has 1 month until he takes the certification examination. He sets up a study group that will meet twice a week to review material. As the month progresses, he grows concerned that he has received four rejection letters from various graduate schools when he has sent eight applications. It is 1 week until the examination, and Mr. Cruze goes to the athletic training room to talk to the AT about his persistent cold, body soreness, and headache. On examination, he has gained 10 lb since the end of swimming season, his blood pressure is 135/75 mm Hg, and he admits to having difficulty sleeping. He is advised to try to reduce his stress (Fig. 20-8) by starting a swimming routine, and he is referred to the campus physician for a possible antibiotic to help with his cold.

1. Based on this scenario, what do you know about Mr. Cruze's situation?
   - ______________________________________

     ____
   - ______________________________________

     ____

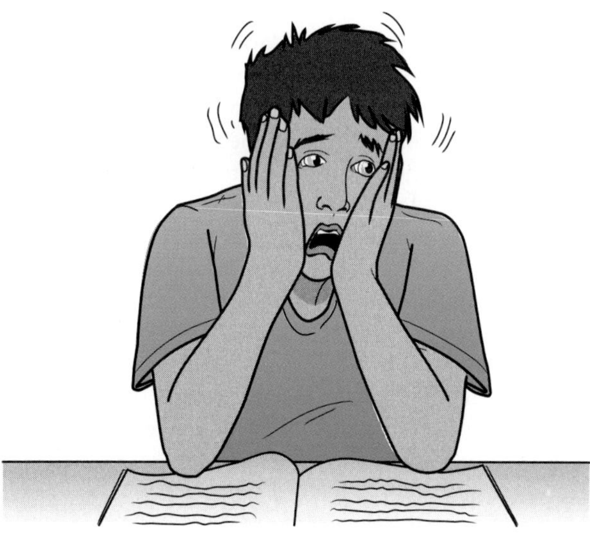

Figure 20-8: Stress.

- ____________________
- ____________________

Brain Jolt
Chronic stress can decrease the immune system and cause many other health problems.

2. Identify key terms and concepts, and research each to broaden your knowledge of psychosocial interventions.
   - What are the different types of stress?

     Answer: ____________________
   - What can happen to the body as a result of chronic stress?

     Answer: ____________________
   - How is general stress different from posttraumatic stress?

     Answer: ____________________
   - Can stress lead to increased risk of injury? If so, how?

     Answer: ____________________
   - What treatments can help treat stress?

     Answer: ____________________

3. Based on the information that you currently have and what was provided by your instructor, what are the possible treatment plans for Mr. Cruze's situation?
   - ____________________
   - ____________________
   - ____________________
   - ____________________

STUDENT SCENARIO 7: DEBBIE POTTS

Debbie Potts is a freshman collegiate cross-country runner. Within the first 6 weeks of school, Ms. Potts has adjusted well to college life. She and her roommate are both runners and seem to be inseparable. One weekend, Ms. Potts returns from a visit home. She becomes concerned that her roommate has not returned by 10:00 p.m. She knew that her roommate was planning to return to campus by 8:00 p.m. for a study session. Ms. Potts contacts her roommate's family only to learn that her roommate was killed in a car accident. Ms. Potts is inconsolable and the campus crisis team, which includes the head athletic trainer, is contacted. The appropriate measures are taken over the next couple of weeks to help Ms. Potts cope with her loss. The cross-country coach contacts the head athletic trainer again 2 weeks after the accident to express his concern that Ms. Potts does not seem to be improving. She is not attending practice and he has received notice that she is not in class either. Fellow teammates notice that she is staying in bed and refusing to join the team for meals. When she does participate in social activities, she seems withdrawn. The head athletic trainer contacts the campus counselor, who takes the necessary steps to contact Ms. Potts to perform an evaluation for depression (Fig. 20-9).

1. Based on this scenario, what do you know about Ms. Potts' situation?
   - ____________________
   - ____________________

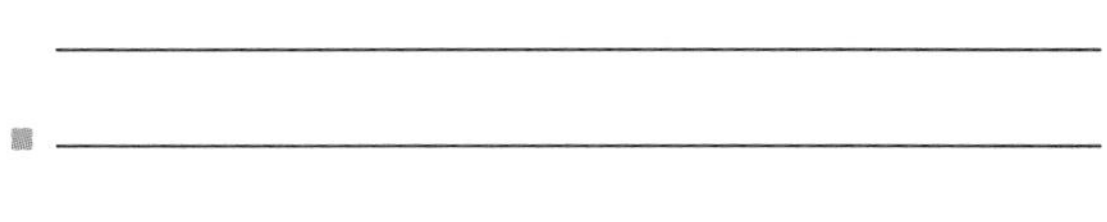

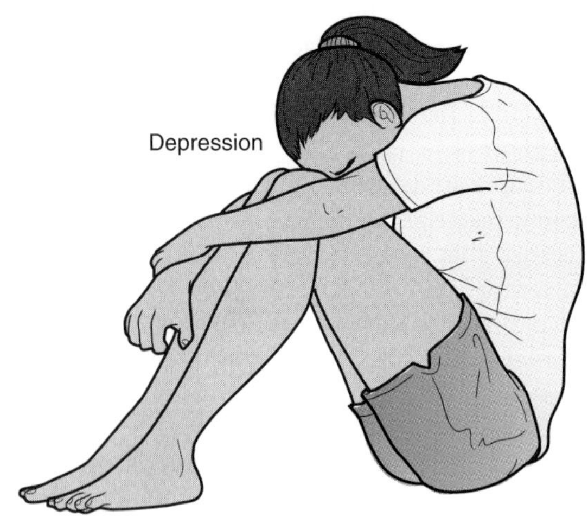

Figure 20-9: Depression.

- ______________________________
  ____
- ______________________________
  ____

Brain Jolt
Severe depression can bring about thoughts of suicide. Referral to a mental health professional and close monitoring is necessary.

2. Identify key terms and concepts, and research each to broaden your knowledge of psychosocial interventions.
   - What is depression?

     Answer: ______________________________
   - What are the signs and symptoms of depression?

     Answer: ______________________________
   - Are there different levels of depression? If yes, elaborate.

     Answer: ______________________________
   - What are the criteria for a diagnosis of clinical depression?

     Answer: ______________________________
   - What are some other increased risks associated with chronic clinical depression?

     Answer: ______________________________
3. Based on the information that you currently have and what was provided by your instructor, what are the possible treatment plans for Ms. Potts' situation?
   - ______________________________
     ____
   - ______________________________
     ____
   - ______________________________
     ____
   - ______________________________
     ____

knowledge checklist

Table 20-1 offers a checklist that can be used by a peer, instructor, or preceptor to evaluate an athlete's treatment plan. Use this checklist as a tool to ensure that the treatment plan is complete and to assess your knowledge of the competencies that apply to this chapter.

TABLE 20-1 ■ Psychosocial Intervention Competency Checklist

	Proficient *Can demonstrate and execute the skill properly*	**Proficient With Assistance** *Can demonstrate and execute the skill with minimal guidance or tips*	**Not Proficient** *Unable to demonstrate and execute the skill properly; need to be reevaluated at another time after further study and practice*
Athlete's Health History			
Medical history			
Current medications			
Medical allergies			
Family history of mental illness			
Psychosocial Intervention Knowledge			
Demonstrates understanding of personality traits			
Demonstrates recognition of abnormal social, emotional, and mental behaviors			
Demonstrates the use of psychological techniques to motivate patients during rehabilitation and return to play (e.g., goal setting, anxiety reduction)			
Demonstrates understanding of the Kübler-Ross reactions to injury			
Identifies warning signs of disordered eating			
Describes the role of various mental health-care providers and demonstrates proper guidelines for referral			
Describes the proper measures to ensure patient confidentiality			

REFERENCES

Arthur-Cameselle, J. N., & Quatromoni, P. A. (2010). Factors related to the onset of eating disorders reported by female collegiate athletes. *The Sport Psychologist, 25*, 1–17.

Ivarsson, A., & Johnson, U. (2010). Psychological factors as predictors of injuries among senior soccer players. A prospective study. *Journal of Sports Science and Medicine, 9*, 347–352.

National Athletic Training Association. (2011). *Athletic training education competencies* (5th ed.). Retrieved from http://www.nata.org/sites/default/files/5th-Edition-Competencies-2011-PDF-Version.pdf

Prentice, W. (2010). *Arnheim's principles of athletic training: A competency-based approach* (14th ed.). New York, NY: McGraw-Hill.

Starkey, C., Brown, S. D., & Ryan, J. (2010). Examination of orthopedic and athletic injuries (3rd ed.). Philadelphia, PA: F.A. Davis.

Thein-Nissenbaum, J. M., et al. (2012). Menstrual irregularity and musculoskeletal injury in female high school athletes. *Journal of Athletic Training, 47*, 74–82.

Venes, D. (Ed.). (2009). *Taber's cyclopedic medical dictionary* (21st ed.). Philadelphia, PA: F.A. Davis.

part five

Personal Performance Enrichment

chapter 21

Sport Nutrition

chapter outline

athletic trainer's corner

Out there in the real world, one athletic trainer experienced the following:

I had my first memorable experience dealing with nutrition during my senior year of college working with my volleyball team. My first encounter occurred when a few of my athletes came to me because they had been feeling more fatigued than usual and wanted some tips on how to improve their energy. I had them give me a list of what they ate each day for a week, and we developed better options to give them more energy based on this list. The second situation I encountered involved one of the smallest girls on the team. It became clear that whenever we had team meals, she rarely ate a reasonable amount of food. The coaching and athletic training staff became concerned that an eating disorder might be the cause. After a few conversations, my supervising athletic trainer and I discovered that she had a problem with eating in front of others. As soon as she returned to her room and was around a smaller crowd of a few close friends, she would eat considerably more. These experiences taught me how to manage young female athletes. Weight and food are commonly sensitive subjects with this group. As an athletic trainer, do not assume things about your athletes before you have gathered all the facts, because things are not always as they seem.

Kristin McQuiniff, AT, ATC
Washington Court House, Ohio

learning outcomes

After working through this chapter, you will be able to:

1. Explain the role of nutrition in maintaining a healthy lifestyle and enhancing performance.
2. Describe nutritional intake recommendations and how these are related to dietary analysis.
3. Explain the current hydration guidelines and describe the risks associated with variation from these standards.
4. Describe the nutritional differences associated with changes in an individual's health, age, and activity level.

introduction

As an athletic trainer, you are responsible for educating your athletes and patients and assisting them with improving their personal performance and health. Throughout this section, you will be presented with various scenarios pertaining to different aspects of personal performance. Using the information given, you are to design a plan to help these athletes and patients improve. These activities will help you fine-tune your skills and develop new and beneficial fitness plans. Before beginning a fitness plan, ensure that you completely understand your athlete's issue or goal and any confounding factors that could affect your decisions. By implementing all the information you have learned in the classroom, you can determine a plan of action to help athletes and patients improve. The Brain Jolts in this chapter are tips to help you bridge the gap from the athlete's issue or goal to the treatment plan. Each Brain Jolt leads you to information that could assist you in improving your athlete's personal performance. You may discover repetitive information; this repetition reinforces important information and aids learning.

MODEL SCENARIO 1: WILLIAM CLUCKNER

William Cluckner is a freshman collegiate football player at his first day of twice daily practices. Before the practices begin, the athletes are required to attend a seminar on hydration. Mr. Cluckner already thinks that he knows enough about hydration, though. He is familiar with how an athlete's urine should appear clear or light colored if he or she is properly hydrated; however, after listening to the seminar, he still does not realize how much of the human body is composed of water (Fig. 21-1). Mr. Cluckner never considered the hydration requirements before, during, and after practice to optimize his energy level and performance. The athletic training staff members provide several recommendations to help the football team optimize their performance. Mr. Cluckner also learns that after practice the athletes are to check their weight to determine any water weight loss. The specific water hydration amount required is conveyed to each athlete in preparation for the next practice. The athletes are not allowed to practice in the next session until all the lost water weight is regained.

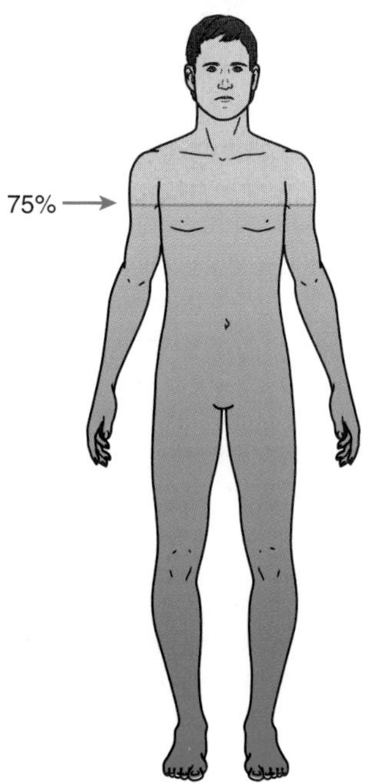

Figure 21-1: How much of the body contains water?

1. Based on this scenario, what do you know about the information given to Mr. Cluckner on hydration?
   - *If the urine is light colored, hydration is achieved.*
   - *Pre-, peri-, and post-hydration requirements affect performance.*
   - *Athletes are weighed before and after practice.*
   - *Water weight lost during activity must be regained.*
2. Identify key terms and concepts, and research each to broaden your knowledge of sport nutrition.
   - Define *hydration*.
     The addition of water to a substance, tissue, or person
   - How many glasses of water on average should athletes consume?
     Players on average should consume 10 glasses of water per day.
   - What are some recommendations for hydration before, during, and after practice?
     Two hours before competition, Mr. Cluckner should drink two additional 8-oz cups of water. During practice, the team should have a water break every 15 min to consume at least half of a cup of cool water.
   - What formula is used to determine the amount of fluid an athlete should drink versus weight lost during a practice?
     For every pound of weight that is lost, the athlete should consume 20 to 24 oz of water.
   - Why are the athletic training staff members focusing on hydration?
     Proper hydration helps to avoid heat-related illnesses that can turn into life-threatening emergencies.
   - What are the signs and symptoms of dehydration?
     Fatigue, dizziness, nausea, and exhaustion

- Should sports drinks be a part of the recovery hydration plan?
  A sports drink is another form of proper hydration that can be consumed in addition to the required amount of water. A sports drink helps to replace essential electrolytes that can be lost during perspiration.

3. Based on the information that you currently have and what was provided by your instructor, what do you need to help Mr. Cluckner remember?
   You need to educate Mr. Cluckner about the importance of hydration. Mr. Cluckner needs to remember the amount of water, given specific to him, before, during, and after practice. Be sure to remind Mr. Cluckner that he will be weighed before and after practice, and he is being held responsible for maintaining his hydration status to avoid an increased risk of illness or injury. If he is unable to monitor his lost fluids and replace them, he could be barred from further practices.

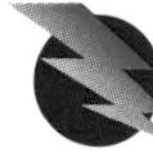

Brain Jolt

Urine color when hydrated is a lighter color. A darker or deeper urine color signifies a greater level of dehydration.

Conversation Buffer

Hydration is an important aspect of athletics. Therefore, it is vital to educate your athletes and coaches about proper hydration. Many coaches view hydration breaks during practice as a waste of time and a practice intended for the weaker players. Impart proper education to the coaches about how hydration can increase athletic performance and prevent injury and illness. Be sure to discuss this with the coaches and athletes during the preseason as well.

MODEL SCENARIO 2: JASON KOHLRUST

Jason Kohlrust is a collegiate sprinter whose track and field program has recently hired a new coach who is also the college's dietitian. Mr. Kohlrust is excited to work with him, because he believes that nutrition can improve his running performance. On the first day of practice, the track and field team has a meeting to review the year's schedule and the required nutrition plan for the team. The coach informs the sprinters that they should eat to lose fat while trying to gain lean muscle mass. By reducing body fat, Mr. Kohlrust will have more explosive power. In addition, sprinters rely on anaerobic energy for performance. As a result, Mr. Kohlrust needs to eat a meal of simple carbohydrates that is low in salt, fiber, and fat and a moderate amount of protein 3 to 4 hours before competition. He also needs to stay well hydrated. After activity, his meal needs to include foods that will replace the muscle glycogen that is lost during activity (Fig. 21-2).

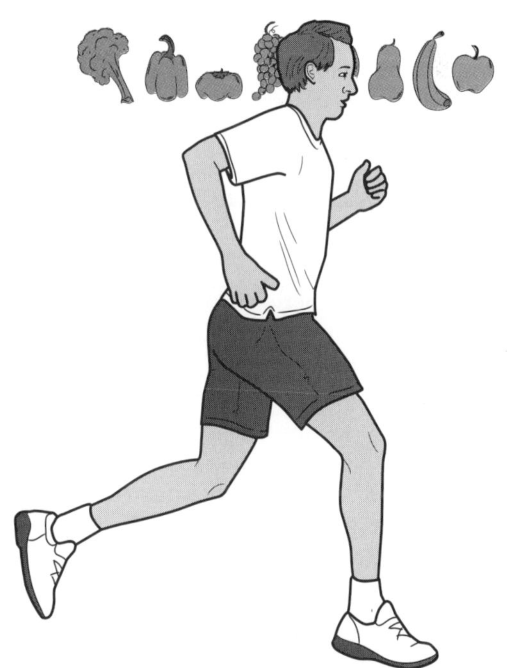

Figure 21-2: Nutrition for sprinters.

1. Based on this scenario, what do you know about Mr. Kohlrust's nutrition recommendations?
   - *Eat to lose weight and fat, but build lean muscle.*
   - *Sprinters need simple carbohydrates for quick bursts of energy.*
   - *Three to four hours before competition, Mr. Kohlrust needs to have a meal of simple carbohydrates low in salt, fiber, and fat and a moderate amount of protein.*
   - *The timing of meals and the foods consumed are important.*
   - *Hydration is mandatory.*
   - *After activity, his meal needs to include foods that will replace the muscle glycogen that is lost during activity.*

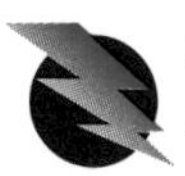

Brain Jolt

Increased protein intake will help an athlete gain lean muscle mass.

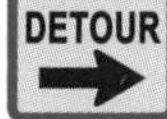

Treatment Detour

A group of authors reviewed 29 studies that explored nutrition knowledge in athletes. They wanted to systematically review the level of knowledge in athletes compared with non-athletes, and determine whether nutritional knowledge affects dietary intake. Although the evidence is weak, they found that athletes have similar general knowledge but potentially greater knowledge in some areas of nutrition compared with non-athletes. General nutrition knowledge was also greater in females compared with males and greater in elite athletes and those with specific nutrition educations. In their review of nutrition knowledge and its effect on dietary intake, the researchers found that there was a weak correlation between better education and good dietary intake. Although better evidence for these findings is needed, even this weak evidence highlights the importance of nutrition education. Athletes require proper nutrition for their active lifestyle. The more knowledge they have, the better they will eat and hydrate for improved performance and health (Heaney, O'Connor, Michael, Gifford, & Naughton, 2011).

2. Identify key terms and concepts, and then research each to broaden your knowledge of nutrition.
   - Define *anaerobic energy*.
     Exercise that takes place in the absence of oxygen
   - How does having a lower body fat percentage allow Mr. Kohlrust to have more explosive power?
     There will be less body mass to overcome and more muscle to create explosive movements.
   - Should Mr. Kohlrust eat anything during activity?
     During competition, Mr. Kohlrust should eat an additional high-carbohydrate snack. A fruit or cereal bar is a good choice.
   - Explain muscle glycogen.
     Muscle glycogen is the excess carbohydrates stored in a muscle that are used as energy during competition. Depending on the length of the competition, the muscle glycogen can be released for energy use or used by the body in a different capacity.
   - What foods does Mr. Kohlrust need to consume after activity to replace muscle glycogen?
     Foods that are rich in carbohydrates, proteins, and electrolytes need to be consumed after activity to help replace any lost nutrients.

3. Based on the information that you currently have and what was provided by your instructor, what are the possible solutions for Mr. Kohlrust's situation?
   Mr. Kohlrust needs to modify his diet to lose body fat and increase his lean muscle mass. He can do this by reducing excess fat in his diet and increasing lean protein intake. Three to four hours before competition, he should eat a meal of simple carbohydrates, low in salt, fiber, and fat, and a moderate amount of protein. In addition, during competition Mr. Kohlrust can eat a fruit or cereal bar. Afterward, he needs to eat foods that are rich in carbohydrates, proteins, and electrolytes to help replace any lost nutrients.

STUDENT SCENARIO 1: IRENE DOLAN

Irene Dolan is a mother of two male high school athletes. She is concerned that she might not be providing the correct nutritional balance for both of her sons' diets. Mrs. Dolan decides to meet with the high school's athletic trainer to discuss the correct calorie breakdown that her boys require. The athletic trainer focuses on the breakdown of the macronutrients and recommends that the daily calorie intake be 55% to 60% from carbohydrates, 25% to 30% from fat, and 15% to 20% from protein. Mrs. Dolan is advised that the boys will most likely need additional calories from carbohydrates during the sport season. Mrs. Dolan and the athletic trainer also discuss which foods are best for each macronutrient category (Fig. 21-3).

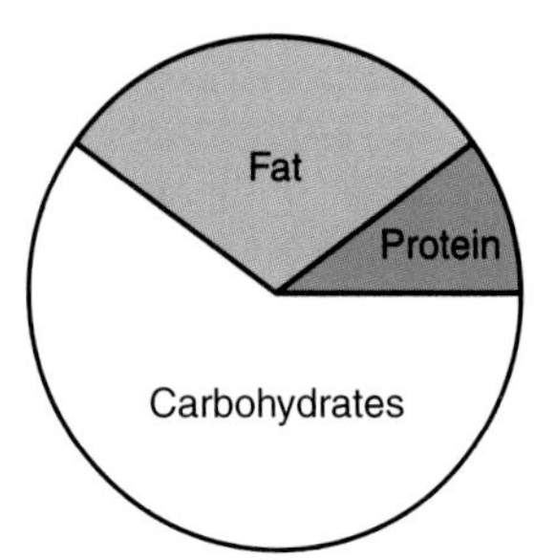

Figure 21-3: Daily calorie intake.

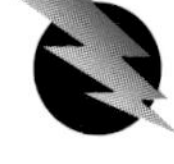

Brain Jolt
Carbohydrates are crucial to an athlete's diet. Be sure that you recommend complex carbohydrates instead of simple carbohydrates to your athletes.

1. Based on this scenario, what do you know about nutrition recommendations for Mrs. Dolan's sons?
   - ____________________
   - ____________________
   - ____________________
   - ____________________

2. Identify key terms and concepts, and research each to broaden your knowledge of sport nutrition.
   - Define *macronutrients*.

     Answer: ____________________

- Why is it important to an athlete's diet to follow these specific food group breakdowns?

  Answer: ______________________________
- Explain carbohydrates and their function.

  Answer: ______________________________
- Explain fats and their function.

  Answer: ______________________________
- Explain proteins and their function.

  Answer: ______________________________
- Why would Mrs. Dolan's sons need extra carbohydrates during a sports season?

  Answer: ______________________________

3. Based on the information that you currently have and what was provided by your instructor, what are possible food recommendations to improve the nutritional intake of Mrs. Dolan's sons?

- ______________________________
- ______________________________
- ______________________________
- ______________________________

STUDENT SCENARIO 2: TERRI STRONG

Terri Strong is a typical American, who is moderately sedentary, eats too much fast food, and would rather choose a cola over a glass of water. Ms. Strong has recently had a health scare and decides that it is time to change her habits. She attends a class that explores proper nutrition and how to turn eating a healthy diet into a habit. Ms. Strong's health can significantly improve with modest changes to her diet and by adding physical activity to her day. During the class, the instructor discusses the breakdown of MyPlate (Fig. 21-4). This government program highlights the recommended breakdown of food groups and the suggested servings. It is a tool that assists individuals in improving their lifestyles. Hydration is another key ingredient to Ms. Strong's health. Because the body is 65% to 75% water, it is a much-needed nutrient. Drinking eight to ten 8-oz glasses of water daily is recommended to help maintain normal body functions. Physical activity is also suggested. Combining physical activity, hydration, and better food choices will keep Ms. Strong on the right path to good health.

Figure 21-4: MyPlate. (Courtesy of http://www.choosemyplate.gov)

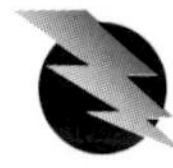

Brain Jolt

Remember to eat in moderation. Eating too much from any food group can cause health issues.

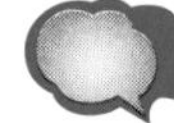

Conversation Buffer

Healthy nutrition is at the center of complete body wellness. It is important to discuss the long-term and short-term health benefits of healthy nutrition with athletes and patients. Because of Ms. Strong's health scare, she is now open to understanding the additional health risks that can be warded off by engaging in a healthy lifestyle. Be sure to discuss the resources available to help athletes and patients with their lifestyle changes.

1. Based on this scenario, what do you know about Ms. Strong?

- ______________________________
- ______________________________
- ______________________________
- ______________________________

2. Identify key terms and concepts, and then research each to broaden your knowledge of sport nutrition.
   - Explain where you can find MyPlate.

     Answer: ______________________________
   - When did it originate?

     Answer: ______________________________
   - Based on MyPlate, what daily food selections and serving amounts would you recommend to Ms. Strong?

     Answer: ______________________________
   - When Ms. Strong begins exercising, should she increase her water intake for optimal hydration?

     Answer: ______________________________
   - Define *moderately sedentary*.

     Answer: ______________________________
   - What are the physical activity recommendations?

     Answer: ______________________________
   - Ms. Strong has been moderately sedentary. What type of exercise plan should she start?

     Answer: ______________________________
3. Based on the information that you currently have and what was provided by your instructor, what are possible physical activities, food recommendations, and hydration amounts for improving Ms. Strong's nutrition?
   - ______________________________
   - ______________________________
   - ______________________________
   - ______________________________

STUDENT SCENARIO 3: **AUDRINA COOK**

Audrina Cook is a 45-year-old weekend-warrior type of athlete. She has just started training for a marathon that is 4 months away. She decides that she wants to improve her eating habits while training. Ms. Cook makes an appointment with a dietitian to discuss food groups and shopping for nutritional foods. One area that is explained to Ms. Cook is the importance of reading food labels. Originally, food labels were seen mainly on processed food containers. Now, food labels are displayed with many fruits, vegetables, and meats and are required by law by the FDA. Food labels provide details about the nutritional information for one serving of that particular food. The content breakdown is based on a diet of 2,000 calories per day. Ms. Cook is advised to look at the calorie content of the foods first. If the calorie content is high, it is usually a good indicator that she should not buy that item. Details to note on a food label are the amount of fat, sodium, sugar, and protein in a serving. Ms. Cook is also shown the daily percentage value on the right hand column of the food label and the meaning of this information (Fig. 21-5).

1. Based on this scenario, what do you know about the advice given to Ms. Cook on how to read food labels?
   - ______________________________
   - ______________________________
   - ______________________________
   - ______________________________

Sample label for macaroni and cheese

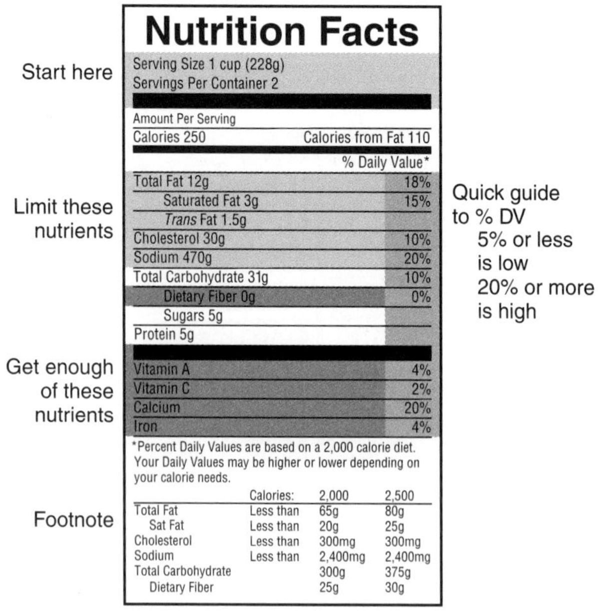

Nutrition Facts

Start here	Serving Size 1 cup (228g) Servings Per Container 2	
	Amount Per Serving	
	Calories 250	Calories from Fat 110
		% Daily Value*
Limit these nutrients	Total Fat 12g	18%
	Saturated Fat 3g	15%
	Trans Fat 1.5g	
	Cholesterol 30g	10%
	Sodium 470g	20%
	Total Carbohydrate 31g	10%
	Dietary Fiber 0g	0%
	Sugars 5g	
	Protein 5g	
Get enough of these nutrients	Vitamin A	4%
	Vitamin C	2%
	Calcium	20%
	Iron	4%

Quick guide to % DV
5% or less is low
20% or more is high

Footnote: *Percent Daily Values are based on a 2,000 calorie diet. Your Daily Values may be higher or lower depending on your calorie needs.

	Calories:	2,000	2,500
Total Fat	Less than	65g	80g
Sat Fat	Less than	20g	25g
Cholesterol	Less than	300mg	300mg
Sodium	Less than	2,400mg	2,400mg
Total Carbohydrate		300g	375g
Dietary Fiber		25g	30g

Figure 21-5: Food label.

2. Identify key terms and concepts, and research each to broaden your knowledge of sport nutrition.
   - Explain what type of services a dietitian can provide for an individual.

     Answer: ______________________
   - Explain each part of the nutritional information on a food label.

     Answer: ______________________
   - If you are not consuming 2,000 calories per day, how do you determine an individual serving?

     Answer: ______________________
   - The dietary recommendations are broken down into three types. Explain what these are.

     Answer: ______________________
   - How does the daily percentage value apply to the dietary recommendations?

     Answer: ______________________
3. Based on the information that you currently have and what was provided by your instructor, what are possible recommendations for Ms. Cook's nutritional diet plan?
   - ______________________
   - ______________________
   - ______________________
   - ______________________

Brain Jolt

Serving sizes are extremely important. When comparing labels, be sure to compare serving sizes as well and determine the accurate nutritional value.

Conversation Buffer

It is important to discuss food labels with athletes and patients and interpret the information. People think many foods are healthy; however, after reviewing the food labels it is apparent that many are not as nutritionally sound as projected. This can be an important factor when trying to make changes for a healthier lifestyle.

STUDENT SCENARIO 4: PAMELA FRANKLIN

Pamela Franklin is a senior collegiate cross-country runner who averages 6 to 7 miles/day. She reports for preseason and is evaluated by the team's orthopedic physician for her yearly physical. She mentions a "hot spot" on her right tibia that has been tender for the majority of the summer. She has a radiograph taken to rule out a stress fracture. The bone scan results are positive, along with the radiograph showing that her right tibia is porous (Fig. 21-6). She talks with the athletic trainer about her calcium intake and menstrual cycle and admits that she does not include milk in her diet because she does not like the taste. She states that she has irregular menstrual cycles, often missing 3 to 4 months at a time. The subject of osteoporosis is discussed with Ms. Franklin, and she is advised to take a calcium supplement and eat a high-calcium diet, while avoiding foods and drinks that can leach calcium from the bones, such as soda.

1. Based on this scenario, what do you know about Ms. Franklin?
   - ______________________
   - ______________________
   - ______________________
   - ______________________

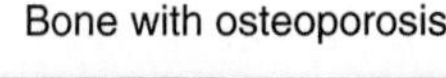
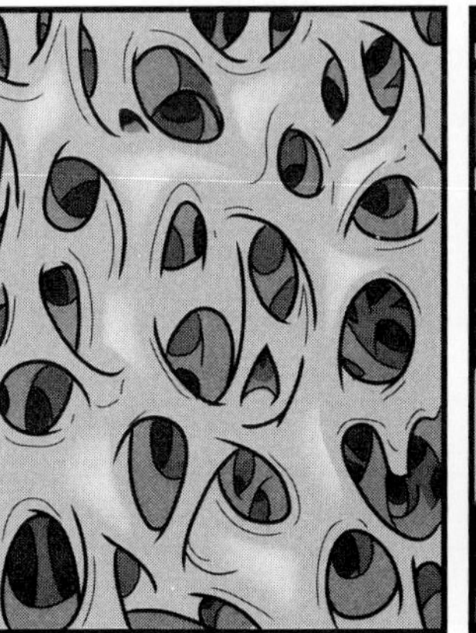

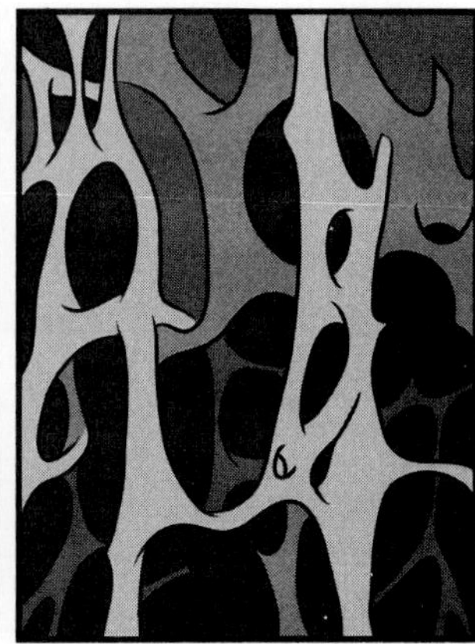

Figure 21-6: Osteoporosis in bone.

Brain Jolt
Calcium is better absorbed with the simultaneous intake of vitamin D.

2. Identify key terms and concepts, and research each to broaden your knowledge of sport nutrition.
   - How do "hot spots" develop?

     Answer: ________________
   - Explain what is meant by a bone being "porous."

     Answer: ________________
   - Why is it important to be aware of Ms. Franklin's menstrual cycles?

     Answer: ________________
   - Define *osteoporosis*.

     Answer: ________________
   - Are there different types of calcium supplements? Explain the benefit of each.

     Answer: ________________
   - What type of diet will increase the excretion of calcium from the body?

     Answer: ________________

3. Based on the information that you currently have and what was provided by your instructor, what are the possible food recommendations that can be made to improve Ms. Franklin's calcium intake?
   - ________________
   - ________________
   - ________________
   - ________________

STUDENT SCENARIO 5: MARCOS HERNANDEZ

Marcos Hernandez is a 35-year-old man who has recently joined a gym. He is encouraged by his fellow coworkers to join them in their morning workout. A few weeks into the 4-day lifting routine, Mr. Hernandez increases his carbohydrate intake to provide more energy. A fellow lifting partner suggests taking a creatine supplement to increase his intensity during his workouts. Mr. Hernandez is not familiar with creatine, so he addresses the topic with the gym's athletic trainer. He learns that creatine does have an important role in energy metabolism. There are two types of creatine and the athletic trainer discusses the functions and benefits of each. Because Mr. Hernandez is interested in taking the supplement, he is instructed on an initial loading phase while being advised of the potential side effects. He also learns that he can obtain creatine by eating certain fish and meats that have a certain number of grams per kilogram (Fig. 21-7).

1. Based on this scenario, what do you know about Mr. Hernandez?
   - ________________
   - ________________
   - ________________
   - ________________

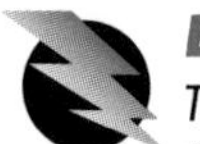

Brain Jolt
The FDA does not regulate supplements.

2. Identify key terms and concepts, and then research each to broaden your knowledge of sport nutrition.
   - Explain creatine. What are the two types?

     Answer: ________________
   - Explain how creatine plays an important role in energy metabolism.

     Answer: ________________

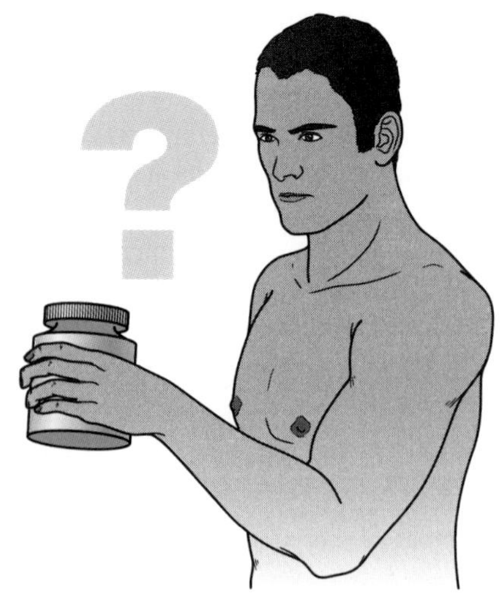

Figure 21-7: Creatine.

- List the steps for the initial loading phase of taking creatine.

  Answer: ___
- What are the potential side effects of creatine?

  Answer: ___
- Is creatine banned by any organizations?

  Answer: ___
- What types of meat and fish could Mr. Hernandez eat?

  Answer: ___
- What is the FDA?

  Answer: ___
- What does it mean if something is not regulated by the FDA?

  Answer: ___

3. Based on the information that you currently have and what was provided by your instructor, what are the possible food recommendations that Mr. Hernandez could consider to increase his energy and weight-lifting performance?
   - ___
   - ___
   - ___
   - ___

STUDENT SCENARIO 6: MARSHA POOLE

Marsha Poole is a high school senior who has been noticing some fatigue 3 hours after her workout. She asks the school's athletic trainer for a post-workout food list. The athletic trainer explains to Ms. Poole that these are known as *recovery foods*. Along with giving the body the right kind of nutrients after a workout, hydration is mandatory. Ms. Poole is advised to avoid sugars and fats. Protein that digests easily after a workout is a good choice for an athlete. Whole grains break down quickly to provide an energy burst. When hydrating, electrolytes need to be replenished as well. If choosing a sports drink, an athlete should choose one that contains sodium and potassium (Fig. 21-8).

1. Based on this scenario, what do you know about Ms. Poole and recovery foods?
   - ___
   - ___
   - ___
   - ___

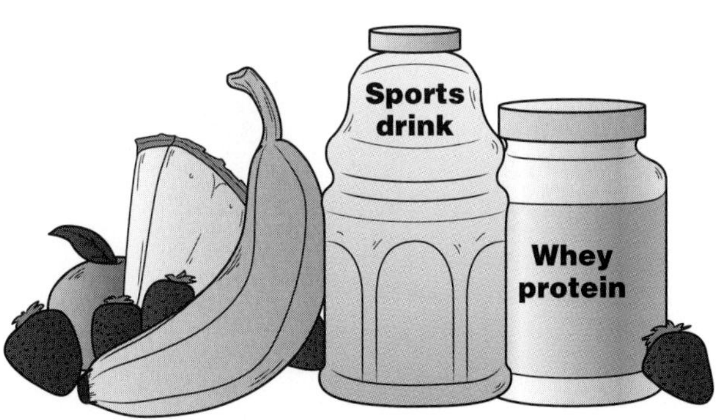

Figure 21-8: Recovery foods.

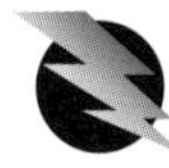

Brain Jolt

Sweat consists of water and electrolytes; therefore, both need to be replaced after physical activity.

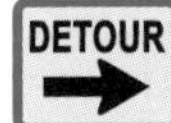

Treatment Detour

Post-exercise recovery is just as important to training goals as the preparation and exercise session itself. Although there are some differences between genders concerning body fat loss and exercise intensity, there appear to be no differences in other nutritional aspects. For example, there is no difference observed in each gender's ability to replenish glycogen stores, the optimal timing required for carbohydrate intake, and the need to consume carbohydrates as soon as possible after exercise. Carbohydrate intake should be proportional to body mass, and carbohydrate-rich meals are recommended for recovery. Adding 0.2 to 0.5 g/day of protein and carbohydrate in a 3:1 ratio per kilogram is recommended. This information helps athletic trainers make recommendations to their athletes and coaches for proper recovery (Hausswirth & Meur, 2011).

2. Identify key terms and concepts, and research each to broaden your knowledge of sport nutrition.
   - Why should athletes stay away from sugar and fat after a workout?

     Answer: ______________________________
   - Explain the importance of having protein after a workout.

     Answer: ______________________________
   - How much sodium and potassium is recommended to consume after physical activity, per serving?

     Answer: ______________________________
   - If you work with an athlete who is diabetic, would you still recommend he or she consume a sports drink for post-workout hydration?

     Answer: ______________________________
   - Define *electrolyte*.

     Answer: ______________________________

3. Based on the information that you currently have and what was provided by your instructor, what are the possible food recommendations that Ms. Poole can choose for the post-workout recovery phase?
   - ______________________________
   - ______________________________
   - ______________________________
   - ______________________________

STUDENT SCENARIO 7: HUNTER KNELLS

Hunter Knells is a collegiate soccer player who has recently approached the college's athletic training staff to discuss proper nutrition. He does not seem to have as much energy after halftime as he did during the first half of a game. When he returns to the game after halftime, he feels sluggish, fatigued, and sometimes dizzy. He started drinking an electrolyte sports drink during the past two games, and the dizziness has since ceased, but he still continues to experience fatigue and sluggishness. He learns that his activity is aerobic because of his activity level and duration. He needs to have a more complex carbohydrate intake before activity along with a protein-based food. He needs to eat specific foods before, during, and after the game for optimal performance (Fig. 21-9).

1. Based on this scenario, what do you know about Mr. Knells?
   - ______________________________
   - ______________________________
   - ______________________________
   - ______________________________

Treatment Detour

Endurance is a main component to many athletic events. Endurance events that last 10 hours or longer are becoming increasingly popular. However, these events pose challenges regarding energy and nutrition during the event. One study analyzed 18 cyclists engaged in a 384-km bicycle race. Upon completion of the race, the participants were asked to recall their food and fluid intakes during the race and supply the researchers with food labels if available. Blood samples were collected, and body mass was calculated for each participant. On average, it took 16 hours and 21 min to complete the race.

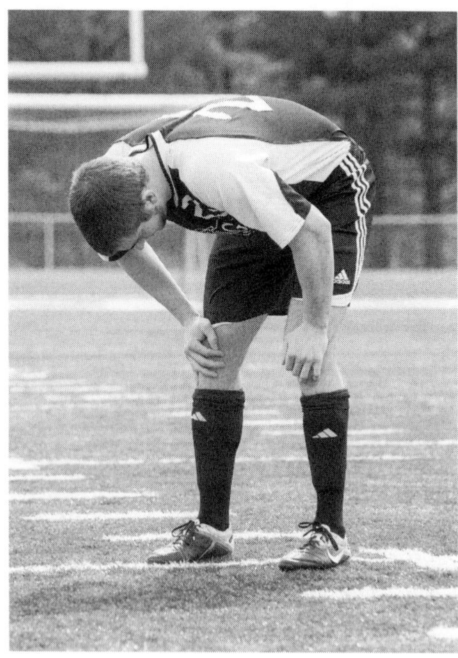

Figure 21-9: Hunter Knells after halftime.

On evaluation, it is evident that the energy intake was significantly lower than the estimated energy requirements for the race. It was also found that there was a significant negative relationship between energy intake and time to complete the race, specifically carbohydrate and fat intake. This research shows that the energy deficit should be minimized and additional energy intake from fat should be investigated, because cyclists already have high carbohydrate intake. Therefore, when working with an ultra-endurance athlete, it is important to properly track and make available the proper nutritional foods and liquids (Black, Skidmore, & Brown, 2012).

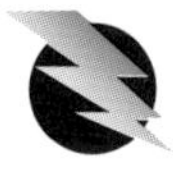

Brain Jolt

Carbohydrate loading is sometimes used before an aerobic endurance event.

2. Identify key terms and concepts, and research each to broaden your knowledge of sport nutrition.
   - Why did the electrolyte sports drink help with Mr. Knells' dizziness?

     Answer: ______________________
   - Define *aerobic*.

     Answer: ______________________
   - What type of carbohydrates should Mr. Knells eat for optimal performance?

     Answer: ______________________
   - What type of proteins should Mr. Knells eat for optimal performance?

     Answer: ______________________
   - Describe meals and snacks that would benefit Mr. Knells before, during, and after each game.

     Answer: ______________________
3. Based on the information that you currently have and what was provided by your instructor, what are the possible food recommendations that Mr. Knell can consider to help with his performance before, during, and after each game?
   - ______________________
     ____
   - ______________________
     ____
   - ______________________
     ____
   - ______________________
     ____

knowledge checklist

Table 21-1 offers a checklist that can be used by a peer, instructor, or preceptor to evaluate an athlete's treatment plan. Use this checklist as a tool to ensure that the treatment plan is complete and to assess your knowledge of the competencies that apply to this chapter.

TABLE 21-1 ■ Sport Nutrition Competency Checklist

	Proficient *Can demonstrate and execute the skill properly*	**Proficient With Assistance** *Can demonstrate and execute the skill with minimal guidance or tips*	**Not Proficient** *Unable to demonstrate and execute the skill properly; need to be reevaluated at another time after further study and practice*
Athlete's Health History			
Medical history			
Current medications			
Medical allergies			
Athlete's nutritional goals			
Sport Nutrition Knowledge			
Demonstrates understanding of sport nutrition and its role in performance enhancement, illness and injury prevention, and a healthy lifestyle			
Demonstrates ability to educate patients and athletes regarding nutrition			
Demonstrates ability to read and understand food labels			
Demonstrates understanding of nutritional intake recommendations			
Identifies warning signs of unhealthy or improper nutrition			
Describes the importance of hydration			
Describes the proper foods required for all phases of activity, including the individual's specific needs			

REFERENCES

Black, K. E., Skidmore, P. M. L., & Brown, R. C. (2012). Energy intakes of ultraendurance cyclists during competition: An observational study. *International Journal of Sport Nutrition and Exercise Metabolism, 22*, 19–23.

Hausswirth, C., & Meur, Y. L. (2011). Physiological and nutritional aspects of post-exercise recovery: Specific recommendations for female athletes. *Sports Medicine, 41*, 861–882.

Heaney, S., O'Connor, H., Michael, S., Gifford. J., & Naughton, G. (2011). Nutrition knowledge in athletes: A systematic review. *International Journal of Sport Nutrition and Exercise Metabolism, 21*, 248–261.

National Athletic Training Association. (2011). *Athletic training education competencies* (5th ed.). Retrieved from http://www.nata.org/sites/default/files/5th-Edition-Competencies-2011-PDF-Version.pdf

Prentice, W. (2010). *Arnheim's principles of athletic training: A competency-based approach* (14th ed.). New York, NY: McGraw-Hill.

Venes, D. (Ed.). (2009). *Taber's cyclopedic medical dictionary* (21st ed.). Philadelphia, PA: F.A. Davis.

chapter 22

Strength Training

chapter outline

athletic trainer's corner

Out there in the real world, one personal trainer experienced the following:

I have had several memorable experiences over the years dealing with personal training. Recently, I had a new client in her early 20s begin training and seek general fitness and nutrition guidance. I learned that she had recently lost more than 50 lb through diet and exercise and had hit a major plateau. Our first few training sessions went well and we were off to a great start as she learned proper form and technique in a variety of exercises. Toward the end of our third session, I asked her to do a brand new exercise. This particular exercise was not that difficult, but it looked intimidating. She immediately told me there was no way she could do it because she was not strong enough or coordinated enough. I continued to encourage her, reassuring her that I would be there every step of the way. She then started to cry! That was the first time I had ever had a client begin to cry from being scared to try something new. Knowing her fitness level and that she was capable of what I was asking, I continued to gently encourage her and reassure her that she could in fact complete the exercise. After a moment, she tried and succeeded. I knew that the exercise was both safe and functional for her; therefore, I was confident that pushing her outside her comfort zone would provide a sense of accomplishment and renew her confidence.

Amy M. Zimmerman, CPT
Personal Trainer
Vital Fitness
Wilmington, Ohio

learning outcomes

After working through this chapter, you will be able to:

1. Compare and contrast the various types of strength-training programs and their expected results.
2. Explain the safety precautions for strength-training programs.
3. Demonstrate the proper technique and body positioning for strengthening exercises and the proper use of equipment.
4. Explain strength-training modifications for an individual's age, fitness level, medical history, and fitness goals.

MODEL SCENARIO 1: KIP HOUSTON

Kip Houston is a collegiate football player, and his team is currently in its offseason weight-lifting program. Three weeks into the program, the certified strength and conditioning specialist (CSCS) talks with the team members about increasing their lifting weight during certain strengthening exercises and varying their lifting routine. The team has reached the point of lifting the first two sets of an exercise with ease. The CSCS wanted to have each individual increase his lifting weight by 2% to 10% from the original weight, depending on whether the lift was an upper-extremity or lower-extremity lift. Mr. Houston finds this instruction discouraging. He was taking pride in being able to finish his current routine and lifting weight with ease. Mr. Houston approaches the CSCS with his frustration, and the CSCS talks with him about the muscle overload principle and progressive resistive exercises. Mr. Houston learns that the team will change its weight room routine periodically because the team should refrain from continually repeating the same exercises week after week (Fig. 22-1).

1. Based on this scenario, what do you know about Mr. Houston's situation?
   - *He is frustrated that he has to change his weight during his lifts and start new exercises.*
   - *He learned that he should refrain from continual repetition of exercises.*
   - *Progressive resistive training will affect strength and fitness.*
   - *He should apply the overload principle when training.*
   - *He needs to increase his lifting weight by 2% to 10% from the original weight, depending on whether the lift is for the upper or lower extremity.*
2. Identify key terms and concepts and then research each to broaden your knowledge of strength training.
   - Define the role of a CSCS.

     According to the National Strength and Conditioning Association, "Certified Strength and Conditioning Specialists (CSCSs) are professionals who apply scientific knowledge to train athletes for the primary goal of improving athletic performance. They conduct sport-specific testing sessions, design and implement safe and effective strength-training and conditioning programs, and provide guidance regarding nutrition and injury prevention. Recognizing that their area of expertise is separate and distinct, CSCSs consult with and refer athletes to other professionals when appropriate."
   - Explain the *overload principle.*

     The body or a muscle must experience a greater load or stress than normal for improvements or adaptations to occur. This can be done by changes in training time, frequency, or intensity.
   - Explain a progressive resistive exercise program.

     A progressive resistive exercise (PRE) program is used to increase the force production in muscles through repetition, number of sets, changing the rest time between sets, or changing the resistance or weight applied.
   - What is the goal of an offseason lifting program?

     To gain strength and muscular endurance for the upcoming season.
   - Why do you increase a PRE program by percentages?

     A PRE program is increased by percentages, from the original lifting weight, to be more efficient for all ages and lifting abilities. Increasing by percentages also ensures safety.
   - Is it important to design a PRE program to be sport-specific or position-specific?

     Yes, specific exercises need to be implemented to strengthen the muscle groups most used in that sport or position. The exercises need to produce the proper muscle fatigue, engage different muscle fibers, and mimic the individual's sport activity. For example, the individual may need endurance, power, or explosivity.

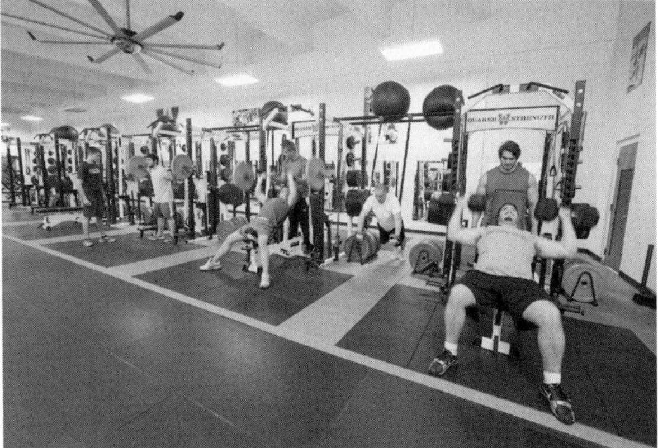

Figure 22-1: Kip Houston's progressive resistive exercise.

3. Based on the information that you currently have and what was provided by your instructor, what do you need to do to help Mr. Houston's situation?

   It needs to be reinforced again to Mr. Houston that, to improve for the upcoming football season, he must continually challenge his body. To do this, he has to increase his lifting weight by percentages, based on his original lifting weight. This will help to increase his strength, but reduce the risk of injury because he is increasing his weight in a progressive way. He also needs to incorporate new exercises that challenge the same muscle groups, but in a different manner. For example, he can go from a leg press to a squat or change the type of bench press from traditional to military press. This way, he is still working on the right muscles but also challenging his body in a safe manner.

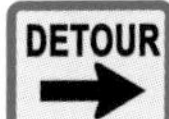

Treatment Detour

The use of strength training to increase strength and power in athletes is a common practice within the sports world. However, another goal of strength-training programs is to increase athletic performance. There is sufficient evidence to show that strength-training programs should continue to be an important part of the athletic preparation of team sports; however, research shows that not all strength programs are equally successful. The best strength programs have individualized specificity to a certain athlete's needs, variation throughout the program, and periodization. This practice becomes challenging when training a team sport that has various positions with different fitness and strength requirements. The athletes with similar goals or positions should do specific training for their needs and then join with the other groups for more general cardiovascular fitness (McGuigan, Wright, & Fleck, 2012).

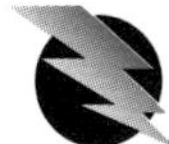

Brain Jolt

In strengthening exercises, never trade proper technique and form for more weight or repetitions. When strengthening with improper form, the athlete loses neuromuscular control and stability of the accessory muscles, possibly resulting in injury.

MODEL SCENARIO 2: JEROME LANGENKAMP

Jerome Langenkamp is a 13-year-old junior high basketball player, and his team has begun a summer weight-lifting program. Mr. Langenkamp's parents have signed a consent form for him to participate in a 3-day weight-training preparation program. The 1-hour session for 3 days will be taught by the high school athletic trainer (AT). The AT has assisted the junior high basketball coaches with a program that will be appropriate for prepubescent adolescents. After this 3-day preparation program, the athletes will continue the summer program with their coaches. During the 3 days, Mr. Langenkamp and his fellow teammates will learn about lifting. He will learn and practice the proper lifting form for the weight machines the team will be using, such as the leg press (Fig. 22-2). The goal of the lifting program is to educate the team on proper form, to use low weight and high repetitions, and to have fun. Throughout his summer lifting, Mr. Langenkamp can expect to have a small increase in the size of his muscles; however, as a result of his developing body systems, the muscle gains will not be like those a high school athlete would experience.

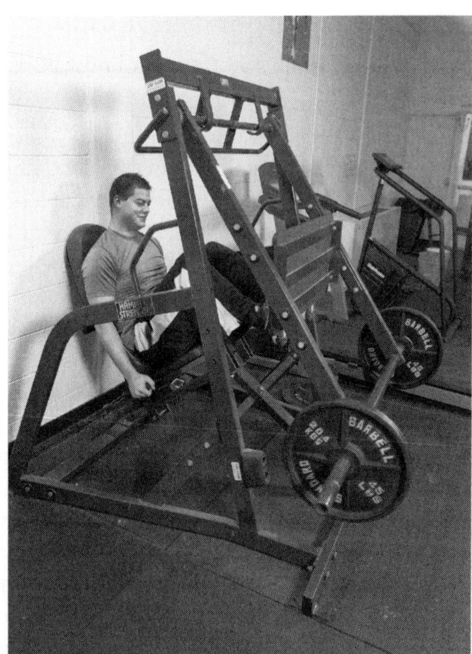

Figure 22-2: Jerome Langenkamp showing proper form on a leg press machine.

1. Based on this scenario, what do you know about Mr. Langenkamp's strength-training program?
   - *The program was developed by the AT and junior high basketball coaches for prepubescent adolescents.*
   - *Mr. Langenkamp's parents have given consent for him to participate.*
   - *The program will consist of 1-hour sessions for 3 days focusing on proper form, low-weight and high-repetition lifting, and having fun.*
   - *With body systems still developing, he can expect some muscle mass increase, but not like what he will see as a high school athlete.*

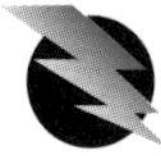

Brain Jolt

It is imperative that young adolescents be taught proper technique for doing safe, age-appropriate, sport-specific exercises.

2. Identify key terms and concepts and then research each to broaden your knowledge of strength training.
   - Define *prepubescent.*
     Being in the period just before puberty

- Why is consent from the athletes' parents needed?
  Because the athletes are minors (younger than 18 years)
- Why is it important for prepubescent adolescent athletes to use low weights and high repetitions?
  The prepubescent adolescent still does not have all 10 body systems fully developed; therefore, adding a great deal of weight could stress the bones and bone growth by damaging the epiphyseal plate.
- Why can Mr. Langenkamp expect only small muscle strength gains?
  Mr. Langenkamp's hormone level, specifically testosterone, is still low. Testosterone is needed to help build muscle.
- Why is it beneficial for adolescents to participate in a weight-lifting program?
  It is beneficial for adolescents to participate in a weight-lifting program because it helps to increase self-esteem, self-confidence, mental discipline, coordination, and general strength to decrease the risk of injury.

3. Based on the information that you currently have and what was provided by your instructor, what are the foundations for Mr. Langenkamp's training program?
Strength training for adolescents is an important part of their conditioning program. Strength training can help to increase bone growth, which means stronger bones. Bones fuse by the early 20s; therefore, gradually increasing an athlete's weight-lifting program is beneficial. After athletes reach puberty, they will have the muscle-building hormones necessary for a more intense weight-lifting program. Muscle mass for boys normally peaks around the age of 18 to 25. Girls normally peak around age 16 to 20. Additional tools that can be added to a strength-training program for adolescents besides just weight machines are core-strengthening exercises, proprioception exercises, and sport-specific exercises.

STUDENT SCENARIO 1: NINA DEBROSSE

Nina Debrosse is a senior high school track and field athlete who competes in shot put. She hopes to reach the state finals this year because she was sidelined last year from a back injury. As part of her offseason training, she has been lifting weights for her upper and lower body along with undergoing cardiovascular training. Two weeks before the first track meet, she notices soreness in her back. She attributes this soreness to the lack of proper stretching during her training warm-up routine. She hopes that, with adding stretching to her warm-up routine and icing after practice, the soreness will go away. Fearful of missing another track season, Ms. Debrosse does not mention the discomfort to the AT for 3 weeks. The pain occurs when she is rotating at her legs, through the hip region, and up to her upper torso when performing the shot put movement. She is evaluated by her AT, and before any type of diagnosis is given, the AT asks to watch Ms. Debrosse throw the shot put. The AT notices that Ms. Debrosse has both mechanical and strength issues throughout her entire shot put movement, which could possibly be causing her back pain. In addition, the AT notes that her core is weak by observing improper plank form (Fig. 22-3) when asked to hold the plank position.

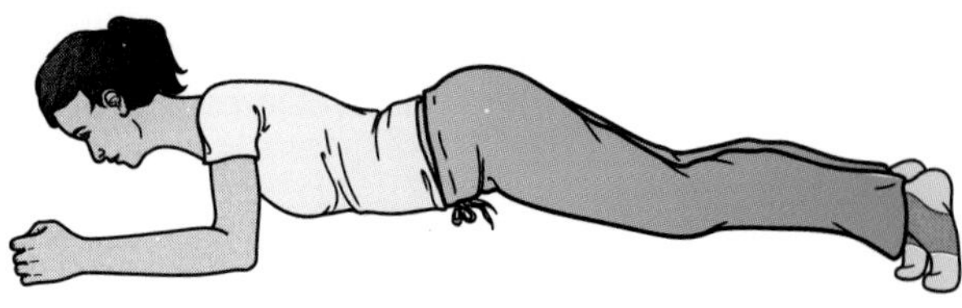

Figure 22-3: Nina Debrosse's improper plank form.

1. Based on this scenario, what do you know about Ms. Debrosse's core stability?

- ______________________________
- ______________________________
- ______________________________
- ______________________________

2. Identify key terms and concepts and then research each to broaden your knowledge of strength training.

- Knowing that Ms. Debrosse has a history of back pain, is it important to know her injury history to help understand her current problem? If so, why?
  Answer: ______________________________
- How else can you determine a weak core?
  Answer: ______________________________
- What type of stretches would be appropriate for Ms. Debrosse during her training warm-up?
  Answer: ______________________________

- How would any strength deficit of her lower body affect Ms. Debrosse's power to throw the shot put?

Answer: ______

- What type of mechanical issues could lead Ms. Debrosse to have low back problems?

Answer: ______

- What is the proper plank position?

Answer: ______

- What core muscles are activated with the plank hold position? Which muscles could be weak, attributing to Ms. Debrosse's back pain?

Answer: ______

- What exercises should Ms. Debrosse add to her current training program to address her strength deficits?

Answer: ______

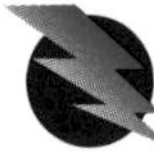

Brain Jolt

Core strength and stability will protect the lumbar spine in all motions.

Conversation Buffer

A core stability program is an important and crucial component of any strength program, as it helps athletes reduce injury caused by improper mechanics. Coaches and athletes need to learn a core program that focuses on good form and proper breathing techniques. These exercises will help to increase strength to the lumbar, abdominal, hip, and pelvic regions, which will improve the athlete's overall performance and reduce the risk of injury.

3. Based on the information that you currently have and what was provided by your instructor, what are the possible solutions for Ms. Debrosse's situation?

- ______
- ______
- ______
- ______

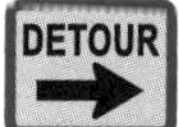

Treatment Detour

Kettlebells have become popular in many gyms and are a part of various training programs. The purpose of one study was to examine the effectiveness of kettlebell training in the transfer of strength and power to weight-lifting and power-lifting exercises and to improve muscular endurance. Thirty-seven participants were assigned to either an experimental group or control group to perform a kettlebell program 2 days per week for 10 weeks. The researchers found that kettlebells did improve power and strength. This is important because kettlebells, which are inexpensive, can be a more realistic method for training because resources are limited for many programs and for individuals training at home (Manocchia, Spierer, Lufkin, Minichiello, & Castro, 2012).

STUDENT SCENARIO 2: VALERIE FRANTZ

Valerie Frantz is a freshman collegiate volleyball player who has been noticing weakness in her right shoulder when making contact with the ball. The weakness occurs when her right shoulder is actively flexed at 180 degrees from extension. Ms. Frantz feels like she is not getting the same explosive power at that joint angle when making contact with the ball (Fig. 22-4). The AT evaluates her to rule out any injury or anatomical issues that may be occurring with her right shoulder. The assessment is positive for bilateral strength differences with flexion, internal rotation, and external rotation of the shoulder. The AT recommends that Ms. Frantz begin a rehabilitation program that will help her increase her general strength in her shoulder and specifically at that joint angle.

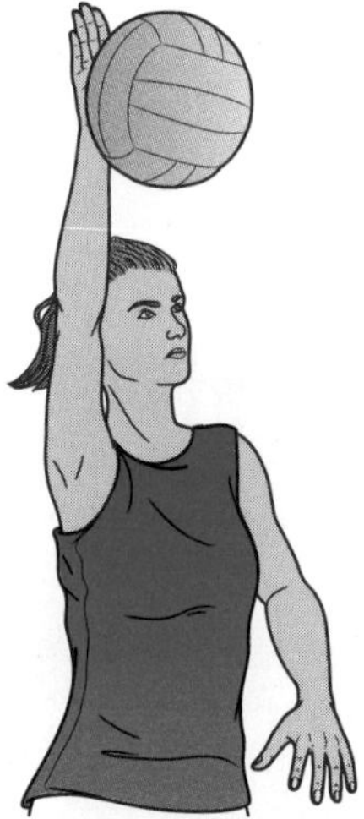

Figure 22-4: Valerie Frantz's position of weakness.

Brain Jolt
The joint angle in this type of strengthening does not change.

1. Based on this scenario, what do you know about Ms. Frantz's situation?
   - ______________________________
   - ______________________________
   - ______________________________
   - ______________________________
2. Identify key terms and concepts and then research each to broaden your knowledge of strength training.
   - Define *explosive power.*

     Answer: ______________________________
   - What are some reasons that Ms. Frantz could be having these types of issues?

     Answer: ______________________________
   - What type of strength training will increase strength at one specific joint angle?

     Answer: ______________________________
   - What are the pros and cons of this type of strengthening?

     Answer: ______________________________
   - Would you also train and strengthen the muscles at different angles?

     Answer: ______________________________
   - What type of strength-training exercises would you recommend to Ms. Frantz?

     Answer: ______________________________
3. Based on the information that you currently have and what was provided by your instructor, what are the possible solutions for Ms. Frantz's situation?
   - ______________________________
   - ______________________________
   - ______________________________
   - ______________________________

STUDENT SCENARIO 3: CLAY RIFE

Clay Rife is a 25-year-old man whose workout routine includes lifting and cardiovascular activity 4 to 5 days/week. He has decided to compete at a bodybuilding show in 12 weeks. He knows that he will need to change his eating habits and his lifting program. His lifting program has mainly focused on his upper body, using the exercise machines only; however, he does not have a lifting partner and feels uncomfortable using free weights (Fig. 22-5). To gain knowledge and to get the most effective workout, Mr. Rife hires a personal trainer to assist him in his training program. He is surprised that his program includes a combination of both free weights and exercise machines. The personal trainer explains that isotonic exercises can be done using either method, and that it is important to use both.

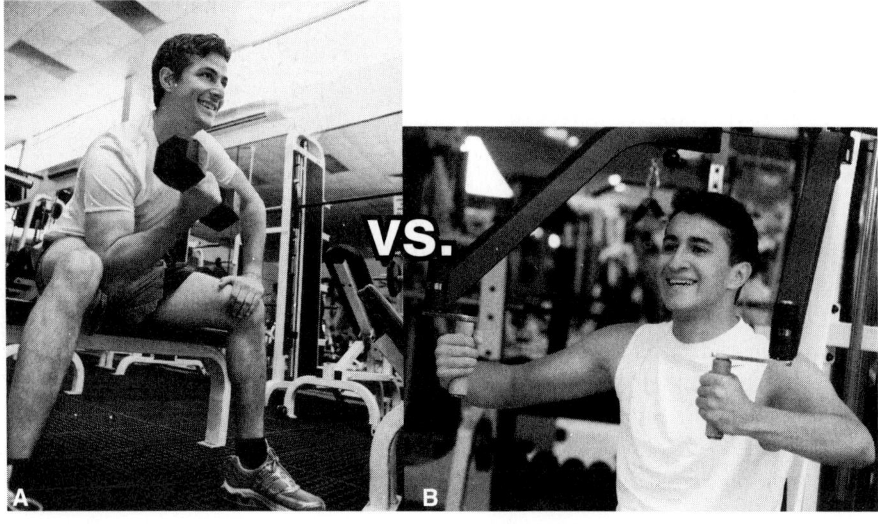

Figure 22-5: Clay Rife's free weights (A) versus weight machines (B). (A. Jupiterimages © Thinkstock B. © Thinkstock)

1. Based on this scenario, what do you know about Mr. Rife's strength-training program?
    - ______________________________
    - ______________________________
    - ______________________________
    - ______________________________
2. Identify key terms and concepts and then research each to broaden your knowledge of athletic strength training.
    - Define *isotonic.*

      Answer: ______________________
    - What are the benefits of using exercise machines?

      Answer: ______________________
    - What are the cons of using exercise machines?

      Answer: ______________________
    - What are the benefits of using free weights?

      Answer: ______________________
    - What are the cons of using free weights?

      Answer: ______________________
    - Why is it important to use a combination of both methods with isotonic exercises?

      Answer: ______________________
    - Which method is the safest while lifting alone?

      Answer: ______________________
    - What is the role of a spotter when lifting free weights?

      Answer: ______________________
    - Is it possible to change the plane of movement when working with free weights?

      Answer: ______________________
3. Based on the information that you currently have and what was provided by your instructor, what are the possible solutions for Mr. Rife's exercise program?
    - ______________________________
    - ______________________________
    - ______________________________
    - ______________________________

Brain Jolt
When designing an exercise program for an individual, you must understand his or her lifting experience, goal for the program, available resources, and the time he or she has to meet that goal.

STUDENT SCENARIO 4: ALMA VORESS

Alma Voress is the secretary in a high school administrative office, and has been talking with the school's CSCS about a personal fitness program. Currently, she walks the school's track 2 to 3 days/week at a brisk pace. She recently read about the importance of strength training for aging females, but is concerned about two things. First, she does not want to gain a large amount of muscle mass. Second, her available time for exercise is limited. She can devote only 1 hour after work. The CSCS would like for Ms. Voress to increase her fitness routine to 5 days/week. If she agrees, 2 of the 5 days would be spent walking as she currently does, and 3 days would be devoted to a circuit weight-training program (Fig. 22-6). This weight-training program will be age appropriate, will fit within her time constraints, and will keep the weight amounts low to tone her body and avoid gaining bulky muscles.

1. Based on this scenario, what do you know about Ms. Voress' strength training?
    - ______________________________
    - ______________________________
    - ______________________________
    - ______________________________

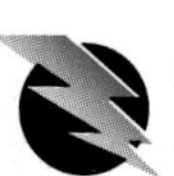

Brain Jolt
Maximal health benefits are achieved through a combination of training techniques and various fitness activities.

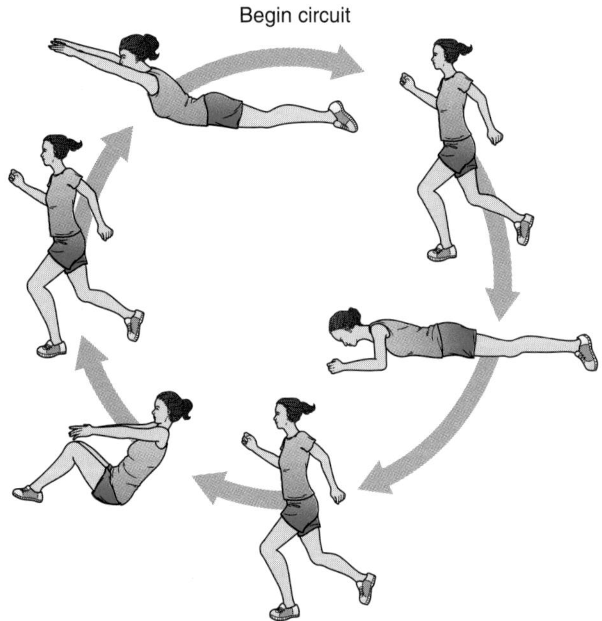

Figure 22-6: Alma Voress' circuit training.

Treatment Detour

One study examined the effect of concurrent muscular strength and high-intensity running interval training on professional soccer players' explosive performances and aerobic endurance. The study included 39 participants who were in an experimental or control group. Both groups participated in 8 weeks of regular soccer training, but the experimental group also participated in additional muscular strength and high-intensity interval training twice per week. Muscular strength training consisted of four sets of six-repetition maximums of high-pull, jump squat, bench press, back half-squat, and chin-up exercises. The high-intensity interval training consisted of 16 intervals each of 15-sec sprints at 120% of individual maximal aerobic speed interspersed with 15 sec of rest. The experimental group had significant changes in vertical jump height, 10-m and 30-m sprint times, and aerobic speed tests. This study shows that high-intensity interval running with high-load muscular strength training can be used in addition to traditional soccer training to enhance soccer players' explosive performances and aerobic endurance. This training combination is highly effective for improving athletic performance (Wong, Chaouachi, Chamari, Dellal, & Wisloff, 2010).

2. Identify key terms and concepts and then research each to broaden your knowledge of strength training.
   - Explain what a CSCS is.

     Answer: ____________________
   - In what types of environments would you expect to see a CSCS work?

     Answer: ____________________
   - Would it be beneficial for an AT to become certified as a CSCS?

     Answer: ____________________
   - What is required to become certified as a CSCS?

     Answer: ____________________
   - Explain circuit weight training.

     Answer: ____________________
   - What are the parameters for a circuit weight-training program?

     Answer: ____________________
   - What are the benefits of this type of program?

     Answer: ____________________
   - Explain some important reasons why women should participate in a weight-lifting program.

     Answer: ____________________
3. Based on the information that you currently have and what was provided by your instructor, what are the possible solutions for Ms. Voress' exercise program?
   - ____________________
   - ____________________
   - ____________________
   - ____________________

STUDENT SCENARIO 5: DOUG WHITTINGTON

Doug Whittington is a sophomore collegiate basketball player. He has always been an athlete who works hard during the season and the offseason. Mr. Whittington believes that for him to succeed, he must eat a well-balanced diet, work hard in the weight room, and always be at the top of his cardiovascular level. He is 6 ft, 5 in. tall and is the team's guard. Mr. Whittington has noticed lately that, from the time he receives the ball on the block, he cannot seem to power up like he used to when attempting to shoot the ball against the backboard and into the net. He begins to worry about his starting position and decides to speak with the athletic training staff members. After talking with Mr. Whittington about his workout regimen, the staff notes that he has been doing the same type of weight room routine and cardiovascular routine for approximately 2 months. The athletic training staff members conclude that Mr. Whittington would benefit from a functional strength-training program, designed to take him through all planes of motion. The program will try to mimic the motions used and required for basketball (Fig. 22-7) while still developing strength and power.

1. Based on this scenario, what do you know about Mr. Whittington's strength training?
   - ______________________________
     ____
   - ______________________________
     ____
   - ______________________________
     ____
   - ______________________________
     ____

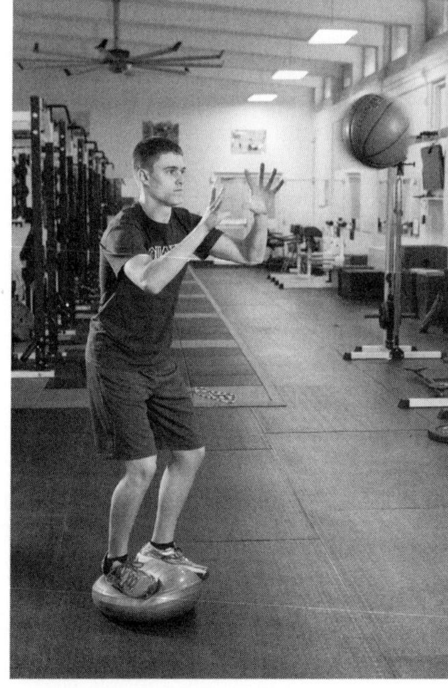

Figure 22-7: Doug Whittington's functional strength exercise.

> **Brain Jolt**
> *After a base of strength has been developed, a functional strength program will help to tailor athletes' skills to their sport's needs.*

2. Identify key terms and concepts and then research each to broaden your knowledge of strength training.
   - Why is Mr. Whittington no longer benefiting from his current weight-lifting and cardiovascular routine?

     Answer: ______________________________
   - Explain functional weight training.

     Answer: ______________________________
   - What is included in this type of program?

     Answer: ______________________________
   - Why is it important to work through all planes of motion?

     Answer: ______________________________
   - How are flexibility and neuromuscular control influenced by a functional weight-training program?

     Answer: ______________________________
   - Why is it important to use sport-specific skills?

     Answer: ______________________________
3. Based on the information that you currently have and what was provided by your instructor, what are the possible solutions for Mr. Whittington's exercise program?
   - ______________________________
     ____
   - ______________________________
     ____
   - ______________________________
     ____
   - ______________________________
     ____

STUDENT SCENARIO 6: GWEN WARWICK

Gwen Warwick is a collegiate soccer player and is the team's goalkeeper. This past season, she felt as though she did not always have the strength to force her way into a group and retrieve the soccer ball. As a result, she decides to talk with the AT, who instructs her to start a more structured weight-lifting program. The new program is designed to overload certain muscle groups to fatigue or failure. She had been doing a circuit weight-training program over the summer, which no longer was beneficial. The AT also tells Ms. Warwick that the amount of body fat versus lean muscle tissue will have a significant role in how her body responds to the weight-lifting program. The AT encourages her to continue a lifting program throughout her life, because of the benefits to her metabolism and bone density level, and reminds her to ensure that she is getting all the important nutrients (Fig. 22-8).

1. Based on this scenario, what do you know about Ms. Warwick's strength training?
   - ______________________
   - ______________________
   - ______________________
   - ______________________

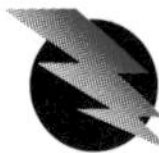

Brain Jolt

Calcium, protein, and iron are important nutritive components in a female strength-training program.

Conversation Buffer

For collegiate athletes, coaches need to stress the importance of healthy food choices and the consumption of the proper vitamins and nutrients. This is especially important for female athletes. Frequently elite female athletes will have already experienced a disrupted menstrual cycle, a change in eating habits, and a lack of nutrients. Discuss the importance of calcium, protein, and iron in the female athlete's diet, and inform athletes about the effects that caffeine and alcohol can have on nutrient absorption and excretion. Coaches of female team members need to discuss the importance of good overall health in gaining peak athletic performance.

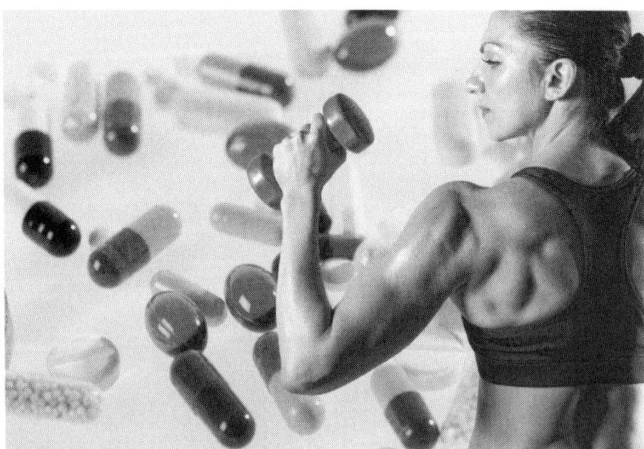

Figure 22-8: Gwen Warwick's nutrition necessities for female athletes. (A and B. © Thinkstock)

2. Identify key terms and concepts and then research each to broaden your knowledge of strength training.
   - What does it mean to overload or fatigue a muscle? Why is it important to do this?

     Answer: ______________________
   - Define *circuit training*.

     Answer: ______________________
   - Why is Ms. Warwick's exercise program no longer beneficial?

     Answer: ______________________
   - How does Ms. Warwick's ratio of body fat to lean muscle tissue affect her weight-lifting program and results?

     Answer: ______________________
   - What is a healthy body fat percentage for women?

     Answer: ______________________
   - Why is it different for men?

     Answer: ______________________
   - Explain how weight lifting affects metabolism.

     Answer: ______________________
   - How does a strength-training program affect bone mineral density?

     Answer: ______________________
3. Based on the information that you currently have and what was provided by your instructor, what are the possible solutions for Ms. Warwick's situation?
   - ______________________
   - ______________________
   - ______________________
   - ______________________

STUDENT SCENARIO 7: RANDELL POORMON

Randell Poormon is a freshman collegiate football player. During the current offseason, the team lifts weights 4 days/week, focusing on different muscle groups. After each lifting session, the athletes are expected to do 30 to 40 min of cardiovascular activity. Mr. Poormon never learned any types of lifting techniques during his high school football career. As a result, when the offensive coach tells him that the timing of his lift is too fast, he does not understand. The offensive coach talks about how Mr. Poormon needs to have a controlled 1- to 2-sec concentric contraction and then a 2- to 4-sec eccentric contraction for fatiguing the muscle (Fig. 22-9). This technique will help to optimize his lifting session. Mr. Poormon is embarrassed that he does not understand the coach, so he talks with the staff AT, who explains concentric versus eccentric phases of motion with weight lifting to build muscular strength. The AT also teaches him that concentric versus eccentric contractions can apply to different muscle groups when talking about joint movement.

1. Based on this scenario, what do you know about Mr. Poormon's strength training?

- ______________________________
- ______________________________
- ______________________________

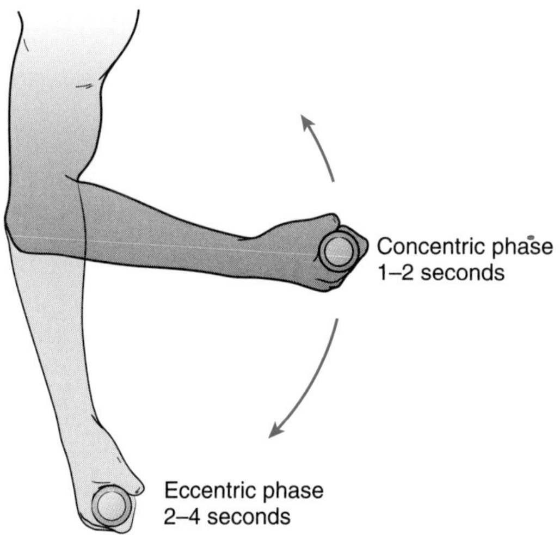

Figure 22-9: Randell Poormon's concentric versus eccentric phase contractions.

- ______________________________

Brain Jolt

Numerous injuries occur in the eccentric phase of motion; therefore, it is important to remember to strengthen muscles both concentrically and eccentrically.

2. Identify key terms and concepts and then research each to broaden your knowledge of strength training.
   - Define *concentric muscle contraction.*

     Answer: ______________________________
   - Define *eccentric muscle contraction.*

     Answer: ______________________________
   - Why should there be a timeframe for performing these types of contractions?

     Answer: ______________________________
   - Why are eccentric contractions more resistant to fatigue than concentric contractions?

     Answer: ______________________________
   - Explain what occurs with an accelerated movement to a specific body part, applying the concentric and eccentric principle.

     Answer: ______________________________
3. Based on the information that you currently have and what was provided by your instructor, what are the possible solutions for Mr. Poormon's exercise program?

- ______________________________
- ______________________________
- ______________________________
- ______________________________

knowledge checklist

Table 22-1 offers a checklist that can be used by a peer, instructor, or preceptor to evaluate an athlete's fitness plan. Use this checklist as a tool to ensure that the fitness plan is complete and to assess your knowledge of the competencies that apply to this chapter.

TABLE 22-1 ■ Strength Training Competency Checklist

	Proficient *Can demonstrate and execute the skill properly*	**Proficient With Assistance** *Can demonstrate and execute the skill with minimal guidance or tips*	**Not Proficient** *Unable to demonstrate and execute the skill properly; need to be reevaluated at another time after further study and practice*
Athlete's Health History			
Medical history			
Strength-training history			
Strength-training goal			
Strength-Training Knowledge			
Demonstrates understanding about isotonic, isometric, and isokinetic strengthening and strengthening principles			
Demonstrates the ability to educate patients or athletes on proper strength-training programs			
Demonstrates the ability to differentiate between various strength-training programs			
Demonstrates an understanding of safety precautions, proper exercise techniques and form, and the use of weight machines			
Identifies improper techniques in clients and how to correct them			
Demonstrates an understanding of proper spotting techniques			

REFERENCES

Baechle, T. R., & Earle, R. W. (Eds.). (2008). *National Strength and Conditioning Association essentials of strength training and conditioning* (3rd ed.). Champaign, IL: Human Kinetics.

Manocchia, P., Spierer, D. K., Lufkin, A. K., Minichiello, J., & Castro, J. (2012). Transference of kettlebell training to strength, power and endurance. *Journal of Strength and Conditioning Research, 27*, 477–484.

McGuigan, M. R., Wright, G. A., & Fleck, S. J. (2012). Strength training for athletes: Does it really help sports performance? *International Journal of Sports Physiology and Performance, 7*, 2–5.

National Athletic Training Association. (2011). *Athletic training education competencies* (5th ed.). Retrieved from http://www.nata.org/sites/default/files/5th-Edition-Competencies-2011-PDF-Version.pdf

Prentice, W. (2010). *Arnheim's principles of athletic training: A competency-based approach* (14th ed.). New York, NY: McGraw-Hill.

Venes, D. (Ed.). (2009). *Taber's cyclopedic medical dictionary* (21st ed.). Philadelphia, PA: F.A. Davis.

Wong, P-L., Chaouachi, A., Chamari, K., Dellal, A., & Wisloff, U. (2010). Effect of preseason concurrent muscular strength and high-intensity interval training in professional soccer players. *Journal of Strength and Conditioning Research, 24*, 653–660.

chapter 23

Fitness Testing

chapter outline

athletic trainer's corner

Out there in the real world, one athletic trainer experienced the following:

As a former high school student, I can remember looking forward to school being out and enjoying my summer. However, as an athlete I learned that I was still going to have to work hard to maintain my muscle strength and endurance. In high school, I participated in two sports and was extremely dedicated to them. Our athletic trainer (AT) took time during his summer break to work with athletes for 6 weeks to improve our speed, strength, flexibility, and endurance. Those early morning training sessions were nothing to look forward to, but I could see the success that came from them in a matter of days. Looking back, it gave me an advantage over athletes who were not involved in any fitness testing. After the 6-week program, the results were incredible; I had numbers to show for it, too. After doing the fitness testing, I had much more confidence in myself and was able to show it on the field.

Currently as an AT, I have firsthand experience and knowledge with fitness testing, and I always stress to coaches that it is important for them to incorporate it in their offseason training. When athletes participate in these types of programs, it lowers their chances of having the minor sprains and strains that ATs typically see. More and more athletes are participating in fitness training programs, and they are the ones who tend to succeed and be more competitive.

Beth Danklefsen, AT, ATC
Sidney High School
Wilson Memorial Sports Medicine
Sidney, Ohio

learning outcomes

After working through this chapter, you will be able to:

1. Describe the standard fitness tests and test equipment used to measure fitness, body composition, flexibility, muscular strength, power, speed, agility, and endurance.
2. Describe testing protocols used to measure fitness, body composition, flexibility, muscular strength, power, speed, agility, and endurance.
3. Interpret results from administering fitness tests to assess an athlete's physical status and fitness level.

MODEL SCENARIO 1: CANDYES CLEARY

Candyes Cleary is a soccer player who is currently in preseason training. Her high school has hired a new athletic trainer (AT) who is implementing preseason fitness testing. With the testing being new and unfamiliar, Ms. Cleary is concerned about her performance. The area of testing today will be static flexibility. The AT explains how important flexibility is for preventing injuries and how it can help to assist the team in soccer. The team will be tested with two types of methods: direct and indirect. The AT gives a description of a direct method using a goniometer and an indirect method using a sit-and-reach test (Fig. 23-1).

1. Based on this scenario, what do you know about Ms. Cleary's situation?
   - *Female soccer player, preseason testing*
   - *Unfamiliar testing and apprehension*
   - *Educated by AT on importance of a flexibility program*
   - *Testing with two types of methods: goniometer and sit-and-reach test*
2. Identify key terms and concepts and then research each to broaden your knowledge of fitness testing.
   - Define *static flexibility*.
     The range of possible movement of a joint and its surrounding muscles during a passive movement

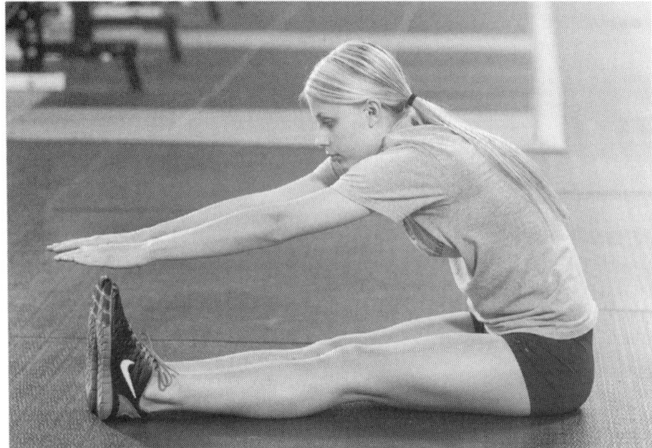

Figure 23-1: Candyes Cleary's sit-and-reach test.

   - Explain the importance of preseason fitness testing.
     Preseason fitness testing is important to assess the athlete's overall fitness level. Flexibility, speed, balance, endurance (cardio/muscular), agility, and body composition are areas that a preseason fitness test should address. Those results should then be used throughout the season as a reference for how the athlete is improving.
   - What is the sit-and-reach method?
     A method that tests the combined flexibility of the low back and hips.
   - Should a postseason flexibility test be performed?
     Yes, to determine what flexibility was gained or lost during the season and to maintain and improve that in the offseason
   - Define the *direct flexibility method*.
     Direct flexibility methods measure angular displacements between adjacent segments or from an external reference.
   - Define *goniometer*.
     An apparatus to measure joint movements and angles
   - Define the *indirect flexibility method*.
     Indirect flexibility tests usually involve the linear measurement of distances between segments or from an external object.
   - Could Ms. Cleary's apprehension influence her testing?
     Yes. Ms. Cleary's apprehension could affect her performance on the test.
3. Based on the information that you currently have and what was provided by your instructor, what do you need to do to implement Ms. Cleary's flexibility test?
   First, have her warm up and stretch before the test. Next, ask her to sit on the floor shoeless with the measuring stick or tape on the floor between her legs, with the zero end toward her body. Ask Ms. Cleary to keep her legs 12 inches apart, her knees fully extended, and her feet in dorsiflexion. Next, have her slowly reach forward with both hands at equal

lengths as far as possible on the measuring stick and hold that position for a couple of seconds. Finally, instruct her to complete this test three times and record the data for the best of the three trials.

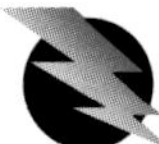

Brain Jolt
In fitness testing, always watch for good form. Substitutions and improper form will alter the test results.

MODEL SCENARIO 2: EMERSON EDGEWATER

Emerson Edgewater is a collegiate football player who has just completed his first football season at the collegiate level. The team will meet again after winter break for its offseason training program. Before break, the freshman football players are required to attend an informative session that outlines the training program. The program will use a periodization approach—an organized training method that involves progressive cycling of various aspects of a training program during a specific period. The information session informs the players that the complete football training program is called a *macrocycle*. The macrocycle is further divided into three or four mesocycles that prepare an athlete through the transition, preparatory, and competition phases. Each mesocycle phase will vary in length of completion time. The goal of the football staff members is to teach the athletes to understand the importance of all phases and to complete each phase to the best of their ability (Fig. 23-2).

1. Based on this scenario, what do you know about Mr. Edgewater's situation?
   - *He is a male collegiate football player.*
   - *He is beginning an offseason training program.*
   - *A complete football training program is a macrocycle.*
   - *This macrocycle has three or four phases called mesocycles.*
   - *Each mesocycle can vary in length.*

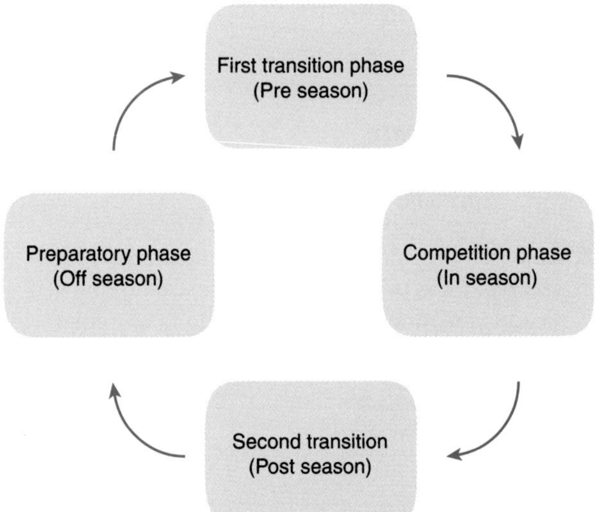

Figure 23-2: Emerson Edgewater's periodization.

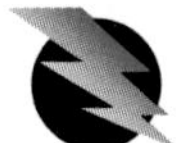

Brain Jolt
In order to have the best performance, a team must follow the guidelines of periodization and the goals of each phase.

2. Identify key terms and concepts and then research each to broaden your knowledge of fitness testing.
   - Explain a macrocycle within a training program.
     A macrocycle is a complete training program of a sport. For seasonal sports, a macrocycle is an entire training year. For an Olympic athlete, a macrocycle would be four years.
   - Explain a mesocycle within a training program.
     A macrocycle is divided into three or four phases known as mesocycles. Within a mesocycle, there are four parts: the preparatory phase, the first transition, the competition phase, and second transition. For a seasonal athlete, this can be offseason, preseason, in season, or postseason.
   - Explain the transition phases of a mesocycle.
     There are two transition phases. This first transition phase is between the preparatory and competition phases. This phase is approximately 1 week long and is the transition from high-volume training and high-intensity training. The second transition phase begins immediately after the last competition phase is completed. This phase is an active rest period; during this period, the athlete is to stay active but not do any type of strenuous activities. An example would be a coed sport or recreational sport. This phase begins the first part of offseason training.
   - Explain the preparatory phase of a mesocycle. Does it have different divisions? If so, explain each.
     The preparatory phase is the time during the offseason and preseason when different sport-related activities are introduced. The preparatory phase has three phases: endurance, strength, and power. The endurance and strength phases are done during the offseason. The power phase occurs during preseason training. The endurance phase is low intensity with high repetitions. The strength phase has the intensity and repetitions increased to a moderate level, while introducing more sport-specific activities. The power phase is primarily the preseason and has a high intensity resembling that of a competition, but with decreased repetitions to allow for a better recovery time.

- Explain the competition phase of a mesocycle.
  The competition phase can be a single event or a sports season. During the competition phase, depending on the length, the focus is on specific sport skills and maintaining cardiovascular endurance.
- Explain a microcycle. Under which phase does it fall?
  A microcycle is typically seen during a sports season. It is a competition phase divided into weeks. Each week starts with high intensity and tapers to low intensity, so that the athlete can recover. The purpose is to peak at the right time for weekly competition.

3. Based on the information that you currently have and what was provided by your instructor, what does Mr. Edgewater need to understand about periodization?
   Mr. Edgewater and his fellow football players need to understand that their training program is broken down because each part has its own importance to gain the best overall athletic performance. Many football players go home over the summer, thus losing much of the offseason endurance and strength work that is completed during the spring. Mr. Edgewater needs to remember that the work required in each phase has a specific purpose. If he fails to complete one phase, the other phases will suffer.

STUDENT SCENARIO 1: AMBROS ROMANOLI

Ambros Romanoli is a junior collegiate soccer player who is about to begin a muscular endurance training program over the summer to help his performance in preseason training. During the first week, he will go through a series of fitness tests to evaluate his physical abilities. Today, he is being evaluated on muscular endurance, which combines strength and stamina (Fig. 23-3). The endurance tests will focus on three different sections of the body: the upper extremity, lower extremity, and core. It is explained to Mr. Romanoli that fatigue is the goal for today, so each exercise will be performed to failure.

1. Based on this scenario, what do you know about Mr. Romanoli's situation?
   - ______________________________
   - ______________________________
   - ______________________________
   - ______________________________

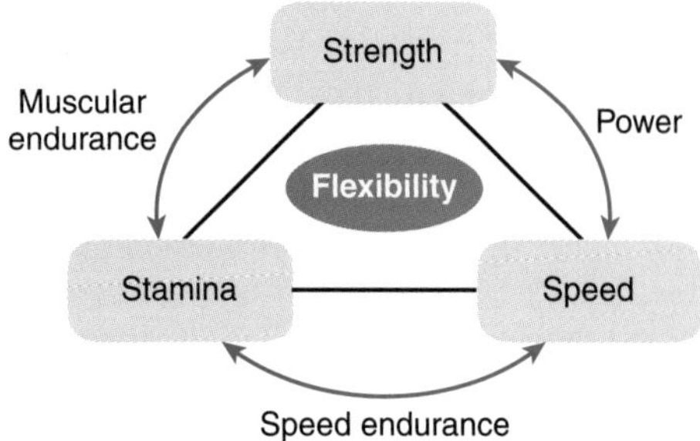

Figure 23-3: Ambros Romanoli's fitness testing paradigm.

2. Identify key terms and concepts and then research each to broaden your knowledge of fitness testing.
   - Define *muscular endurance.*

     Answer: ______________________________
   - What would be included in a muscular endurance program?

     Answer: ______________________________
   - Which three sections of the body will be evaluated? Give examples of the types of exercises that could be applied to each body section, focusing on muscular endurance.

     Answer: ______________________________
   - Why is fatigue a goal for this testing?

     Answer: ______________________________
   - Is the muscular strength endurance testing specific to a muscular group? Explain.

     Answer: ______________________________
   - Are fast-twitch or slow-twitch muscle fibers used for endurance?

     Answer: ______________________________

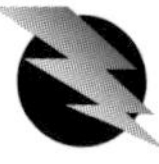

Brain Jolt
When training for muscular endurance, use high repetitions with low weight.

3. Based on the information that you currently have and what was provided by your instructor, how would you administer Mr. Romanoli's muscular endurance tests?
   - ______________________________
   - ______________________________

- ______________________________

- ______________________________

STUDENT SCENARIO 2: JO LYNN ROTTERMAN

Jo Lynn Rotterman is a senior on the girl's high school basketball team. Today at practice, a guest speaker is going to be talking about explosive power and how it relates to basketball. The team learns that not only does explosive power assist with jumping; it can also apply to hitting and throwing. The guest speaker, who wants the team to use as much maximum force as possible when playing basketball, introduces a piece of equipment called the Vertec. It is the machine on which Ms. Rotterman will be tested for vertical jumps after the presentation (Fig. 23-4).

Brain Jolt

Fitness should always be tested and retested at the same time of day, because inconsistent timing can decrease the accuracy of the test results.

Treatment Detour

Fitness tests are used all the time to determine fitness; however, it is unknown how reliable these tests can be in real-world situations. One study examined the reliability of six fitness tests: dynamic balance, Harvard step test, handgrip, vertical jump, pull-ups, and the 60-second jump test. These were evaluated on 238 Cirque du Soleil performers in Las Vegas at baseline, 6-month, 12-month, and 18-month checkpoints. It was found that all the tests except the dynamic balance test were reliable and that the Harvard step and 60-second jump tests had a learning effect. The study also showed that the tests are restricted in their ability to detect conditioning changes in individuals over time; therefore, clinicians must be sure to plan on how the data collected will be used before deciding which tests to include (Burnstein, Steele, & Shrier, 2011).

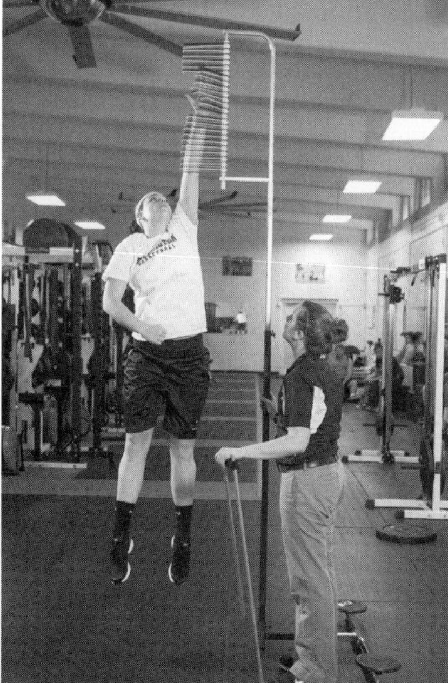

Figure 23-4: Jo Lynn Rotterman's power.

1. Based on this scenario, what do you know about Ms. Rotterman's situation?

- ______________________________
- ______________________________
- ______________________________
- ______________________________

2. Identify key terms and concepts and then research each to broaden your knowledge of fitness testing.

- What is a Vertec?

  Answer: ____________________

- Define *power*.

  Answer: ____________________

- Are fast-twitch muscle fibers or slow-twitch muscle fibers used for power?

  Answer: ____________________

- Explain the stretch-shortening cycle.

  Answer: ____________________

- How does this relate to power?

  Answer: ____________________

- What types of exercises will improve power?

  Answer: ____________________

3. Based on the information that you currently have and what was provided by your instructor, how would you administer Ms. Rotterman's power test?

- ______________________________
- ______________________________

- ____

  ____
- ____

  ____

Conversation Buffer

Be sure to emphasize with your coaches or testing administrator the importance of the sequencing of fitness tests. To ensure testing reliability, it is crucial to administer the fitness tests in an order that ensures optimal performance and to give the proper rest periods between tests.

STUDENT SCENARIO 3: KURT VON NEIDA

Kurt Von Neida is a collegiate cross-country runner starting his junior year. He has the possibility of going to nationals based upon his race times from last year. He is currently running 1 mile in 4 min, 15 sec, and he would like to reduce that by up to 15 sec. He decides to talk with the AT about how to improve his time. The AT talks with him about the need to improve his cardiovascular endurance and to implement maximal aerobic drills into his running regimen. The AT wants to meet Mr. Von Neida the next day to do a VO_2 Max test (Fig. 23-5). This will give the AT information on the types of aerobic drills that would benefit Mr. Von Neida the most for improving his running time.

1. Based on this scenario, what do you know about Mr. Von Neida's situation?
   - ____

     ____
   - ____

     ____
   - ____

     ____
   - ____

     ____

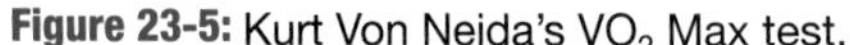

Figure 23-5: Kurt Von Neida's VO_2 Max test.

2. Identify key terms and concepts and then research each to broaden your knowledge of sport fitness testing.
   - Explain cardiovascular endurance.

     Answer: ______________________________
   - Define *aerobic*.

     Answer: ______________________________
   - Define *cardiac output*.

     Answer: ______________________________
   - Define *stroke volume*.

     Answer: ______________________________
   - Define *VO_2 Max*.

     Answer: ______________________________
   - Explain the VO_2 Max test. How can it benefit a training program?

     Answer: ______________________________
   - Explain maximum aerobic drills. Give some examples.

     Answer: ______________________________
3. Based on the information that you currently have and what was provided by your instructor, how will you administer Mr. Von Neida's cardiovascular endurance test?
   - ____

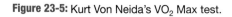

     ____
   - ____

     ____
   - ____

     ____
   - ____

     ____

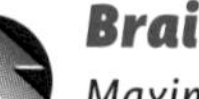

Brain Jolt

Maximal oxygen uptake is the most widely accepted measure of cardiorespiratory fitness.

STUDENT SCENARIO 4: JACKIE WALENDZIK

Jackie Walendzik is a freshman in college. She is 6 ft, 6 in. tall and weighs 150 lb. She has always been tall, lanky, and uncoordinated. Today, the team is seeing the team physician for their yearly physicals, along with performing functional baseline testing. The athletic training staff members want to measure each team member's balance and coordination. Ms. Walendzik is put through static and dynamic balance movements as well as timed coordination drills. She struggles with the drills, but is glad to see that all her teammates have trouble with the beam walk and the wall toss test (Fig. 23-6).

1. Based on this scenario, what do you know about Ms. Walendzik's situation?
   - ______________________________
   ____
   - ______________________________
   ____
   - ______________________________
   ____
   - ______________________________
   ____

Brain Jolt

It is beneficial to test balance and coordination because this will help you identify muscle imbalances, and you can improve these weaknesses through training.

Conversation Buffer

Balance and coordination are two areas often overlooked in young athletes. They are practiced skills. It would be beneficial to discuss with your coaches in junior high and high school the benefits of having drills that focus on balance and coordination. Because an adolescent body is still developing, balance and coordination should be addressed and repeatedly practiced to increase athletic performance and decrease the risk of injury.

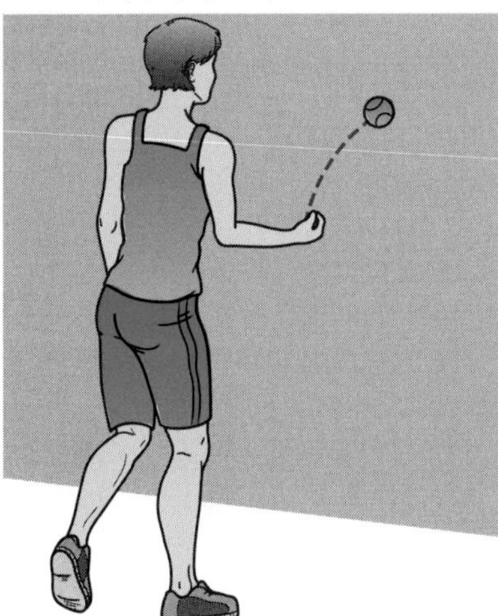

Figure 23-6: Jackie Walendzik's wall toss test.

2. Identify key terms and concepts and then research each to broaden your knowledge of balance and coordination.
   - What could be included in a balance and coordination test?

   Answer: ______________________________
   - Define *static balance.*

   Answer: ______________________________
   - Define *dynamic balance.*

   Answer: ______________________________
   - Define *coordination.*

   Answer: ______________________________
   - Explain the beam walk. What does it test for?

   Answer: ______________________________
   - Explain the wall toss. What does it test for?

   Answer: ______________________________
   - What exercises or activities can be used to improve balance and coordination?

   Answer: ______________________________
3. Based on the information that you currently have and what was provided by your instructor, how will you administer Ms. Walendzik's balance and coordination test?
   - ______________________________
   ____
   - ______________________________
   ____
   - ______________________________
   ____
   - ______________________________
   ____

STUDENT SCENARIO 5: CRAIG MUNTEAN

Craig Muntean is a 30-year-old man who has been referred to an AT for help with beginning a workout regimen. He is considered obese with a body mass index (BMI) of 31, and his physician wants him to lower his BMI below 25. He has an initial visit with the AT to have his body composition measured. The AT will measure Mr. Muntean's body composition using the skinfold method (Fig. 23-7). His body fat percentage will also be determined using the Siri equation, and the results from the initial visit will be used as a reference for his workout program.

1. Based on this scenario, what do you know about Mr. Muntean's situation?
   - ______________________________
   - ______________________________
   - ______________________________
   - ______________________________

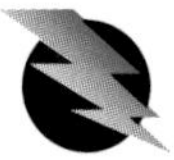

Brain Jolt
Remember that the recommended body fat percentage is higher for women than for men.

2. Identify key terms and concepts and then research each to broaden your knowledge of body composition testing.
   - Define *body composition.*

     Answer: ______________________________
   - Define *body mass index (BMI).*

     Answer: ______________________________
   - How do you determine BMI, and what are the levels?

     Answer: ______________________________
   - How is BMI used for an athlete versus a non-athlete? Can the accuracy of the BMI vary for a heavily muscled athlete or non-athlete?

     Answer: ______________________________
   - Explain the skinfold method. What type of equipment is used?

     Answer: ______________________________
   - Are the skinfold sites the same for men and women? What are the sites?

     Answer: ______________________________
   - Define and explain the *Siri equation.*

     Answer: ______________________________
   - What other types of body composition methods can be used? Which method is the most accurate?

     Answer: ______________________________
   - What is the recommended range of body fat percentage for males?

     Answer: ______________________________

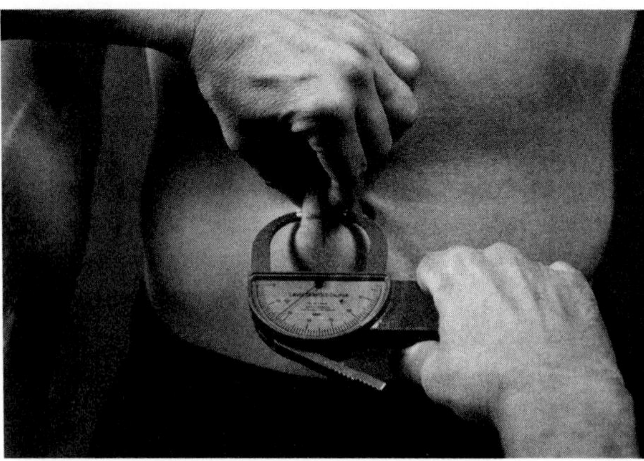

Figure 23-7: Craig Muntean's skinfold method. From Brehm, B. (2013). (*The psychology of health and fitness: Applications for behavior change.* Philadelphia, PA: F.A. Davis)

3. Based on the information that you currently have and what was provided by your instructor, how will you measure Mr. Muntean's body composition?
   - ______________________________
   - ______________________________
   - ______________________________
   - ______________________________

STUDENT SCENARIO 6: LIONEL ROYER

Lionel Royer is a senior collegiate soccer player who plays forward on the team. During preseason conditioning, Mr. Royer and his fellow teammates are working with a CSCS to help with their speed. He will be timed on a variety of speed drills to help the CSCS gauge his improvement throughout preseason conditioning. He is instructed to do the Loughborough Intermittent Shuttle Test (LIST; Fig. 23-8). During the test, he and his teammates will simulate the speed necessary during a soccer match. Before the speed testing begins, Mr. Royer must attach a foot pod to his shoelace.

1. Based on this scenario, what do you know about Mr. Royer's situation?
   - ____________________
   - ____________________
   - ____________________
   - ____________________

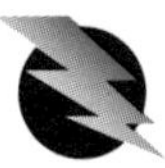

Brain Jolt

With running speed, there is a direct correlation between stride frequency and stride length.

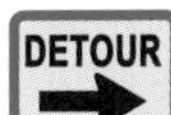

Treatment Detour

Fitness tests are often used for athlete training at institutions across the world. However, not all institutions have the budgets to supply electrical timing systems for these fitness tests. One study examined the reliability of trained and untrained raters and the validity of manual and automatic timing of speed-agility tests, such as the 4 × 10-m shuttle run and the 30-m running speed test in adolescents. It was found that manual measurements by a trained rater using a stopwatch are a valid and reliable measure to assess speed and agility. Therefore, institutions are not required to purchase expensive timing systems, but they do need to invest in training their testing administrators (Vicente-Rodriguez et al., 2011).

2. Identify key terms and concepts and then research each to broaden your knowledge of speed testing.
   - Define *speed*.

     Answer: ____________________
   - What is the purpose of speed testing?

     Answer: ____________________
   - Explain what the LIST shuttle drill is.

     Answer: ____________________

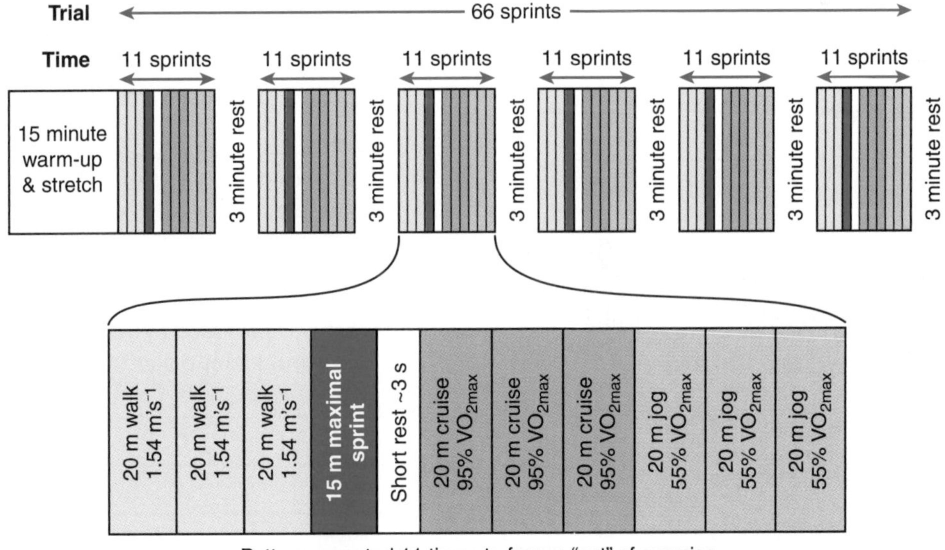

Figure 23-8: Lionel Royer's Loughborough Intermittent Shuttle Test.

- Explain what a foot pod is. Why would it be important for a competitive athlete to use a foot pod for speed testing rather than a pedometer?

  Answer: ______________________
- Give examples of other speed tests that Mr. Royer might be asked to do.

  Answer: ______________________
- Can the surrounding environment affect the speed test results?

  Answer: ______________________

3. Based on the information that you currently have and what was provided by your instructor, explain the process of administering Mr. Royer's speed test.

- ______________________
- ______________________
- ______________________
- ______________________

STUDENT SCENARIO 7: **THOMAS MAUST**

Thomas Maust is a collegiate football running back. The coach tells his players that agility is a core component when playing that position. In order to succeed as a running back, the player must be able to change his speed and direction quickly. Therefore, running backs are given the agility T-test (Fig. 23-9) during the preseason, at midseason, and during the postseason to see the improvements that result from their training regimen.

1. Based on this scenario, what do you know about Mr. Maust's situation?

- ______________________
- ______________________
- ______________________
- ______________________

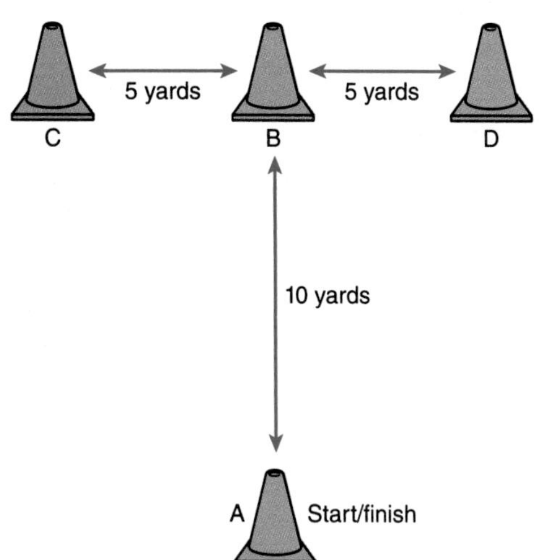

Figure 23-9: Thomas Maust's pro agility T-test.

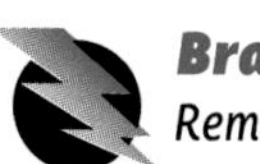

Brain Jolt
Remember to train agility with anticipated and unanticipated changes in speed and direction.

2. Identify key terms and concepts and then research each to broaden your knowledge of agility testing.

- Define *agility*.

  Answer: ______________________
- Can different playing surfaces affect agility?

  Answer: ______________________
- What other fitness tests gauge agility?

  Answer: ______________________
- Why is it important to train agility with anticipated and unanticipated changes?

  Answer: ______________________
- What types of activities or drills will help to improve agility?

  Answer: ______________________

3. Based on the information that you currently have and what was provided by your instructor, explain how you would administer Mr. Maust's agility test.

- ______________________
- ______________________
- ______________________
- ______________________

knowledge checklist

Table 23-1 offers a checklist that can be used by a peer, instructor, or preceptor to evaluate an athlete's fitness-testing plan. Use this checklist as a tool to ensure that the fitness-testing plan is complete and to assess your knowledge of the competencies that apply to this chapter.

TABLE 23-1 ■ Fitness Testing Competency Checklist

	Proficient *Can demonstrate and execute the skill properly*	**Proficient With Assistance** *Can demonstrate and execute the skill with minimal guidance or tips*	**Not Proficient** *Unable to demonstrate and execute the skill properly; need to be reevaluated at another time after further study and practice*
Athlete's Health History			
Medical history			
Strength training and fitness history			
Fitness goal			
Fitness testing history			
Fitness-Testing Knowledge			
Demonstrates understanding about fitness testing guidelines and procedures and the equipment needed			
Demonstrates ability to educate patients or athletes on proper fitness testing techniques and procedures			
Demonstrates the ability to differentiate between various fitness tests			
Demonstrates ability to administer fitness tests for fitness, body composition, flexibility, muscular strength, power, speed, agility, and endurance			
Demonstrates an understanding of and ability to interpret results of various fitness tests			

REFERENCES

Baechle, T. R., & Earle, R. W. (Eds.). (2008). *National Strength and Conditioning Association essentials of strength training and conditioning* (3rd ed.). Champaign, IL: Human Kinetics.

Burnstein, B. D., Steele, R. J., & Shrier, I. (2011). Reliability of fitness tests using methods and time periods common in sport and occupational management. *Journal of Athletic Training, 46*, 505–513.

National Athletic Training Association. (2011). *Athletic training education competencies* (5th ed.). Retrieved from http://www.nata.org/sites/default/files/5th-Edition-Competencies-2011-PDF-Version.pdf

Prentice, W. (2010). *Arnheim's principles of athletic training: A competency-based approach* (14th ed.). New York, NY: McGraw-Hill.

Starkey, C., Brown, S. D., & Ryan, J. (2010). *Examination of orthopedic and athletic injuries* (3rd ed.). Philadelphia, PA: F.A. Davis.

Venes, D. (Ed.). (2009). *Taber's cyclopedic medical dictionary* (21st ed.). Philadelphia, PA: F.A. Davis.

Vicente-Rodríguez, G., Rey-López, J. P., Ruíz, J. R., Jiménez-Pavón, D., Bergman, P., Ciarapica, D., Heredia, J. M., Molnar, D., Gutierrez, A., Moreno, L. A., & Ortega, F. B.; HELENA Study Group. (2011). Interrater reliability and time management validity of speed-agility field tests in adolescents. *Journal of Strength and Conditioning Research, 25*, 2059–2063.

chapter 24

Exercise Prescription

chapter outline

athletic trainer's corner

Out there in the real world, one certified strength and conditioning specialist experienced the following:

One day in March, an athlete came to our facility in need of training to prepare for college football camps in June. The athlete told us the most important area for improvement was the 40-yard dash. This is a common theme for most athletes coming to our program, but most of the time the athletes need much more than an improved 40-yard dash time, so this situation was rare. We went through a variety of tests; he could run a 40-yard dash in 4.85 sec, but we expected much better because he had a 36-in. vertical jump and a 9.5-ft broad jump. Clearly, the athlete was powerful but not efficient in his ability to produce force through the ground while running. We worked him through our program so that he would peak for his camp in June, but everything changed when he grasped the concept of pushing through the ground while running instead of reaching out and pulling his way through when he ran. When the athlete tested at his college camps in June, he consistently ran between 4.45 and 4.48 sec in the 40-yard dash and ran a personal best of 4.39 sec. Needless to say, this athlete went from having no interest from colleges to earning several Division I scholarship offers.

Andrew Winkler, CSCS
Director
Fast-Twitch Performance Enhancement
Dayton, Ohio

learning outcomes

After working through this chapter, you will be able to:

1. Describe the role of exercise in the maintenance of a healthy weight and lifestyle.
2. Design fitness programs for individuals to meet their personal health and fitness needs and goals and educate them about their program.
3. Explain the fundamentals and principles for different components of a fitness program, and differentiate between various fitness methods.

MODEL SCENARIO 1: GUNNAR WERWICK

Gunnar Werwick is a collegiate basketball player who plays guard. His playing time was limited as a freshman, and he attributes this to his low vertical jump. He is 6 ft, 1 in. tall, whereas his fellow guards are 5 inches taller, and they are able to jump much higher for rebounds. Mr. Werwick meets with the athletic trainer (AT) to discuss a program to help him increase his vertical jump. The AT states that they will first test his vertical jump to measure his progress throughout the program. They also discuss exercises that will be included in his program like plyometrics, including depth jumps (Fig. 24-1) and other strengthening exercises like squats. Mr. Werwick and the AT discuss the frequency of this program, noting that he is currently in season. The intensity and duration of the activities are also important.

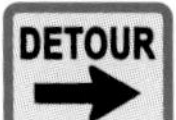

Treatment Detour

Athletes and coaches are always looking for ways to improve force production and power. Plyometrics are often used to attain this goal. In one study, 21 volleyball players, ages 12 to 19 years, went through a 16-week period of plyometric training. The purpose of this study was to determine the efficiency of a chosen plyometric training protocol on youth volleyball players' force capabilities during their usual training period. These participants were tested at baseline, 4 weeks, and the conclusion of the program. These tests included standing long jump, depth leap long jump, medicine ball throws up in 10 sec, medicine ball throws forward against a wall in 10 sec, maximal vertical jump height, and maximal vertical jumps to the maximal height in 10 sec. Each participant had four training sessions per week, two of which included plyometric training. During this training, the plyometric exercises included squat jumps, depth jumps, lateral box push-offs, overhead throws, power drops, and plyometric push-ups. The results showed that this protocol within this study increased speed force production rather than power. Therefore, these types of exercises should be used with athletes to increase speed force skills instead of power (Vassil & Bazanovk, 2012).

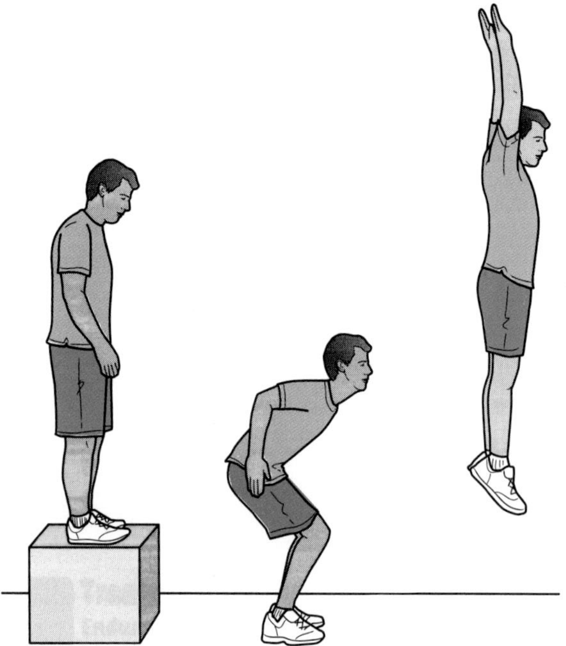
Figure 24-1: Gunnar Werwick's depth jump.

1. Based on this scenario, what do you know about Mr. Werwick's situation?
   - *Collegiate basketball player, male, in season*
   - *Wants to increase vertical jump in hopes of improving playing time*
   - *Program discussed between AT and Mr. Werwick*
   - *Program to include strengthening and plyometric training*
2. Identify key terms and concepts and then research each to broaden your knowledge of exercise prescription.
   - Define *plyometric exercise*.
     An eccentric contraction of a muscle followed by an explosive movement of the same muscle
   - Why are plyometric exercises important?
     Plyometrics are performed to increase a muscle's ability to generate an explosive force. The vertical jump is performed by the lower-body muscles. Training those muscles to do explosive movement will help Mr. Werwick to jump higher and farther.
   - How would you test Mr. Werwick's vertical jump?
     Instruct Mr. Werwick to face a wall while holding a piece of chalk. Have him squat down and explode up, marking the wall with the chalk at the highest point of his jump. Measure the jump with a tape measure and use that chalk line as a starting point for his program. You can also test this using a Vertec device.
   - Why would squats be included in Mr. Werwick's program?
     A vertical jump recruits many muscle groups to make the movement happen. The lower body, core, and back muscles all have a part in this movement. Squats are a strengthening technique that can be addressed as just one area to help assist with the explosive movement needed in a vertical jump.
   - What are depth jumps?
     Depth jumps are recommended only for mature athletes. Depth jumps involve using a platform that is 0.5 to 0.8 m off the ground. The athlete stands on the platform with his feet shoulder-width apart. Keeping his head up and

facing forward, he steps slightly off the platform, and as soon as he feels the ground underneath the balls of his feet, he explodes back up with a vertical jump. Depth jumps are a great exercise to work both concentric and eccentric contracts of the same muscle group.

- Define *frequency*.
  How often the program will be repeated or performed in a week
- Define *duration*.
  The time from the beginning to the end of an exercise program
- Define *intensity*.
  The amount of exertion that an athlete will give to an exercise program, based on his maximum heart rate (MHR)

Conversation Buffer

It is critical to discuss the importance of safety with your athletes when they are doing plyometric training. Athletes are usually thinking of the next motion explosively; however, emphasize that they have to finish one phase of an exercise safely and with proper mechanics before exploding to the next phase. This technique will ensure they have a lower injury risk and gain the most benefits from the exercise.

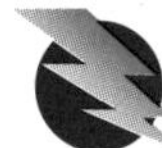

Brain Jolt

Train your core and lower body to help with your vertical jump.

3. Based on the information that you currently have and what was provided by your instructor, which exercise program would be beneficial for Mr. Werwick? Include the mode, frequency, and duration of the program.
   To increase his vertical jumping, Mr. Werwick should perform the following functional drills: vertical jumps, depth jumps, on-box jumps, standing broad jumps, and ankle jumps. Strengthening exercises also need to be a part of this program. Dead lifts, box squats, gluteal muscle and hamstring exercises, and single-leg squats are just a few examples of strengthening exercises to incorporate into a plyometric vertical jump program. If an athlete is currently in season, the frequency of the plyometric training should only be 2 days/wk and 30 min in duration. There should be at least 48 hours between each plyometric training session for muscle recovery. The intensity of the program will be based on Mr. Werwick's MHR range and whether low intensity or high intensity is the focus for the session.

MODEL SCENARIO 2: DAMON SCHMERMUND

Damon Schmermund is a collegiate football player who plays wide receiver. This year during the twice daily conditioning sessions, the offensive coach is having the receivers work on agility drills. The agility drills are added to the program to help the receivers with the speed, coordination, and explosive movement needed when changing movements and directions quickly. The coach talks with the players about a shuttle run drill (Fig. 24-2) that they will be performing. This drill, done with variations, will be added to their conditioning program 2 days/wk. The duration of the agility session will depend on the intensity the coach wants the athletes to achieve.

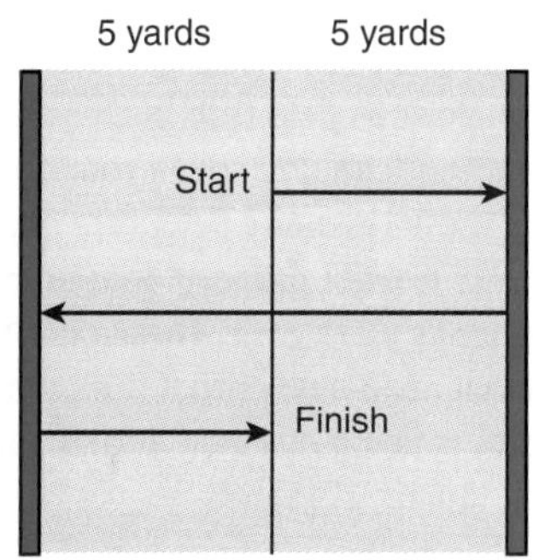

Figure 24-2: Damon Schmermund's shuttle run drill.

1. Based on this scenario, what do you know about Mr. Schmermund's situation?
   - *Male football player*
   - *Doing wide receiver agility drills*
   - *Agility program occurring 2 days/wk*
   - *Session duration determined by coach's intensity goal for the athlete*

Conversation Buffer

You must talk with athletes about the importance of deceleration. Agility involves quick changes in direction. However, athletes must learn to decelerate before they can change directions. Discuss and teach proper braking mechanics to help your athletes reduce the risk of injury from trying to change direction explosively without proper deceleration.

2. Identify key terms and concepts and then research each to broaden your knowledge of exercise prescription.
   - Explain *agility drills*.
     Agility drills are drills that an athlete will perform to work on speed, coordination, and explosive power when changing directions.

- What is speed and how does it apply to an agility program?
  Speed in a program that is working the lower body is usually seen as quick foot or leg speed. An agility program works by putting the lower body through different drills that focus on quick movements.
- What is coordination and how does it apply to an agility program?
  Coordination is the ability to keep one's balance when having to change movements or direction with a sport-specific activity.
- What are explosive movements, and how do they apply to an agility program?
  Explosive movements are those that require a quick change in direction or movement. Eccentric versus concentric contractions have a role in these types of movements and drills within an agility program.
- How can the intensity of the athlete alter or affect the duration of the program?
  If the athlete is doing a high-intensity agility program, which usually means that his heart rate will be at approximately 90% of his MHR range, he will fatigue much faster than if he kept the program at 60% of his MHR range.

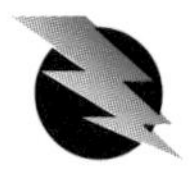

Brain Jolt
It helps to be sport-specific with agility drills to increase athlete motivation.

3. Based on the information that you currently have and what was provided by your instructor, what exercise program would be beneficial for Mr. Schmermund? Include the mode, frequency, and duration of the program.
Mr. Schmermund will be a part of an agility program 2 days/wk. The duration will be no more than 1 hour, based on the intensity that he puts forth. The higher the intensity of the drill, the longer he should rest between drills and the shorter each drill should be. It is important to monitor the fatigue factor as a way to prevent injuries. Always be sure to know the athlete's MHR range for the best performance. The shuttle drill is one in which two cones are placed approximately 25 yards apart. The athlete will sprint from one cone to the next and then back; this is considered one repetition. Variations that can be done are side-to-side cone drills, forward-backward run drills, and forward run–touch the line drills. All these activities can be timed for speed. The explosive power is demonstrated at the start of the timing and then at the quick return or movement coming back to the starting cone. Coordination will be demonstrated when the athlete is asked to change from frontline running to sideline running or backwards running.

STUDENT SCENARIO 1: GLENN FOLCK

Glenn Folck is a collegiate cross-country runner who has been having trouble cutting seconds off his race times and is concerned about the intensities of his training sessions. His cross-country coach has asked the AT to meet with him to discuss the benefits of reaching his desired heart rate range to effectively work the heart and lungs. The AT informs Mr. Folck that, by monitoring the intensity of his work via heart rate, he and the coaches can determine whether his pace is too slow or fast. The AT wants him to find his MHR initially, and then he can help Mr. Folck identify his target heart rate (Fig. 24-3) and an appropriate intensity for his workout.

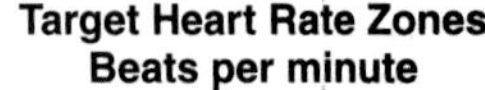

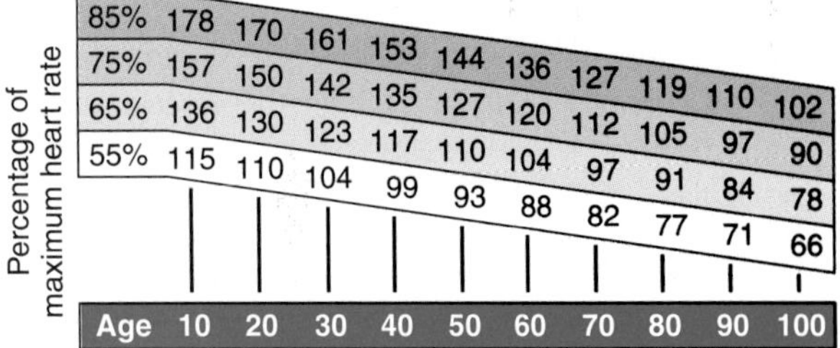

Figure 24-3: Glenn Folck's target heart rates.

Treatment Detour

Athletes frequently wonder how they can get the best workout in the most effective time frame. The best way for athletes to gain the most benefit is to train at the proper intensity during their workouts. It is important for athletes to train at their target heart rate, and a great way to achieve this is to wear a heart rate monitor. This device will quantify their workout by giving them valid heart rate information, and they will then be able to attain their training goal for that workout. To identify an athlete's zone in which he or she has been training, the clinician can perform various field tests such as the 2 × 4-min test and the "can you speak comfortably?" test. During these tests, the peak rate and the average heart rate are the primary data used to determine the patient's work zone. These data can be useful for clinicians to ensure that the proper training intensity is being attained during each training session (Sachs, 2011).

1. Based on this scenario, what do you know about Mr. Folck's situation?
   - ____
   - ____
   - ____
   - ____

2. Identify key terms and concepts and then research each to broaden your knowledge of exercise prescription.
   - Define *intensity*.

     Answer: ______________________
   - Define *heart rate*.

     Answer: ______________________
   - Explain MHR.

     Answer: ______________________
   - Explain target heart rate.

     Answer: ______________________
   - Explain resting heart rate.

     Answer: ______________________
   - Why is it important to know the athlete's MHR?

     Answer: ______________________
   - What is the formula for MHR?

     Answer: ______________________
   - Is using this formula the most accurate method to find the MHR?

     Answer: ______________________
   - Why is it important to know the athlete's resting heart rate?

     Answer: ______________________
   - What is another name for the "can you speak comfortably" test?

     Answer: ______________________

Brain Jolt
Intensity is measured by target heart rate percentages.

3. Based on the information that you currently have and what was provided by your instructor, what exercise program would be beneficial for Mr. Folck when using his heart rate information?
   - ____
   - ____
   - ____
   - ____

STUDENT SCENARIO 2: DWAINE NICODEMUS

Dwaine Nicodemus is a professor who has had a recent health scare. He suffered a cardiac emergency and since then has been taking beta-blockers. His physician also recommended that he begin a workout program and improve his diet and overall health. Currently, Mr. Nicodemus has a sedentary lifestyle. He meets with the campus head AT to discuss a program that will fit his schedule. The AT discusses the importance of starting a program specific to his cardiac recovery and with a low or manageable frequency and duration. The AT would like for Mr. Nicodemus to do some type of exercise to see an increase in cardiovascular endurance and some light strength training. However, in addition to exercise, Mr. Nicodemus needs to change his eating habits and stop eating fast food (Fig. 24-4).

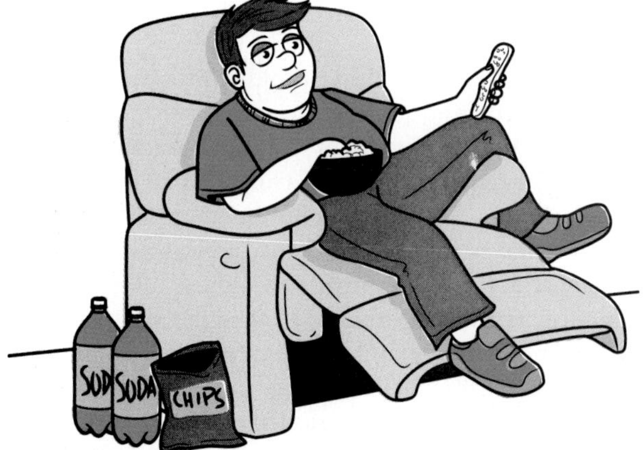

Figure 24-4: Dwaine Nicodemus' sedentary lifestyle.

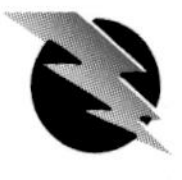
Brain Jolt
Be mindful of medication that could affect an exercise program. A complete patient history will guide you.

Conversation Buffer
It is difficult for career-oriented people to find time to exercise. Explain to them that small bouts of exercise are also beneficial for their health. They do not have to spend hours in the gym to

gain health benefits. Many believe that if they do not devote a major part of their day to exercise, then it is useless, and they forgo exercise completely. An exercise program can be created to fit any lifestyle. People just need to choose an activity that they enjoy and determine how it can fit into their daily schedule. A program that is 30 to 40 minutes long and done three to four times per week is the normal recommended amount of exercise to help improve health.

1. Based on this scenario, what do you know about Mr. Nicodemus' situation?
   - ____________________
   - ____________________
   - ____________________
   - ____________________
2. Identify key terms and concepts and then research each to broaden your knowledge of exercise prescription.
   - Define *sedentary*.

     Answer: ____________________
   - Why is it important to know the types of medication and the precautions when creating an exercise program?

     Answer: ____________________
   - Why is it important to begin with a low-intensity program for an individual who has a sedentary lifestyle?

     Answer: ____________________
   - Define *frequency* and how it relates to a workout program.

     Answer: ____________________
   - Define *duration* and how it relates to a workout program.

     Answer: ____________________
   - Why is it important for Mr. Nicodemus to modify his diet? What foods would be recommended as part of his lifestyle change?

     Answer: ____________________
3. Based on the information that you currently have and what was provided by your instructor, what exercise program would be beneficial for Mr. Nicodemus? Include mode, frequency, and duration of the program.
   - ____________________
   - ____________________
   - ____________________
   - ____________________

STUDENT SCENARIO 3: ANGELA GOLDSTEIN

Angela Goldstein is a 12-year-old who is entering the seventh grade and joining the volleyball team. She is excited to begin the summer workout program that will be 2 to 3 days/wk. When Ms. Goldstein arrives at conditioning, she notices cones on the floor, different-size wooden boxes, and squares taped to the floor. This is not what Ms. Goldstein had envisioned for a summer practice. The coach explains to the girls that the team will do plyometric training 2 days/wk. Because of their age, certain drills will be avoided, and the team will only do age-appropriate plyometric activities. They will focus on footwork drills and low-intensity double-leg hops and jumps (Fig. 24-5).

1. Based on this scenario, what do you know about Ms. Goldstein's situation?
   - ____________________

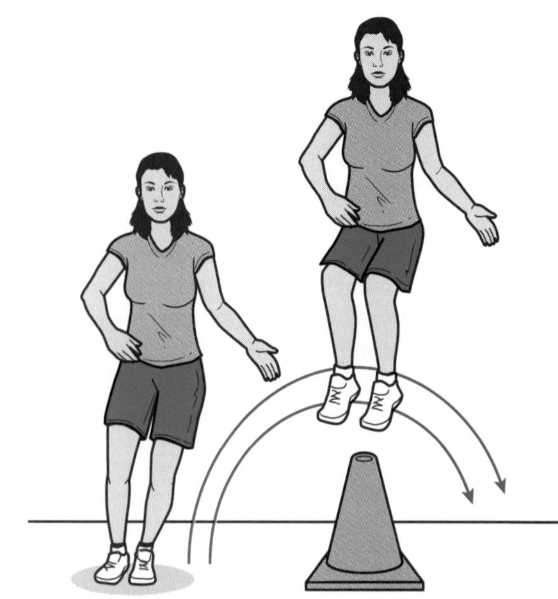

Figure 24-5: Angela Goldstein's double-leg jumps.

- ____

  ____
- ____

  ____
- ____

  ____

2. Identify key terms and concepts and then research each to broaden your knowledge of sport exercise prescription.
   - Define *plyometrics*.

     Answer: ______________________________
   - Is plyometric training beneficial and safe for adolescents? Why is constant supervision necessary?

     Answer: ______________________________
   - What drills should be avoided with adolescents in a plyometric program? Explain why.

     Answer: ______________________________
   - Should the type of plyometric exercises implemented in a program be different for boys and girls? What body changes could hinder this decision?

     Answer: ______________________________
   - Give one example of a drill that would use cones, a drill that would use wooden boxes, and a drill that would use squares on the floor.

     Answer: ______________________________
   - What is the recommended duration, frequency, and intensity for a junior high plyometric training session?

     Answer: ______________________________
3. Based on the information that you currently have and what was provided by your instructor, what exercise program would be beneficial for Ms. Goldstein? Include the mode, frequency, and duration of the program.
   - ____

     ____
   - ____

     ____
   - ____

     ____
   - ____

     ____

Brain Jolt

Adolescents are still developing and maturing. If the proper precautions are not followed, they could damage areas of their bodies that are not fully developed.

STUDENT SCENARIO 4: JACLYN MOZER

Jaclyn Mozer is a collegiate basketball player. During the fall semester, her team will meet with the coaching staff to review its yearly workout program. The AT designs a program that will benefit them during different phases of their season using periodization. The preseason, mid-season, and postseason workout routines will consist of different cardiovascular and strengthening exercises. The mode, frequency, intensity, and duration will also vary with each season (Fig. 24-6).

1. Based on this scenario, what do you know about Ms. Mozer's situation?
   - ____

     ____
   - ____

     ____
   - ____

     ____

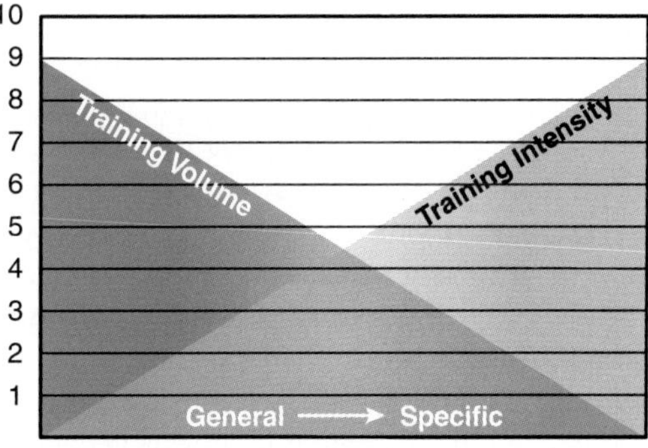

Figure 24-6: Jaclyn Mozer's periodization.

- ____

  ____

2. Identify key terms and concepts and then research each to broaden your knowledge of exercise prescription.
   - Explain periodization training.

     Answer: ____________________
   - List and describe each phase of the periodization cycle.

     Answer: ____________________
   - Define *mode*.

     Answer: ____________________
   - Define *frequency*.

     Answer: ____________________
   - Define *duration*.

     Answer: ____________________
   - What types of cardiovascular and strengthening exercises would you do during a preseason program? Incorporate mode, frequency, and duration.

     Answer: ____________________
   - What types of cardiovascular and strengthening exercises would you do during a midseason program? Incorporate mode, frequency, and duration.

     Answer: ____________________
   - What types of cardiovascular and strengthening exercises would you do during a postseason program? Incorporate mode, frequency, and duration.

     Answer: ____________________
   - Explain overtraining.

     Answer: ____________________
   - How can overtraining be avoided?

     Answer: ____________________

Brain Jolt

Improper periodization will lead to overtraining and burnout for your athletes.

3. Based on the information that you currently have and what was provided by your instructor, what exercise program in each phase would be beneficial for Ms. Mozer? Include the mode, frequency, and duration of the program.
   - ____________________
   - ____________________
   - ____________________
   - ____________________

Conversation Buffer

When developing an exercise program, one component that can be beneficial to incorporate with periodization is exercise that challenges the fast twitch and slow twitch muscles. Each muscle fiber needs to be focused on separately when developing a program. The different phases of an athlete's physical training cycle will demand different physical responses from the muscle groups. Be sure to research the sport, the major muscle groups for the functional movements, and which muscle fibers are recruited during the physical activity. Next, discuss these findings with your athletes and coaches to ensure the most efficient training program.

STUDENT SCENARIO 5: RAYMOND RUSSO

Raymond Russo is a collegiate swimmer. Training for the swim season can be long and sometimes monotonous. As a result, he and his teammates are rather familiar with long swims and tempo swims. Mr. Russo is reporting for conditioning today and is told that the team will do Fartlek training once per week for the next month. The goal of this training program is to provide variation from their typical training program, work all the body systems, and help to increase the lactate threshold (Fig. 24-7).

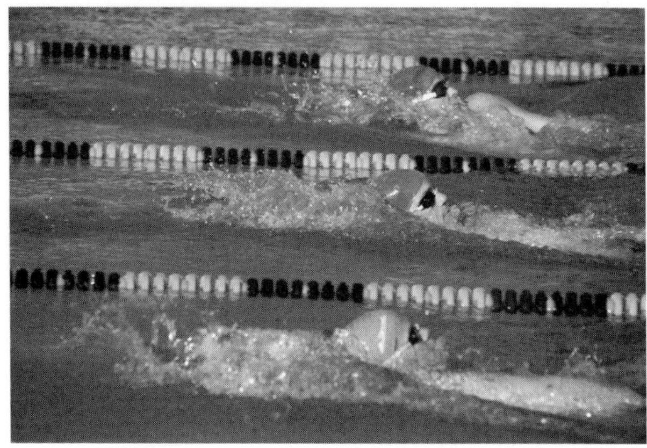

Figure 24-7: Raymond Russo's swim training. © Thinkstock

1. Based on this scenario, what do you know about Mr. Russo's situation?
   - ____________________

- ____
  ____
- ____
  ____
- ____
  ____

Brain Jolt
Fartlek training is typically used for running, cycling, and swimming; however, it can be integrated into any athlete's program.

2. Identify key terms and concepts and then research each to broaden your knowledge of exercise prescription.
   - Define *Fartlek training*.

     Answer: ______________________________
   - What are the benefits of Fartlek training?

     Answer: ______________________________
   - Explain lactate threshold. How does it benefit performance?

     Answer: ______________________________
   - Can you do Fartlek training on different terrains? Explain.

     Answer: ______________________________
   - When should Fartlek training be implemented in a program? What should the duration be?

     Answer: ______________________________
   - Can Fartlek training help race performance by cutting race times? Explain.

     Answer: ______________________________
3. Based on the information that you currently have and what was provided by your instructor, how would you conduct Mr. Russo's Fartlek training? Include the mode, frequency, and duration of the program.
   - ____
     ____
   - ____
     ____
   - ____
     ____
   - ____
     ____

STUDENT SCENARIO 6: RODNEY PARKS

Rodney Parks is a collegiate wrestling coach. He is a new hire for the college, and after seeing the team's fitness level, he has determined that the team needs more intense training to improve its performance. After discussing it with the AT, Mr. Parks decides to have his team do interval training to help with their cardiovascular level, lactic acid threshold, and weight loss. Each team member is required to find his MHR. The team will work at 60% of the MHR and then will increase up to 90% for a short time during the training. The recovery period between training sets needs to be timed and can be either a complete rest or activity at a low level. The wrestling team will do interval training twice per week on the soccer field (Fig. 24-8).

1. Based on this scenario, what do you know about Mr. Parks' situation?
   - ____
     ____
   - ____
     ____

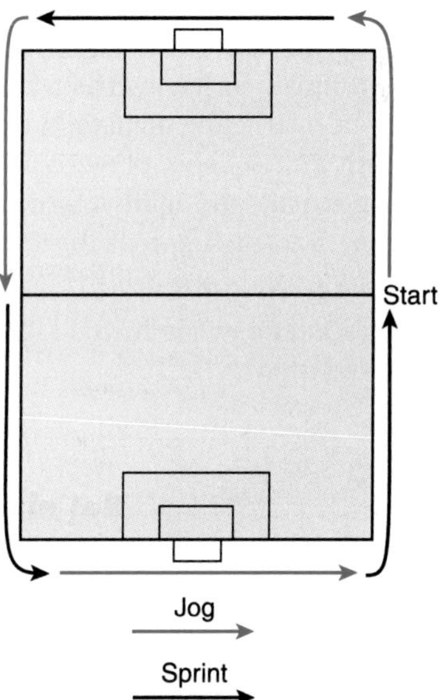

Figure 24-8: Rodney Parks' interval training.

- ______________________________

  ____
- ______________________________

  ____

Brain Jolt
This type of exercise should be done only once the athlete has good aerobic endurance.

2. Identify key terms and concepts and then research each to broaden your knowledge of exercise prescription.
   - Explain interval training.

     Answer: ______________________________
   - What type of sport would benefit from internal training? In what season should it be implemented?

     Answer: ______________________________
   - Explain lactic acid threshold.

     Answer: ______________________________
   - How can interval training assist with lactic acid threshold?

     Answer: ______________________________
   - Why is interval training more effective at weight loss than continuous training?

     Answer: ______________________________
   - How long should the high-intensity phase last?

     Answer: ______________________________
   - How long should the low-intensity phase last?

     Answer: ______________________________
   - Explain how you determine the MHR.

     Answer: ______________________________
3. Based on the information that you currently have and what was provided by your instructor, how should Mr. Parks conduct his interval training? Include the mode, frequency, and duration of the program.
   - ______________________________

     ____
   - ______________________________

     ____
   - ______________________________

     ____
   - ______________________________

     ____

STUDENT SCENARIO 7: TRISH BURDISS

Trish Burdiss is a freshman collegiate volleyball player. She is reporting for the beginning of twice-daily training sessions. The coach is first having the team meet with the AT, who will be instructing them on their conditioning program. With the frequency of twice-daily practices and the resulting fatigue, the agility training will occur 3 days/wk. The AT wants to improve the team's foot and leg speed with ladder and cone drills (Fig. 24-9).

1. Based on this scenario, what do you know about Ms. Burdiss' situation?
   - ______________________________

     ____
   - ______________________________

     ____
   - ______________________________

     ____
   - ______________________________

     ____

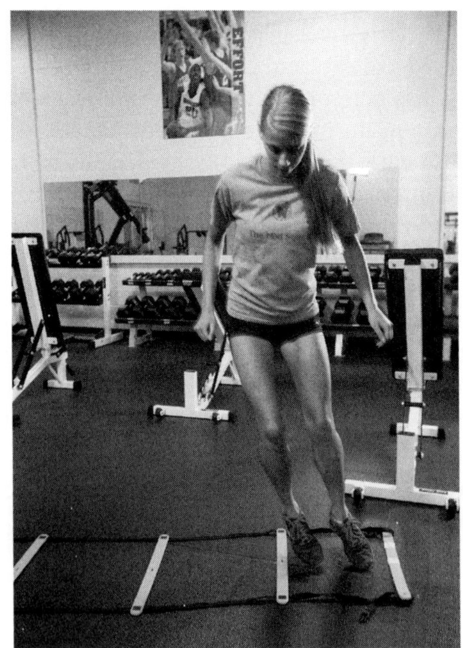

Figure 24-9: Trish Burdiss' ladder drill.

2. Identify key terms and concepts and then research each to broaden your knowledge of exercise prescription.
   - Define *frequency*.

     Answer: ______________________
   - Explain agility training.

     Answer: ______________________
   - What are the benefits of agility training?

     Answer: ______________________
   - Why does fatigue from twice-daily practices need to be considered when deciding the frequency and duration of the agility training for Ms. Burdiss and her team?

     Answer: ______________________
   - Give two examples of a ladder drill for Ms. Burdiss.

     Answer: ______________________
   - Give two examples of a cone drill for Ms. Burdiss.

     Answer: ______________________
   - How long should the duration of each agility session be?

     Answer: ______________________

Brain Jolt

Maximal effort and quickness are crucial for performance improvement from agility ladder training.

3. Based on the information that you currently have and what was provided by your instructor, how would you conduct Ms. Burdiss' agility training? Include the mode, frequency, and duration of the program.
   - ______________________
   - ______________________
   - ______________________
   - ______________________

knowledge checklist

Table 24-1 offers a checklist that can be used by a peer, instructor, or preceptor to evaluate an athlete's fitness plan. Use this checklist as a tool to ensure that the fitness plan is complete and to assess your knowledge of the competencies that apply to this chapter.

TABLE 24-1 ■ Exercise Prescription Competency Checklist

	Proficient *Can demonstrate and execute the skill properly*	**Proficient With Assistance** *Can demonstrate and execute the skill with minimal guidance or tips*	**Not Proficient** *Unable to demonstrate and execute the skill properly; need to be reevaluated at another time after further study and practice*
Athlete's Health History			
Medical history			
Strength training and fitness history			
Fitness goal			
Fitness testing history			
Exercise Prescription Knowledge			
Demonstrates understanding about the role of exercise in the maintenance of a healthy weight and healthy lifestyle			
Demonstrates the ability to differentiate between various methods of fitness training			
Demonstrates ability to design fitness programs for individuals that meet their personal health and fitness needs and goals			
Demonstrates ability to educate patients or athletes about fitness programs			

REFERENCES

Baechle, T. R., & Earle, R. W. (Eds.). (2008). *National Strength and Conditioning Association essentials of strength training and conditioning* (3rd ed.). Champaign, IL: Human Kinetics.

National Athletic Training Association. (2011). *Athletic training rducation competencies* (5th ed.). Retrieved from http://www.nata.org/sites/default/files/5th-Edition-Competencies-2011-PDF-Version.pdf

Prentice, W. (2010). *Arnheim's principles of athletic training: A competency-based approach* (14th ed.). New York, NY: McGraw-Hill.

Sachs, L. (2011). Heart rate training: Exercise results can be improved with proper use of a heart rate monitor. *IDEA Fitness Journal, June,* 28–31.

Vassil, K., & Bazanovk, B. (2012). The effect of plyometric training program on young volleyball players in their usual training period. *Journal of Human Sport and Exercise,* 7 (Proc, 1), S34–S40.

Venes, D. (Ed.). (2009). *Taber's cyclopedic medical dictionary* (21st ed.). Philadelphia, PA: F.A. Davis.

part six

Organization and Administration

chapter 25

Ethics

chapter outline

athletic trainer's corner

Out there in the real world, one athletic trainer experienced the following:

When thinking about ethical issues in the real world, one example comes to mind. I have worked in a clinical setting as an athletic trainer for numerous years now. There was a situation that I witnessed in one of my previous clinics that I believed was a violation of the NATA Code of Ethics and would be a violation of any other professional code of ethics. A patient was progressing well through her rehabilitation with a shoulder injury; however, the main clinician continually encouraged that patient to return for treatment after she had recovered sufficiently to be discharged. It seemed that the clinician was having her do simple exercises for no good reason except that he was able to bill for additional sessions. In order to protect the patient and the clinic as a whole, I brought the situation to my supervisor so the issue could be resolved.

Jennifer H. Ross, AT, PTA
Commonwealth Orthopedic Centers
Edgewood, Kentucky

learning outcomes

After working through this chapter, you will be able to:

1. Describe the National Athletic Trainers' Association (NATA) Code of Ethics and identify violations.
2. Describe the Board of Certification (BOC) Standards of Professional Practice and identify violations.
3. Describe steps to take to avoid ethical violations.
4. Identify possible consequences for ethical violations.

introduction

As an athletic trainer (AT), you are responsible for everything that is involved in the organization and administration of athletic training. Throughout this section, you will be presented with various scenarios pertaining to different aspects of the profession including ethics, risk management, legal aspects, professional development, and management. From the information given, you are to identify whether anything has been done wrong in the scenario and devise solutions to correct these issues or to handle a situation. These activities will help you fine-tune your professional skills, but be sure that you completely understand the issue at hand and any confounding factors that could affect your decisions. By implementing all the information you have learned in the classroom and then applying it to each scenario, you can determine a plan of action.

MODEL SCENARIO 1: JULIAN PERRY

Julian Perry is an AT at a Division I university. He has been there approximately 5 years as the head AT for football. Because it is a Division I university, there is a lot of pressure on Mr. Perry to return injured players to play as fast as possible. Today at practice, the starting quarterback was running a play and inverted his ankle. Mr. Perry evaluates the injury immediately. He does not think that the athlete fractured anything or that he tore any ligaments. Knowing that they have a big game on Saturday, Mr. Perry calls the team doctor and sends the athlete for imaging. The radiograph shows no fracture, and the doctor sees no signs of torn ligaments. The doctor wants the athlete to do rehabilitation with Mr. Perry three times per day the entire week to be able to play on Saturday, and they have rush-ordered an ankle brace for the athlete to wear for the game. This all happened on Monday. On Tuesday, an athlete on the scout team who does not play in games inverted his ankle as well. Again, Mr. Perry evaluated his ankle and did not conclude that there was any fracture or torn ligament. He gave the athlete ice, removed him from practice for the day (Fig. 25-1), and told him to come to the athletic training room the next day for a recheck. Each athlete ultimately had the same severity of inversion ankle sprain.

Treatment Detour

The NATA Code of Ethics and the BOC Standards of Professional Practice are documents with which each AT must comply in order to safely practice within the profession. These documents outline the proper principles to follow and the professional responsibility to report any violations in order to maintain a professional reputation. The documents are available at http://www.nata.org/codeofethics and http://www.bocatc.org, respectively.

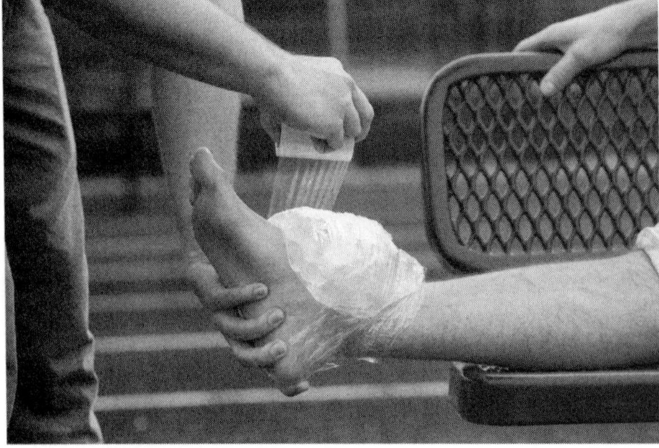

Figure 25-1: Julian Perry with football athlete.

1. Based on this scenario, what do you know about Mr. Perry's actions?
   - *Head AT for Division I football*
   - *Worked there for 5 years*
   - *Head quarterback inverted his ankle*
   - *Negative evaluation; called the team doctor and got the athlete a radiograph, started extensive rehabilitation, and rush-ordered an ankle brace*
   - *An athlete on the scout team who does not play often inverted his ankle*
   - *Negative evaluation; athlete removed from practice to ice the injury and instructed to return the next day for a recheck*
   - *Same severity of injury for both*
2. Identify key terms and concepts and then research each to broaden your knowledge of ethical issues.
   - Do you see any violations of the NATA Code of Ethics or BOC Standards of Professional Practice?
     Yes.
   - If yes, what are the violations?
     Each athlete had similar injuries with the same severity; however, the starting quarterback got immediate care from the team doctor, a radiograph, and extensive rehabilitation, and Mr. Perry rush-ordered an ankle brace for the game on Saturday. This violates principle 1 of the NATA Code of Ethics: "Members shall respect the rights, welfare, and dignity of all." If this is the necessary treatment for the injuries, then the second athlete who does not play should receive the same medical treatment.
3. Based on the information that you currently have and what was provided by your instructor, what needs to be done now and in the future regarding Mr. Perry's situation?
   Mr. Perry needs to realize that his actions are not ethical. Every athlete must receive the same medical

treatment and be given the same opportunities for medical treatment. He must remember that the AT is there for the health of the athletes and is not to make decisions influenced by a certain athlete's role on the team. Each evaluation should be done independently and without regard for a player's team status. The administration or Mr. Perry's superior could address this with him, or Mr. Perry could be reported to the NATA ethical board by another AT. As a result, there could be an investigation and consequences determined by the ethical board.

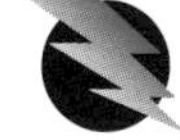

Brain Jolt

Ethical violations can be reported to your professional organization anonymously.

STUDENT SCENARIO 1: MONICA ARNOLD

Monica Arnold is an AT and a certified strength and conditioning specialist (CSCS) at the collegiate level. She is working with the wrestling team, which has historically been highly competitive within its conference. This year, Ms. Arnold has two athletes who are predicted to go to nationals to compete if they do well throughout the season. One of the athletes is having trouble with weigh-ins because he is always a few tenths of a pound off from his proper weight. Ms. Arnold knows that her institution has a low budget and can drug test only one athlete per sport per season. Because another wrestler has already been tested this year, she knows that the rest of the wrestling team will not be tested for drugs until the national competition. Therefore, she recommends a supplement for her athlete to help him lose weight faster. She knows that the U.S. Food and Drug Administration does not regulate these supplements, so there could be a banned substance in them. Regardless, the athlete will not be tested until the national competition, and she will instruct him to stop using the supplement in time to avoid a positive test result. Ultimately, if he does not make his weight now and win, he will never get to nationals (Fig. 25-2).

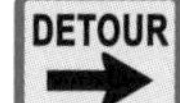

Treatment Detour

The *National Strength and Conditioning Association Professional Standards and Guidelines* is a document with which each CSCS or certified personal trainer must comply in order to safely practice the profession. This document outlines the proper principles to follow and the professional responsibility to report any violations in order to maintain a professional reputation. These documents are available at www.nsca-lift.org.

1. Based on this scenario, what do you know about Ms. Arnold's actions?
   - ______________________________
   - ______________________________
   - ______________________________

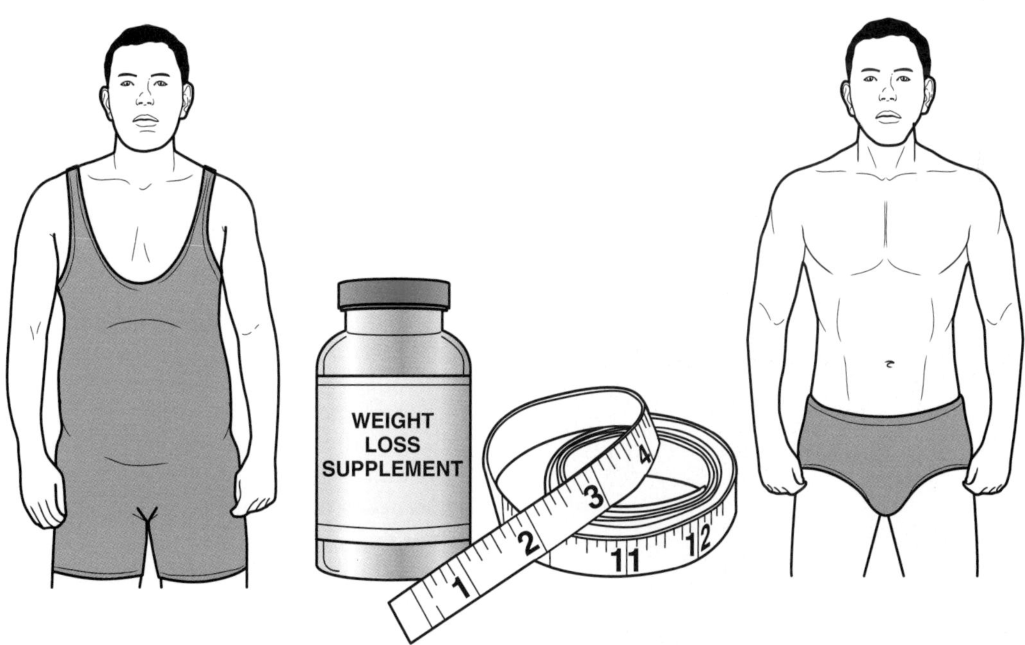

Figure 25-2: Monica Arnold's wrestler weight loss.

- ______________________________

  ____

2. Identify key terms and concepts and then research each to broaden your knowledge of ethical issues.
   - Do you see any violations of the NATA Code of Ethics, BOC Standards of Professional Practice, or the National Strength and Conditioning Association Professional Standards and Guidelines?

   Answer: ______________________________
   - If yes, what are the violations?

   Answer: ______________________________

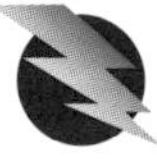

Brain Jolt

Most schools have their own drug-testing policy. Make sure you know your school's policy, but also understand that there can always be additional drug tests if suspicion is warranted.

3. Based on the information that you currently have and what was provided by your instructor, what needs to be done regarding Ms. Arnold's situation?
   - ______________________________

     ____
   - ______________________________

     ____
   - ______________________________

     ____
   - ______________________________

     ____

STUDENT SCENARIO 2: PERCY POWELL

Percy Powell is a new AT in the National Basketball Association. During his first game, the starting center on his team tears the anterior cruciate ligament (ACL) in his left knee after rebounding a shot. Following an immediate evaluation, Mr. Powell is certain that it is a torn ACL because of positive results of a Lachman test and an anterior drawer test for laxity. Mr. Powell sends the athlete for magnetic resonance imaging (MRI) of his knee to verify the initial evaluation. The results of the MRI are not back by the time the game ends. After the game, the media approach Mr. Powell regarding the injured athlete and inquire about his playing status (Fig. 25-3). They are concerned about the star player and ask Mr. Powell about details of the injury and the foreseen outcome. Mr. Powell explains his evaluation and injury assessment, but says that he is waiting for the MRI results. He also states that the athlete will most likely be on the injured list for the rest of the season.

1. Based on this scenario, what do you know about Mr. Powell's actions?
   - ______________________________

     ____

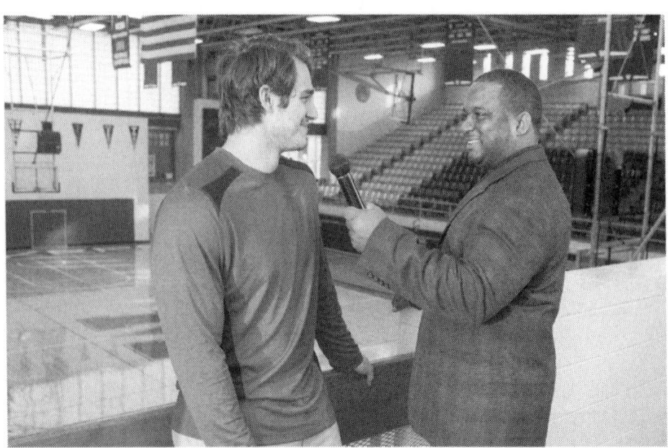

Figure 25-3: Percy Powell talking with the media.

   - ______________________________

     ____
   - ______________________________

     ____
   - ______________________________

     ____

2. Identify key terms and concepts and then research each to broaden your knowledge of ethical issues.
   - Do you see any violations of the NATA Code of Ethics or BOC Standards of Professional Practice?

   Answer: ______________________________
   - If yes, what are the violations?

   Answer: ______________________________

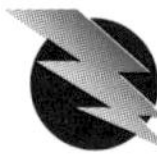

Brain Jolt

Many privacy acts, such as the Health Insurance Portability and Accountability Act of 1996 (HIPAA) and the Family Educational Rights and Privacy Act of 1974 (FERPA), limit communication to certain people. Be sure to understand what privacy policies are enforced at your place of practice.

3. Based on the information that you currently have and what was provided by your instructor, what needs to be done regarding Mr. Powell's situation?
   - ______________________________

     ____

- ____
  ____
- ____
  ____
- ____
  ____

Conversation Buffer
Be sure to emphasize with your coaches and athletes the importance of these privacy acts. With your coaches, if they are privy to medical information, ensure that they are aware of the need to comply with privacy acts. Depending on the setting, coaches might not be allowed to talk to media, professors, or parents. When conversing with athletes, ask them who should know about the injury or condition and be sure to have them sign the proper documentation, if they have not already done so, to allow you to share the information.

STUDENT SCENARIO 3: ALEXIA LEMUIEX

Alexia Lemuiex is an AT in the collegiate setting. Her college is fairly small, and there are only two ATs on campus; the other is male. Recently, Ms. Lemuiex has noticed some inappropriate actions and conversations initiated by her male colleague with some of the female athletes. She has tried to address these actions with him, pointing out that he is not maintaining a professional boundary with the athletes. He assures her that he is just trying to fit in with them and make them feel comfortable, so that they will tell him when they are injured. He has also become friends with them on many social networking sites and is talking about their nights out partying and drinking. Ms. Lemuiex has overheard him telling some athletes where he was hanging out after work and has seen him flirting in the athletic training room during their rehabilitations (Fig. 25-4). Ms. Lemuiex concludes that she has tried to talk to him and cannot do anything else to help the situation.

1. Based on this scenario, what do you know about Ms. Lemuiex's actions?
   - ____
     ____

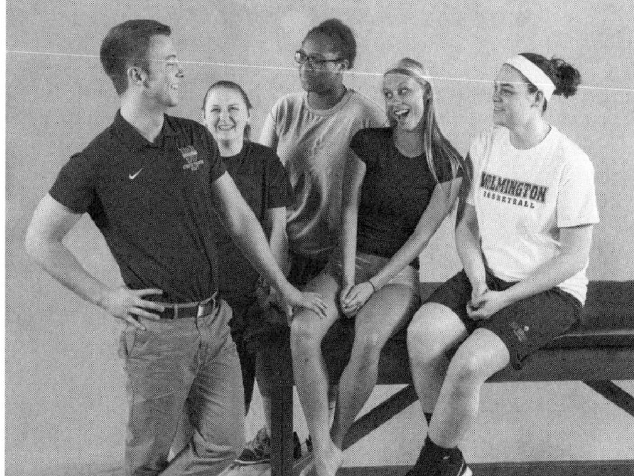

Figure 25-4: Alexia Lemuiex's male colleague with female athletes.

   - ____
     ____
   - ____
     ____
   - ____
     ____

2. Identify key terms and concepts and then research each to broaden your knowledge of sport ethical issues.
   - Do you see any violations of the NATA Code of Ethics or BOC Standards of Professional Practice?

     Answer: ____
   - If yes, what are the violations?

     Answer: ____
3. Based on the information that you currently have and what was provided by your instructor, what needs to be done regarding Ms. Lemuiex's situation?
   - ____
     ____
   - ____
     ____
   - ____
     ____
   - ____
     ____

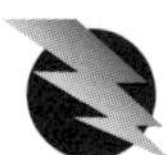

Brain Jolt
Even if you are not the offender breaking the Code of Ethics, you still can have a professional responsibility.

STUDENT SCENARIO 4: BRANDON REIMAN

Brandon Reiman has recently finished graduate school, where he was a graduate assistant in athletic training with a collegiate track team in West Virginia. As graduation approached in May, Mr. Reiman started applying for jobs. He accepted a new job at a small college in Ohio—a position that had to be filled immediately so that he could cover the college's summer camps in June. He began working 2 weeks after moving to Ohio, and as a result of the quick move, he did not apply for an Ohio Athletic Trainer's License. He was unfamiliar with the state regulation because he never had to obtain a license in West Virginia to work as an AT (Fig. 25-5).

1. Based on this scenario, what do you know about Mr. Reiman's actions?

   - ______________________________
   - ______________________________
   - ______________________________
   - ______________________________

Brain Jolt

Each state has its own requirements for practicing as an AT. Be sure to check with your state's regulatory or licensing agency.

2. Identify key terms and concepts and then research each to broaden your knowledge of ethical issues.
   - Do you see any violations of the NATA Code of Ethics or BOC Standards of Professional Practice?

     Answer: ______________________________
   - If yes, what are the violations?

     Answer: ______________________________
3. Based on the information that you currently have and what was provided by your instructor, what needs to be done regarding Mr. Reiman's situation?
   - ______________________________
   - ______________________________
   - ______________________________
   - ______________________________

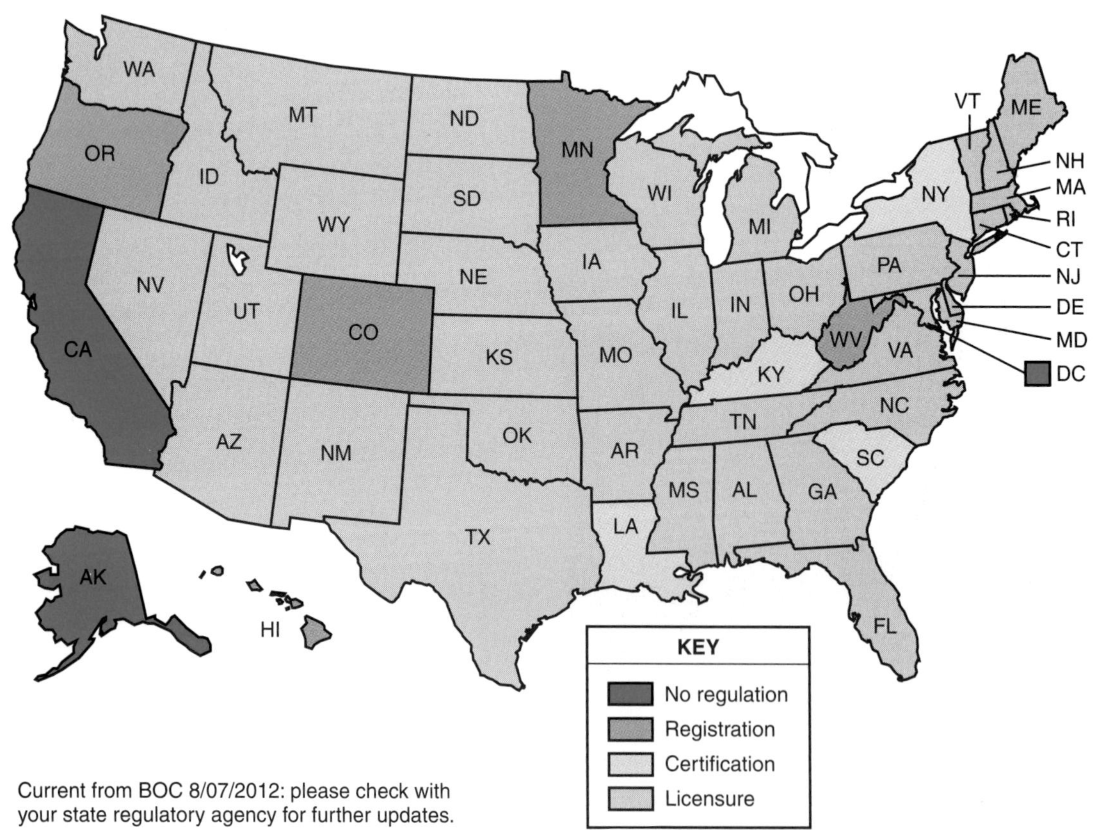

Figure 25-5: Brandon Reiman's map of state regulations.

STUDENT SCENARIO 5: TAY BRAUNSTEIN

Tay Braunstein is an AT at a college that offers health insurance coverage for every student athlete. It covers injuries and illnesses related to athletic performance. A men's basketball player comes to the athletic training room on Sunday morning complaining of pain in his foot. On evaluation, it appears that the athlete may have broken his great toe and first metatarsal. After talking with the athlete, it seems odd to Mr. Braunstein that he did not hear about this injury after the game on Saturday. Finally, after further discussion, the athlete tells Mr. Braunstein that he hurt his foot Saturday night at a party and that he does not have other health insurance. He asks whether they could just pretend that the injury happened during the game so that the school insurance will cover the radiographs and doctor's visit. Mr. Braunstein agrees and sends him for medical treatment (Fig. 25-6).

1. Based on this scenario, what do you know about Mr. Braunstein's actions?

- ____________________
- ____________________
- ____________________
- ____________________

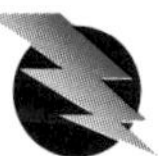

Brain Jolt

It is important to understand your school's insurance coverage and what an athlete's secondary policy covers. This information will help you to find the proper treatment within one of the two insurance plans.

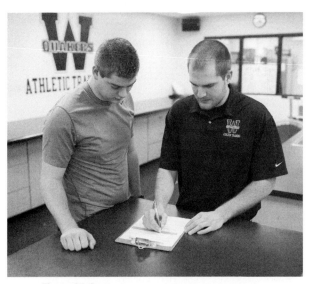

Figure 25-6: Tay Braunstein's health insurance.

Conversation Buffer

It is extremely important to have a good rapport with your athletes so that they will be truthful about their injuries and illnesses. An evaluation can be difficult if the mechanism of injury is wrong. Try to make athletes understand that honesty is the best policy, and you must know what really happened in order to provide the best treatment.

Treatment Detour

Ethics and decision making are sometimes situational. Athletic trainers cannot prepare for every situation. As a result, ATs need to be educated on ethics and ethical decision making in order to make the correct decision when faced with that issue. One qualitative study interviewed ATs with extensive experience working with athletes and confronting the most common ethical issues seen. The top themes identified were interdisciplinary conflicts, including miscommunication about roles, conflicts of interest due to divided loyalties, conflicts in acting in the athlete's best interest, and pressure to return to play from the coach, parent, supervisor, administration, or athlete. Because each situation cannot be rehearsed, it is important to understand the foundation of your profession's code of ethics and basic concepts in applied ethics (Greenfield & West, 2012).

2. Identify key terms and concepts and then research each to broaden your knowledge of ethical issues.

- Do you see any violations of the NATA Code of Ethics or BOC Standards of Professional Practice?

  Answer: ____________________

- If yes, what are the violations?

  Answer: ____________________

3. Based on the information that you currently have and what was provided by your instructor, what needs to be done regarding Mr. Braunstein's situation?

- ____________________
- ____________________
- ____________________
- ____________________

STUDENT SCENARIO 6: DAIVYA KHAN

Daivya Khan is an AT who has been practicing in the profession for more than 20 years. She was successful in her early years of practicing, but recently she has been criticized for her outdated methods. Ms. Khan believes that her methods work fine and does not understand why she should learn new treatment methods and spend money to go to a workshop or conference when she already knows how to evaluate and rehabilitate injuries. In addition, during the past reporting cycle for the BOC, she did not have enough continuing education credits to meet the requirement for her athletic training certification (Table 25-1). As a result, she has received a letter from the BOC regarding her failure to comply with the regulations.

1. Based on this scenario, what do you know about Ms. Khan's actions?
   - ____________________
   - ____________________
   - ____________________

TABLE 25-1 ■ Categories of Continuing Education Opportunities

Category A: Provider programs approved by the Board of Certification
Category B: Professional development
Category C: Post-certification college or university coursework
Category D: Individualized options

- ____________________

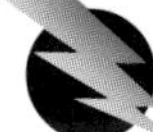

Brain Jolt

Attending large symposiums creates an opportunity to see a wide range of presentations. A continuing education opportunity is what you make of it. If you have years of experience, relate your experiences with questions to the speaker for further discussion, making it more interesting for you and those attending.

2. Identify key terms and concepts and then research each to broaden your knowledge of ethical issues.
   - Do you see any violations of the NATA Code of Ethics or BOC Standards of Professional Practice?

     Answer: ____________________
   - If yes, what are the violations?

     Answer: ____________________
3. Based on the information that you currently have and what was provided by your instructor, what needs to be done regarding Ms. Khan's situation?
   - ____________________
   - ____________________
   - ____________________
   - ____________________

STUDENT SCENARIO 7: ELMO COSTA

Elmo Costa is an AT with a history of alcoholism who has experienced some recent family turmoil. His colleagues suspect that he is having trouble with his alcoholism again after being in control of it for 2 years. Mr. Costa has been coming into work late and showing up at his sport assignment reeking of alcohol. He has been out sick a lot in the last month as well. There have also been reports of Mr. Costa in the local college bar drinking with students and wearing his university athletic training polo shirt from work (Fig. 25-7).

1. Based on this scenario, what do you know about Mr. Costa's situation?
   - ____________________

Fall and Rise from Alcoholism
Sober
Occasional drink
Frequent drinking
Behavior changes
Family/work problems
Obsessive drinking
Rock bottom
Desire for help
Learns alcoholism is an illness
Stops alcohol
Improved behavior
New life
Sober

Figure 25-7: Elmo Costa's alcoholism.

- ______________________________
- ______________________________
- ______________________________

Brain Jolt
Do not ignore a colleague's or peer's atypical behavior because, if not recognized and addressed, it could become hazardous to an athlete's health.

2. Identify key terms and concepts and then research each to broaden your knowledge of ethical issues.
   - Do you see any violations of the NATA Code of Ethics or BOC Standards of Professional Practice?

     Answer: ______________________________

   - If yes, what are the violations?

     Answer: ______________________________

3. Based on the information that you currently have and what was provided by your instructor, what needs to be done regarding Mr. Costa's situation?
   - ______________________________
   - ______________________________
   - ______________________________
   - ______________________________

knowledge checklist

Table 25-2 offers a checklist that can be used by a peer, instructor, or preceptor to evaluate a student's understanding of the profession. Use this checklist as a tool to assess your knowledge of the competencies that apply to this chapter.

TABLE 25-2 ■ Ethics Competency Checklist

	Proficient *Shows understanding of content*	**Proficient With Assistance** *Shows understanding of content with prompting*	**Not Proficient** *Is unclear about content and needs to be reevaluated at another time after further review*
Governing Bodies			
Can locate the NATA Code of Ethics			
Can locate the BOC Standards of Professional Practice			
Administrative Standards			
Demonstrates understanding of the Code of Ethics and the Standards of Professional Practice			
Demonstrates ability to recognize violations			
Demonstrates understanding of the consequences of violations			
Can identify steps that can be taken to avoid violations			

BOC, Board of Certification; NATA, National Athletic Trainers' Association.

REFERENCES

Greenfield, B. H., & West, C. R. (2012). Ethical issues in sports medicine: A review and justification for ethical decision making and reasoning. *Sports Health, 4,* 475–479.

National Athletic Training Association. (2011). *Athletic training education competencies* (5th ed.). Retrieved from http://www.nata.org/sites/default/files/5th-Edition-Competencies-2011-PDF-Version.pdf

Prentice, W. (2010). *Arnheim's principles of athletic training: A competency-based approach* (14th ed.). New York, NY: McGraw-Hill.

Venes, D. (Ed.) (2009). *Taber's cyclopedic medical dictionary* (21st ed.). Philadelphia, PA: F.A. Davis.

chapter 26

Risk Management

chapter outline

athletic trainer's corner

Out there in the real world, one athletic trainer experienced the following:

The word *concussion* has become popular among people of all ages, life events, and levels of sport. I have found that many coaches are being educated more thoroughly on concussions in the courses they must attend as part of their coaching training. Whether at the high school or collegiate level, guidelines have been addressed by the governing sport associations about ways to manage an athlete who sustains a concussion. To ensure consistency within our program, I have recently proposed a concussion policy for the local hospital. This policy is a detailed return-to-play guideline for the area high school athletic trainers. The medical director of the hospital was consulted regarding concussion protocols that were important to implement into this policy. A computer-based program and a list of possible symptoms caused by functional sport-specific drills are just a couple of areas addressed within the policy. Because of the frequent occurrence of concussions, it is important for every organization to have a policy in place to consistently and properly care for athletes who sustain a concussion.

Melissa Noble, AT, ATC
Head AT, Fairlawn High School
Assistant AT, Sidney High School
Wilson Memorial Hospital
Sidney, Ohio

learning outcomes

After working through this chapter, you will be able to:

1. Identify risk-management procedures involved in athletic training.
2. Identify the steps needed to follow through with the risk-management procedures that have been established.
3. Develop emergency action plans (EAPs) and identify changes that need to be made in existing EAPs.
4. Identify the necessary components of preparticipation physicals and describe the importance of these physicals.

MODEL SCENARIO 1: JOHN WRECK

John Wreck is employed by a hospital as an athletic training program coordinator who oversees eight high school athletic trainers (ATs). The hospital administration approaches him about creating a concussion policy in line with current guidelines that the high school ATs will follow when a concussion is suspected or diagnosed. Mr. Wreck wants the policy to be a concussion-management plan directed by the team physician that will outline the roles and responsibilities of the athletic training staff. He also researches the state's high school athletic association rules and guidelines on concussion management. The high schools will now be required to purchase ImPACT (Fig. 26-1), a computerized neurocognitive assessment program. In addition, with the new program, Mr. Wreck wants to be sure that the topic of concussion management is thoroughly addressed with the athletes and their parents before the season begins. An acknowledgment statement must be signed by the coaches, athletes, and parents during the preseason.

1. Based on this scenario, what do you know about Mr. Wreck's situation?
   - *Male, athletic training program coordinator*
   - *Oversees eight high schools*
   - *Implementing a concussion policy*
   - *Researches state athletic association's rules on concussions*
   - *Mandates that high schools purchase ImPACT, a computerized neurocognitive assessment program*
2. Identify key terms and concepts and then research each to broaden your knowledge of risk management in athletic training.
   - Explain the ImPACT program.
     The neurocognitive assessment program is an immediate postconcussion measuring tool for cognitive functions. This program has a baseline test that is done before the start of the sports season and is used later only if an athlete suffers a concussion. The testing information is compared with that individual's preseason and postconcussion results. Athletes take the preseason test every 2 years.
   - Outline what information needs to be included in the concussion policy.
     The signs and symptoms of a concussion, the medical personnel authorized to treat the athlete, the return-to-play guidelines, and baseline testing are important topics to cover in a concussion policy.
   - Should coaches be a part of the concussion-management plan?
     Coaches need to be educated on the concussion-management plan. They need to know their role and responsibilities if one of their athletes suffers a concussion.
   - Why is it important to know the state athletic association's views on concussion management?
     The state athletic association is the governing body for high school athletes.
   - What information pertaining to concussions should be addressed on the acknowledgement statement for athletic participation? Why is it important for athletes to sign this?
     The information on a concussion acknowledgement form should include a list of symptoms that an athlete might experience if he or she suffers a concussion, an outline of the dangers of not reporting these symptoms, and a postconcussion protocol that must be followed. It is important for athletes to sign this form to show that they accept responsibility for reporting the signs and symptoms of a concussion to the AT. This holds athletes accountable for their own safety.
3. Based on the information that you currently have and what was provided by your instructor, what needs to be done regarding Mr. Wreck's situation?
   Mr. Wreck needs to research the appropriate guidelines and governing bodies that would have influence over his high schools' athletes. He just needs to be sure to communicate all information to the necessary parties, have a routine check at the schools on the concussion procedures, and ensure that appropriate paperwork is being filled out. As long as Mr. Wreck has his staff members performing the duties within their scope of practice when handling a concussion, the staff is not at risk of legal issues.

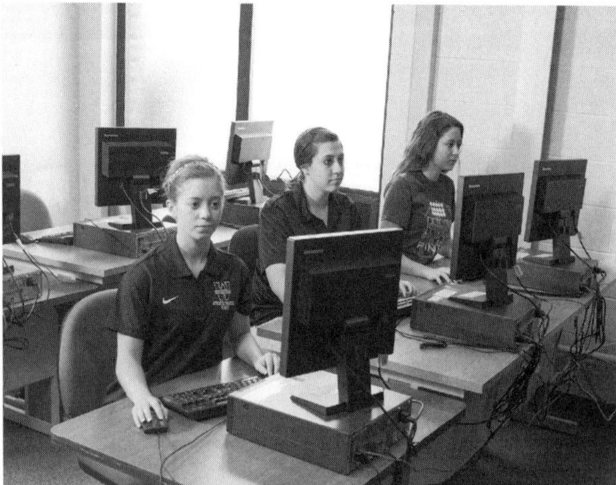

Figure 26-1: John Wreck's ImPACT.

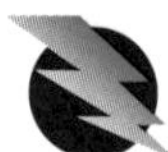

Brain Jolt

When writing a concussion policy, it is recommended that a physician be consulted to ensure the best protocol.

STUDENT SCENARIO 1: TINA AUZENNE

Tina Auzenne is a high school AT employed at a hospital that has recently acquired two new high schools for athletic training services. Neither school had preexisting athletic training coverage for athletic events. Ms. Auzenne is assigned to one of the high schools where she will provide athletic training services. She discusses with the athletic director the different areas of focus that will be needed to make services successful. These necessities include athletic coverage guidelines, budget parameters, and athlete and parent education. Ms. Auzenne's first task before athletic coverage begins is to develop an EAP (Fig. 26-2). She knows that this is extremely important for providing timely, concise medical care and that everyone involved needs to be aware of the contents of the EAP.

1. Based on this scenario, what do you know about Ms. Auzenne's situation?
   - ______________________________________
   - ______________________________________
   - ______________________________________
   - ______________________________________

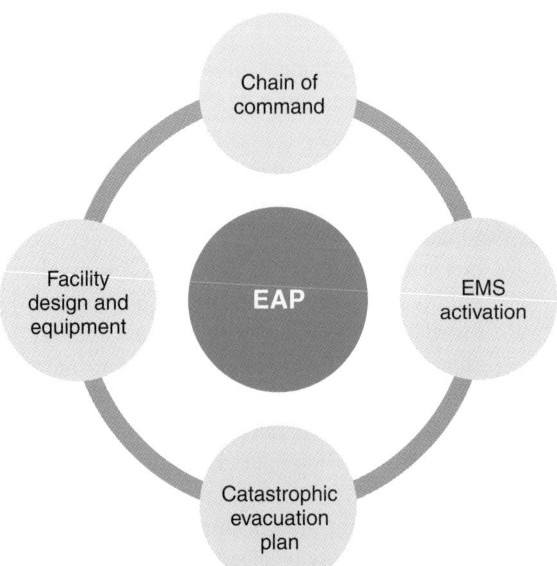

Figure 26-2: Tina Auzenne's components of an emergency action plan.

2. Identify key terms and concepts and then research each to broaden your knowledge of risk management in athletic training.
   - What is an EAP?

     Answer: ______________________________
   - Why is an EAP important to athletic training services?

     Answer: ______________________________
   - What information should be included in an EAP?

     Answer: ______________________________
   - Who should be a part of the EAP?

     Answer: ______________________________
   - Where should the EAP be posted?

     Answer: ______________________________

Brain Jolt

An EAP must be concise and facility specific for the most efficient plan in the event of an emergency.

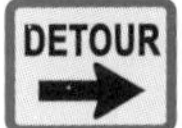

Treatment Detour

Sudden death is a horrible and oftentimes unpredictable catastrophe in sports. There are numerous causes for sudden death in physically active people. Asthma, heat illness, sudden cardiac arrest, cervical spine injuries, and lightning are just a few. However, research shows that certain factors can decrease the risk of catastrophic loss. Although the list is not all-inclusive, understanding the reasons for sudden death can help in preventing the situation when possible. Research shows that an EAP is one way to reduce risk. Every organization that sponsors athletic events should have an EAP, and it should be developed in cooperation with local EMS, school public safety officials, onsite first responders, school medical staff, and school administrators. In addition, evidence shows that the EAP needs to be venue specific and reviewed annually with those involved. Casa et al. (2012) also state that the success rate of an EAP is higher when an AT is present at school athletic contests. Although coaches and administrators are trained in first aid and cardiopulmonary resuscitation, training will not prepare them for all of the causes of sudden death. It is impossible to prevent every sudden death, but the number can be greatly decreased when the best plan is in place and an AT is available to take charge of an emergency medical situation (Casa et al., 2012).

3. Based on the information that you currently have and what was provided by your instructor, what needs to be done regarding Ms. Auzenne's situation?
   - ______________________________
   - ______________________________
   - ______________________________
   - ______________________________

STUDENT SCENARIO 2: DANIEL TAVERNIER

Daniel Tavernier is a collegiate head AT. Ten minutes into football warm-ups, Mr. Tavernier contacts the equipment manager and discusses with him the potential for an accident involving improper field setup. He points out that the goalposts are not ready for the game (Fig. 26-3) and that this is dangerous for the players. The equipment manager explains that he was interrupted from the pregame field setup to help with a helmet fitting in the building. While he was fitting the football helmet, his work-study students arrived to help with the field setup, and he failed to tell them where he stopped when he was interrupted.

1. Based on this scenario, what do you know about Mr. Tavernier's situation?
   - ______________________________
   - ______________________________
   - ______________________________
   - ______________________________

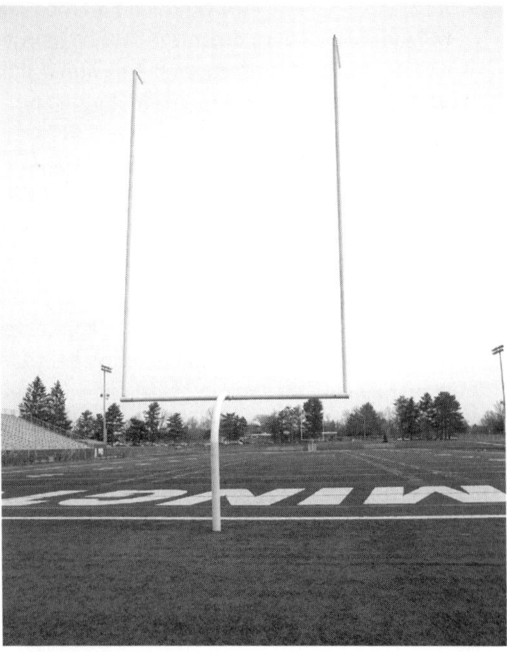

Figure 26-3: Daniel Tavernier's unsafe goal post.

2. Identify key terms and concepts and then research each to broaden your knowledge of risk management in athletic training.
   - Define *accident*.

     Answer: ______________________________
   - Could Mr. Tavernier be found negligent if an accident occurred? If yes, explain.

     Answer: ______________________________
   - Could the equipment manager be found negligent if an accident occurred? If yes, explain.

     Answer: ______________________________
   - What procedures can be put in place to avoid this issue in the future?

     Answer: ______________________________

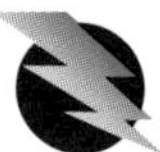

Brain Jolt

Recheck all equipment on and off the field as well as facility conditions before the game to reduce the risk of injury.

Conversation Buffer

Whether you are the equipment manager, the AT, a coach, grounds crew, or an official, we all have a duty to prevent any hazards to an athlete. Everyone has to take part in keeping athletes safe. Athletes who participate in a high-contact sport already have a greater chance of being injured. Athletes do not need the added possibility of being injured because of a broken, unprotected, or uncertified piece of equipment. Be sure that the lines of communication are open between all those involved and that there are checks and balances in place to ensure safety. This could include a pregame meeting with all involved or even checklists separated for each party, all of which are given to one person to ensure that everything has been checked.

3. Based on the information that you currently have and what was provided by your instructor, what needs to be done regarding Mr. Tavernier's situation?
   - ______________________________
   - ______________________________
   - ______________________________
   - ______________________________

STUDENT SCENARIO 3: KIM PUTNAM

Kim Putnam is the AT at a local high school and has been contacted by the school nurse because a wrestler has methicillin-resistant *Staphylococcus aureus* (MRSA) infection. Ms. Putnam was not notified by the athlete because he lacked knowledge of the signs and symptoms of MRSA. He thought his sore was an infected follicle. Upon further discussion with the athlete, the wrestler mentions that the wrestling mats are cleaned every other day to save money on disinfectant, and they had been sharing towels that the coach provides to wipe off excess sweat during practice. The school wants to take the necessary steps to prevent the risk of MRSA spreading to other teammates. Ms. Putnam first wants to perform a skin check on all wrestlers to rule out any other cases. Any open wounds will need to be covered for participation. Ms. Putnam is also recommending that the wrestling team wash their hands frequently and shower immediately after practice (Fig. 26-4).

1. Based on this scenario, what do you know about Ms. Putnam's situation?
   - ______________________________
   - ______________________________
   - ______________________________
   - ______________________________

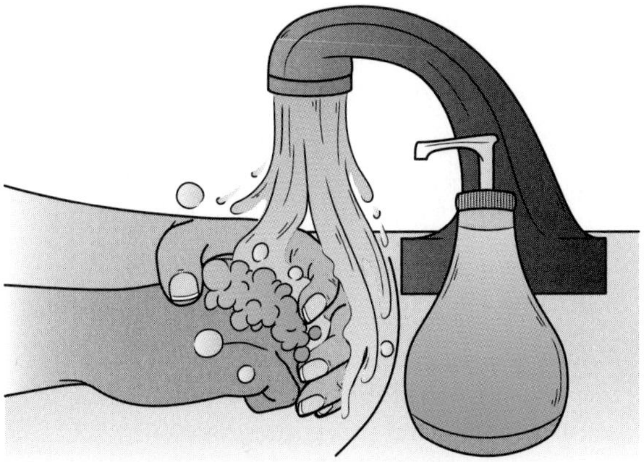

Wash Your Hands and Shower

Figure 26-4: Kim Putnam's proper hygiene.

2. Identify key terms and concepts and then research each to broaden your knowledge of risk management in athletic training.
   - Was the wrestling coach negligent with his care for the wrestling mats?

     Answer: ______________________________
   - Could the wrestling coach be held liable for the spread of MRSA through the wrestling team and potentially the school?

     Answer: ______________________________
   - Will the wrestler with MRSA infection be cleared to return to activity if the wound is covered?

     Answer: ______________________________
   - What type of documentation is required if a wrestler is suspected of a skin disease?

     Answer: ______________________________
   - How does this document lower the risk of spreading an infectious disease?

     Answer: ______________________________
3. Based on the information that you currently have and what was provided by your instructor, what needs to be done regarding Ms. Putnam's situation?
   - ______________________________
   - ______________________________
   - ______________________________
   - ______________________________

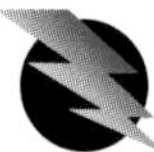

Brain Jolt

Equipment cleanliness is important for reducing the risk of spreading infectious disease. Be sure to use the proper cleaning products to ensure athletes' safety.

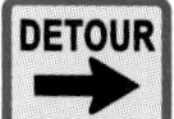

Treatment Detour

One study assessed the knowledge of ATs regarding MRSA and the use of disinfectants used to control infection in athletic training facilities. A survey of 163 ATs employed in the high school and college settings was taken. The survey included questions regarding knowledge of MRSA, knowledge of common disinfectants, reported practices for disinfecting hard surfaces, and personal hygiene habits and individual experiences with MRSA. It was found that 57% of respondents thought that MRSA was a problem in their practice setting, and 92% perceived MRSA to be a national problem. There was discrepancy in respondents' knowledge of disinfectants and the most effective ways to clean surfaces. Many respondents could not correctly identify effective cleaning solutions for MRSA. In addition, it was found that 10% of the respondents did not know that whirlpools can be potential sources of contaminants.

This study also emphasized the importance of AT hygiene. Thirty percent reported that they frequently or sometimes washed their hands before treating an athlete. However, 35% reported that they sometimes, occasionally, or never cleaned their hands between working with different athletes. Athletic trainers are responsible for decreasing the risk of spreading disease; therefore, this information about hygiene practices can help ATs to be more diligent about their actions. By using the recommended disinfectant and proper hygiene guidelines, the risk of contamination can be reduced and contained (Kahanov, Gilmore, Eberman, Roberts, Semerjian, & Baldwin, 2011).

STUDENT SCENARIO 4: SANDRA DUELL

Sandra Duell is the administrative coordinator at a Division II college. It is brought to her attention that for the past month the athletic training staff has been faced with a policy and procedures issue. They have been noticing campus administrators and people in the community requesting athletic training services without a signed physician referral. For information on how to handle this situation, the athletic training staff referred to the policy and procedures manual. However, the existing manual does not have a basic rule on how to handle this liability concern. Ms. Duell consults with the college's lawyer about the school's liability insurance contact. She wants to know to whom it dictates services can be provided. Ms. Duell educates the athletic training staff on the procedure that will now be implemented when providing athletic training services to outside individuals. She will be revising the policy and procedures manual on this particular topic (Fig. 26-5).

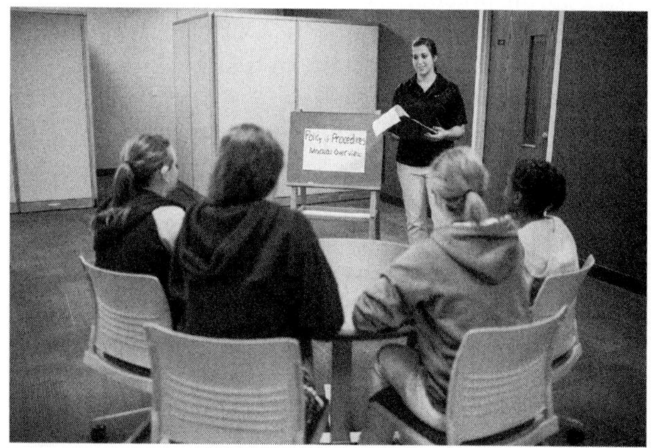

Figure 26-5: Sandra Duell's policy and procedures manual.

1. Based on this scenario, what do you know about Ms. Duell's situation?
   - ____________________
   - ____________________
   - ____________________
   - ____________________

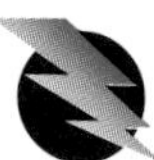

Brain Jolt

The more specific the information in this manual, the more protection the staff will have for making decisions in uncharted territory.

2. Identify key terms and concepts and then research each to broaden your knowledge of risk management in athletic training.
   - Explain a policy and procedures manual. Why is it important?

     Answer: ____________________
   - Who has responsibilities outlined in an athletic training policy and procedures manual?

     Answer: ____________________

- Give a few examples of the areas that can be covered in a policy and procedures manual.

  Answer: ____________________

- How often should a policy and procedures manual be updated?

  Answer: ____________________

3. Based on the information that you currently have and what was provided by your instructor, what needs to be done regarding Ms. Duell's situation?
   - ____________________
   - ____________________
   - ____________________
   - ____________________

STUDENT SCENARIO 5: **PETE WIXSON**

Pete Wixson is a dual-credentialed AT and certified strength and conditioning specialist at a local high school. He has been talking to the high school about the risks involved with its weight room equipment. Many pads on the Nautilus machines are cracked or split, or the padding is missing. A stability bar on the squat rack was severed by rust and welded back together. The seat on the leg extension no longer adjusts at the back, and a person has to use a piece of padding from an old seat to move it forward. In addition, a cable on one of the cable weight machines is frayed (Fig. 26-6). Mr. Wixson is concerned for the safety of anyone who might use these pieces of equipment.

1. Based on this scenario, what do you know about Mr. Wixson's situation?

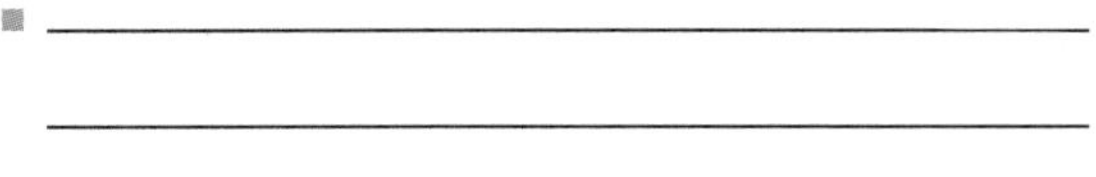

   - ____________________
   - ____________________
   - ____________________

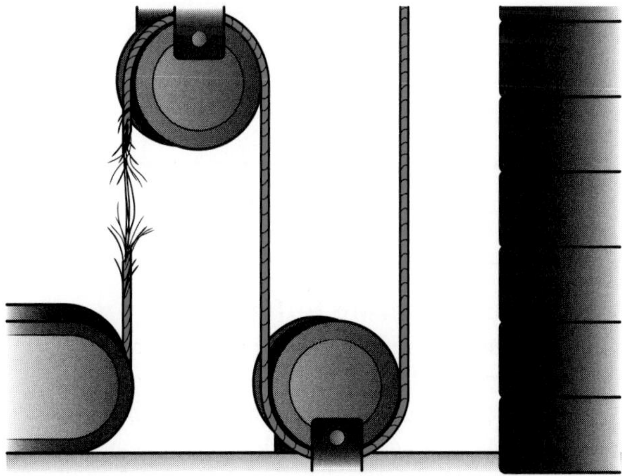

Figure 26-6: Pete Wixson's unsafe cable on a weight machine.

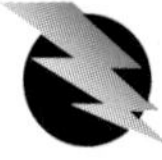

Brain Jolt
The intended functioning of fitness equipment is a direct responsibility of the facility or organization.

2. Identify key terms and concepts and then research each to broaden your knowledge of risk management in athletic training.
   - Is Mr. Wixson or the school liable for any injury that might occur on the damaged equipment? Explain.

     Answer: ____________________

   - Should documentation be posted warning people about the faulty equipment?

     Answer: ____________________

   - What should Mr. Wixson do if a team wants to use the weight room equipment? List some actions that he could consider taking.

     Answer: ____________________

3. Based on the information that you currently have and what was provided by your instructor, what needs to be done regarding Mr. Wixson's situation?
   - ____________________
   - ____________________

- ______________________________

  ____

- ______________________________

  ____

STUDENT SCENARIO 6: TROY SIMROSE

Troy Simrose is an assistant AT at the local college. As a result of inadequate treatment from another AT, the head AT tells Mr. Simrose that he and the team physician would like him to take over an athlete's rehabilitation on the lacrosse team. The lacrosse player injured his left knee 3 weeks ago and is not making significant strides in his rehabilitation program. The AT who covers the lacrosse team misdiagnosed the injury and has not been keeping proper documentation. As a result, improper decisions regarding the athlete's rehabilitation program have been made. Mr. Simrose looks through the lacrosse player's file and notices that the injury report is not complete and daily progress notes (Fig. 26-7) are missing. Mr. Simrose is known for being thorough with his files.

1. Based on this scenario, what do you know about Mr. Simrose's situation?
   - ______________________________

     ____
   - ______________________________

     ____
   - ______________________________

     ____

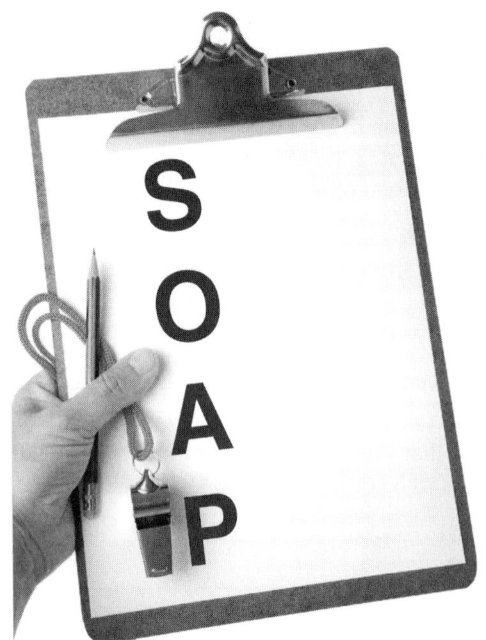

Figure 26-7: Troy Simrose's SOAP notes.

- ______________________________

  ____

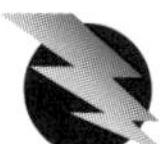

Brain Jolt

Proper documentation can be done in many formats and either on hard copy or electronically. Be sure to be familiar with your employer's protocols.

2. Identify key terms and concepts and then research each to broaden your knowledge of risk management in athletic training.
   - Why is it important to keep accurate documentation of an athletic injury?

     Answer: ______________________________
   - Should Mr. Simrose complete the unfinished injury report?

     Answer: ______________________________
   - Would it be beneficial to go through the entire file on the lacrosse player and make sure that all forms are up-to-date?

     Answer: ______________________________
   - Could the lacrosse AT be found negligent with his/her care from the time of the initial injury?

     Answer: ______________________________
3. Based on the information that you currently have and what was provided by your instructor, what needs to be done regarding Mr. Simrose's situation?
   - ______________________________

     ____
   - ______________________________

     ____
   - ______________________________

     ____
   - ______________________________

     ____

Conversation Buffer

Keeping accurate records can help to avoid any type of liability concern or issue. However, many ATs see injuries on the field, where a computer is not always accessible. Athletic trainers must be organized to complete the necessary information for all injuries, whether they are on or off the field. Injury evaluations, daily treatment logs, and SOAP notes are just a few examples of documents they must complete accurately and in a timely manner and then file in the proper location. To prevent problems, ATs must be sure to discuss these expectations and guidelines with the staff and hold people accountable to keep records consistent.

STUDENT SCENARIO 7: MARCIE GUMP

Marcie Gump is a high school AT. The school's athletic director approaches her about organizing a mass physical examination day. The athletic director would like the preparticipation physical examination day to be open to grades 7 through 12. There are approximately 150 athletes at the school. Ms. Gump decides to use stations (Fig. 26-8) to organize the examinations. She believes that this type of format will be most efficient for the large number of athletes involved. Ms. Gump needs to have a team of 10 to 12 medical examiners to help evaluate the physical, orthopedic, general, and wellness sections. This will allow the athletes to receive a detailed examination in a short amount of time.

1. Based on this scenario, what do you know about Ms. Gump's situation?
   - ______________________________
   - ______________________________
   - ______________________________
   - ______________________________

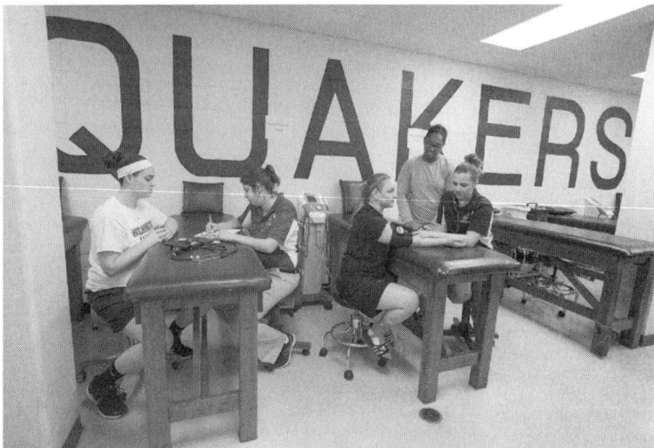

Figure 26-8: Marcie Gump's preparticipation physical examinations.

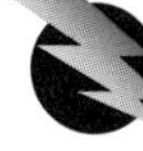

Brain Jolt
An athlete has to be cleared by a physician, via a preparticipation physical, to participate in an athletic event.

2. Identify key terms and concepts and then research each to broaden your knowledge of risk management in athletic training.
   - Explain the importance of a preparticipation physical examination.

     Answer: ______________________________
   - How often should a physical examination be updated?

     Answer: ______________________________
   - Why is a detailed medical history of an athlete important?

     Answer: ______________________________
   - List which type of trained medical personnel could help assist each section.

     Answer: ______________________________
   - What is the importance of each section or station of the examination? What are the key things to be evaluated and why?

     Answer: ______________________________
3. Based on the information that you currently have and what was provided by your instructor, what needs to be done regarding Ms. Gump's situation?
   - ______________________________
   - ______________________________
   - ______________________________
   - ______________________________

knowledge checklist

Table 26-1 offers a checklist that can be used by a peer, instructor, or preceptor to evaluate a student's understanding of risk management in the profession. Use this checklist as a tool to assess your knowledge of the competencies that apply to this chapter.

TABLE 26-1 ■ Risk Management Competency Checklist

	Proficient *Can demonstrate and execute the skill properly*	**Proficient With Assistance** *Can demonstrate and execute the skill with minimal guidance or tips*	**Not Proficient** *Unable to demonstrate and execute the skill properly; need to be reevaluated at another time after further study and practice*
Risk Management			
Identify risk-management procedures			
Identify steps needed to follow through with the risk-management procedures			
Administrative Responsibilities			
Develop EAPs			
Critique and modify existing EAPs			
Identify components needed for preparticipation physical examinations			
Explain and demonstrate preparticipation setup and facilitation			
Identify the importance of preparticipation physicals and what information should be gathered from the examinations			

EAP, emergency action plan.

REFERENCES

Casa, D. J., Guskiewicz, K. M., Anderson, S. A., Courson, R. W., Heck, J. F., Jimenez, C. C., McDermott, B. P., Miller, M. G., Stearns, R. L., Swartz, E. E., & Walsh, K. M. (2012). National athletic trainers' association position statement: Preventing sudden death in sports. *Journal of Athletic Training, 47,* 96–118.

Kahanov, L., Gilmore, E. J., Eberman, L. E., Roberts, J., Semerjian, T., & Baldwin, L. (2011). Certified athletic trainers' knowledge of methicillin-resistant *Staphylococcus aureus* and common disinfectants. *Journal of Athletic Training, 46,* 415–423.

National Athletic Training Association. (2011). *Athletic training education competencies* (5th ed.). Retrieved from http://www.nata.org/sites/default/files/5th-Edition-Competencies-2011-PDF-Version.pdf

Prentice, W. (2010). *Arnheim's principles of athletic training: A competency-based approach* (14th ed.). New York, NY: McGraw-Hill.

Venes, D. (Ed.). (2009). *Taber's cyclopedic medical dictionary* (21st ed.). Philadelphia, PA: F.A. Davis.

chapter 27

Legal Aspects

chapter outline

athletic trainer's corner

Out there in the real world, one athletic trainer experienced the following:

I was introduced to the real potential of legal liability early in my career. At the end of a private high school lacrosse game, a sore loser took his frustrations out on one of my athletes. The opposing athlete flung the ball at our athlete as he was removing his helmet. The ball struck our athlete in the jaw line. Besides a painful jaw, no other signs or symptoms were displayed. Still, the mechanism of injury was a high-velocity object thrown at close range, and I suggested that the athlete be examined. The athlete's parents were not present, but his girlfriend's parents were. They said his father was playing golf, and they were happy to take the athlete to the emergency department and pick up his father on the way. Note that this occurred before everyone had a mobile phone. On Monday morning, I was called into the Dean's office. Present were the Dean, the school's attorney, the father of the athlete, his attorney, and the girlfriend's parents. I was asked to explain my actions and why I had let the girlfriend's parents take his son to the hospital. At the end of the conversation, the athlete's father was extremely upset that his golf game had been interrupted for a minor injury because his son's jaw was not fractured. He demanded compensation for his round of golf. All parties agreed to this settlement, and I was taught the valuable lesson of always having professional liability insurance in the event that legal proceedings should arise.

A. S. Woody Goffinett, MBA, ATC, AT, EMT-T, FF
Dayton Sports Medicine Institute
Dayton, Ohio

learning outcomes

After working through this chapter, you will be able to:

1. Identify the laws that govern athletic training.
2. Identify the consequences of violating the laws of athletic training.
3. Describe the basic terminology and legal aspects of athletic training and practicing as an athletic trainer (AT).
4. Identify and describe precautions that can be taken to avoid legal issues when practicing as an AT.

MODEL SCENARIO 1: TIM GILLFOIL, JR.

Tim Gillfoil, Jr., is a 17-year-old junior football player. Three weeks into the football season, his father dies. His father was his biggest supporter so, when returning to football 2 weeks later, it is a big adjustment for him. At that week's Friday night home game, Mr. Gillfoil suffers a concussion. He has minor symptoms but is unable to return to the game. The following Monday, the AT gives Mr. Gillfoil an ImPACT test to assess his condition. These results will be compared with baseline scores obtained before the beginning of football season. Two weeks after the concussion, Mr. Gillfoil is scoring normal on the ImPACT test, but he continues to have a mild headache. It has been noted that he is now exhibiting mild symptoms of depression. The death of his father and now the lingering symptoms of the concussion are leaving him feeling defeated. That Friday morning, Mrs. Gillfoil, his mother, brings in a written consent to the AT assuming all liability for Mr. Gillfoil and the risk that he takes returning to activity immediately (Fig. 27-1a). The AT tells Mrs. Gillfoil that he recommends holding Mr. Gillfoil from any activity until he is free of symptoms. However, because Mrs. Gillfoil provided written consent and signed a release of liability and assumption of risk form (Fig. 27-1b), the AT allowed Mr. Gillfoil to participate in that evening's game. That evening, he receives another blow to the head and has to be transported to the hospital after sustaining another concussion.

1. Based on this scenario, what do you know about Mr. Gillfoil's situation?
   - *17-year-old football player*
   - *Father died recently*
   - *Sustains a concussion*
   - *Symptoms not subsiding*
   - *Having depression symptoms*
   - *Against medical recommendation, guardian provides a written letter of assumption of risk to return him to play immediately*
2. Identify key terms and concepts and then research each to broaden your knowledge of the legal aspects of athletic training.
   - Do you see any legal violations?
     Yes.
   - If yes, what are the violations?
     The AT should not return the athlete to play unless the athlete is asymptomatic. By returning the athlete to play too soon, the AT runs the risk of further injury and possible legal action by the athlete. However, with the parent taking and signing for full liability, this takes the responsibility off the AT.
   - Define *assumption of risk*.
     A doctrine of law whereby the plaintiff assumes the risk of medical treatment or procedures and cannot recover damages for injuries sustained as a result of the known and described dangers and risks.
   - Why is Mrs. Gillfoil, his mother, able to accept that responsibility?
     Ms. Gillfoil is able to assume the risk for Mr. Gillfoil because he is a minor and she is his legal guardian.
   - Because the ImPACT testing no longer showed cognitive postconcussion symptoms, should the AT have accepted the risk and returned Mr. Gillfoil back to activity?
     The AT should not assume the risk of returning Mr. Gillfoil back to activity. The ImPACT test should be viewed as another part of a concussion return-to-play scenario. All physical and cognitive symptoms need to be considered. An athlete has to be asymptomatic before returning to activity.
3. Based on the information that you currently have and what was provided by your instructor, what needs to be done regarding Mr. Gillfoil's situation?
   The conversation with Mrs. Gillfoil needs to be documented. The AT needs to note that he voiced his concerns for Mr. Gillfoil returning to activity while he still exhibited physical signs of a concussion. The written assumption of risk and the ImPACT test results should be included in Mr. Gillfoil's file. In addition, the AT needs to contact the team physician responsible for the care of that athlete, to inform him of the assumption of risk that Mrs. Gillfoil has accepted through written documentation.

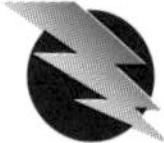

Brain Jolt
Legal decisions for a minor fall in the hands of the parent or guardian.

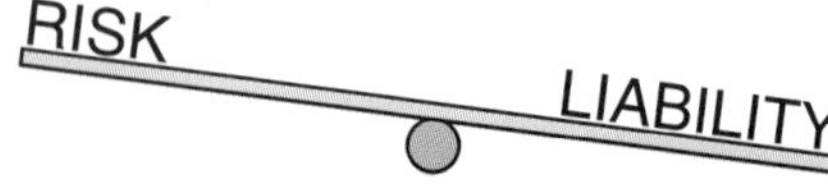

Figure 27-1a: Tim Gillfoil, Jr.'s risk.

RELEASE OF LIABILITY AND ASSUMPTION OF RISK

In consideration of being allowed to participate in any way in the above listed activity, I, the undersigned, acknowledge, appreciate, and agree that:

1. The risk of injury from the activities involved in these sport events is significant, including the potential for major injuries such as injuries to the eyes, loss of sight, joint injuries, back injuries, heart attacks, concussions, paralysis, and even death, and while particular rules, equipment, and personal discipline may reduce this risk, the risk of serious injury does exist; and

2. I assume all of the risks that may or can arise out of participating in the activities, both known and unknown, including but not limited to the athletic activity itself, use of the equipment, field, or facilities, the acts of others, or the unavailability of emergency care, and assume full responsibility for my participation; and

3. I willingly agree to comply with the stated instructions and policies and customary terms and conditions for participation. If, however, I observe any unusual significant hazard during my presence or participation, I will remove myself from participation and bring such to the attention of the nearest official immediately; and

4. I, for myself and on behalf of my heirs, assigns, personal representatives, and next of kin, hereby release, indemnify, and hold *enter institution*, and their officers, officials, agents, and/or employees, other sort participants, sponsoring agencies, sponsors, advertisers, and, if applicable, owners and lessors of premises used to conduct the event or activity ("Releases") harmless with respect to any and all injury, disability, death, or loss or damage to person or property, to the fullest extent permitted by law; and

5. I understand and acknowledge that I am surrendering valuable legal rights in this agreement; and

6. I understand and expressly agree that this agreement is intended to be as broad and inclusive as permitted by the law of the State for which it is used and that if any portion of this agreement is held invalid, it is agreed that the balance of the agreement shall continue in full force and effect and that whatever portion is held invalid shall be interpreted and construed to afford as much protection to *enter institution* as permitted by the applicable law.

I HAVE READ THIS RELEASE OF LIABILITY AND ASSUMPTION OF RISK AGREEMENT, FULLY UNDERSTAND ITS TERMS, UNDERSTAND THAT I HAVE GIVEN UP SUBSTANTIAL RIGHTS BY SIGNING IT, AND SIGN IT FREELY AND VOLUNTARILY WITHOUT ANY INDUCEMENT.

Signature ______________________________________ Date ____________________
(Parent/Guardian if under 18 years old)
Printed Name ___________________________________

Figure 27-1b: Tim Gillfoil, Jr.'s release of liability and assumption of risk form.

STUDENT SCENARIO 1: TANIA STOLLE

Tania Stolle is a high school AT. She is in the athletic training room when a female basketball player is brought in to see her. Ms. Stolle is familiar with this particular player because of attention-seeking behaviors she exhibits regularly. The athlete explains the mechanism of injury to Ms. Stolle, revealing that she inverted her right ankle and has point tenderness over the lateral malleolus. Ms. Stolle notices mild edema on the lateral aspect of the ankle, but the athlete has a history of right ankle sprains. Ms. Stolle believes that this is an attempt to get attention; therefore, she does not continue her evaluation and decides to tape the right ankle (Fig. 27-2) and return the athlete to activity. She receives a telephone call later that evening from her athletic director. He informs Ms. Stolle that the athlete's parents took her for an examination of her ankle because of pain, and the radiographs revealed a right lateral malleolus fracture. The neglected care is in question, and the athletic director would like to meet with Ms. Stolle tomorrow.

1. Based on this scenario, what do you know about Ms. Stolle's situation?
   - ______________________________
   - ______________________________
   - ______________________________
   - ______________________________

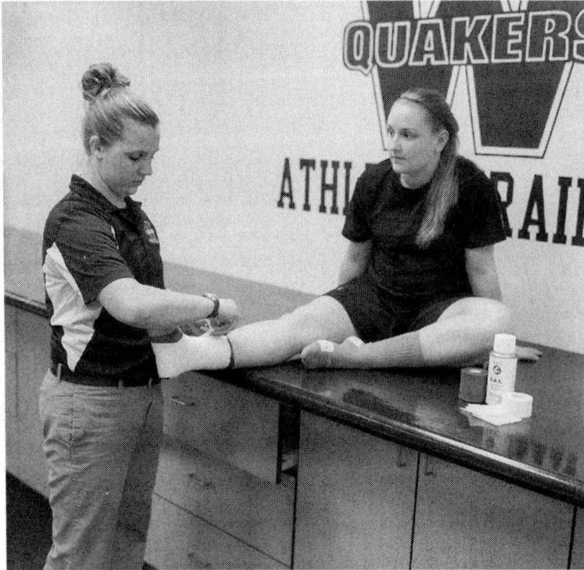

Figure 27-2: Tania Stolle taping athlete's ankle.

2. Identify key terms and concepts and then research each to broaden your knowledge of the legal aspects of athletic training.
   - Do you see any legal violations?

     Answer: ______________________________
   - If yes, what are the violations?

     Answer: ______________________________
   - Define *negligence*. Does this apply to this situation?

     Answer: ______________________________
   - Was Ms. Stolle wrong in viewing the injured athlete as a malingerer?

     Answer: ______________________________
   - What was Ms. Stolle's first mistake?

     Answer: ______________________________

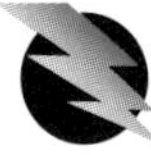

Brain Jolt

To provide the best medical care, always treat every injury and athlete as though it is his or her first time in the athletic training room.

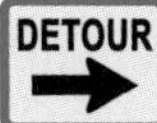

Treatment Detour

Mr. Ramsey is a former football player from Auburn University, and he is suing Mr. Gamber for negligence regarding a back injury. Mr. Ramsey's complaint is that, when he had a back injury, he was further injured by Mr. Gamber's lack of supervision with his rehabilitation and, as a result, lost his chances of furthering his football career. Mr. Ramsey claims that he was injured while lifting weights as part of his rehabilitation program. He also claims that he was doing exercises that were not part of the plan set by his doctor. Mr. Ramsey claims in his testimony that the weight room assistant had him do weighted box squats that were not allowed by his doctor. When the assistant was questioned, this claim was denied, and he testified that Mr. Ramsey did leg curls and arm curls on an incline bench. The outcome of this case was that there was not enough evidence to prove negligence against Mr. Gamber. It is important to keep good documentation of doctors' notes and communication with any professional involved in a case. All medical treatment should be supervised and documented per a doctor's recommendation.

Austin Chaz Ramsey, Plaintiff, *v* Arnold Gamber, Defendant
Civil Action No: 3:09cv919-MHT (WO)
U.S. District Court for the Middle District of Alabama, Eastern Division
2011 U.S District Lexis 90133
August 12, 2011

Conversation Buffer

Many ATs would agree that there are always one or two athletes who frequently malinger. Frequently, these athletes' injuries are treated negligently. Every athlete and every injury needs to be treated with fresh eyes. The injuries that you overlook will be the ones that could cost you your licensure. Be sure to talk with each athlete about every injury, inquiring about every aspect of your typical evaluation, and do not dismiss anything before you have all the information.

3. Based on the information that you currently have and what was provided by your instructor, what should have been done regarding Ms. Stolle's situation?

- ______________________________
- ______________________________
- ______________________________
- ______________________________

STUDENT SCENARIO 2: HELEN VESCIO

Helen Vescio is the head AT at a college and is currently covering soccer during the fall season. At practice today, a midfielder takes a direct hit to his left side. Mrs. Vescio has to assist the player off the field. Upon initial evaluation, the player is having difficulty breathing and has point tenderness over ribs 5 to 7. The soccer player also has rebound tenderness and palpable crepitus near ribs 5 to 7 (Fig. 27-3). Because the player does not want to risk losing his starting position, he asks Mrs. Vescio not to refer him on for further evaluation until tomorrow. Against Mrs. Vescio's better judgment, she decides to wait until tomorrow. She will reevaluate him at that point and decide whether radiographs are needed. Mrs. Vescio is told later that evening by the head soccer coach that the athlete had to be taken to the hospital after practice because he had labored breathing. The head soccer coach discusses his concern with Mrs. Vescio regarding her lack of judgment and how she failed by not referring her athlete for further evaluation.

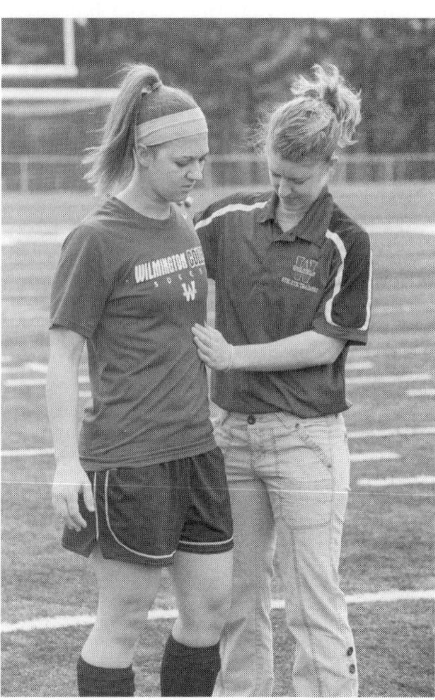

Figure 27-3: Helen Vescio's evaluation of injury.

1. Based on this scenario, what do you know about Mrs. Vescio's situation?

- ______________________________
- ______________________________
- ______________________________
- ______________________________

2. Identify key terms and concepts and then research each to broaden your knowledge of the legal aspects of athletic training.
   - Do you see any legal violations?

     Answer: ______________________________
   - If yes, what are the violations?

     Answer: ______________________________
   - Define *nonfeasance*. Does this apply to this situation?

     Answer: ______________________________

- What legal action could be taken?

Answer: ______________________________

Brain Jolt
You have an unbiased legal duty to act consistently for every athlete regardless of the athlete's request or his or her role on the team.

3. Based on the information that you currently have and what was provided by your instructor, what should have been done regarding Mrs. Vescio's situation?
   - ______________________________
   - ______________________________
   - ______________________________
   - ______________________________

STUDENT SCENARIO 3: THOMAS BALTES

Thomas Baltes is a high school AT in Ohio. The state of Ohio OTPTAT Board (Occupational Therapy/Physical Therapy/Athletic Training; Fig. 27-4) has provisions in place for a team traveling without a team physician or AT and the athletic training services that can be provided to them. A hosting AT can provide only first aid or emergency care and routine care to a visiting team. Mr. Baltes is providing home athletic coverage for today's soccer game. An opposing player goes down, and Mr. Baltes has to assist the player off the field. He decides to do an evaluation of the player at the request of the opposing team's coach. The opposing team's head coach is Mr. Baltes' wife. Mr. Baltes believes that the soccer player has a mild medial collateral ligament sprain. If taped, the player could return to activity. The opposing coach trusts Mr. Baltes' evaluation and returns the player to the game.

1. Based on this scenario, what do you know about Mr. Baltes' situation?
   - ______________________________
   - ______________________________
   - ______________________________
   - ______________________________

Figure 27-4: Thomas Baltes' malfeasance. (© Thinkstock)

2. Identify key terms and concepts and then research each to broaden your knowledge of the legal aspects of athletic training.
   - Do you see any legal violations?

     Answer: ______________________________
   - If yes, what are the violations?

     Answer: ______________________________
   - Define *malfeasance*. Does this apply to this situation?

     Answer: ______________________________
   - Can Mr. Baltes evaluate the athlete?

     Answer: ______________________________
   - Was Mr. Baltes' decision to evaluate and treat the opposing player influenced by his relationship with the opposing team's head coach?

     Answer: ______________________________
   - What are your state licensure laws for providing care to visiting teams?

     Answer: ______________________________
3. Based on the information that you currently have and what was provided by your instructor, what should have been done regarding Mr. Baltes' situation?
   - ______________________________
   - ______________________________

- ______________________________
- ______________________________

Brain Jolt
An AT is to perform only those duties allowed by his or her state's governing board.

STUDENT SCENARIO 4: EUGENE YANKEL

Eugene Yankel is a 35-year-old man. He has completed his daily workout routine and proceeds into the locker room to shower. When entering the locker room, Mr. Yankel comes upon a male who is supine on the floor. Mr. Yankel immediately surveys the scene. He approaches the supine male and begins his assessment. Mr. Yankel calls 9-1-1.The supine male is unresponsive and has no pulse. Mr. Yankel begins cardiopulmonary resuscitation (CPR; Fig. 27-5). Upon the arrival of emergency medical services (EMS), the man has a pulse and is breathing. Mr. Yankel is certified in CPR by the American Red Cross as a lay person. He gets his certification card out just in case the EMS technicians would like to see it, which is when he notices that his certification expired 1 month ago. He is concerned that he might be liable because his CPR certification is not current, but then he remembers the Good Samaritan Law.

1. Based on this scenario, what do you know about Mr. Yankel?
   - ______________________________
   - ______________________________
   - ______________________________
   - ______________________________

Figure 27-5: Eugene Yankel beginning cardiopulmonary resuscitation.

Brain Jolt
Good Samaritans are protected as long as they are giving reasonable care or assistance.

2. Identify key terms and concepts and then research each to broaden your knowledge of the legal aspects of athletic training.
   - Do you see any legal violations?

     Answer: ______________________________
   - If yes, what are the violations?

     Answer: ______________________________
   - Define *Good Samaritan Laws.* Do these apply to this situation?

     Answer: ______________________________
   - Have there ever been any lawsuits against a Good Samaritan for performing an emergency duty?

     Answer: ______________________________
   - Does Mr. Yankel need to consult a lawyer because he performed an act for which he was not certified?

     Answer: ______________________________
3. Based on the information that you currently have and what was provided by your instructor, what needs to be done regarding Mr. Yankel's situation?
   - ______________________________
   - ______________________________
   - ______________________________
   - ______________________________

STUDENT SCENARIO 5: MARY SHERIDAN

Mary Sheridan is a collegiate softball player. Each preseason, Ms. Sheridan gives the softball AT an EpiPen device (Fig. 27-6) prescribed by the team physician to keep in the medical kit. During a game, Ms. Sheridan is in center field, when she signals to the head coach that she needs assistance. The head coach and the AT approach Ms. Sheridan and notice immediately that she is short of breath. She states that she has been stung by a bee in her right arm and needs her EpiPen. The AT runs to get the EpiPen from the medical kit. Ms. Sheridan is supine on the ground when the AT returns. The AT injects the device into Ms. Sheridan's right bicep, just below the bee sting. The AT holds the device for 30 sec at the right bicep and then removes it. 9-1-1 has to be called because Ms. Sheridan's breathing has become more labored and she is now unconscious.

1. Based on this scenario, what do you know about Ms. Sheridan's situation?
   - ______________________________
   - ______________________________
   - ______________________________
   - ______________________________

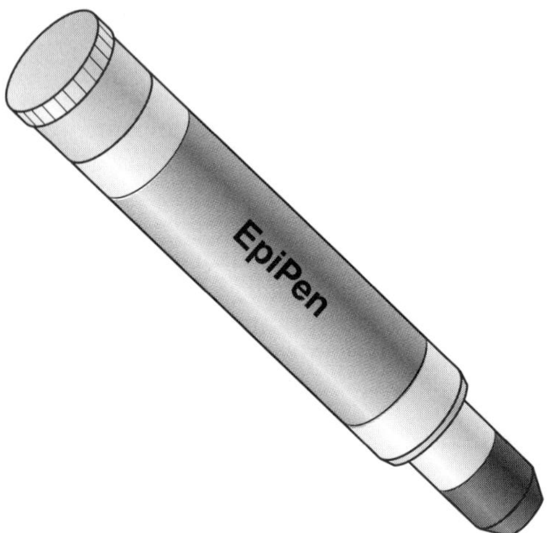

Figure 27-6: Mary Sheridan's EpiPen.

Brain Jolt

Improper care can cause a medical situation to turn into a life-threatening emergency.

2. Identify key terms and concepts and then research each to broaden your knowledge of the legal aspects of athletic training.
   - Do you see any legal violations?

     Answer: ______________________________
   - If yes, what are the violations?

     Answer: ______________________________
   - Define *misfeasance*. Does this apply to this situation?

     Answer: ______________________________
   - What can be viewed as the AT's first oversight to provide immediate care?

     Answer: ______________________________
   - Does an AT have to be certified in administering an EpiPen?

     Answer: ______________________________
   - Explain the proper procedure for administering an EpiPen.

     Answer: ______________________________
3. Based on the information that you currently have and what was provided by your instructor, what needs to be done regarding Ms. Sheridan's situation?
   - ______________________________
   - ______________________________
   - ______________________________
   - ______________________________

STUDENT SCENARIO 6: LYNN IVORY

Lynn Ivory is a high school AT who is employed by the area local hospital and is being sued by a family from an opposing school. Ms. Ivory was the hosting AT for a basketball tournament at her high school. She was sitting with a parent and discussing an ankle injury because her team had finished playing. Two local teams were playing when a basketball player slid into the bleachers headfirst. Ms. Ivory noticed the incident but did not get up to check on the player because it was not someone from her team. The opposing team's coach had to assist the player off the court. Ms. Ivory did not think much of the incident until 1 month later when she was contacted by her employer. The player who Ms. Ivory neglected to assist suffered a concussion and a vertebral fracture at C5. The player was not cleared to return to basketball for the rest of the season. The hospital director told Ms. Ivory that, because of her negligence, the parents of the opposing player were seeking legal representation. The hospital director discussed the amount of liability coverage that they would provide, but also wanted to know whether Ms. Ivory carried her own professional liability insurance (Fig. 27-7).

1. Based on this scenario, what do you know about Ms. Ivory's situation?

- ______________________________
- ______________________________
- ______________________________
- ______________________________

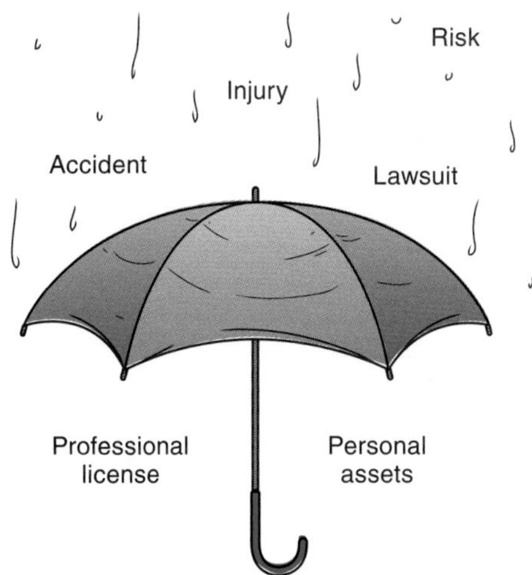

Figure 27-7: Lynn Ivory's professional liability insurance.

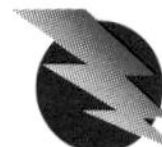

Brain Jolt

Know the limits and the financial coverage of your employer's liability insurance and your own professional liability insurance.

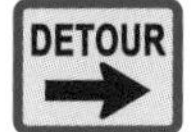

Treatment Detour

In one court case, Mr. Howard sued Mr. Templin, an AT employed at the Missouri Bone and Joint Center, for causing injury to his back in a workout. Mr. Howard went to the center for treatment after an ankle injury to improve his football skills. During the workout, Mr. Howard felt intense pain in his back. Mr. Templin simply said "no pain, no gain" and suggested that he "push through it." After pushing through the pain, Mr. Howard's pain immediately went from a 6 to a 10 on the pain scale. It was later determined that he had herniated a disk. Mr. Templin was accused of doing an incomplete evaluation and not heeding Mr. Howard's complaints of pain. The jury found Mr. Templin negligent on all accounts and awarded Mr. Howard $175,000. The Missouri Bone and Joint Center appealed this case but the appeal request was denied. This case shows that ATs need to listen to their athletes and, although they should encourage their athletes to work hard, they cannot push them too hard because doing so might increase the risk of injury or intensify a current injury.

Alvin Howard, Appellee, v Missouri Bone and Joint Center, Inc., Appellant; No. 09-2914; U.S. Court of Appeals for the Eighth Circuit; 615 F.3d 991; 2010 U.S. App. Lexis 16699; April 12, 2010.

Conversation Buffer

Documentation is the key to protecting yourself legally. If legal action is ever brought against you, you must have written documentation of the injury evaluation, treatment, and pertinent conversations regarding the incident that you have with the athlete, parents, coaches, administrators, and others. This documentation and your professional liability insurance are the best ways to protect yourself from liability.

2. Identify key terms and concepts and then research each to broaden your knowledge of the legal aspects of athletic training.

- Do you see any legal violations?

Answer: ______________________

- If yes, what are the violations?

Answer: ______________________

- Define *professional liability insurance.*

  Answer: ____________________
- Should Ms. Ivory carry professional liability insurance in addition to her employer's liability insurance coverage?

  Answer: ____________________
- Do you see any violation of the National Athletic Trainers' Association or Board of Certification standards of professional practices?

  Answer: ____________________
- What care could Ms. Ivory have provided to the injured opposing player?

  Answer: ____________________

3. Based on the information that you currently have and what was provided by your instructor, what needs to be done regarding Ms. Ivory's situation?

- ____________________
- ____________________
- ____________________
- ____________________

STUDENT SCENARIO 7: CARL MAGEE

Carl Magee is a clinical AT with a company that does not employ any other clinical ATs. Mr. Magee is excited to show the physical therapy staff the value that an AT can bring to patients and benefits through reimbursements. He asks the director of the physical therapy department whether all the reimbursement forms pertaining to third-party payers have been submitted (Fig. 27-8). Mr. Magee is reassured that this has been done. Two months into his employment, Mr. Magee is contacted by the billing department. They ask him to complete the necessary forms for insurance companies to get approval for athletic training services or care. Mr. Magee consults the director, who states that he did not realize that an AT had specific billing codes. He thought that, because Mr. Magee was paired with a physical therapist, he could use the physical therapy billing codes.

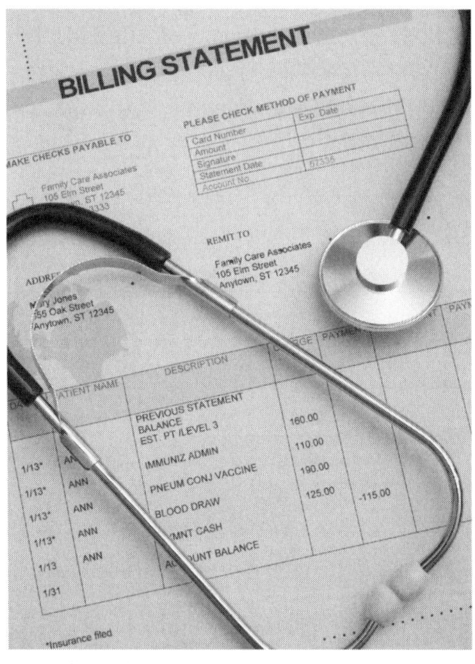

Figure 27-8: Carl Magee's third-party reimbursement. (© Thinkstock)

1. Based on this scenario, what do you know about Mr. Magee's situation?

- ____________________
- ____________________
- ____________________
- ____________________

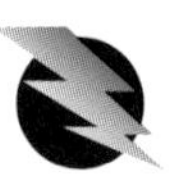

Brain Jolt

Using the proper codes, ATs can be reimbursed for their services from certain insurance companies.

2. Identify key terms and concepts and then research each to broaden your knowledge of the legal aspects of athletic training.

- Do you see any legal violations?

  Answer: ____________________
- If yes, what are the violations?

  Answer: ____________________
- Explain third-party reimbursement.

  Answer: ____________________

- Does third-party reimbursement apply to a clinical AT or only to physical therapists and physical therapy assistance?

  Answer: ____________________

- What forms need to be completed for third-party reimbursement for athletic training?

  Answer: ____________________

3. Based on the information that you currently have and what was provided by your instructor, what needs to be done regarding Mr. Magee's situation?

- ____________________
- ____________________
- ____________________
- ____________________

knowledge checklist

Table 27-1 offers a checklist that can be used by a peer, instructor, or preceptor to evaluate a student's understanding of the legal aspects of the profession. Use this checklist as a tool to assess your knowledge of the competencies that apply to this chapter.

TABLE 27-1 ■ Legal Aspects Competency Checklist

	Proficient *Shows understanding of content*	**Proficient With Assistance** *Shows understanding of content with prompting*	**Not Proficient** *Is unclear about content and needs to be reevaluated at another time after further review*
Professional Governance			
Identify the laws that govern athletic training			
Identify the consequences of violating the laws of athletic training			
Legal Aspects of Profession			
Describe the basic terminology and legal aspects of athletic training and practicing as an athletic trainer			
Identify and describe the precautions that can be taken to avoid issues when practicing as an athletic trainer			

REFERENCES

National Athletic Training Association. (2011). *Athletic training education competencies* (5th ed.). Retrieved from http://www.nata.org/sites/default/files/5th-Edition-Competencies-2011-PDF-Version.pdf

Prentice, W. (2010). *Arnheim's principles of athletic training: A competency-based approach* (14th ed.). New York, NY: McGraw-Hill.

Starkey, C., Brown, S. D., & Ryan, J. (2010). *Examination of orthopedic and athletic injuries* (3rd ed.). Philadelphia, PA: F.A. Davis.

Venes, D. (Ed.). (2009). *Taber's cyclopedic medical dictionary* (21st ed.). Philadelphia, PA: F.A. Davis.

chapter 28

Professional Development

chapter outline

athletic trainer's corner

Out there in the real world, one athletic trainer experienced the following:

I have often discussed developmental options with prospective athletic trainers (ATs) and typically give one major piece of advice: diversify your knowledge. I have often witnessed recently graduated and certified ATs contemplate their next step in professional development. There are many choices for those looking to expand their knowledge. They can choose to expand their knowledge in athletic training specifically or choose various other educational avenues. This choice depends on their personal career goals.

Here is my story. I graduated with my undergraduate degree in kinesiology (exercise science), but had finished all the core curriculum requirements for physical therapy and athletic training. I knew from the beginning that I wanted to work within an athletic population. During my last year, I had the opportunity to become a certified massage therapist (CMT) over a 6-month training program. When I graduated from my undergraduate program, I was already a CMT with my bachelor's degree. Interestingly, I was drawn to law enforcement and stood at the crossroads of the academy or physical therapy assistant (PTA) school. I was accepted into a physical therapy assistant program and completed my associate's degree in 7 months in an aggressive program within a nationally ranked physical therapy program. I learned from the beginning that getting employed as a PTA with a bachelor's degree and CMT certification set me apart from other candidates and opened opportunities that otherwise would have been unattainable. I worked as a teaching assistant (TA) and CMT for approximately 3 years.

While working at a small outpatient physical therapy company, I was offered an opportunity to complete my athletic training degree, complete my certified strength and conditioning specialist endeavor, and start a new sports medicine division. The sports medicine division allowed me the opportunity to establish an athletic training program for a large high school and a professional baseball organization. I was rewarded with the title of Director of Sports Medicine, and my administrative responsibilities expanded.

During the time that I was Director of Sports Medicine, the United States Olympic Committee (USOC) Sports Medicine Team had a program to bring in professionals to assist the full-time staff members. I was originally brought in as a massage therapist and evolved into a dual-role professional: AT and CMT for the USOC. Through this organization, I have experienced and seen some wonderful international sporting events. Although being an AT and CMT was fulfilling, I continued to have an interest in law enforcement. I had often contemplated how I could merge my passion for this profession and my skills as a health-care provider. Fortunately for me, my new employer had the same thing in mind. I became a certified tactical medic through an intensified training program to gain the knowledge and skills of tactical combat casualty care. My team was no longer the typical sporting team; instead, it was a civilian combat team (e.g., special weapons and tactics [SWAT], special response team [SRT]). Because of my experience in sports medicine and as a CSCS, this job led to my eventually becoming a police academy instructor and primary fitness, health, and wellness consultant and instructor for the State Attorney General's Office and its law enforcement regulatory agency.

Through all my different paths, I am fortunate to have accepted a management position with a new hospital and helped to implement an entirely new sports medicine division for the hospital and the entire community. I continue to work as a tactical medic, consult for the State Attorney General's Office law enforcement agency, teach at the police academy, service a local high school full time, travel for the USOC Olympic Athletes, and perform my hospital administration duties.

The moral of the story is to continue to work hard and know what you want to accomplish with your career. Professional development requires effort, desire, and the willingness to never stop learning.

Travis Snyder, AT, ATC, PTA, CMT, CSCS, NREMT-B, EMT-T
Manager, Sports Medicine Services
Fort Hamilton Hospital

learning outcomes

After working through this chapter, you will be able to:

1. Describe the importance and role of the National Athletic Trainers' Association (NATA), the Board of Certification (BOC), and the Commission on Accreditation of Athletic Training Education (CAATE).
2. Explain the process of obtaining and maintaining the required state and national credentials for practicing as an AT.
3. Describe the roles of other health-care professionals, their scope of practice, and how they differ from the practice of athletic training.
4. Identify ways to promote the profession of athletic training and ways to encourage lifelong learning among those in the profession.

MODEL SCENARIO 1: DAKOTA TURNER

Dakota Turner is a collegiate AT, and he is trying to determine what he needs to do to complete the necessary number of continuing education units (CEUs) for the BOC. He has 70 CEUs and needs to find a symposium to attend that will complete the remaining CEUs for his reporting period ending in 2013. He also checks his state licensure CEU reporting sheet to determine whether he has the correct number for his state licensure. Mr. Turner practices athletic training in the state of Ohio, and he keeps a reporting sheet for the BOC and the state because the yearly reporting periods and the CEU amounts required are different for the state of Ohio and for the BOC. Therefore, he must check both reporting requirements to stay in compliance for each entity. This will be the last time Mr. Turner needs to follow these BOC requirements because, starting in January 2014, a new guideline will go into effect (Fig. 28-1).

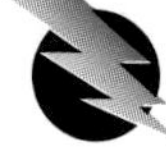

Brain Jolt

There are different categories in which CEUs can be obtained, and sometimes limits are set for certain categories.

1. Based on this scenario, what do you know about Mr. Turner's situation?
   - *Male, certified collegiate AT in state of Ohio*
   - *Trying to determine what he needs to do to complete CEUs for BOC reporting period*

Looking Ahead to 2014

The following chart provides the CE requirements as of 2014, which marks the beginning of two-year reporting periods:

CURRENT		
CE Accumulation Period	**Expiration Date**	**CEUs Due**
1/1/2013 – 12/31/2015 or 1/1/2014 – 12/31/2016 or 1/1/2015 – 12/31/2017	12/31/2015 or 12/31/2016 or 12/31/2017	75

➧

AS OF 2014		
CE Accumulation Period	**Expiration Date**	**CEUs Due**
1/1/2014 – 12/31/2015	12/31/2015	50

Figure 28-1: Dakota Turner's continuing education requirement change. (With permission from BOC. http://www.bocatc.org/-bocatc/images/stories/boc_newsletter/cu_winter11.pdf. Accessed January 28, 2013.)

- *Has completed 70 CEUs for 2013 period*
- *Keeping a CEU reporting sheet for both NATA and state because of different reporting time frames*
- *Requirements for BOC changing in 2014*

2. Identify key terms and concepts and then research each to broaden your knowledge of professional development in athletic training.

- What is the BOC CEU reporting term? How many CEUs are required each term?

  As long as the AT is not a recent graduate, the BOC reporting period for CEUs ending in 2013 is 3 years. The BOC requires 75 CEUs and proof of a current certification in CPR or first aid.

- Give examples of the categories in which CEUs can be obtained.

  There are four main categories: Category A is approved provider programs, Category B is professional development and holds a CEU maximum, Category C is postcertification college or university coursework, and Category D is individualized options and holds a CEU maximum. Some of the options include symposiums, seminars, workshops, presenting at a conference, authoring a research article, and postgraduate coursework.

- If you attend a symposium that is not certified by NATA or BOC, can you still report those? Explain.

  Any CEUs that are reported to the NATA or BOC have to be from an approved provider. If you attend an athletic training event that is not approved by the NATA or BOC, those CEUs cannot be included on the reporting sheet.

- If your state requires licensure, how many CEUs do you need to complete in a reporting term? What is the state licensure's CEU reporting term?

  Mr. Turner practices in the state of Ohio, which does require a license to practice as an AT. The reporting period for the state of Ohio is 25 CEUs every 2 years.

3. Based on the information that you currently have and what was provided by your instructor, what needs to be done in Mr. Turner's situation?

Mr. Turner can check the BOC-approved provider list at http://www.bocatc.org to see which providers in his area are approved. The NATA, regional, and state organizations will also have a list of future conferences and symposiums that he can attend. Mr. Turner can then contact the provider of the event and obtain any necessary information, such as how many CEUs are approved for that symposium, who the presenters are, and what topics will be addressed at the event.

STUDENT SCENARIO 1: LANCE HUELSCAMP

Lance Huelscamp is a graduating athletic training student and has just taken the BOC examination. While he is waiting for his results and looking for a job, pending his certification, Mr. Huelscamp has decided to return to his previous summer employment at an automotive factory where he works on the assembly line (Fig. 28-2). As part of a new initiative at his employer, he is attending a required wellness program. Mr. Huelscamp is surprised that the wellness instructor is an AT. This type of employment is not a traditional setting for an AT but is becoming more popular. Mr. Huelscamp remembers a coworker getting hurt while on the job, and he did not realize that his care was provided by a certified AT.

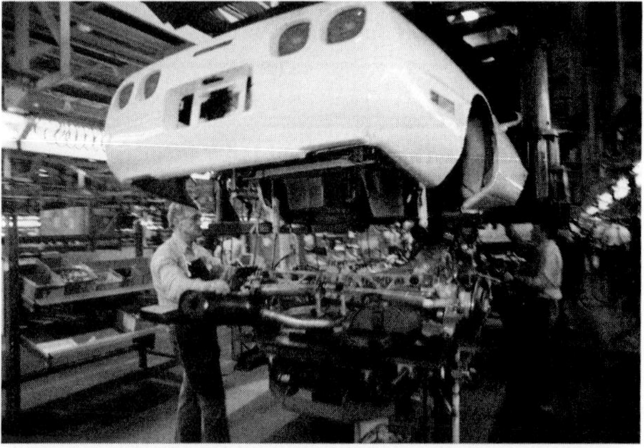

Figure 28-2: Lance Huelscamp's automotive assembly line. (© Thinkstock)

1. Based on this scenario, what do you know about Mr. Huelscamp's situation?

- ______________________________
  ____
- ______________________________
  ____
- ______________________________
  ____
- ______________________________
  ____

2. Identify key terms and concepts and then research each to broaden your knowledge of professional development in athletic training.

- Give examples of other nontraditional athletic training settings.

  Answer: ______________________________

- Which traditional athletic training setting primarily employs most ATs? Why?

  Answer: ______________________________

- Could Mr. Huelscamp work for the automotive factory as an AT while waiting for his examination results? Explain.

  Answer: ______________________________
- Explain the job description for an industrial AT.

  Answer: ______________________________
- In the nontraditional industrial setting, would the rules governing an AT be different from those of a traditional athletic training setting?

  Answer: ______________________________

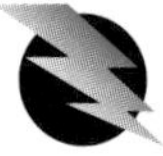

Brain Jolt

Broad knowledge of a workplace's equipment and function is necessary for an industrial AT.

Treatment Detour

Within the profession of athletic training, there are the traditional settings such as the clinic, high school, or college. However, the industrial setting is beginning to emerge as a favorable option for graduates. A qualitative study was done surveying seven ATs who are employed in only the industrial-occupational setting and graduated from a CAATE-accredited athletic training education program (ATEP) between May 2007 and May 2009. The goal of this study was to determine whether there is successful preparation in education programs for the industrial-occupational setting. This is critical information for ATEPs, continuing education, and postgraduate work. The author found that most of the entry-level ATs believed that they were well-prepared for this setting, with the only identified weakness being in the knowledge of ergonomics. Overall, job satisfaction was high regarding fewer and better hours, higher salaries, and the satisfaction of helping people. This is important to learn. Hopefully in the future, more emphasis can be placed on learning proper ergonomics because this is a growing opportunity for ATs (Schilling, 2011).

3. Based on the information that you currently have and what was provided by your instructor, what can be done about being an AT in Mr. Huelscamp's employment setting?

- ______________________________
- ______________________________
- ______________________________
- ______________________________

STUDENT SCENARIO 2: ABIGAIL DUCKRO

Abigail Duckro is a recent athletic training graduate. She has passed her BOC and licensure examinations and has accepted an athletic training job with a high school. Her employer is actually a local hospital that has a contract with a high school for athletic training services. She is new to the state, and her employer wants her to take an active role in the NATA (Fig. 28-3) and the state athletic training organization. This will allow Ms. Duckro the opportunity to stay current with ongoing changes in the athletic training profession and allow her to become familiar with state laws. Belonging to the state athletic training organization is another way for Ms. Duckro to broaden her athletic training knowledge and career network. She has also expressed an interest to her new employer regarding obtaining other memberships or certifications in fitness organizations that would benefit both her and her employer.

1. Based on this scenario, what do you know about Ms. Duckro's situation?

- ______________________________

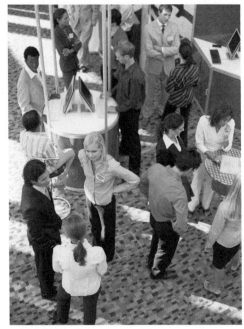

Figure 28-3: Abigail Duckro's membership. © George Doyle (© Thinkstock)

- ____
____
- ____
____
- ____
____

Brain Jolt
The ACSM and NSCA are popular fitness organizations for ATs.

2. Identify key terms and concepts and then research each to broaden your knowledge of professional development in athletic training.
   - What does ACSM stand for? Explain what the organization does.

   Answer: ____
   - What does NSCA stand for? Explain what the organization does.

   Answer: ____
   - Which state and local professional organizations are available to you for membership?

   Answer: ____
   - As a member of the NATA, are you automatically enrolled in the NATA district organizations? In which district is your state? Name the other states that are in that district.

   Answer: ____
   - Is the NATA membership the same as the BOC membership? Explain.

   Answer: ____
3. Based on the information that you currently have and what was provided by your instructor, what memberships can Ms. Duckro obtain with her interest in fitness?
   - ____
   ____
   - ____
   ____
   - ____
   ____
   - ____
   ____

STUDENT SCENARIO 3: MIRANDA SWANK

Miranda Swank is a clinical and secondary certified AT. She is required to split her 40-hour workweek between the two athletic training settings (Fig. 28-4a and 28-4b). Ms. Swank has an injured athlete coming to the clinic for rehabilitation. He has 1 week left before a recheck visit with the physician. In the clinical setting, Ms. Swank reports to a physical therapist. Any changes or new rehabilitation exercises for the athlete must be implemented by the physical therapist. The physician's initial prescription was for physical therapy services. Upon the athlete's recent visit to his physician, he is now cleared for functional sport activities and has been discharged from physical therapy. As a result, the athlete can begin sport-specific exercises with Ms. Swank at the high school. She is now able to treat the athlete because the physician specified athletic training services on the prescription. Therefore, Ms. Swank is able to evaluate, increase or decrease weight for exercises, and change various exercises to help return the athlete to play.

1. Based on this scenario, what do you know about Ms. Swank's situation?
   - ____
   ____
   - ____
   ____

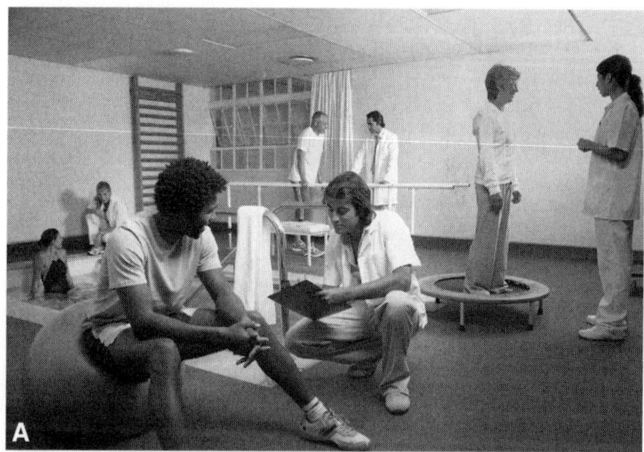

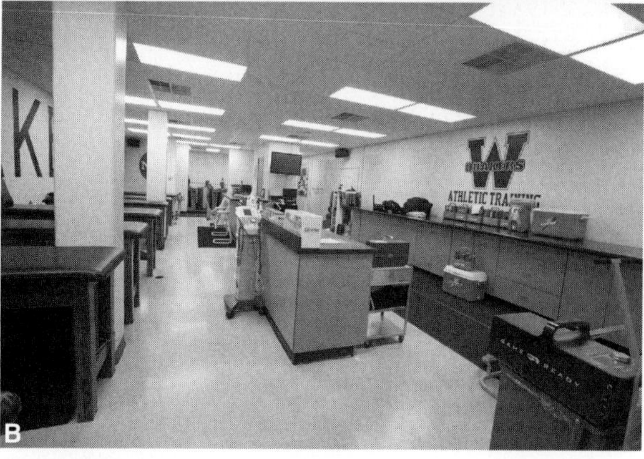

Figure 28-4: Miranda Swank's physical therapy clinic versus athletic training room. (© Thinkstock)

- ____

____

- ____

____

Brain Jolt
The role of the AT in each employment setting is dictated by governing laws.

2. Identify key terms and concepts and then research each to broaden your knowledge of professional development in athletic training.
- What are the laws for athletic training services in a clinical setting versus a secondary setting such as a high school?

Answer: ___________________________________
- Why does Ms. Swank have to report to a physical therapist in her employment setting?

Answer: ___________________________________
- Why does a physician have to specify the type of services and who can treat that individual? Does billing for services provided to the athlete affect this decision?

Answer: ___________________________________
- Because the athlete is one of Ms. Swank's students, why is she not permitted to provide more treatment for him in the physical therapy clinic? Why, on the other hand, is Ms. Swank able to supervise the athlete's rehabilitation program at the high school?

Answer: ___________________________________

3. Based on the information that you currently have and what was provided by your instructor, what differences are there in Ms. Swank's employment settings?
- ____

____

- ____

____

- ____

____

- ____

____

STUDENT SCENARIO 4: MASON LIEMPNER

Mason Liempner is a 45-year-old AT who received his athletic training degree in 1987. The athletic training program from which he graduated was an internship program, under the supervision of the Committee on Allied Health Education and Accreditation. Mr. Liempner now works as a high school AT. His employer has mandated that all ATs attend a workshop to become a preceptor for the ATEP. The local university, as part of its CAATE (Fig. 28-5) reaccreditation self-study, is implementing an off-campus rotation for the athletic training students. Mr. Liempner reviews the accredited curriculum and notices that the rotations and academic requirements are very different from when he was in college.

1. Based on this scenario, what do you know about Mr. Liempner's situation?
- ____

____

- ____

____

- ____

____

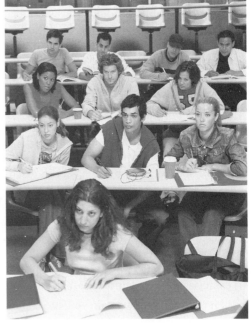

Figure 28-5: Mason Liempner's reaccreditation. (© Thinkstock)

- ______________________________
____

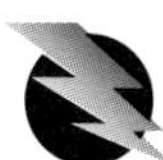

Brain Jolt
Professional (i.e., entry-level) ATEPs must be accredited by CAATE.

2. Identify key terms and concepts and then research each to broaden your knowledge of professional development in athletic training.
   - Explain CAATE and its role in athletic training.

   Answer: ______________________________
   - Explain the history of the athletic training profession.

   Answer: ______________________________
   - As a preceptor for the program, Mr. Liempner would have certain responsibilities to the students. Explain.

   Answer: ______________________________
   - Describe the evolution of athletic training with accreditation.

   Answer: ______________________________
   - Explain the history and difference between an internship athletic training program and an accredited program. Are there currently two routes of education?

   Answer: ______________________________
   - How often does a CAATE athletic training program perform a self-study? Explain.

   Answer: ______________________________
3. Based on the information that you currently have and what was provided by your instructor, what does Mr. Liempner need to know about ATEPs?
   - ______________________________
   ____
   - ______________________________
   ____
   - ______________________________
   ____
   - ______________________________
   ____

STUDENT SCENARIO 5: ANTHONY WOOTEN

Anthony Wooten is a high school AT and has been with his current employer for 15 years. The athletic training coordinator at his employer oversees 10 high school ATs and is planning to resign. Mr. Wooten would like to be considered for the position; however, it requires a master's degree. Mr. Wooten has worked in both the clinical and high school settings, and he also holds a certified strength and conditioning specialist (CSCS) credential. The highest education Mr. Wooten has is a bachelor's degree, but he hopes that his years of experience will outweigh his lack of graduate education. Mr. Wooten has considered getting his master's degree, but he always thought that he did not have time for this commitment. He was unsure whether he could devote the necessary time to do the research that a master's degree requires. Mr. Wooten is disappointed to see that his advancement within his athletic training program is not possible without a graduate education; therefore, he is looking into programs to complete his master's degree to advance his career (Fig. 28-6).

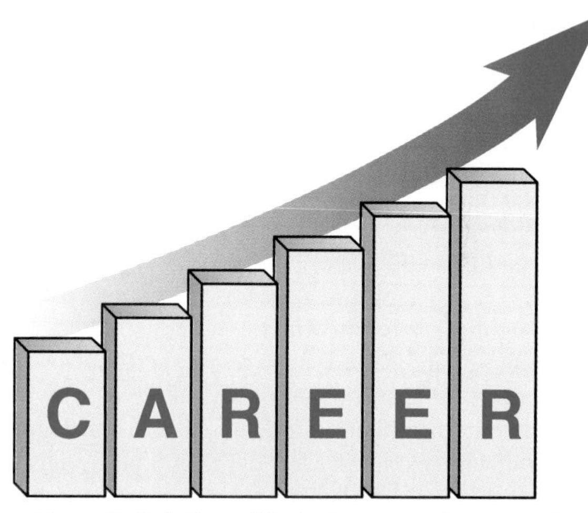

Figure 28-6: Anthony Wooten's career advancement.

1. Based on this scenario, what do you know about Mr. Wooten's situation?
   - ______________________________
   ____
   - ______________________________
   ____
   - ______________________________
   ____
   - ______________________________
   ____

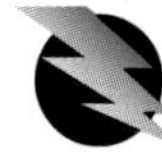

Brain Jolt
Graduate level work is a requirement for many career settings within the profession.

Conversation Buffer

It is important to link your career desires with your education. Think about the setting in which you wish to work and be aware of the education requirements. In addition, talk with your advisors and mentors about the direction of graduate work. This can help you broaden your résumé and can lead to employment in the setting of your choice. It is also a good idea to try to find an internship within this setting to ensure that it aligns with your career goals before investing your time in that direction of study.

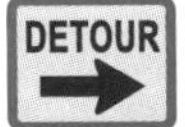

Treatment Detour

A qualitative study was undertaken to identify the reasons why graduating undergraduate students chose a postprofessional program in athletic training (PPAT) accredited by NATA. The study included 19 first-year PPAT students representing 13 of the 16 accredited PPAT programs. It was found that students chose to get an advanced degree in athletic training based on their long-term career goals. In addition, they chose a program that would help them gain more experience while still having support. They looked for an academic program that will advance their knowledge base, offer assistantships with financial support, and provide mentorship that will help them secure a career (Mazerolle & Dodge, 2012).

2. Identify key terms and concepts and then research each to broaden your knowledge of professional development in athletic training.
- Should Mr. Wooten be considered for the athletic training coordinator position without meeting all the necessary requirements?

  Answer: ____________________
- Why is graduate education important for an AT?

  Answer: ____________________
- In which areas of concentration could Mr. Wooten have focused his master's degree to benefit his career?

  Answer: ____________________
- Explain evidence-based learning. How is it incorporated into the athletic training profession?

  Answer: ____________________

3. Based on the information that you currently have and what was provided by your instructor, what can be done in Mr. Wooten's situation?
- ____________________
- ____________________
- ____________________
- ____________________

STUDENT SCENARIO 6: COREY HIGHLEY

Corey Highley is a recent athletic training graduate. He has completed and passed the necessary certification examinations, but is still unsure about the type of work environment in which he prefers to use his degree. Mr. Highley has explored a few of the options under the sports medicine umbrella. He has considered the high school setting, one of the most common settings in athletic training, but is unsure that the evening hours would work in the future with a family. A physician extender has also been an area of interest for Mr. Highley. He has spoken with the team physician with whom he worked as an athletic training student, but he is concerned about working with the older population. Mr. Highley has recently completed his CSCS certification and is thinking that he could use his ATC and CSCS credentials at a sports performance enhancement facility (Fig. 28-7). The diversity of athletic training employment has left Mr. Highley with a difficult decision.

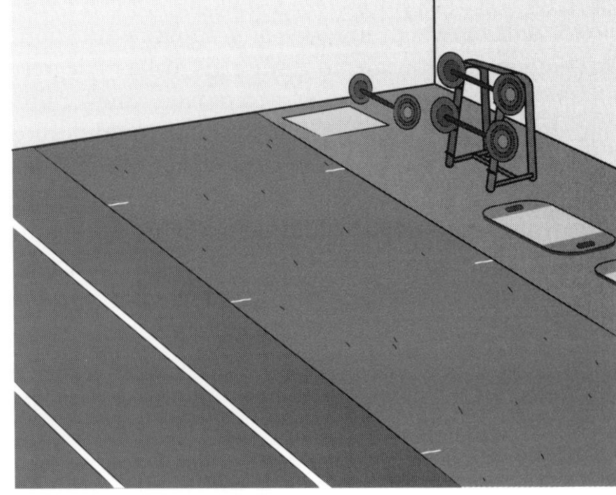

Figure 28-7: Corey Highley's sports performance enhancement facility.

1. Based on this scenario, what do you know about Mr. Highley's situation?
   - ______________________________________
   - ______________________________________
   - ______________________________________
   - ______________________________________

Brain Jolt

Athletic training has evolved into a profession with many employment options and numerous avenues to your career goals.

Conversation Buffer

Entering the workforce can be an intimidating experience for newly certified ATs. To help ease that intimidation, be sure to expose athletic training students to many different work environments in which an AT can be employed. Nontraditional settings can be just as rewarding to an AT as traditional settings. Athletic training students should step out of their comfort zones and explore all the possibilities that the field has to offer.

2. Identify key terms and concepts and then research each to broaden your knowledge of professional development in athletic training.
   - Explain the duties of a high school AT.

     Answer: ______________________________________
   - Explain the duties of an AT as a physician extender.

     Answer: ______________________________________
   - How would a certified AT be beneficial in a sports performance enhancement facility?

     Answer: ______________________________________
   - Give examples of other athletic training employment opportunities.

     Answer: ______________________________________
3. Based on the information that you currently have and what was provided by your instructor, what are the options for Mr. Highley's situation?
   - ______________________________________
   - ______________________________________
   - ______________________________________
   - ______________________________________

STUDENT SCENARIO 7: CLARE BORSCHT

Clare Borscht is a clinical education coordinator for an athletic training program at a Division III college. She would eventually like to move up within the program to become the athletic training program director; therefore, she wants to pursue a doctoral degree. Ms. Borscht recognizes that athletic training is moving toward an evidence-based practice model (Fig. 27-8) and wants to enhance her knowledge in this area. If she focused her doctorate on an area pertaining to this approach, it would enhance her résumé and make her more suited for a program director position, because this is a part of the accreditation standards. However, Ms. Borscht is unsure how to pursue this goal and which area of study and research would be best.

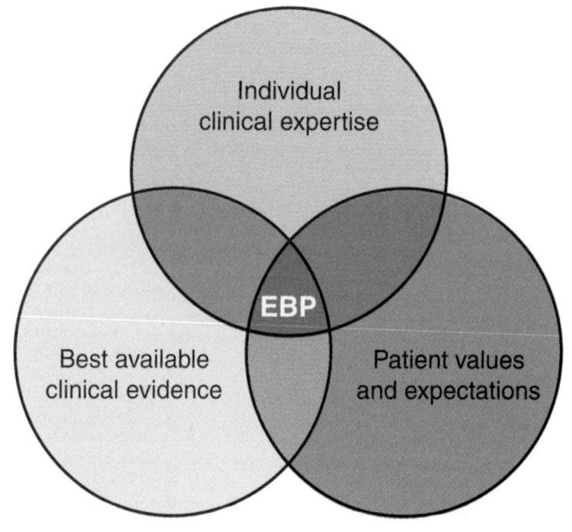

Figure 28-8: Clare Borscht's evidence-based practice.

1. Based on this scenario, what do you know about Ms. Borscht's situation?
   - ______________________________________

- ______________________________
  ____
- ______________________________
  ____
- ______________________________
  ____

Brain Jolt
As allied health professionals, ATs need to pursue evidence-based research to help the profession grow.

2. Identify key terms and concepts and then research each to broaden your knowledge of professional development in athletic training.
   - Explain how acquiring a doctorate would enhance Ms. Borscht's résumé.

     Answer: ______________________________
   - What types of doctoral programs exist, and what are the time commitments for these programs?

     Answer: ______________________________
   - Can any AT, regardless of employment setting, pursue research?

     Answer: ______________________________
   - What are the benefits of research?

     Answer: ______________________________
3. Based on the information that you currently have and what was provided by your instructor, what are the reasons for pursuing a doctorate in Ms. Borscht's situation?
   - ______________________________
     ____
   - ______________________________
     ____
   - ______________________________
     ____
   - ______________________________
     ____

knowledge checklist

Table 28-1 offers a checklist that can be used by a peer, instructor, or preceptor to evaluate a student's understanding of the profession. Use this checklist as a tool to assess your knowledge of the competencies that apply to this chapter.

TABLE 28-1 ■ Professional Development Competency Checklist

	Proficient *Shows understanding of content*	**Proficient With Assistance** *Shows understanding of content with prompting*	**Not Proficient** *Is unclear about content and needs to be reevaluated at another time after further review*
Professional Governance			
Identify laws that govern athletic training			
Describe the importance and role of the NATA, the BOC, and the CAATE			
Career Advancement			
Explain the process of obtaining and maintaining the required state and national credentials for practicing as an athletic trainer			
Identify and describe the roles of other health-care professionals, their scope of practice, and the differences between the scopes of athletic training			
Identify ways to promote the profession of athletic training and to encourage lifelong learning among those in the profession			

BOC, Board of Certification; CAATE, Commission on Accreditation of Athletic Training Education; NATA, National Athletic Trainers' Association.

REFERENCES

Mazerolle, S. M., & Dodge, T. M. (2012). National Athletic Trainers' Association-accredited postprofessional athletic training education: Attractors and career intentions. *Journal of Athletic Training, 47*, 467–476.

National Athletic Training Association. (2011). *Athletic training education competencies* (5th ed.). Retrieved from http://www.nata.org/sites/default/files/5th-Edition-Competencies-2011-PDF-Version.pdf

Prentice, W. (2010). *Arnheim's principles of athletic training: A competency-based approach* (14th ed.). New York, NY: McGraw-Hill.

Schilling, J. F. (2011). Educational preparation and experiences in the industrial-occupational setting: A qualitative study of athletic training graduates' perspectives. *Athletic Training Education Journal, 6*, 99–106.

Venes, D. (Ed.). (2009). *Taber's cyclopedic medical dictionary* (21st ed.). Philadelphia, PA: F.A. Davis.

chapter 29

Athletic Training Management

chapter outline

athletic trainer's corner

Out there in the real world, one athletic trainer experienced the following:

I have been fortunate in my career to have worked as an athletic trainer (AT) for two different high schools—one small and one big—and to have served as the head AT for a Division III college. One thing I can be certain of is that no matter the size of an organization, careful budgeting is crucial, regardless of your budget. The task of managing a large budget and inventory can seem daunting, but you have to be just as careful—if not more creative—with a tiny budget as well. Regardless of your budget, my advice is to get to know your suppliers well and determine how they can help you with your needs. Also, keep meticulous records to help with ordering from year to year. You might not feel prepared to manage your first supply budget, but with careful planning you can make those dollars stretch. If you are taking over a program, ask the athletic director (or your supervisor) for a copy of the athletic training budget expenditures from the previous year. This information can be a helpful guide for what you need to order and keep you from struggling with what and how much to order.

Erika Smith-Goodwin, PhD, ATC
Interim Vice President for Academic Affairs and Dean of Faculty
Professor of Athletic Training
Wilmington College
Wilmington, Ohio

learning outcomes

After working through this chapter, you will be able to:

1. Describe the components in designing a safe and efficient athletic training facility.
2. Identify and explain the components of capital and operational budgets.
3. Explain the statutes that regulate the privacy and security of medical records.
4. Identify the components involved with maintaining accurate medical records and ways of managing patient files.

MODEL SCENARIO 1: EDDIE SCOTLAND

Every 2 years, Eddie Scotland, a head AT, collects the athletic training documentation sheets for revisions. Mr. Scotland knows the importance of documentation and therefore views this task as one way to help make program improvements. He will revise the documents to coincide with the format that is used in the new computer software program that was recently purchased for patient file management (Fig. 29-1). The new injury progress sheets will follow more of a subjective, objective, assessment, and plan (SOAP) note format, and the daily treatment log will be broadened to include the treatment instead of just the athletes' names and the sports in which they participate. Mr. Scotland wants the athletic training students to understand the importance of thorough records and documentation and will hold a training session with them at the start of the new semester. However, a colleague is insisting that there is no longer a need for paper documentation.

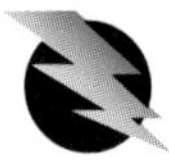

Brain Jolt

Accurate documentation will help to ensure proper and consistent rehabilitation when there are multiple ATs in the facility.

1. Based on this scenario, what do you know about Mr. Scotland's situation?
   - *Head AT revising documentation sheets*
   - *Revising occurs every 2 years*
   - *Change to SOAP note format*
   - *Daily treatment log revised*
   - *New software program for patient file management*
2. Identify key terms and concepts and then research each to broaden your knowledge of athletic training management.
   - Why is accurate documentation important?

     Proper patient care is often questioned, especially in a world where lawsuits are common. Having accurate documentation of any treatments provided or documentation of a conversation about a patient's care is just one more step to help defend an AT's actions if there are accusations of wrongdoing. In addition, this documentation will help an AT progress with rehabilitation properly, especially when there are multiple ATs working with an athlete.
   - **Give examples of other forms of documentation that must occur daily in the athletic training room.**

     Other types of daily documentation that occur in the athletic training room include the daily treatment log, injury evaluation sheets, SOAP notes, cleaning logs, and the supply and equipment list or inventory.
   - **Explain the importance of a computer software program for an athletic training room. Give one example of a software program.**

     A computer software program for athletic training and patient file management can be a useful tool. Software programs can assist with tracking athletic injuries and producing injury lists, daily treatments, preparticipation physical information, and SOAP notes. Team rosters can also be formatted along with supply and equipment inventories. An example of a computer program that is widely used is SportsWare2011.
   - **Name some items that are important to remember when doing medical documentation.**

     You should always write in blue or black ink, the athlete's name and injury should be clearly noted, all documentation should include a date and signature of the treating AT, any mistakes should be initialed, and the documentation will typically include medical shorthand.
3. **Based on the information that you currently have and what was provided by your instructor, what needs to be done in Mr. Scotland's situation?**

   There always has to be a paper trail. In an educational environment, athletic training students need to understand the importance of taking the time to complete documentation on paper. This process then carries over into the professional world of athletic training. The athletic training environment is one that does not always allow the time to sit down at the computer and input information in a timely manner. The convenience of a computer software program is not available out on the football field or baseball diamond; however, paper and pen can be readily available, and the information can be entered later into the software program when it is available.

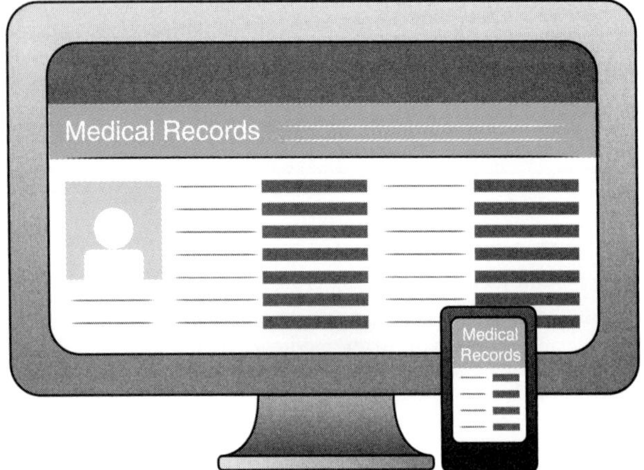

Figure 29-1: Eddie Scotland's patient file-management software.

STUDENT SCENARIO 1: BROOKE LOCHARD

Brooke Lochard is a high school AT, and her school is constructing a new athletics building. The school administrators have contacted Ms. Lochard about the design of the new athletic training room. It would be centrally located near the locker rooms and the gymnasium. Ms. Lochard advises the school administrators that the layout and size of the athletic training room needs to accommodate all sports teams, while also providing space for the various stations needed for patient care. She provides the school administrators with an outline of the proposed athletic training room design (Fig. 29-2) and the equipment needed to adequately provide athletic training care to the athletes.

1. Based on this scenario, what do you know about Ms. Lochard's situation?
   - ______________________________
   ____
   - ______________________________
   ____
   - ______________________________
   ____
   - ______________________________
   ____

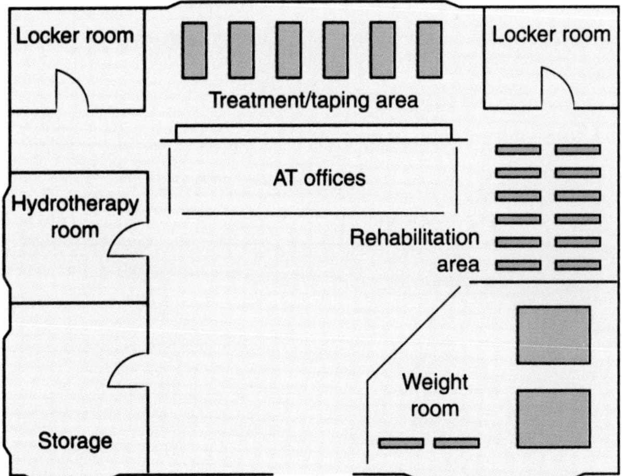

Figure 29-2: Brooke Lochard's athletic training room design layout.

2. Identify key terms and concepts and then research each to broaden your knowledge of athletic training management.
   - What size athletic training room would accommodate a Division I high school athletic training program?

     Answer: ______________________________
   - What is the minimum size recommendation for an athletic training room?

     Answer: ______________________________
   - What athletic training stations should be included within the athletic training room design?

     Answer: ______________________________
   - What safety measures need to be considered when designing this facility?

     Answer: ______________________________
   - What equipment is needed for each athletic training station?

     Answer: ______________________________
   - Design a Division I high school athletic training room that Ms. Lochard could submit to the school administrators.

     Answer: ______________________________

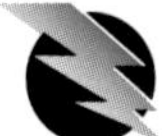

Brain Jolt

When designing an athletic training room, positioning as it pertains to locker room access and facility access is a major component to consider.

3. Based on the information that you currently have and what was provided by your instructor, what should be done in Ms. Lochard's situation?
   - ______________________________
   ____
   - ______________________________
   ____
   - ______________________________
   ____
   - ______________________________
   ____

STUDENT SCENARIO 2: LIAM MCAFEE

Liam McAfee provides athletic training coverage at a Division III high school. The program is in its second year, and he cares for approximately 150 athletes. The athletic director has given Mr. McAfee a $2,000 supply budget. The previous year, the school had not budgeted for athletic training expenses, and Mr. McAfee could purchase only five boxes of tape, gauze, and adhesive bandages. Much of Mr. McAfee's supply list is used to purchase expendable items (Fig. 29-3). However, this year, he needs to make a large nonexpendable purchase: a complete vacuum splint kit. When Mr. McAfee completes the supply list, he will e-mail it to various athletic training suppliers to get a bid from those companies.

1. Based on this scenario, what do you know about Mr. McAfee's situation?

- ______________________________
- ______________________________
- ______________________________
- ______________________________

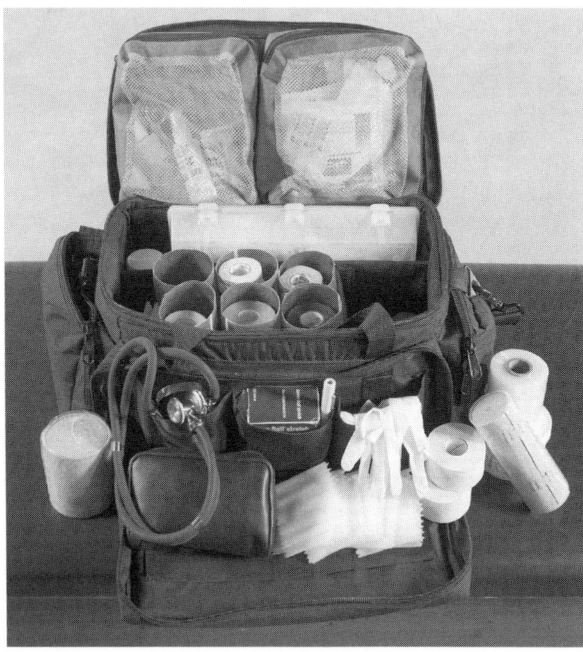

Figure 29-3: Liam McAfee's athletic training supplies.

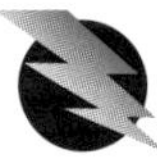

Brain Jolt
Competitive bidding of supplies is a way to help save money for schools with limited budgets.

2. Identify key terms and concepts and then research each to broaden your knowledge of athletic training management.
   - Define *expendable item*. Give examples.

     Answer: ______________________________
   - Define *nonexpendable item*. Give examples.

     Answer: ______________________________
   - Which items do you believe are the bare-minimum necessities?

     Answer: ______________________________
   - Create a supply list with a $2,000 budget and assume that the prior expendable inventory has been depleted.

     Answer: ______________________________
   - Research the athletic training suppliers in your area. To whom would you submit your inventory list?

     Answer: ______________________________
3. Based on the information that you currently have and what was provided by your instructor, what should be done in Mr. McAfee's situation?
   - ______________________________
   - ______________________________
   - ______________________________
   - ______________________________

STUDENT SCENARIO 3: CASSY KASSEL

Cassy Kassel is a 29-year-old unemployed certified AT. She has a master's degree in athletic training management and 5 years of experience at a small college as the assistant AT. She is preparing for an interview with her alma mater, and the job description for the Division III head AT position includes overseeing football and wrestling, teaching duties, and supervising the athletic training room. Two weeks after the interview, Ms. Kassel is told that she did not receive the position. She learns that the athletic director would prefer to have a male head AT working with football. Ms. Kassel believes that she was not given equal consideration for the position based on her gender, which is a violation of the EEOC (Equal Employment Opportunity Commission) (Fig. 29-4).

1. Based on this scenario, what do you know about Ms. Kassel's situation?

- ______________________________
- ______________________________
- ______________________________
- ______________________________

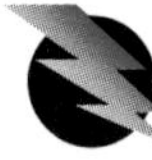

Brain Jolt

By law, all qualified individuals have to be given equal consideration for a job opening.

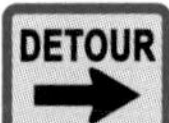

Treatment Detour

Graduate assistantships are a great way to bridge your undergraduate education to the real world. Whether you are a student looking to pursue a graduate education or the head AT looking to fill an assistantship spot, there are a few things that are extremely important for easing the transition from a student to a professional AT. The first is to learn the policies and procedures of the institution. There are many things to learn when getting a new position or hiring a new graduate assistant. The most critical things to learn are the important policies such as insurance coverage; administration of medications; information pertaining to emergency care planning, including the location of the nearest hospital and the emergency action plan of each facility; and procedures in the athletic training facility, such as supply inventory and cleaning procedures. The next strategy to help the transition is locating the inventory and identifying physical resources. The third strategy is creating a time-management plan by making a schedule. Finally, the last strategy is building solid professional relationships. These steps will help students become more confident as professional ATs and will also help the head AT educate the new graduate assistants to make the transition easier (Rogers, Hampton, & Barringer, 2012).

2. Identify key terms and concepts and then research each to broaden your knowledge of athletic training management.

- What is the EEOC?

  Answer: ______________________________
- Can a job description state that a position is for a male head AT? Explain.

  Answer: ______________________________
- What questions cannot be asked in an interview in order to comply with the law?

  Answer: ______________________________
- Does the termination of an employee follow the same laws? Explain.

  Answer: ______________________________

3. Based on the information that you currently have and what was provided by your instructor, what should be done in Ms. Kassel's situation?

- ______________________________
- ______________________________
- ______________________________
- ______________________________

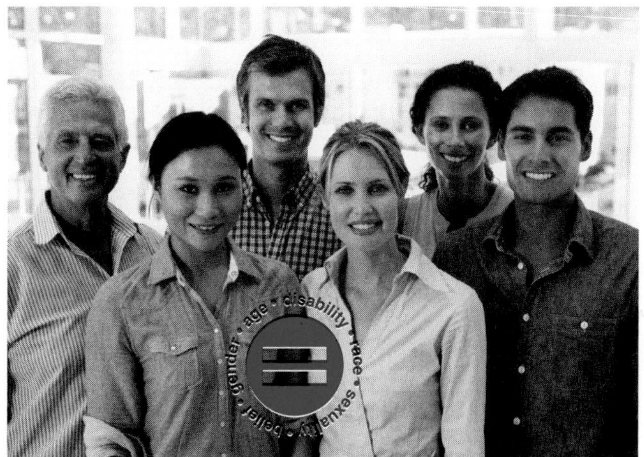

Figure 29-4: Cassy Kassel's equal employment opportunity. (© Thinkstock)

STUDENT SCENARIO 4: BRANDI DANKLEFSEN

Brandi Danklefsen is the new head AT for a Division II college. She is concerned that the workstation that the athletic training students use to record athletic injuries and rehabilitations is not private and secure. The workstation is located in the middle of the athletic training room (Fig. 29-5) and is visible and accessible from each side to anyone walking through the room. The daily treatment log, SOAP notes, and initial evaluations are completed at this workstation. Currently, the patient files are kept in an unlocked filing cabinet in Ms. Danklefsen's office. The cabinet is unlocked so that athletic training students can access it more easily. Ms. Danklefsen is concerned that the program is at risk for a Health Insurance Portability and Accountability Act (HIPAA) violation.

1. Based on this scenario, what do you know about Ms. Danklefsen's situation?
   - ______________________________
   - ______________________________
   - ______________________________
   - ______________________________

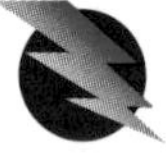

Brain Jolt
HIPAA protects the medical privacy of an individual.

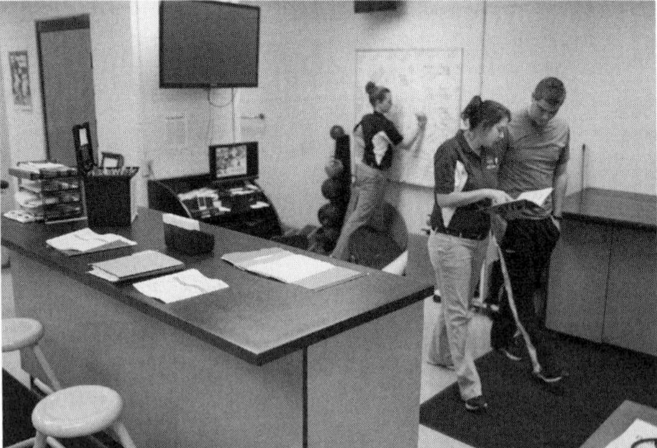

Figure 29-5: Brandi Danklefsen's workstation in the athletic training room.

Conversation Buffer
It is important to remind any students you supervise or coaches who are privy to medical information that only those given permission to have medical information can remain informed. For students, this means that they cannot talk to their roommates and friends. For coaches, it means that they cannot talk to other players or the media without permission from the patient. This information is confidential and should be kept that way.

2. Identify key terms and concepts and then research each to broaden your knowledge of athletic training management.
   - Explain HIPAA.

     Answer: ______________________________
   - Is there a privacy violation in this scenario?

     Answer: ______________________________
   - Does the workstation need to be relocated?

     Answer: ______________________________
   - Are the files kept in Ms. Danklefsen's office considered secure?

     Answer: ______________________________
   - Can the athletic training students and Ms. Danklefsen discuss an athlete's medical information with anyone? Explain.

     Answer: ______________________________
3. Based on the information that you currently have and what was provided by your instructor, what should be done in Ms. Danklefsen's situation?
   - ______________________________
   - ______________________________
   - ______________________________
   - ______________________________

STUDENT SCENARIO 5: TAYLOR CARNES

Taylor Carnes is the athletic training coordinator for the local hospital. She oversees seven high schools of different sizes. Ms. Carnes is putting together the yearly reports for the hospital board, because each year the board examines the revenue generated by the athletic training program referrals (Fig. 29-6). The athletic training services that the hospital provides to the local high schools are viewed as a community service. On a monthly basis, the athletic training staff members are required to compile a list of their school's physician and radiology visits for their athletes.

1. Based on this scenario, what do you know about Ms. Carnes' situation?
   - ______________________________
   - ______________________________
   - ______________________________
   - ______________________________

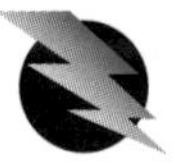

Brain Jolt

Documentation on your referral list should include every initial doctor's visit and follow-up visits.

2. Identify key terms and concepts and then research each to broaden your knowledge of athletic training management.
   - Define *referral*.

   Answer: ______________________________

Referral Form

Name ______________________________ Date ____________
Diagnosis ______________________________
Instructions:
- ☐ Emergency Room (ER)
- ☐ Physician
- ☐ Physical Therapy
- ☐ Athletic Training Services

Comments: ______________________________
Restrictions: ______________________________

Figure 29-6: Taylor Carnes' referral form.

- Why does each school need to compile a list of referrals for the board?

  Answer: ______________________________
- Give examples of different types of referrals that an AT can use for an athletic injury. Explain each referral.

  Answer: ______________________________
- What type of revenue would be generated for the hospital when using hospital-based physicians or facilities?

  Answer: ______________________________
- Would the revenue generated at each school be the same or different?

  Answer: ______________________________

Conversation Buffer

Many high schools have athletic training services provided to them by local hospitals. Hospitals are viewing the relationship with high schools as a community service. The hospital will supply the AT to the school in exchange for exclusive promotional services. Therefore, if your local high school does not have athletic training coverage, be sure to communicate with the local hospital about developing a business relationship.

Treatment Detour

There are many things that go into the administration of athletic training services. With anything that is done regarding these services, the physical and mental welfare of the athletes must be the highest priority of the AT. There are a few things that should be done to help attain this goal. There should always be a medical director to help oversee the athletic training services and to coordinate care within a network of physicians. Therefore, the AT must always practice within the written or verbal instructions given by the physician or by the standing orders approved by the medical director. In addition, it is important that the AT, in an administrative role, also communicate with the coaches that they cannot act outside of these approved guidelines and can only act upon what is within their training. Finally, it is important to have an administrative structure that minimizes conflicts of interest in which the well-being of an athlete could be jeopardized. These steps will help to facilitate the best athletic training services ("Ten Principles," 2012).

3. Based on the information that you currently have and what was provided by your instructor, why does Ms. Carnes require these schools' lists in this situation?

   ■ ______________________________

   ____

   ■ ______________________________

   ____

   ■ ______________________________

   ____

   ■ ______________________________

   ____

STUDENT SCENARIO 6: **ODIE SHRUNK**

Odie Shrunk has an operating budget of $25,000 for the collegiate athletic training program that he oversees. The bulk of the operating budget goes to supplies and equipment for the athletic training room. Supplies and equipment should be broken into four categories when evaluating an operating budget. Mr. Shrunk keeps a log in which athletes sign for nonexpendable supplies when they are injured or recovering after treatment or surgery. Keeping track of these supplies and recollecting them allows for Mr. Shrunk to save and spend more money purchasing pieces of capital equipment each year. Every few years, Mr. Shrunk can submit a request to purchase nonconsumable capital equipment that needs to be replaced to keep the athletic training room in safe working condition. This year, he would like to purchase a new whirlpool (Fig. 29-7), because the current one is leaking and not running properly.

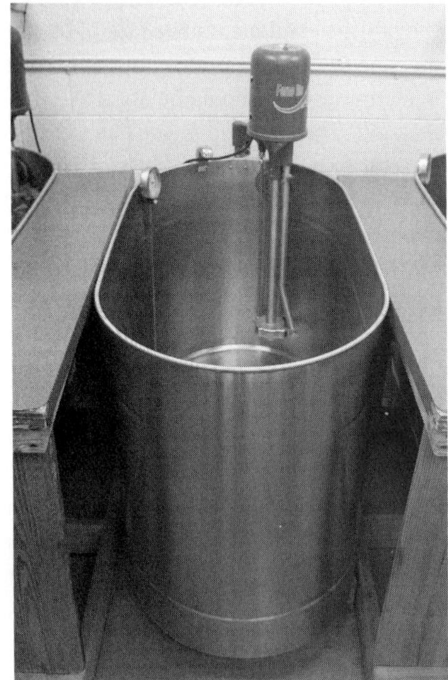

Figure 29-7: Odie Shrunk's whirlpool used in an athletic training room.

1. Based on this scenario, what do you know about Mr. Shrunk's situation?

   ■ ______________________________

   ____

   ■ ______________________________

   ____

   ■ ______________________________

   ____

   ■ ______________________________

   ____

Brain Jolt

By monitoring supplies and inventory, you can potentially find extra money to purchase equipment that will be used in the athletic training room for many years.

2. Identify key terms and concepts and then research each to broaden your knowledge of athletic training management.
   - Define *supplies* within athletic training.

     Answer: ______________________________
   - Define *equipment* within athletic training.

     Answer: ______________________________
   - What are nonexpendable supplies? Give an example.

     Answer: ______________________________
   - What are expendable supplies? Give an example.

     Answer: ______________________________
   - Explain nonconsumable capital equipment. Give an example.

     Answer: ______________________________
   - Explain what would be listed on a capital equipment list.

     Answer: ______________________________

3. Based on the information that you currently have and what was provided by your instructor, what are the options for Mr. Shrunk's situation?

   - ____

     ____

   - ____

     ____

   - ____

     ____

   - ____

     ____

knowledge checklist

Table 29-1 offers a checklist that can be used by a peer, instructor, or preceptor to evaluate a student's understanding of the profession. Use this checklist as a tool to assess your knowledge of the competencies that apply to this chapter.

TABLE 29-1 ■ Athletic Training Management Competency Checklist

	Proficient *Shows understanding of content*	**Proficient With Assistance** *Shows understanding of content with prompting*	**Not Proficient** *Is unclear about content and needs to be reevaluated at another time after further review*
Administrative Responsibilities			
Explain the statutes that regulate the privacy and security of medical records			
Identify the components involved with maintaining accurate medical records and ways of managing patient files			
Operational Procedures			
Describe the components involved in designing a safe and efficient athletic training facility			
Identify and explain the components of capital and operational budgets			

REFERENCES

National Athletic Training Association. (2011). *Athletic training education competencies* (5th ed.). Retrieved from http://www.nata.org/sites/default/files/5th-Edition-Competencies-2011-PDF-Version.pdf

Prentice, W. (2010). *Arnheim's principles of athletic training: A competency-based approach* (14th ed.). New York, NY: McGraw-Hill.

Rogers, S. D., Hampton, C. E., & Barringer, S. (2012). Transition from student to clinician in a scholastic sport setting. *International Journal of Athletic Therapy and Training, 17,* 45–48.

Ten principles to guide administration of sports medicine athletic training services. (2012, July). *International Journal of Athletic Therapy and Training* [on-line serial], *17,* 3.

Venes, D. (Ed.). (2009). *Taber's cyclopedic medical dictionary* (21st ed.). Philadelphia, PA: F.A. Davis.

Index

part seven

Flashcards

Shock

Frostbite

Anaphylaxis

External Hemorrhage: Laceration

Seizure

Diabetic Emergency

Internal Hemorrhage: Kidney

Epidural Hematoma

Sickle Cell Trait

Asthma Attack

Waxy, white appearance
Tingling, pain
Prolonged exposure
★

Rapid, weak pulse
Cool, clammy skin
Elevate legs
★

Scraping/tearing of tissue
Minimal bleeding
★

Trouble breathing
Cool, clammy skin
Injector held 10 sec.
★

Confusion
Pale, bluish lips
Fruity breath
★

Sweating
Posturing
Disorientation
★★

Direct blow
Initially asymptomatic
Symptoms deteriorate rapidly
Unequal pupils
Life-threatening emergency
★★

Direct blow
Rigid muscles
Hematuria
★★

Trouble breathing
Chest tightness
Wheezing
★

Severe pain in limbs
Flu-like symptoms
Upper right quadrant rigid
Abnormal blood cells
★★

Traction Splint	AED
Airway Adjunct	Conscious Choking Sequence
Administer Oxygen	C-Spine Stabilization and Backboarding
Bag-Valve Mask	Recovery Position
Check/Call/Care	Unconscious Choking Sequence

Portable
No metal or water
Analyze heart rhythm

★★

Direct blow
Leg length discrepancy
Long bone stabilizing
Equipment post femoral fracture

★★

Encourage coughing
Gasping for air
Obtain consent

★

Jaw thrust maneuver
Gag reflex absent
Device to administer oxygen

★★

Limp but conscious
Stabilize victim
Log roll
Facemask removal

★★

Used with breathing difficulty
Supplemental
Flowrate important

★

Signs of life present
Responder must leave the scene
or patient vomiting
Modified technique available

★

Two-person technique
Delivers higher concentration
of oxygen

★

Unconscious victim
Ventilation unsuccessful
Reposition head but same result

★

Emergency action sequence
Required response different per
age group

★

Helmet Fitting

Acclimation

Knee Brace

Ankle Taping

Orthotics

Preparticipation Physical

Sling Psychrometer

McConnell Taping

Hip Pointer Padding

Lisfranc Injury

Weight chart
Practice gear regulations and modifications
Staggered practices
★★

Two fingers above the eyebrow
Thin object at cheek and ear
Injury prevention
★

Prevention or post injury
Support ligaments
Anchors
Inversion/eversion pull
★

Post injury or prevention
Correct alignment required
6" above and 6" below patella
★★

Family history
Identify medical issues
Orthopedic evaluation
★

To assist with pes planus
Examine shoe wear pattern
Customized
★★

Corrective technique
Patella tracking
Typical lateral to medial realignment
★★

Assists with environmental conditions
Humid air
Dry air
★

Forceful hyperplantar flexion of forefoot
Dorsal foot pain
Unable to bear weight
Unstable forefoot
★★★

Doughnut shape
Ecchymosis at the iliac crest
Ace wrap to secure
★

Lateral Ankle Sprain
Anterior Talofibular
Ligament

Achilles Tendon
Rupture

Fibula Fracture

Retrocalcaneal Bursitis

Syndesmotic Ankle
Sprain

Sever's Disease

Morton's Neuroma

Sesamoiditis

Jones Fracture

LCL Tear

Gross deformity
Positive Thompson test

★★

Positive anterior drawer test
Laxity in sinus tarsi

Chronic
Watery edema
Painful while wearing shoes

Direct blow to lower leg
Pain laterally
No increased pain with weight-bearing

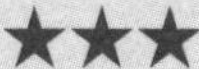

Posterior calcaneal pain
Adolescent athlete
Pain with activity

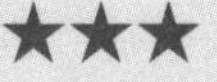

Pain is more proximal
Hyperdorsiflexion and external rotation of ankle
Positive Kleiger's test
Negative compression test

Repetitive hyperextension
Plantar foot edema
Pain with push-off mechanism

Plantar nerve affected
Numbness near third and fourth metatarsals

Negative McMurray's (IR)
Positive varus test @ 0°
Negative apprehension test

Excessive inversion and plantar flexion of foot
High nonunion rate
Positive tap/percussion test

★★

Unhappy Triad

Osgood-Schlatter Disease

Patella Dislocation

Chondromalacia

ACL Tear

Pes Anserine Bursitis

Medial Meniscus Tear

Patella Femoral Syndrome

MCL Sprain

Hip Pointer

Anterior tibial tuberosity deformity
Tight quadriceps muscle
Rapid growth spurt

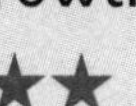

Positive McMurray's (ER)
Buckling
Positive valgus @ 0/20/30°

Negative patella apprehension test
Positive patella grind test
Positive patella compression test

Negative varus test
Edema on lateral side
Positive apprehension test

Runner's knee
Edema
Medial irritation at muscle insertion

Negative apprehension test
Positive anterior drawer test (neutral)
Negative anterior drawer @ 30°(IR)

Irregular patella tracking
Weak VMO
General knee pain/soreness

Catching
Positive Apley's grind
Positive McMurray's (ER)

Direct blow
Moderate to severe ecchymosis
Unable to flex hip without localized pain

★★

Negative Lachman test
Negative anterior drawer @ 15° (ER)
Positive valgus @ 30°

Myositis Ossificans

Groin Strain

Shin Splints

Femur Fracture

Tibia/Fibula Fracture

Hamstring Rupture

Hip Flexor Strain

ITB Syndrome

Acute Compartment Syndrome

Carpal Tunnel

Pain with active and resistive movements
Adductor magnus pain

★★

Decreased muscle function
Hematoma
Calcification

★★

Leg-length discrepancy
Traction splint needed
Leg position: external rotation

★★

Diffuse lower anterior leg pain
Tight gastrocnemius
Overuse injury

★★

Posterior thigh internal hemorrhaging
Palpable divot or mass
Complete loss of function

★★

Direct blow lower leg
Positive compression test
Positive percussion test

★★

Lateral knee pain
Palpable lateral tightness
Positive Ober test

★★

Anterior hip pain
Pain over rectus femoris
Ace wrap

★★

Positive Tinel sign
Positive Phalen test

Direct blow
Anterior lower-leg tightness and numbness
Decreased dorsal pedal pulse

Lateral Epicondylitis: Tennis Elbow

Boxer Fracture

Scaphoid Fracture

Gamekeeper's Thumb

UCL Tear

Forearm Fracture

Colles Fracture

Elbow Dislocation

Subungual Hematoma

Pectoralis Major Tear

Direct axial force
Fifth metacarpal

★★

Overuse
Pain with resistive wrist extension
Pain over extensor carpi radialis longus origin

Forceful abduction of the IP joint
Point tenderness/edema on medial aspect of thumb
Laxity

★★

Edema over carpal bones
Point tenderness in anatomical snuff box
Preiser's disease

Deformity of radius and ulna
False joint
Moderate to severe edema/pain

★★

Pain over medial side of elbow
Positive valgus stress test

Deformity at medial/lateral epicondyle
Never reduce

Fall on outstretch hand
Distal radius displaced
Dinnerfork deformity

Pop/tearing sensation
Anterior shoulder deformity
Immense pain
Unable to horizontally adduct arm

★★

Accumulation of blood
Creates pressure on nail bed

Thoracic Outlet Syndrome

Winging Scapula

SLAP Lesion

Glenohumeral Instability

AC Separation

Sternoclavicular Separation

Bicipital Tendonitis

Humerus Fracture

Impingement

Orbital Fracture

Nerve involvement
Scapular retraction deformity
Muscular weakness

Numbness
Paraesthesia in arm
Diminished radial pulse
Positive Roos test

Inferior, posterior, anterior instability
"Popping out" sensation
Positive sulcus test

Active horizontal adduction painful
Pinching feeling with adduction of shoulder
Point tenderness around bicipital groove
Negative Yergason's test

Deformity near sternum
Pain with horizontal adduction @ clavicle
Localized edema

Shoulder abduction painful
Distal clavicle deformity
Positive piano key test

Immediate effusion over localized deformity
Diminished radial pulse
Applied traction decreases pain

Active forward flexion of shoulder painful
Tendon edema in groove
Positive Yergason's test

Direct blow
Downward eye movement difficult
Diplopia

Point tenderness and pain near coracoacromial arch
Popping sensation with active ROM
Positive empty can test

Epidural Hematoma

Tooth Dislocation

Cervical Fracture

Cauliflower Ear

Solar Plexus Injury

TMJ

Nasal Fracture

Abdominal Strain

Brachial Plexus Injury
Burner

Concussion

Exposed roots
Milk or saline

★

Headache
Deteriorating symptoms
Arterial bleed

★★★

Hematoma
Shear force
Keloid

★★

Axial loading
Common with 4th, 5th, 6th
Point tender on spinous process

★★

Clicking when opening and closing
Lateral pain when eating

★★

Paralysis of diaphragm
Shortness of breath

★★

Dynamic twisting, shortening, stretching motion
Pain with flexion of core

★★

Direct blow
Epistaxis
Crepitus
Abnormal mobility of the bridge

★★

Possible LOC
No C-spine tenderness
Headache
Blurred vision
Possible amnesia

★★

Stretching of structure
Pain and numbness radiating into fingers
Deltoid weakness

★★

Anatomical Leg-Length Discrepancy

L4 Disc Herniation

Anterior Pelvic Tilt

Spondylolysis

SI Dysfunction

Sciatica

Piriformis Syndrome

Osteitis Pubis

Weak Gluteus Medius

Lumbar Strain

Low back pain with mild numbness
and pain
Positive pain with prone press-up
Positive well straight-leg raise

★★★

Dip with pelvis when walking
Genetic or prior history
Bilateral malleolus alignment issue

Forced extreme hyperextension
Positive single-leg stork stance
Scotty dog

★★★

Low back pain
Lordotic curve
Positive Thomas test
Leg-length discrepancy

★★★

Sharp, shooting pain
Numbness/paraesthesia
Positive bowstring test

★★

Uneven PSIS
Positive distraction test
Often unilateral low back pain

★★★

Groin pain
Pain located near pubis symphysis
Repetitive stress

★★★

Pain with leg extension
and abduction
Hip and buttock pain/tightness
Occasional numbness/paraesthesia
in posterior leg

★★

General low back soreness
Pain lateral to spinous process
No radiating pain

★★

Unsupported pelvic drop
Positive Trendelenburg

Syndesmotic Ankle Sprain

Achilles Tendon Rupture

Plantar Fasciitis

Fibula Fracture

Sesamoiditis

Lisfranc Injury

Jones Fracture

Morton's Neuroma

Grade 1 Lateral Ankle Sprain

Syndesmotic Ankle Sprain

Involves triceps surae
Complete surgical repair
Casted 6 to 8 weeks
Limited gastrocnemius and soleus stretching
Ankle ROM exercises

Proximal ankle injury like medial/lateral sprain
Extended immobilization/walking boot
Control proximal edema

★★

Non-weight-bearing bone
Casted 6 to 8 weeks
PNF
Restore ankle mobility
Alphabet/tubing

Inflamed structure that results in painful walking after periods of rest
Static gastrocnemius and soleus stretch
Night splint
Massage plantar side of foot with tennis ball

★★

Tarsometatarsal instability
Open reduction
Six weeks immobilization
Scar tissue mobilizations
Decrease pain, edema post-surgery

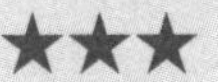

Pain in ball of foot
Three point gait to decrease pressure to great toe
Metatarsal pad/bar
Limit activity to decrease edema
Anti-inflammatory

Nerve affected
Teardrop pad
Change shoe selection
Decrease pain and edema

Involves landmark on 5th metatarsal
Casting/immobilization of foot
Possible bone stimulator
Ankle ROM after 6- to 8-week period
Stretch calf

Ankle injury with slow healing rate
Restore active/passive ROM
BAPS board
Foam pad, single leg
Cutting will irritate high injury

MOI is inversion
Limited activity for a week
Resistive tubing four-way
Alphabet
Toe raises

Lisfranc Injury

Unhappy Triad

PCL Tear

Pes Anserine Bursitis

Patella Tendonitis

Grade 2 MCL Sprain

Medial Meniscus Tear

Patella Femoral Syndrome

Patella Dislocation

Grade 2 ACL Tear

Includes three structures
Surgical intervention
Patella mobilizations
Passive motion machine
Heel slides
SLR

★★★

Forefoot injury
Screws/plates removed if gait altered
NWB—towel scrunches
FWB—toe-ups
Towel stretch

★★

Insertion site of three muscles
NSAIDs
Correct foot alignment
Decrease medial tibial edema
Compression pad/Ace wrap

★★

"Dashboard" injury
Rare surgical intervention
Posterior translation
Strengthen quadriceps

★★

MOI is valgus stress
Decrease medial pain/edema
Hinge brace
Crutches until no apparent limp
Quad sets/SLR

★★

Anterior tendon pain
Overuse injury
Ice massage
Strengthen quadriceps/hamstrings
Iontophoresis
Ultrasound
Patella tendon strap

★★

General knee pain with atrophy of VMO
Decrease edema
Increase VMO strength
SAQ
Increase hamstring flexibility

★★★

Catching/locking
Structure for shock absorption
MRI
Decrease pain/edema
Increase VMO strength
TKEs

★★

Positive anterior drawer test
Moderate instability
Control horseshoe edema
Electrical stimulation
Compression pad/wrap
Maintain quadriceps strength

★★

Can reduce spontaneously
Knee immobilization
Crutches
Horseshoe pad/brace
Avoid excessive knee flexion
SLRs

★★

Unhappy Triad

Hip Flexor Strain

PCL Injury/Surgery

Myositis Ossificans

Medial Meniscus Tear

Tibial Stress Fracture

Patella Femoral Syndrome

Hip Pointer

Medial Tibial Stress Syndrome

Quadriceps Contusion

Anterior hip pain with hip flexion
Decrease pain/anti-inflammatory
Evaluate/compare bilaterally
hip ROM
Iliopsoas stretch
Hip spica

★★

Three structures are affected
in the knee
Weight-bearing by 4 weeks without
brace
Stationary bike for ROM
Running program at 4 months

★★★

Bony deposit
Ice with knee in full flexion
Ultrasound
Deep tissue massage
Achieve knee flexion

★★

Injured structure prevents posterior
translation of tibia
Full extension 6 weeks post-surgery
FWB on crutches
After 6 weeks begin passive ROM
4 months PRE

★★★

Positive bone scan for tibial
"hot spot"
Overuse
Crutches
Non–weight-bearing

★★

The inner two-thirds of this structure
has limited blood supply so healing
is slow
Arthroscopic surgery
PWB/FWB with crutches post-surgery
Heels slides
SLRs

★★

Excessive ecchymosis
Ice massage
Anti-inflammatory
RTP with crest padded

★★

Irregular patellar tracking
McConnell taping
Electrical stimulation to control pain/
edema
TKE with resistive bands
Wall-slides/step-ups

★★

Direct blow to quadriceps
Decrease pain
Electrical stimulation for pain/edema
Ice quadriceps in full flexion
Compression pad

★★

Runner's lower-leg overuse injury
Bone scan/x-ray
Ice massage
Stretch gastrocnemius/soleus
Limit activity until pain free

IT Band Syndrome

Jersey Finger

Hamstring Rupture

Olecranon Bursitis

Groin Strain

Lateral Epicondylitis

Quadriceps Contusion

Ulnar Collateral Ligament Tear Grade 1

IT Band Syndrome

Colles Fracture

Rupture of flexor digitorum profundus
Splint
Ice
Refer for possible surgical intervention

★★

Friction injury on lateral side of knee
Decrease lateral knee pain
Ice massage
Examine for leg-length discrepancy
Limit activity to flat terrain only

★★

Watery elbow edema
Compression pad
Ace wrap
Ice
Possible aspiration

★★

Pop and complete loss of function in posterior thigh
Crutches
Ace wrap
Loss of knee flexion
Excessive ecchymosis
Control pain/edema

★★

Tennis elbow
Ice massage
Strengthen wrist extensors once decreased inflammation

★★

Hip adductor pain
RICE
Hip spica
Limit activity until pain-free

★★

Medial stress injury of elbow
Analyze throwing mechanics
Ice
Strengthen wrist/forearm/shoulder complex

★★

RTP with orthoplast over contused area
Quad sets/SLR
Limit squatting and incline running until completely pain-free

★★

Displaced radius
Surgical intervention
Two weeks post-surgery ROM wrist exercises
FWB on hand 8 to 10 weeks

★★

Foam roller
Ultrasound
Iontophoresis
Address hip abnormalities

Gamekeeper's Thumb

UCL Tear
Grade 3

Forearm Fracture

Sternoclavicular Joint
Sprain

Elbow Dislocation

Pectoralis Major Tear

Jersey Finger

Anterior Shoulder
Dislocation

Lateral Epicondylitis

Thoracic Outlet
Syndrome

Complete elbow ligament tear
Tommy John surgery
Throwing program 6 months post-surgery
RTP 9 months post-surgery

Sprain UCL at MCP joint
Gross laxity
Surgical intervention
Splint up to 3 weeks
RTP, thumb spica taping

Upper medial chest pain
Positive piano key sign
Shoulder ROM exercises once out of sling

Fracture of ulna and radius
Six to eight weeks long arm plaster cast
Removal of cast, wrist/elbow ROM

Deformity near axilla
Lack of horizontal adduction
Resistance tubing for ROM in transverse plane

Reduction of elbow
Elbow immobilized into flexion
Hand grip exercises
Shoulder exercises

Palpable anterior shoulder deformity
Positive apprehension test
Rhythmic stabilization

Surgical intervention to restore flexion at DIP joint
Restore ROM of DIP/PIP joint
Grip exercises
Putty

Numbness and paraesthesia
Swollen hand
Stretch the scalenes

Evaluate activity that caused irritation/repetitiveness
Neoprene elbow sleeve
Ultrasound
Iontophoresis

★★★

Impingement

Bicipital Tendonitis

Labrum Tear

Multidirectional Instability

Bicipital Tendonitis

Thoracic Outlet Syndrome

Multidirectional Instability

Impingement Syndrome

AC Joint Separation

Rib Fracture

Point tender over the groove of the shoulder
Chronic pain with throwing
Thermal ultrasound

Pain with shoulder ROM above 90 degrees
Point tender over subacromial space
Body blade

Hypermobile joints
Strengthen RTC
Strengthen scapular stabilizers

Clicking with shoulder ROM
Positive clunk test
Wall walks

Positive Roos test
Correct shoulder posture
Row exercises
Stretch pectoralis muscles

Positive speed's test
Use bands with low resistance and high repetitions

Inflammation in subacromialbursae
Iontophoresis
Scapular retraction exercises

Shoulder feels "loose"
Positive sulcus test
Extreme ROM in all planes
Serratus punches

Sharp pain with inspiration
Point tenderness
Often in collision sports
Wrap with elastic bandage

Step-off deformity
In a sling, dependent on severity
PROM in all directions

Brachial Plexus Neuropraxia

TMJ Dysfunction

Concussion

Concussion

Whiplash

Spondylolisthesis

Orbital Fracture

Sacroiliac Joint Dysfunction

Epidural Hematoma

Sciatica

Clicking with jaw movement
Ear pain
Limiting chewy foods
NSAIDs and thermal therapy

★★★

Compression or traction mechanism
Results in paralysis
Decreased horizontal abduction

★★★

Once indicated, exertional testing
ImPACT results
If symptoms return, no participation

★★

Tinnitus
Headache
Asymptomatic 24 hours before
RTP protocol

★★★

Bilateral back pain
Pain with extension
Negative straight-leg raise test
Core strengthening

★★★

Point tender over cervical spinous
and transverse processes
Negative cervical compression test
Sudden change in direction
Stretching of SCM

★★★

Asymmetrical PSIS
Low back pain
Positive FABER test
Use of belt
Kinesiotape

★★★

"Blowout" fracture
Diplopia
Refer for x-rays

★★★

Radiating pain down leg
Positive piriformis muscle test
Accompanies chronic low back pain
Figure 4 stretch

★★★

One dilated pupil
Rapid deterioration
Medical emergency

★★★

Disc Herniation

Anatomical Leg-Length Discrepancy

Lumbar Strain

Sciatica

Nerve Root Impingement

Sacroiliac Joint Dysfunction

Spondylolysis

Detached Retina

Functional Leg-Length Discrepancy

Appendicitis

ASIS to medical malleolus
Heel lift
Stretching

★★★

Positive straight-leg raise test
Altered posture
Increased pain with sneezing
Traction

★★★

Radiating pain in posterior leg
Need to correct posture
Increase flexibility
NSAIDs to reduce inflammation

★★

Muscle spasms
Lateral
Sudden extension and trunk rotation
Cat/camel

★★★

Joint is too mobile or immobile
Low back pain
NSAIDs and heat can help
Muscle energy

★★★

History of disc herniation
Numbness/paraesthesia
Positive Milgram test
Neural tension release

★★★

Direct blow to eye
Falling curtain
Immediate referral

★★★

Precursor to spondylolisthesis
Typically unilateral pain
Core strengthening

★★★

Pain in lower right quadrant
Rigidity
Vomiting

★★★

Muscle energy technique to correct
Stretching
Core strengthening

Pink Eye (Conjunctivitis)

Antifungal Medication

Diabetes

Drug Distribution Policy

Spleen Rupture

Analgesics

Kidney Contusion

Supplements

Impetigo

Asthma

Treats tinea pedis
Infection of skin, hair, or nails

★★

Yellow discharge
Pruritus
Erythema

★★★

Caution with minors
Proper documentation
Administered in single-dose pack

★★

Polyuria
Polydipsia
Blurred vision

★★★

Acetaminophen
Ibuprofen
Aspirin

★★

Direct blow upper left quadrant
Kehr's sign
Vomiting

★★★

Not regulated by FDA
Could include banned substances
Performance enhancing

★★

Low back pain
Hematuria
Nausea/vomiting

★★★

Albuterol
Different types of conditions
Can be triggered by allergies
Bronchodilator

★★

Bacterial infection
Itching
In body folds subject to friction

★★★

Drug Testing

Anxiety

Anabolic Steroid Abuse:
"Roid Rage"

Bipolar Depression

Anorexia Nervosa

Depression

Bulimia Nervosa

Stress

Female Athlete Triad

Hydration

Sweaty palms
Shortness of breath
Sleep disruption
Weight loss

Urinalysis
Testing for masking agents
Random selection of athletes

Intermittent episodes of rowdiness in class
Lack of interest in things you love
Headaches
Irritable

Uncharacteristic aggressive behavior
Elevated blood pressure
Decreased testosterone
Acne

Skipping appointments/classes
Excessive sleep
Withdrawn and isolated

Primary amenorrhea
Fainting episodes
Low energy
When eating, pushes food around plate

Persistent colds
Body soreness
Headaches
Increased blood pressure

Often seen going to restroom after meals
Dental issues

Required post-activity
Dark-colored urine
Lost through perspiration

Frequent stress fractures
Secondary amenorrhea
Disordered eating

Anaerobic Athlete (Sprinter)

Eat Complex Carbohydrates and Protein Pre-game and Maintain Proper Hydration

What Are the Daily Intake Recommendations for Nutrition?

Core Stability Training

Needs a Healthy Lifestyle Including Moderate Physical Activity, Proper Hydration, and a Balanced Diet

Isometric Exercises

Calcium Intake

Free Weights

Replace Electrolytes, Avoid Fats and Sugar, and Eat Protein

Strengthening Machines

Athlete is dizzy and sluggish and complains of low energy in the second half of the soccer game.
Proper nutrition recommendations

Nutrition goal to reduce body fat
Eat protein 3–4 hours before activity
Meals include simple carbohydrates low in salt and fat
Recommendations for this particular individual

Exercises to protect the vertebral column
Helps posture
Can train daily

55%–60% from carbohydrates
25%–30% from fats
15%–20% from protein

Exercises often used post-operatively
Need maximal effort
No joint movement

This person is sedentary, lacks water intake, mainly drinks soda, and eats fast food regularly.
Recommendations for this particular individual

Equipment that uses isotonic contractions
Open kinetic chain
Uses stabilizers

Female
Doesn't eat dairy
Has frequent stress fractures
Irregular menstrual cycle
Nutrient missing from athlete's diet

Equipment good for beginners
Single joint strengthening
Expensive

★

Steps taken nutritionally to recover from a high-intensity workout?

Circuit Training

Muscular Endurance Testing

Functional Strength Training

Power Testing

Concentric Contractions

Cardiovascular Endurance Testing

Eccentric Contractions

Coordination/Balance Testing

Abdominal Exercises

Body Composition Testing

Testing combines strength
and stamina
Performed to failure
Each muscle group

★

Mixed method fitness
Involves strength and cardio
Cycles of high intensity and recovery

★★

Testing uses Vertec
Maximum force
Relatable to many sports

★★

Sport-specific fitness
Necessary for return to play from
injury
Mimics biomechanics for activities

★★

Testing may include VO_2 Max
Maximal aerobic drills

★★

Isotonic
Contraction where muscle shortens

★

Functional baseline taken
Static and dynamic
Wall toss test

★★

Isotonic
Contraction where muscle lengthens

★

Siri equation
Skinfold is one method
Different healthy ranges for male
and female

★★

Planks
Using a Swiss ball
Russian twists

★

Speed Testing	Interval Training
Agility Testing	Agility Training
Maximum Heart Rate	Target Heart Rate
Plyometrics	Yes, Because That Supplement Could Include Banned Substances
Periodization	Yes, All Medical Information Is Confidential

Intensity close to VO_2 Max
Combination of high intensity and recovery
Advanced type of training

★★

Loughborough Intermittent Shuttle Test
Stride length
Stride frequency

★★

Quick change in directions or velocity
T-test

★★

Change mode quickly
T-test
Train with anticipated and unanticipated changes

★★

Desired training level
Method to monitor intensity of exercise

★★

220 – age
Point of exhaustion
Intensity of workout

★★

AT tells athlete to take a supplement to lose weight faster, knowing that her wrestling team won't be drug tested until nationals. Ethical violation?

★★★

Explosive exercises
Precautions for adolescents

★★

AT releases medical information to the media without permission from the athlete. Ethical violation?

★★★

Different time periods
Training varies per cycle

★★

Yes, Inappropriate Professional Behavior

Documentation

Yes, Required to Maintain CEUs for State License and Certification

Preparticipation Physicals

Emergency Action Plan

Negligence

Policy and Procedure Manual

Nonfeasance

Equipment Safety

Malfeasance

Reduces liability risk
Ensures proper progression
Kept confidential

AT becomes too friendly with students and is seen drunk at the local bar wearing the university's athletic training polo shirt. Ethical violation?

Identifies high-risk individuals
Includes waiver forms
Involves different examinations

AT has been complacent with continuing education and argues that her "old" methods of treating athletes are still best. Ethical violation?

Student with attention seeking behaviors, who presents with an ankle injury, is returned to play after abbreviated evaluation and is later confirmed by ER to have sustained a right lateral malleolus fracture. Any legal violation? If so, what?

Limits risk
Specific per facility
Activates EMS

AT delays care of a rib injury by request of athlete, who has labored breathing and palpable crepitus. Any legal violation? If so, what?

Limits risk
Directs daily actions
Staff regulations

AT doesn't follow state law regulating a hosting AT's rights in treating opposing team's players as a result of a personal relationship. Any legal violation? If so, what?

★★★

Inspect per manufacturer guidelines
Disinfect regularly
Supervises

Good Samaritan Law	Sports Medicine Umbrella
Professional Liability Insurance	Athletic Training Room Design
High School, Collegiate, & Professional Athletics; Clinic Setting; Industrial; Military; Performing Arts	Supply Bids
Professional Organizations (NATA, etc.)	Budgeting
Commission on Accreditation of Athletic Training Education (CAATE)	Security/ Privacy of Medical Records

Group of different health-care providers that care for and treat physically active populations; scope of practice can vary by profession

★

An individual begins CPR on someone and is concerned because his certification for the lay responder is expired. Any legal violation? If so, what?

★

Specific areas for injury evaluation and treatment, rehabilitation, administration, hydrotherapy, storage, taping and bandaging; consider how to be used, number of athletes, design elements, etc.

★★

AT hosting a basketball tournament treats her player's injury while avoiding evaluation of an injury for the opposing team. Legal action is taken by the opposing player. What does AT need for professional protection?

★★★

Allows ATC to get supplies at cheapest amount by companies competing for their business

★★★

Multiple areas for athletic trainers to find employment; traditional and nontraditional

★

Itemized list of expected/estimated income and expenses; systematic way to plan and execute different classifications

★★★

National, district, and state levels; way for athletic trainers to stay current on AT knowledge and career networking

★★

Must maintain confidentiality with all patient records; purpose of HIPAA; penalties for violating HIPAA; have secure storage for all patient records

★★★

The accrediting body for undergraduate athletic training education programs

★★